COVID-19: A Multidisciplinary Approach

Editorial Advisor

JOEL J. HEIDELBAUGH

T0229077

ELSEVIER

1600 John F. Kennedy Boulevard • Suite 1800 • Philadelphia, Pennsylvania, 19103-2899

http://www.theclinics.com

CLINICS COLLECTIONS
ISSN 2352-7986, ISBN-13: 978-0-323-93871-6

Editor: Katerina Heidhausen (k.zaliva@elsevier.com)

© **2022 Elsevier Inc. All rights reserved.**

This periodical and the individual contributions contained in it are protected under copyright by Elsevier, and the following terms and conditions apply to their use:

Photocopying
Single photocopies of single articles may be made for personal use as allowed by national copyright laws. Permission of the Publisher and payment of a fee is required for all other photocopying, including multiple or systematic copying, copying for advertising or promotional purposes, resale, and all forms of document delivery. Special rates are available for educational institutions that wish to make photocopies for non-profit educational classroom use. For information on how to seek permission visit www.elsevier.com/permissions or call: (+44) 1865 843830 (UK)/(+1) 215 239 3804 (USA).

Derivative Works
Subscribers may reproduce tables of contents or prepare lists of articles including abstracts for internal circulation within their institutions. Permission of the Publisher is required for resale or distribution outside the institution. Permission of the Publisher is required for all other derivative works, including compilations and translations (please consult www.elsevier.com/permissions).

Electronic Storage or Usage
Permission of the Publisher is required to store or use electronically any material contained in this periodical, including any article or part of an article (please consult www.elsevier.com/permissions). Except as outlined above, no part of this publication may be reproduced, stored in a retrieval system or transmitted in any form or by any means, electronic, mechanical, photocopying, recording or otherwise, without prior written permission of the Publisher.

Notice
No responsibility is assumed by the Publisher for any injury and/or damage to persons or property as a matter of products liability, negligence or otherwise, or from any use or operation of any methods, products, instructions or ideas contained in the material herein. Because of rapid advances in the medical sciences, in particular, independent verification of diagnoses and drug dosages should be made.

Although all advertising material is expected to conform to ethical (medical) standards, inclusion in this publication does not constitute a guarantee or endorsement of the quality or value of such product or of the claims made of it by its manufacturer.

Clinics Collections (ISSN 2352-7986) is published by Elsevier Inc., 360 Park Avenue South, New York, NY 10010-1710. Business and editorial offices: 1600 John F. Kennedy Boulevard, Suite 1800, Philadelphia, PA 19103-2899. **POSTMASTER:** Send address changes to *Clinics Collections*, Elsevier Health Sciences Division, Subscription Customer Service, 3251 Riverport Lane, Maryland Heights, MO 63043. **Customer Service: Telephone: 1-800-654-2452** (U.S. and Canada); **1-314-447-8871** (outside U.S. and Canada). **Fax: 314-447-8029.** E-mail: **journalscustomerserviceusa@elsevier.com** (for print support); **journalsonlinesupport-usa@elsevier.com** (for online support).

Reprints. For copies of 100 or more of articles in this publication, please contact the Commercial Reprints Department, Elsevier Inc., 360 Park Avenue South, New York, NY 10010-1710. Tel.: 212-633-3874; Fax: 212-633-3820; E-mail: reprints@elsevier.com.

Contributors

EDITOR

JOEL J. HEIDELBAUGH, MD, FAAFP, FACG
Departments of Family Medicine and Urology, University of Michigan Medical School, Ann Arbor, Michigan, USA; Ypsilanti Health Center, Ypsilanti, Michigan, USA

AUTHORS

SURYA KIRAN AEDMA, MD
Department of Medicine, Carle Foundation Hospital, Urbana, Illinois, USA; HCA Midwest Health, Overland Park, Kansas, USA

RITESH AGNIHOTHRI, MD
Complex Medical Dermatology Fellow, Department of Dermatology, University of California San Francisco, San Francisco, California, USA

ADNAN AHMED, MD
Kansas City Heart Rhythm Institute, HCA Midwest Health, Overland Park, Kansas, USA

LINDSEY R. BADEN, MD
Division of Infectious Diseases, Brigham and Women's Hospital, Harvard Medical School, Boston, Massachusetts, USA

DAVID B. BANACH, MD, MPH, MS
Associate Professor of Medicine, Department of Medicine, University of Connecticut School of Medicine, Farmington, Connecticut, USA

DANIEL BARROWS, LCSW, MHA, FACHE
Telehealth Program Analyst, Spinal Cord Injuries and Disorders, National Program Office, Veterans Health Administration, Washington, DC, USA

GIACOMO BELLANI, MD, PhD
Department of Medicine and Surgery, University of Milano-Bicocca, Department of Emergency and Intensive Care, San Gerardo Hospital, Monza, Italy

ANKEET S. BHATT, MD, MBA
Division of Cardiovascular Medicine, Brigham and Women's Hospital, Boston, Massachusetts, USA

GIUSEPPE BIONDI-ZOCCAI, MD
MStat, Division of Cardiology, Santa Maria Goretti Hospital, Department of Medical-Surgical Sciences and Biotechnologies, Sapienza University, Latina, Italy; Mediterranea Cardiocentro, Naples, Italy

NEIL BLUMBERG, MD
Director of Transfusion Medicine/Blood Bank, Department of Transfusion Medicine/Blood Bank, University of Rochester Medical Center, Rochester, New York, USA

MICAH BRICKHILL-ATKINSON
Medical Student, Department of Family Medicine, University of Virginia School of Medicine, Charlottesville, Virginia, USA

SAMUEL M. BROWN, MD, MS
Division of Pulmonary and Critical Care Medicine, Department of Medicine, University of Utah School of Medicine, Salt Lake City, Utah, USA; Division of Pulmonary and Critical Care Medicine, Department of Medicine, Intermountain Medical Center, Murray, Utah, USA

CHRISTINE CAHILL, RN, MS
Nurse Coordinator, Department of Transfusion Medicine/Blood Bank, Patient Blood Management, University of Rochester Medical Center, Rochester, New York, USA

MARIA PAOLA CANALE, MD
Department of Systems Medicine, University of Rome Tor Vergata, Center for Atherosclerosis, Policlinico Tor Vergata, Rome, Italy

ANNA M. CERVANTES-ARSLANIAN, MD
Clinical Vice Chair, Chief of Neurocritical Care, Department of Neurology, Assistant Professor, Departments of Neurology, and Neurosurgery, and Medicine (Infectious Disease), Boston University School of Medicine, Boston Medical Center, Boston, Massachusetts, USA

RISHI CHARATE, MD
Kansas City Heart Rhythm Institute, HCA Midwest Health, Overland Park, Kansas, USA

GAETANO CHIRICOLO, MD
Division of Cardiology, "Tor Vergata" University Hospital, Department of Biomedicine and Prevention, "Tor Vergata" University of Rome, Rome, Italy

FRANCESCA CONWAY, MD
Msc Candidate, London School of Hygiene and Tropical Medicine, London, United Kingdom

MATTHEW DALE, MD, PhD
Surgical Resident, Department of Surgery, Creighton University, School of Medicine, Omaha, Nebraska, USA

FRANCESCO DE FELICE, MD
Division of Cardiology, San Camillo Hospital, Rome, Italy

ARMANDO DEL PRETE, MD
Division of Cardiology, Santa Maria Goretti Hospital, Latina, Italy; Department of Systems Medicine, University of Rome "Tor Vergata," Rome, Italy

MICHAËL DESJARDINS, MD
Division of Infectious Diseases, Brigham and Women's Hospital, Harvard Medical School, Boston, Massachusetts, USA; Division of Infectious Diseases, Centre Hospitalier de l'Université de Montréal, Montreal, Quebec, Canada

ELIZABETH DIMMOCK, MSN
Center for LGBTQ+ Health, Cleveland Clinic Foundation, Lakewood, Internal Medicine, Cleveland Clinic Community Care, Cleveland, Ohio, USA

PEZAD N. DOCTOR, MBBS
Department of Pediatrics, Children's Hospital of Michigan, Detroit, Michigan, USA

PETER D. FABRICANT, MD, MPH
Department of Orthopaedic Surgery, Hospital for Special Surgery, New York, New York, USA

MASSIMO FEDERICI, MD
Department of Systems Medicine, University of Rome Tor Vergata, Center for Atherosclerosis, Policlinico Tor Vergata, Rome, Italy

BAILEY FERGUSON, MBA
Center for LGBTQ+ Health, Cleveland Clinic Foundation, Lakewood, Ohio, USA

THOMAS FORD, MD
Department of Neurology, Boston University School of Medicine, Boston, Massachusetts, USA

LINDY P. FOX, MD
Professor, Department of Dermatology, University of California San Francisco, San Francisco, California, USA

PHOEBE E. FREER, MD, FSBI
Section Chief, Breast Imaging, Associate Professor of Radiology, Department of Radiology and Imaging Sciences, University of Utah Health/Huntsman Cancer Institute, Salt Lake City, Utah, USA

CASEY E. GODSHALL, MD
Assistant Professor, Department of Medicine, University of Connecticut, Farmington, Connecticut, USA

WILLIAM CHRISTOPHER GOLDEN, MD
Associate Professor, Eudowood Neonatal Pulmonary Division, Department of Pediatrics, Johns Hopkins School of Medicine, Baltimore, Maryland, USA

BARRY GOLDSTEIN, MD, PhD
Deputy Executive Director, Spinal Cord Injuries and Disorders, National Program Office, Veterans Health Administration, Washington, DC, USA; Professor, Department of Rehabilitation Medicine, University of Washington, Seattle, Washington, USA

RAKESH GOPINATHANNAIR, MD
Kansas City Heart Rhythm Institute, HCA Midwest Health, Overland Park, Kansas, USA

GIACOMO GRASSELLI, MD
Department of Pathophysiology and Transplantation, University of Milan, Department of Anesthesia, Intensive Care and Emergency, Fondazione IRCCS Ca' Granda Ospedale Maggiore Policlinico, Milan, Italy

RICHARD HARLAN, MD
Center for LGBTQ+ Health, Cleveland Clinic Foundation, Lakewood, Obstetrics, Gynecology & Women's Health Institute, Cleveland Clinic Foundation, Cleveland, Ohio, USA

FERN R. HAUCK, MD, MS, FAAFP
Spencer P. Bass, MD Twenty-First Century Professor of Family Medicine, Professor of Public Health Sciences, Director of Research and Faculty Development, Director,

International Family Medicine Clinic, Department of Family Medicine, University of Virginia Health System, Charlottesville, Virginia, USA

JAMES HEKMAN, MD
Center for LGBTQ+ Health, Cleveland Clinic Foundation, Lakewood, Internal Medicine & Geriatrics, Cleveland Clinic Community Care, Cleveland, Ohio, USA

KATHRYN W. HENDRICKSON, MD
Division of Pulmonary and Critical Care Medicine, Department of Medicine, University of Utah School of Medicine, Salt Lake City, Utah, USA; Division of Pulmonary and Critical Care Medicine, Department of Medicine, Intermountain Medical Center, Murray, Utah, USA

DENISSE S. HOLCOMB, MD
Assistant Professor, Department of Obstetrics and Gynecology, The University of Texas Southwestern Medical Center, Dallas, Texas, USA

JACOB HOOFMAN, MS
Wayne State University School of Medicine, Detroit, Michigan, USA

DEEPAK KAMAT, MD, PhD
Department of Pediatrics, UT Health Science Center, UT Health San Antonio, San Antonio, Texas, USA

KYLE N. KUNZE, MD
Department of Orthopaedic Surgery, Hospital for Special Surgery, New York, New York, USA

DHANUNJAYA LAKKIREDDY, MD, FACC, FHRS
Executive Medical Director, Kansas City Heart Rhythm Institute, HCA Midwest Health, Overland Park, Kansas, USA; Professor of Medicine, University of Missouri-Columbia, Columbia, Missouri, USA

DALGISIO LECIS, MD
Division of Cardiology, "Tor Vergata" University Hospital, Rome, Italy

ORLY LEIVA, MD
Department of Medicine, Brigham and Women's Hospital, Boston, Massachusetts, USA

AURORA MAGLIOCCA, MD, PhD
Department of Medicine and Surgery, University of Milano-Bicocca, Monza, Italy

EUGENIO MARTELLI, MD
Department of General and Specialist Surgery "P. Stefanini", Sapienza University of Rome, Rome, Italy; Division of Vascular Surgery, S. Anna and S. Sebastiano Hospital, Caserta, Italy

EUGENIO MARTUSCELLI, MD
Division of Cardiology, "Tor Vergata" University Hospital, Department of Biomedicine and Prevention, "Tor Vergata" University of Rome, Rome, Italy

ROBERT G. MARX, MD, MSc
Department of Orthopaedic Surgery, Hospital for Special Surgery, New York, New York, USA

DEBRA MASEL, MT, (ASCP) SBB
Chief Supervisor, Department of Transfusion Medicine/Blood Bank, University of Rochester Medical Center, Rochester, New York, USA

GIANLUCA MASSARO, MD
Division of Cardiology, "Tor Vergata" University Hospital, Rome, Italy

JILL MEADE, PhD
Assistant Professor, Department of Pediatrics, Wayne State University, Psychologist, Children's Hospital of Michigan, Detroit, Michigan, USA

ROSSELLA MENGHINI, PhD
Department of Systems Medicine, University of Rome Tor Vergata, Rome, Italy

KLAUS MERGENER, MD, PhD, MBA
Affiliate Professor of Medicine, Division of Gastroenterology, University of Washington, Seattle, Washington, USA

IAN MONROE, MD
Surgical Resident, Department of Surgery, Creighton University, School of Medicine, Omaha, Nebraska, USA

CARMINE MUSTO, MD, PhD
Division of Cardiology, San Camillo Hospital, Rome, Italy

ANDREA NATALE, MD, FACC, FHRS
Executive Medical Director, Texas Cardiac Arrhythmia Institute, St. David's Medical Center, Austin, Texas, USA; Consulting Professor, Division of Cardiology, Stanford University, Palo Alto, California, USA; Adjunct Professor of Medicine, Heart and Vascular Center, Case Western Reserve University, Cleveland, Ohio, USA; Director, Interventional Electrophysiology, Scripps Clinic, San Diego, California, USA; Senior Clinical Director, EP Services, California Pacific Medical Center, San Francisco, California, USA

AISHWARYA NAVALPAKAM, MD
Fellow-in-Training, Division of Allergy and Immunology, Department of Pediatrics, Pediatric Specialty Center, Children's Hospital of Michigan, Detroit, Michigan, USA

HENRY NG, MD, MPH
Center for LGBTQ+ Health, Cleveland Clinic Foundation, Lakewood, Internal Medicine & Geriatrics, Primary Care Pediatrics, Cleveland Clinic Community Care, Cleveland, Ohio, USA

ANDY NGO, MD
Transfusion Medicine Fellow, Department of Transfusion Medicine/Blood Bank, University of Rochester Medical Center, Rochester, New York, USA

BENEDICT U. NWACHUKWU, MD, MBA
Department of Orthopaedic Surgery, Hospital for Special Surgery, New York, New York, USA

HIBA OBEID, MD
Center for LGBTQ+ Health, Cleveland Clinic Foundation, Lakewood, Internal Medicine & Geriatrics, Cleveland Clinic Community Care, Cleveland, Ohio, USA

MILIND PANSARE, MD
Associate Professor, Department of Pediatrics, Division of Allergy and Immunology, Pediatric Specialty Center, Children's Hospital of Michigan, Central Michigan University, Detroit, Michigan, USA

ITHAN D. PELTAN, MD, MSc
Division of Pulmonary and Critical Care Medicine, Department of Medicine, University of Utah School of Medicine, Salt Lake City, Utah, USA; Pulmonary Division, Department of Medicine, Intermountain Medical Center, Murray, Utah, USA

ANTONIO PESENTI, MD
Department of Pathophysiology and Transplantation, University of Milan, Department of Anesthesia, Intensive Care and Emergency, Fondazione IRCCS Ca' Granda Ospedale Maggiore Policlinico, Milan, Italy

MARCO PICICHÈ, MD
Department of Cardiac Surgery, San Bortolo Hospital, Vicenza, Italy

NAGA VENKATA K. POTHINENI, MD
Kansas City Heart Rhythm Institute, HCA Midwest Health, Overland Park, Kansas, USA; Section of Electrophysiology, Division of Cardiovascular Medicine, University of Pennsylvania, Philadelphia, Pennsylvania, USA

WILLIAM F. RAYBURN, MD, MBA
Adjunct Professor, Department of Obstetrics and Gynecology, College of Graduate Studies, Medical University of South Carolina, Charleston, South Carolina, USA; Associate Dean, Continuing Medical Education and Professional Development, Distinguished Professor and Emeritus Chair, Professor, Maternal Fetal Medicine, Department of Obstetrics and Gynecology, University of New Mexico School of Medicine, Albuquerque, New Mexico, USA

MAJED A. REFAAI, MD
Associate Director of Transfusion Medicine/Blood Bank, Department of Transfusion Medicine/Blood Bank, University of Rochester Medical Center, Rochester, New York, USA

EMANUELE REZOAGLI, MD, PhD
Department of Medicine and Surgery, University of Milano-Bicocca, Department of Emergency and Intensive Care, San Gerardo Hospital, Monza, Italy

DOMENICO G. DELLA ROCCA, MD, PhD
Texas Cardiac Arrhythmia Institute, St. David's Medical Center, Austin, Texas, USA

GIUSEPPE MASSIMO SANGIORGI, MD
Division of Cardiology, "Tor Vergata" University Hospital, Department of Biomedicine and Prevention, "Tor Vergata" University of Rome, Rome, Italy

PAUL J. SCHENARTS, MD, FACS
Department of Surgery, Professor of Surgery, Creighton University, School of Medicine, Omaha, Nebraska, USA

RACHEL SCHENKEL, MD
Surgical Resident, Department of Surgery, Creighton University, School of Medicine, Omaha, Nebraska, USA

MICHAEL SCHWABE, MD
Surgical Resident, Department of Surgery, Creighton University, School of Medicine, Omaha, Nebraska, USA

ELIZABETH SECORD, MD
Professor of Pediatrics, Division Chief for Allergy and Immunology, Wayne State University School of Medicine, Professor, Pediatric Allergy and Immunology, Wayne State University, Wayne Pediatrics, Detroit, Michigan, USA

AMY C. SHERMAN, MD
Division of Infectious Diseases, Brigham and Women's Hospital, Harvard Medical School, Boston, Massachusetts, USA

JULIE G. SHULMAN, MD
Department of Neurology, Boston University School of Medicine, Boston, Massachusetts, USA

PATRICIA R. SLEV, PhD, D(ABCC)
Section Chief, Immunology Division, ARUP Laboratories, Associate Professor, Department of Pathology, University of Utah School of Medicine, Salt Lake City, Utah, USA

LYNN C. SMITHERMAN, MD
Associate Professor, Vice Chair of Medical Education, Department of Pediatrics, Wayne State University School of Medicine, Detroit, Michigan, USA

BEENA G. SOOD, MD, MS
Department of Pediatrics, Wayne State University School of Medicine, Detroit, Michigan, USA

MUTHIAH VADUGANATHAN, MD, MPH
Division of Cardiovascular Medicine, Brigham and Women's Hospital, Boston, Massachusetts, USA

FRANCESCO VERSACI, MD
Division of Cardiology, Santa Maria Goretti Hospital, Latina, Italy

JENNIFER R. WALTON, MD, MPH
Assistant Professor, Division of Developmental Behavioral Pediatrics, Department of Pediatrics, Nationwide Children's Hospital, The Ohio State University College of Medicine, Columbus, Ohio, USA

LYNDSAY ZIMMERMAN, BSN
Center for LGBTQ+ Health, Cleveland Clinic Foundation, Lakewood, Ohio, USA

Contents

> Pandemic preparedness is a key function of any health care facility. Activities pertaining to pandemic preparedness should be developed and maintained within a broader emergency management plan. The use of a Hospital Incident Command System can centralize coordination of the response and facilitate internal and external communication. This review addresses several components of pandemic preparedness, including incident management, health care personnel safety, strategies to support ongoing clinical activities, and organizational communication during a pandemic. Preparations addressing potential ethical challenges and the psychological impact associated with pandemic response are also reviewed.

> Italy was the first western country facing an outbreak of coronavirus disease 2019 (COVID-19). The first Italian patient diagnosed with COVID-19 was admitted, on Feb. 20, 2020, to the intensive care unit (ICU) in Codogno (Lodi, Lombardy, Italy), and the number of reported positive cases increased to 36 in the next 24 hours, and then exponentially for 18 days. This triggered a response that resulted in a massive surge in ICU bed capacity. The COVID19 Lombardy Network organized a structured logistic response and provided scientific evidence to highlight information on COVID-19 associated respiratory failure.

> In 2019, an emerging coronavirus, SARS-COV-2, was first identified. In the months since, SARS-CoV-2 has become a global pandemic of unimaginable scale. In 2021, SARS-CoV-2 continues to be a huge public health burden and a dominating issue in health care. In addition, SARS-CoV-2 has placed a spotlight on laboratory medicine and its key role in infectious disease management. The SARS-CoV-2 antibody testing landscape is vast and consists of dozens of antibody tests that have received EUA. The laboratory is faced with choosing the right test, staying current with the rapidly evolving recommendations, and updating test information for

interprofessional, and multidisciplinary approach. The authors offer references for best practices set forth by organizations and thought leaders in transgender health and describe the key processes they developed to respectfully deliver affirming care to transgender and nonbinary patients.

Andy Ngo, Debra Masel, Christine Cahill, Neil Blumberg, and Majed A. Refaai

SARS-CoV-2 (also known as COVID-19) has been an unprecedented challenge in many parts of the medical field with blood banking being no exception. COVID-19 has had a distinctly negative effect on our blood collection nationwide forcing blood banks, blood centers, and the US government to adopt new policies to adapt to a decreased blood supply as well as to protect our donors from COVID-19. These policies can be seen distinctly in patient blood management and blood bank operations. We are also faced with developing policies and procedures for a nontraditional therapy, convalescent plasma; its efficacy and safety is still not completely elucidated as of yet.

Gianluca Massaro, Dalgisio Lecis, Eugenio Martuscelli, Gaetano Chiricolo, and Giuseppe Massimo Sangiorgi

COVID-19 is an acute respiratory disease of viral origin caused by SARS-CoV-2. This disease is associated with a hypercoagulable state resulting in arterial and venous thrombotic events. The latter are more frequent, especially in patients who develop a severe form of the disease and are associated with an increased mortality rate. It is therefore essential to identify patients at higher risk to initiate antithrombotic therapy. Hospitalized patients treated with treatment dose of anticoagulants had better outcomes than those treated with prophylactic dose. However, several trials are ongoing to better define the therapeutic and prevention strategies for this insidious complication.

Maria Paola Canale, Rossella Menghini, Eugenio Martelli, and Massimo Federici

Coronavirus-19 disease (COVID-19) affects more people than previous coronavirus infections and has a higher mortality. Higher incidence and mortality can probably be explained by COVID-19 causative agent's greater affinity (about 10–20 times) for angiotensin-converting enzyme 2 (ACE2) receptor compared with other coronaviruses. Here, the authors first summarize clinical manifestations, then present symptoms of COVID-19 and the pathophysiological mechanisms underlying specific organ/system disease. The worse clinical outcome observed in COVID-19 patients with diabetes may be in part related to the increased ADAM17 activity and its unbalanced interplay with ACE2. Therefore, strategies aimed to inhibit ADAM17 activity may be explored to develop new effective therapeutic approaches.

COVID-19 has afflicted the health of children and women across all age groups. Since the outbreak of the pandemic in December 2019, various epidemiologic, immunologic, clinical, and pharmaceutical studies have been conducted to understand its infectious characteristics, pathogenesis, and clinical profile. COVID-19 affects pregnant women more seriously than nonpregnant women, endangering the health of the newborn. Changes have been implemented to guidelines for antenatal care of pregnant women, delivery, and newborn care. We highlight the current trends of clinical care in pregnant women and newborns during the COVID-19 pandemic.

The coronavirus disease 2019 (COVID-19) pandemic has caused severe economic and health impacts in the United States, and the impact is disproportionately more in socially disadvantaged areas. The available data, albeit limited in children, suggest that the initial concerns of the potential impact of COVID-19 illness in children with asthma are unproven thus far. The reduction in asthma morbidities is due to improved adherence, COVID-19 control measures, school closures, and decreased exposure to allergens and viral infections in children. During the pandemic, asthma guidelines were updated to guide physicians in asthma care. Due to the unpredictable nature of COVID-19, it is important to be vigilant, adhere to treatment guidelines, and implement preventive measures to eradicate the virus and improve outcomes in children with asthma.

Coronavirus disease 2019 (COVID-19), an emergent disease caused by severe acute respiratory syndrome coronavirus 2 (SARS-CoV-2), has rapidly spread since its discovery in 2019. This article reviews the broad spectrum of cutaneous manifestations reported in association with SARS-CoV-2 infection. The most commonly reported cutaneous manifestations associated with COVID-19 infection include pernio (chilblain)-like acral lesions, morbilliform (exanthematous) rash, urticaria, vesicular (varicella-like) eruptions, and vaso-occlusive lesions (livedo racemosa, retiform purpura). It is important to consider SARS-CoV-2 infection in the differential diagnosis of a patient presenting with these lesions in the appropriate clinical context.

As the world clamored to respond to the rapidly evolving coronavirus 2019 (COVID-19) pandemic, health care systems reacted swiftly to provide uninterrupted care for patients. Within obstetrics and gynecology, nearly every facet of care was influenced. Rescheduling of office visits, safety of labor and delivery and in the operating room, and implementation of telemedicine are examples. Social distancing has impacted academic centers in the education of trainees. COVID-19 vaccine trials have increased awareness of including pregnant and lactating women. Last, the pandemic has reminded us of issues related to ethics, diversity and inclusiveness, marginalized communities, and the women's health workforce.

The Covid-19 pandemic of 2020 caused great disruption to breast imaging and breast cancer care. Screening mammography was deferred nationwide (and internationally) for a period of weeks to months. Patients and some breast centers delayed diagnostic imaging and biopsies leading to a decrease in the incidence of cancer detected. Additionally, there were significant changes to breast cancer care algorithms. Practices were greatly affected financially as well as in terms of workflow logistics and educational methods. The many reaching effects of the pandemic on breast imaging are reviewed.

The unprecedented COVID-19 pandemic and its rapid global shutdowns have posed tremendous challenges for GI practices, including sudden delays in endoscopic procedures. As full reopening approaches, practices are wrestling with completely retooling their operations to ensure the resumption of high-quality, safe, and effective patient care. The pandemic's long-term effects on practice operations must be assessed: What will postpandemic GI care look like? Will some aspects of our work be changed forever, and if so, what are the practice management implications? This chapter surveys the pandemic's impact on US-based GI practices and discusses key "lessons learned" for future operations.

Acute respiratory distress syndrome (ARDS) is a heterogeneous syndrome of high morbidity and mortality with global impact. Current epidemiologic estimates are imprecise given differences in patient populations, risk factors, resources, and practice styles around the world. Despite improvement in supportive care which has improved mortality, effective targeted therapies remain elusive. The Coronavirus Disease 2019 pandemic has resulted in a large number of ARDS cases that, despite less heterogeneity than multietiologic ARDS populations, still exhibit wide variation in physiology and outcomes. Intensive care unit rates of death have varied widely in studies to date because of a variety of patient and hospital-level factors. Despite some controversy, the best management of these patients is likely the same supportive measures shown to be effective in classical ARDS. Further epidemiologic studies are needed to help characterize the epidemiology of ARDS subphenotypes to facilitate identification of targeted therapies.

The COVID-19 Patient in the Surgical Intensive Care Unit   339

Ian Monroe, Matthew Dale, Michael Schwabe, Rachel Schenkel, and Paul J. Schenarts

COVID-19 continues to rampage around the world. Noncritical care–trained physicians may be deployed into the intensive care unit to manage these complex patients. Although COVID-19 is primarily a respiratory disease, it is also associated with significant pathology in the brain, heart, vasculature, lungs, gastrointestinal tract, and kidneys. This article provides an overview of COVID-19 using an organ-based, systematic approach.

Perspectives on the Impact of the COVID-19 Pandemic on the Sports Medicine Surgeon: Implications for Current and Future Care   361

Kyle N. Kunze, Peter D. Fabricant, Robert G. Marx, and Benedict U. Nwachukwu

As the COVID-19 (Coronavirus disease 2019) pandemic continues, the paradigm of treatment continues to rapidly evolve, especially for sports medicine surgeons, because treatment before the pandemic was considered predominantly elective. This article provides subjective and objective data on the changes implicated by the COVID-19 pandemic with regard to the interactions and practices of sports medicine surgeons. This perspective also considers the potential impact on the patients and athletes treated by sports medicine surgeons.This article discusses the impact of the COVID-19 pandemic on sports medicine and provides thoughts on how the landscape of the field may continue to change.

Virtual Care in the Veterans Affairs Spinal Cord Injuries and Disorders System of Care During the COVID-19 National Public Health Emergency   369

Daniel Barrows and Barry Goldstein

Telehealth reduces disparities that result from physical disabilities, difficulties with transportation, geographic barriers, and scarcity of specialists, which are commonly experienced by individuals with spinal cord injuries and disorders (SCI/D). The Department of Veterans Affairs (VA) has been an international leader in the use of virtual health. The VA's SCI/D System of Care is the nation's largest coordinated system of lifelong care for people with SCI/D and has implemented the use of telehealth to ensure that Veterans with SCI/D have convenient access to their health care, particularly during the restrictions that were imposed by the COVID-19 pandemic.

Preface

COVID. COVID-19. The pandemic. Whatever we choose to call this great disrupter of our lives, the medical field has been forced to rapidly adapt, respond, and innovate with respect to clinical care, education, and research. This issue of *Clinics Collections* highlights many aspects of what we have learned thus far during the COVID-19 pandemic. In this nascent field of medicine, by the time this issue is in print, there will already be substantial additional research available to guide health care professionals. Nonetheless, the articles herein serve as a formidable blueprint for guiding health care across many domains.

The issue begins with a review of pandemic preparedness and the development of a critical response plan when Italy was suffering as one of the initial epicenters of COVID-19. As testing became available, and eventually vaccines, health care providers had to quickly augment their knowledge of relevant pathology and immunology. Telehealth became a necessity for ensuring continuity of care and as a portal to urgent care across all fields of medicine. Similarly, novel paradigms for teaching learners from medicine and nursing to pharmacy and allied health professionals developed and evolved out of rapid innovation and necessity. Key articles herein highlight elements of mental health, health disparities, and the impact of COVID-19 on special populations, including refugees and transgender patients. Clinicians have witnessed many unforeseen consequences of the pathophysiologic effects of COVID-19 spanning hypercoagulability, cardiovascular effects, pulmonary disease, dermatology, and neurologic effects across pediatric and adult populations. Protocols quickly developed to guide clinicians in procedures, endoscopy, the critical care setting, and the operating room.

I would like to extend my gratitude to the many authors who have created these incredibly informative articles—likely at one of the most stressful and demanding times in their careers—to provide such timely education for all of us. I would also like to acknowledge my colleagues at Elsevier for championing this issue of *Clinics Collections*, and I trust that our readers will benefit in reading it as much as I have.

Joel J. Heidelbaugh, MD, FAAFP, FACG
Departments of Family Medicine and Urology
University of Michigan Medical School
Ann Arbor, MI 48103, USA

Ypsilanti Health Center
200 Arnet, Suite 200
Ypsilanti, MI 48198, USA

E-mail address:
jheidel@umich.edu

Clinics Collections 12 (2022) xix
https://doi.org/10.1016/j.ccol.2022.03.001
2352-7986/22/© 2022 Published by Elsevier Inc.

Pandemic Preparedness

Casey E. Godshall, MD, David B. Banach, MD, MPH, MS*

KEYWORDS

- Pandemic • Occupational health and safety • Incident management • Ethics
- Wellness

KEY POINTS

- Pandemic preparedness is an essential function of any health care facility. An Emergency Management Program can guide a facility through a pandemic response, and the Hospital Incident Command System can centralize communication and coordination to rapidly respond to a crisis.
- Plans for staffing and utilization of space to prepare for the continued provision of routine inpatient and outpatient care, as well as the surge of pandemic-related patients, must be developed and be reviewed and revised routinely.
- Consideration should be given to the ethical challenges inherent to a pandemic in which there may be a scarcity of resources.
- The maintenance of psychological health and well-being of health care workers making difficult treatment decisions under highly stressful conditions and potentially putting their own health at risk should be incorporated into pandemic preparedness planning.

INTRODUCTION

The coronavirus disease 2019 (COVID-19) pandemic has illustrated the ways in which many health care facilities and health systems were not adequately prepared for the crisis conditions caused by a rapidly emerging respiratory virus. Major challenges faced early on during the pandemic included shortages of personal protective equipment (PPE), health care personnel frequently being exposed to or infected with severe acute respiratory syndrome coronavirus 2 (SARS-CoV-2), and insufficient preparations for the surge of patients.[1] Although a discussion of all aspects of pandemic preparedness is beyond the scope of this review, we address several aspects of pandemic preparedness focused on health care facilities to provide clinicians and facility administrators guiding principles in preparation for future pandemics.

This article previously appeared in *Infectious Disease Clinics*, Volume 35, Issue 4, December 2021.

The authors have no disclosures relevant to this article.

Department of Medicine, University of Connecticut School of Medicine, Farmington, CT, USA

* Corresponding author. University of Connecticut School of Medicine, 263 Farmington Avenue, Farmington, CT 06030.

E-mail address: dbanach@uchc.edu

2352-7986/22/© 2021 Elsevier Inc. All rights reserved.

INCIDENT MANAGEMENT DURING A PANDEMIC

Previously published guidance for outbreak management and response has recommended the incorporation of an Emergency Management Program (EMP) to provide guidance through the 4 phases of incident management: preparedness, mitigation, response, and recovery.[2] The use of an all-hazards self-assessment can help facility leadership prepare in fulfilling its core mission of patient care during a pandemic. The National Incident Management System provides guidance to government, nongovernmental organizations, and the private sector to work together to prevent, protect against, mitigate, and respond to incidents, including infectious diseases pandemics.[3] The Hospital Incident Command System (HICS) is a structure within the EMP that coordinates the hospital command functions that have been identified during incident management and describes how responsibility is distributed within the management team in a facility (**Fig. 1**). This group may operate out of a single Incident

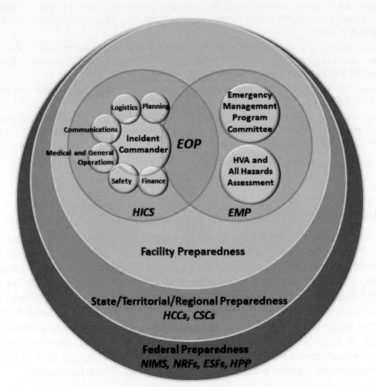

Fig. 1. Diagram of incident management preparedness structures and frameworks. This diagram was created by the authors of the Society of Healthcare Epidemiology of America Outbreak Response Training Program expert guidance document to illustrate how US preparedness structures and frameworks relate, starting at the federal level and moving to the facility level. CSC, Crisis Standards of Care; EMP, Emergency Management Program; EOP, Emergency Operations Plan; ESF, Emergency Support Function; HCC, Health Care Coalition; HICS, Hospital Incident Command System; HPP, Hospital Preparedness Program, NIMS, National Incident Management System; HVA, hazard vulnerability analysis; NRF, National Response Framework. (*From* Banach DB, Johnston BL, Al-Zubeidi D, et al. Outbreak response and incident management: SHEA guidance and resources for healthcare epidemiologists in United States acute-care hospitals. Infect Control Hosp Epidemiol. 2017;38(12):1393-419. https://doi.org/10.1017/ice.2017.212; with permission.)

Command Center (ICC) in a physical location at the facility, or through teleconference or video communication systems, as necessary. Depending on the nature of the pandemic event and the associated operations required to respond, a facility may need to activate either the entire HICS system or various components. Familiarity with the facility's HICS is required for rapid, effective, and sustained function of the system, which requires training team members and the deployment of exercises that use the system to identify any gaps or challenges. Institutional experiences during the initial COVID-19 crisis have further delineated specific roles of key administrative leadership in the incident management response, and they have reported effective strategies for coordinating members of the incident management team within a facility.[4–6]

In pandemic preparedness planning activities, the membership of the ICC should be frequently revisited and updated as new individuals join the organization's pandemic response team and as roles change within the structure of the HICS. One of the key roles of the HICS is to identify the key internal and external stakeholders required in pandemic response.[1] Internal stakeholders can be divided into 4 categories: direct care providers, administrative leadership, patient care support services, and facility services. External stakeholders may include a broader group, depending on the nature and impact of the outbreak/pandemic. This group would likely include local, regional, or national public health agencies; regional health care facilities and collaborative networks; and local municipalities. Understanding the local and regional infrastructures for emergency response and establishing a system to rapidly communicate and coordinate with the key stakeholders is a critical component of pandemic preparedness.

HEALTH CARE PERSONNEL PROTECTION AND SAFETY

Occupational health and safety among the health care workforce is a central priority in pandemic preparedness. The prevention of infection among those working in health care and other essential industries provides the ability to sustain the delivery of medical care and other essential services to the population during a pandemic. The understanding of infection transmission for the organism of concern coupled with the hierarchy of infection controls provides the basis for designing appropriate infection prevention strategies in health care settings.

Previous experiences with SARS, and most recently the COVID-19 pandemic, have highlighted the disproportionate impact of high-consequence respiratory viruses on health care personnel. During the early phases of the SARS epidemic in Toronto, Canada, health care personnel represented a large proportion of total infected individuals, more than 30% in a high infection incidence setting.[7] Most infections occurred in situations in which infection control precautions had not been initiated or were not implemented successfully.[8] During the COVID-19 pandemic, health care personnel were infected at a higher rate than the general population,[9] particularly in the early phases of the pandemic.[10] Health care personnel have also been infected at disproportionately higher rates in the setting of the recent Ebola and Marburg virus disease outbreaks over the past decade, generally in the setting of inadequate infection prevention measures and caring for patients with unsuspected infection.[11]

In the setting of a pandemic the optimal strategy for preventing infections among health care personnel depends on the organism of concern and its characteristics, particularly the route and mechanism of infection transmission. A strategy using the hierarchy of controls, frequently used in occupational medicine, has been used as a means of determining how to implement feasible and effective control solutions. This approach can guide pandemic preparedness programs, in developing strategies to protect health care personnel in the event of an infectious disease pandemic[12] (**Fig. 2**). The hierarchy of controls includes 3 components: engineering controls, administrative controls, and behavioral controls, each of which can be implemented in the context of infectious diseases pandemic response.

Engineering controls involve separating the health hazard (the patient with suspected or confirmed infection) from the health care worker, and when not possible, reduce the amount of contact between an infected patient and the organism of concern and the potentially infected health care worker. In the setting of an infectious disease pandemic, this may include specific wards or areas dedicated to patients with suspected or confirmed infection and creating a patient care environment that reduces transmission. Creating such an environment may include improving ventilation, use of negative pressure airborne isolation rooms and the use of high-efficiency particulate air (HEPA) filtration.[13] During the COVID-19 pandemic, indoor transmission in poorly ventilated environments was an important factor that facilitated transmission. Although most hospital facilities are generally well-ventilated, when nontraditional health care environments are involved in the care of infectious patients, as occurred during the COVID-19 pandemic, ensuring adequate ventilation is an important engineering control to address in pandemic preparation. HEPA filtration is highly effective in preventing the spread of organisms of 0.3 μm diameter or higher,[14] thus ensuring access to these devices may be warranted in pandemic planning. A layered approach to engineering controls in the prevention of SARS-CoV-2 transmission is

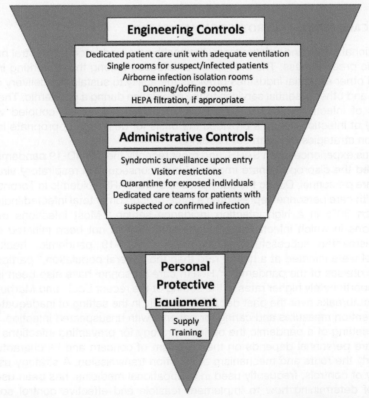

Fig. 2. Hierarchy of infection controls and components in pandemic preparedness.

recommended by Centers for Disease Control and Prevention (CDC) and can be supported for future pandemics in which airborne or droplet transmission occurs.[15]

Administrative controls, policies and procedures, and accompanying education are critical in preventing the spread of infectious diseases during pandemics. As part of the development of a pandemic preparedness plan, health care facility leadership should ensure that policies and protocols are designed to ensure rapid identification and isolation of potentially infectious patients and diagnostic testing and clinical management occurs in a setting that reduces the potential for exposure of others in the health care facility. This process includes detailed descriptions of movement within the facility and cleaning and disinfection of potentially contaminated surfaces. Although the details of these processes may need to be adjusted based on the organism of concern, pandemic preparation plans should identify locations and routes of patient movement that minimize spread of infection to health care personnel and others in the health care setting. These administrative controls may also include syndromic surveillance of all individuals entering the facility, visitor restrictions, and quarantining exposed personnel, all of which have been recommended in the COVID-19 pandemic response.[16] Importantly, health care personnel should be educated on these plans and easy, real-time access to the planning documents, when needed, should be ensured.

PPE, a barrier to protect individuals from exposure to the infectious agent, is an important part of the prevention strategy but remains the most prone to failure because it does not eliminate the hazard but rather reduces the risk of infection. Depending on the route of infection for a given pathogen, PPE will need to be adjusted. For many respiratory infections, PPE has focused primarily on the use of facemasks, and in some cases, higher-level filtration respiratory protection. The COVID-19 pandemic highlighted the role of eye protection in preventing infection.[17] Nonetheless, ensuring access to PPE, including a variety of sizes to accommodate all health care personnel, and education on how to properly don, doff, and wear PPE is a critical component of pandemic preparedness.

SUPPORTING INPATIENT CLINICAL ACTIVITIES DURING A PANDEMIC

The provision of inpatient clinical care and the associated supportive health care activities during a pandemic poses unique challenges. Guided by the emergency management plan, facility leadership within the incident command structure needs to continually evaluate the delivery of clinical services to patients and how this can be done in a safe and effective manner. The diversion of resources to provide care for infected patients may significantly impair the ability to provide care to those not infected by the organism of concern, resulting in deferral of care, particularly preventive and elective care.[18]

Surge capacity refers to the ability to evaluate and care for a markedly increased volume of patients that challenges or exceeds normal operating capacity, and there are public health principles that guide medical surge capacity and capability outlined by the United States Department of Health and Human Services.[19] Given the uncertainty surrounding the rate at which this increase can occur, preparations to respond to varying level of medical surge can guide decisions regarding resource allocation. Although most surge planning centers on ensuring sufficient hospital beds, personnel, pharmaceuticals, supplies, and equipment to provide care to patients, it is important to realize that flexibility will be needed to address the specific organism and disease epidemiology of concern. For instance, in the SARS-CoV-2 pandemic based on the frequency of critical illness,[20] expansion of critical care beds into areas of facilities such as operating rooms and perioperative areas was needed.[21] With these transitions, staff that are not typically responsible for the clinical management of critically ill patients need additional education and specialized training on how to safely provide standardized care to critically ill patients.

Beyond ensuring available space for patients, maintaining sufficient qualified health care personnel to provide care can be a primary challenge during a pandemic. During a pandemic, care services can be streamlined into focusing on the expanded numbers of patients who are impacted by the organism of concern and the deferral of elective care. Staffing will need to be rapidly expanded to adequately provide care to the increased number of patients in the facility. Thus, staffing modeling for the pandemics will need to be rapidly adjusted to accommodate this increase in clinical care needs, likely requiring frequent, potentially daily review by facility leadership. An additional challenge lies in the direct impact of the pandemic on the health care workforce,[22] including health care personnel who become infected and ill from exposure at work and in the community and those who are required to quarantine due to exposure to the infectious agent, as occurred during the COVID-19 pandemic. Thus, HICS leadership needs to work closely with nursing and human resource leaders to identify opportunities to adjust staffing scheduling and potentially expand the pool of available, adequately trained staff that can be rapidly deployed to provide clinical services. This process may involve measures such as rapidly hiring new staff and activating staff that may have training in clinical care but may not be engaged in direct care responsibilities. Expansion of the health care workforce at a regional level and the associated measures to address staffing needs during the COVID-19 pandemic have been described.[23] Notably, specialized expertise in certain areas, such as infectious diseases, emergency medicine, or critical care, may be limited. Thus, in pandemic preparedness, planning for the ability to mobilize clinical and technical expertise and coordinate collaboration with facility expertise in education and communication to provide real-time education and training to others to support these efforts is needed.

ROLE OF AMBULATORY CARE IN A PANDEMIC

In a pandemic due to a rapidly spreading contagious pathogen, health care focus naturally shifts to ensuring the ability to care for a surge of patients requiring hospitalization. However, health systems need to prepare for continued ambulatory care of patients with chronic illnesses, as well as care for those with mild to moderate pandemic-related infections who do not require hospitalization. The consequences of deferred care of chronic illnesses, as well as missed opportunities for preventive health care, create significant challenges for the health care system and increase overall costs.[24] In addition, ambulatory care services can be used to offload emergency department (ED) and urgent care settings by providing treatment to mild to moderately infected patients.

Telehealth is critical to providing continued routine care, and this technology can be leveraged to deliver a variety of services. Routine follow-ups and urgent visits for noninfectious complaints can temporarily be done via telehealth. During the COVID-19 pandemic, institutions that had little to no experience with telehealth were able to successfully convert to majority telehealth services and conduct thousands of billable visits using this platform.[25,26] Beyond these standard virtual visits, providers may choose to perform proactive population care, such as compiling registries of patients with certain poorly controlled health problems or conditions that place them at high risk for morbidity and mortality and reaching out to these vulnerable populations regularly to both ensure that chronic issues are being addressed and monitor for exposures to, or symptoms of, the emerging contagion.[27]

Telehealth tools, such as mobile device applications and interactive Web sites, can also be used for outpatients with mild to moderate infections. Apps or Web sites allowing patients to enter symptoms and self-triage can allow for streamlined outpatient care, offload some visits or calls to EDs and urgent care, and provide patients with education and guidance regarding treatment and quarantine.[28–30] Continued outpatient monitoring through interactive technology can permit care providers to track sick patients while they quarantine and guide them to higher levels of care as needed.[31]

During the COVID-19 pandemic, many outpatient offices were able to increase their capacity to offer acute care visits, screening, and diagnostic testing by performing these services in a walk-up or drive-through setting. An outdoor setting allows for additional distancing, as well as an open-air atmosphere that ensures additional safety for patients and staff by preventing transmission of a respiratory virus, especially during specimen collection for testing.[32]

As part of the effort to offload EDs during a pandemic surge, staff who typically work in an outpatient setting can be deployed to the ED to see noninfectious emergencies within their field. Physicians within surgical subspecialties, including obstetrics and gynecology, will likely not be performing elective procedures during this time and can potentially be deployed to assist in this fashion.[33]

Telehealth, outdoor screenings, and redeployment efforts are key ways to deliver care during a pandemic; however, ambulatory offices must also have plans for providing safe in-person care once it is deemed possible. The COVID-19 pandemic demonstrated the lack of preparedness that most ambulatory offices have to safely provide care during a pandemic with a respiratory pathogen. Most offices are not designed to have separate entrances and exits for patients, enough space for physical distancing in waiting rooms and lines, or proper ventilation systems or other engineering infection control measures.[34] It is critical that outpatient offices give thought to these renovations and system modifications to prepare for the next pandemic.

COMMUNICATION STRATEGIES

Given the rapidly changing conditions of a pandemic, a health care facility and its staff will need effective and efficient methods of internal and external communication to internal and external stakeholders. Keeping health care workers fully informed is a key component of providing adequate support to staff during a crisis to enable continued confidence in job performance. The CDC provides training for methods of communication during an emergency through their Crisis and Emergency Risk Communication (CERC) tool (**Table 1**). The most important principles outlined in this training are be first, be right, be credible, express empathy, promote action, and show respect. Members of the ICC should train themselves in CERC methods of communication for both internal and external messages sent during a pandemic.[35]

In terms of modes of communication, many options exist and using a variety of formats will increase impact and effectiveness of communication activities. Daily e-mails with important updates to all internal stakeholders, including health care personnel, can be an effective way to provide updated information on the pandemic response activities. Creating a living document or Web page that is frequently updated with protocols and procedures for staff to use as a daily resource is a way to have all important information that health care workers will reference in a centralized location.[32] Other options for daily updates and managing questions from staff include a text group or online chat board monitored by a content expert.[4] Hospitals can consider taking advantage of newer formats and platforms to keep staff updated, like creating a mobile phone app or starting a weekly or daily podcast on which

Table 1
Crisis and emergency risk communication

The Six Principles of CERC	The Five Pitfalls to Avoid
1. Be first: In a time-sensitive crisis, communicating early and quickly is crucial. The first source of information often becomes the preferred source	1. Mixed messages from multiple experts
2. Be right: Accuracy establishes credibility Information can include what is known, what is unknown, and what is being done to fill the gaps	2. Information released late
3. Be credible: Do not compromise honesty and truthfulness, even in a crisis	3. Paternalistic attitudes
4. Express empathy: Acknowledge harm and suffering created by the crisis. Address what people are feeling and the challenges being faced. This builds trust and rapport	4. Not countering rumors and myths in real time
5. Promote action: Give people meaningful things to do to calm anxiety, restore order, and promote a sense of control	5. Public power struggles and confusion
6. Show respect: Respectful communication promotes cooperation and rapport when people feel vulnerable	

Adapted from Office of Public Health Preparedness and Response (OPHPR). Crisis & Emergency Risk Communication (CERC). Centers for Disease Control and Prevention website. https://emergency.cdc.gov/cerc/. Accessed February 2021.

physicians and other subject matter experts, as well as administrators and managers, can share information.[36] Infectious disease physicians can contribute by creating content regarding the latest scientific information available. Disseminating scientific information in an easily accessible manner can provide necessary education and, importantly, reduce confusion and combat any online misinformation that may occur during a crisis or a pandemic.

Communication with facility leaders should be bidirectional, easy to access, and frequent. Feedback and questions must be welcomed, encouraged, and sought out on a continuous basis. To this end, a facility may elect to set up a unique e-mail address to which all questions, concerns, and issues can be sent. A method of giving anonymous feedback via phone or e-mail should be created to prevent staff from being afraid to offer negative feedback.[3] Daily or weekly open forums welcoming discussion should be arranged either in person or virtually.[37] In large group sessions, it is a good idea to devote some time to a positive experience or outcome and to find time to praise staff. This focus on good news, rather than letting any discussion simply devolve into talk about what is going poorly, can build morale and refocus efforts.[4]

ETHICAL CONSIDERATIONS

During pandemic conditions, many elements of health care are likely to be stretched to capacity, including hospital beds and ventilators; PPE; diagnostic, therapeutic, or preventative interventions; and health care workers themselves. Consideration must be given to how a hospital and its staff will respond when faced with a scarcity of resources.[38]

In times of austerity, a hospital may decide to shift their ethical framework from one of promoting and working toward the health of each individual patient to a plan to maximize benefits with limited resources. Maximizing public health benefit means taking into consideration a patient's ability to recover fully if treated and prioritizing scarce resources for these patients over those who are unlikely to survive if treated, as well as those who are likely to survive even without treatment.[39] This determination can be problematic and not clear-cut in many circumstances, because speculating about a patient's prognosis can be challenging even when resources are abundant. Undoubtedly, making these determinations would be complex, emotional, and potentially traumatic for all health care workers involved. In addition, there are legal considerations as the shift away from individual rights occurs, and as providers are faced with the unfortunate potential to make determinations based solely on discriminatory factors such as age.[40] Individuals with expertise in biomedical ethics and legal considerations in these determinations can be essential in providing guidance in decision-making. When surveyed about their ability and preparedness to make these determinations during a crisis situation, one group of physicians in Canada indicated feeling only partially prepared, with most reporting that this situation would be considerably difficult to experience.[41]

As such, it is imperative that hospitals create an ethical framework for the possible shift of resources during times of pandemic-associated scarcity. Clear, transparent, and consistent protocols for the use of resources must be drafted ahead of any pandemic, so that appropriate and sound stewardship of supplies can occur at the earliest onset of any shortage, to preempt physicians from having the difficult task of deciding which patients are offered life-saving measures during a crisis. Ideally, the triage of sick patients and determinations about the use of resources such as intensive care unit beds and ventilators would not be made by the treating team. These determinations should be made based on the framework already in place, and final decisions could be made by a team led by those with training in ethics, legal matters, and palliative care.[42]

Consideration may also need to be given to ethical questions regarding health care workers' obligations to continue to put themselves at risk for infection during a pandemic involving an infectious contagion. Doctors and nurses have a right to protect themselves and members of their family from illness. Shortages of PPE and staffing may lead to situations in which health care workers are potentially asked to care for patients without having all of the necessary equipment or support to do so while preventing disease transmission. Every effort should be made to ensure that health care workers, who have the specialized training to provide care and without whom operations would not be able to continue, are prioritized with regard to PPE distribution. An ethics team may consider having prepandemic discussions regarding a health care worker's right to discharge their duty in a situation in which resources are lacking. Collaboration with health care workers regarding expectations of duty during a pandemic should be undertaken before any such scenario.[43]

PREVENTING PSYCHOLOGICAL INJURY

Health care facilities have an obligation to make preparations to look out for the well-being of their staff during a pandemic. Health care workers will be asked to potentially put themselves in harm's way and to treat patients in times of medical uncertainty and scarcity of resources, during which poor outcomes are likely. Prevention of emotional distress and mitigation of its causative factors should be the goal, rather than only providing posttraumatic psychological services.[44] Preserving emotional wellness and resilience from the start of a pandemic achieves the goal of maintaining stable health care services and ideally preventing staff shortages from absenteeism.

Giving health care personnel the knowledge and tools to feel fully prepared to face pandemic conditions is the first and most essential step to preventing psychological and moral injury; this means keeping all staff well-informed and providing sufficient supplies of PPE. Staff who feel fully supported in their duties and properly prepared to face all challenges are less likely to suffer mental health problems after a crisis.[45]

Depending on the experiences of staff and the degree of moral injury or psychological damage that may occur during a pandemic, stress may manifest in different ways in health care workers, ranging from signs and symptoms of acute stress reactions to development of posttraumatic stress disorder.[46] Staff should be educated to recognize these symptoms in themselves, and leaders and managers should evaluate their staff regularly, as well. Regular counseling or debrief sessions held among health care worker cohorts with shared experiences can be one way to monitor staff for development of stress reactions, allow an outlet for emotions, and offer additional help when needed.[46]

Additional sources of stress during a pandemic include uncertainty about maintaining employment and income, as well as fear of bringing a contagion home from work and infecting family members. To whatever extent possible, income should be ideally guaranteed to frontline staff who are asked to put themselves at risk every day. For staff with significant exposures to infected individuals, testing should be offered quickly and free of charge. To allay fears of transmitting an infection to family, hospitals may make use of nearby hotels or other sites for quarantine accommodations for sick or isolated personnel.[47]

When a staff member presents with signs of mental health problems during or after a pandemic, hospitals should offer psychological support services in the form of counseling or even referral for psychiatric care. An organization's mental health providers could be redeployed to treat staff and provide counseling and therapy sessions. Required and regularly scheduled check-ins with peer support counselors or trained therapists for all frontline staff can help normalize the act of seeking psychological support.[48]

SUMMARY

The high likelihood of future pandemics from emerging or reemerging infectious pathogens is widely accepted.[49] The increasing interrelatedness of our world, the changing climate, antibiotic misuse, and animal exposures are all reasons why novel pathogens are likely to increasingly crossover to infect humans with pandemic potential. Despite diligent efforts in emergency preparedness, the COVID-19 pandemic found many health care facilities underprepared for several aspects of pandemic readiness. We must learn from this experience and use this time to better prepare for continued high-quality health care delivery and for the continued well-being and safety of health care personnel before the next pandemic.

REFERENCES

1. Cavallo JJ, Donoho DA, Forman HP. Hospital capacity and operations in the coronavirus disease 2019 (COVID-19) pandemic—planning for the Nth patient. JAMA Health Forum 2020;1(3):e200345.

2. Banach DB, Johnston BL, Al-Zubeidi D, et al. Outbreak response and incident management: SHEA guidance and resources for healthcare epidemiologists in United States acute-care hospitals. Infect Control Hosp Epidemiol 2017;38(12): 1393–419.
3. Federal Emergency Management Agency (FEMA). Emergency Management Institute (EMI). National Incident Management. System (NIMS) website. Available at: https://training.fema.gov/nims/. Accessed March 31, 2021.
4. Gupta S, Federman DG. Hospital preparedness for COVID-19 pandemic: experience from department of medicine at Veterans Affairs Connecticut Healthcare System. Postgrad Med 2020;132(6):489–94.
5. Orsini E, Mireles-Cabodevila E, Ashton R, et al. Lessons on outbreak preparedness from the cleveland clinic. Chest 2020;158(5):2090–6.
6. Zorn CK, Pascual JM, Bosch W, et al. Addressing the challenge of COVID-19: one health care site's leadership response to the pandemic. Mayo Clin Proc Innov Qual Outcomes 2021;5(1):151–60.
7. Varia M, Wilson S, Sarwal S, et al. Hospital Outbreak Investigation Team. Investigation of a nosocomial outbreak of severe acute respiratory syndrome (SARS) in Toronto, Canada. CMAJ 2003;169(4):285–92.
8. Centers for Disease Control and Prevention (CDC). Cluster of severe acute respiratory syndrome cases among protected health-care workers–Toronto, Canada, April 2003. MMWR Morb Mortal Wkly Rep 2003;52(19):433–6.
9. Galanis P, Vraka I, Fragkou D, et al. Seroprevalence of SARS-CoV-2 antibodies and associated factors in healthcare workers: a systematic review and meta-analysis. J Hosp Infect 2021;108:120–34.
10. Sahu AK, Amrithanand VT, Mathew R, et al. COVID-19 in health care workers - A systematic review and meta-analysis. Am J Emerg Med 2020;38(9):1727–31.
11. Selvaraj SA, Lee KE, Harrell M, et al. Infection rates and risk factors for infection among health workers during ebola and marburg virus outbreaks: a systematic review. J Infect Dis 2018;218(suppl_5):S679–89.
12. Thorne CD, Khozin S, McDiarmid MA. Using the hierarchy of control technologies to improve healthcare facility infection control: lessons from severe acute respiratory syndrome. J Occup Environ Med 2004;46(7):613–22.
13. Morawska L, Tang JW, Bahnfleth W, et al. How can airborne transmission of COVID-19 indoors be minimised? Environ Int 2020;142:105832.
14. United States Environmental Protection Agency. Indoor Air Quality: What is a HEPA Filter?. Available at: https://www.epa.gov/indoor-air-quality-iaq/what-hepa-filter-1. Accessed March 31, 2021.
15. Centers for Disease Control and Prevention (CDC). Ventilation in buildings. Available at: https://www.cdc.gov/coronavirus/2019-ncov/community/ventilation.html. Accessed March 31, 2021.
16. Centers for Disease Control and Prevention (CDC). Infection Control Guidance for Healthcare Professionals about Coronavirus (COVID-19). Available at: https://www.cdc.gov/coronavirus/2019-ncov/hcp/infection-control.html. Accessed March 31, 2021.
17. Chu DK, Akl EA, Duda S, et al. COVID-19 systematic urgent review group effort (SURGE) study authors. Physical distancing, face masks, and eye protection to prevent person-to-person transmission of SARS-CoV-2 and COVID-19: a systematic review and meta-analysis. Lancet 2020;395(10242):1973–87.
18. Whaley CM, Pera MF, Cantor J, et al. Changes in health services use among commercially insured US populations during the COVID-19 pandemic. JAMA Netw Open 2020;3(11):e2024984.

19. U.S. Department of Health and Human Services. Medical surge capacity and capability handbook, chapter 1, what is medical surge?. Available at: https://www.phe.gov/Preparedness/planning/mscc/handbook/chapter1/Pages/whatismedicalsurge.aspx. Accessed March 31, 2021.
20. Abate SM, Ahmed Ali S, Mantfardo B, et al. Rate of Intensive Care Unit admission and outcomes among patients with coronavirus: a systematic review and meta-analysis. PLoS One 2020;15(7):e0235653.
21. Griffin KM, Karas MG, Ivascu NS, et al. Hospital preparedness for COVID-19: a practical guide from a critical care perspective. Am J Respir Crit Care Med 2020;201(11):1337–44.
22. Chou R, Dana T, Buckley DI, et al. Epidemiology of and risk factors for coronavirus infection in health care workers: a living rapid review. Ann Intern Med 2020; 173(2):120–36.
23. Keeley C, Jimenez J, Jackson H, et al. Staffing up for the surge: expanding the New York city public hospital workforce during The COVID-19 Pandemic. Health Aff (Millwood) 2020;39(8):1426–30.
24. Rawaf S, Allen LN, Stigler FL, et al. Global forum on universal health coverage and primary health care. Lessons on the COVID-19 pandemic, for and by primary care professionals worldwide. Eur J Gen Pract 2020;26(1):129–33.
25. Lau J, Knudsen J, Jackson H, et al. Staying connected in the COVID-19 pandemic: telehealth at the largest safety-net system In The United States. Health Aff (Millwood) 2020;39(8):1437–42.
26. Lonergan PE, Washington SL Iii, Branagan L, et al. Rapid utilization of telehealth in a comprehensive cancer center as a response to COVID-19: cross-sectional analysis. J Med Internet Res 2020;22(7):e19322.
27. Krist AH, DeVoe JE, Cheng A, et al. Redesigning primary care to address the COVID-19 pandemic in the midst of the pandemic. Ann Fam Med 2020;18(4): 349–54.
28. Judson TJ, Odisho AY, Neinstein AB, et al. Rapid design and implementation of an integrated patient self-triage and self-scheduling tool for COVID-19. J Am Med Inform Assoc 2020;27(6):860–6.
29. Galmiche S, Rahbe E, Fontanet A, et al. Implementation of a self-triage web application for suspected COVID-19 and its impact on emergency call centers: observational study. J Med Internet Res 2020;22(11):e22924.
30. Schrager JD, Schuler K, Isakov AP, et al. Development and usability testing of a web-based COVID-19 self-triage Platform. West J Emerg Med 2020;21(5): 1054–8.
31. Ford D, Harvey JB, McElligott J, et al. Leveraging health system telehealth and informatics infrastructure to create a continuum of services for COVID-19 screening, testing, and treatment. J Am Med Inform Assoc 2020;27(12):1871–7.
32. Kwon KT, Ko JH, Shin H, et al. Drive-through screening center for COVID-19: a safe and efficient screening system against massive community outbreak. J Korean Med Sci 2020;35(11):e123.
33. Yaffee AQ, Peacock E, Seitz R, et al. Preparedness, adaptation, and innovation: approach to the COVID-19 pandemic at a decentralized, quaternary care department of emergency medicine. West J Emerg Med 2020;21(6):63–70.
34. Garg S, Basu S, Rustagi R, et al. Primary health care facility preparedness for outpatient service provision during the COVID-19 pandemic in india: cross-sectional study. JMIR Public Health Surveill 2020;6(2):e19927.
35. Office of Public Health Preparedness and Response (OPHPR). Crisis & Emergency Risk Communication (CERC). Centers for Disease Control and Prevention

website. Available at: https://emergency.cdc.gov/cerc/. Accessed March 31, 2021.

36. Anyanwu EC, Ward RP, Shah A, et al. A mobile app to facilitate socially-distanced hospital communication during the COVID-19 pandemic: implementation experience. JMIR Mhealth Uhealth 2021.

37. Chowdhury JM, Patel M, Zheng M, et al. Mobilization and preparation of a large urban academic center during the COVID-19 pandemic. Ann Am Thorac Soc 2020;17(8):922–5.

38. Leider JP, Debruin D, Reynolds N, et al. Ethical guidance for disaster response, specifically around crisis standards of care: a systematic review. Am J Public Health 2017;107(9):e1–9.

39. Sese D, Ahmad MU, Rajendram P. Ethical considerations during the COVID-19 pandemic. Cleve Clin J Med 2020.

40. Farrell TW, Francis L, Brown T, et al. Rationing limited healthcare resources in the COVID-19 era and beyond: ethical considerations regarding older adults. J Am Geriatr Soc 2020;68(6):1143–9.

41. Dewar B, Anderson JE, Kwok ESH, et al. Physician preparedness for resource allocation decisions under pandemic conditions: a cross-sectional survey of Canadian physicians, April 2020. PLoS One 2020;15(10):e0238842.

42. Emanuel EJ, Persad G, Upshur R, et al. Fair allocation of scarce medical resources in the time of covid-19. N Engl J Med 2020;382(21):2049–55.

43. Bakewell F, Pauls MA, Migneault D. Ethical considerations of the duty to care and physician safety in the COVID-19 pandemic. CJEM 2020;22(4):407–10.

44. Walton M, Murray E, Christian MD. Mental health care for medical staff and affiliated healthcare workers during the COVID-19 pandemic. Eur Heart J Acute Cardiovasc Care 2020;9(3):241–7.

45. Greenberg N, Docherty M, Gnanapragasam S, et al. Managing mental health challenges faced by healthcare workers during covid-19 pandemic. BMJ 2020;368:m1211.

46. Zaka A, Shamloo SE, Fiorente P, et al. COVID-19 pandemic as a watershed moment: a call for systematic psychological health care for frontline medical staff. J Health Psychol 2020;25(7):883–7.

47. Almaghrabi RH, Alfaraidi HA, Al Hebshi WA, et al. Healthcare workers experience in dealing with Coronavirus (COVID-19) pandemic. Saudi Med J 2020;41(6):657–60.

48. Carmassi C, Foghi C, Dell'Oste V, et al. PTSD symptoms in healthcare workers facing the three coronavirus outbreaks: what can we expect after the COVID-19 pandemic. Psychiatry Res 2020;292:113312.

49. Morens DM, Fauci AS. Emerging pandemic diseases: how we got to COVID-19. Cell 2020;182(5):1077–92.

Development of a Critical Care Response - Experiences from Italy During the Coronavirus Disease 2019 Pandemic

Emanuele Rezoagli, MD, PhD[a,b],*, Aurora Magliocca, MD, PhD[a],
Giacomo Bellani, MD, PhD[a,b], Antonio Pesenti, MD[c,d],
Giacomo Grasselli, MD[c,d]

KEYWORDS

- Critical care • Pandemic • Coronavirus disease 19 • COVID19 Lombardy Network
- Organizational response • Helmet continuous positive airway pressure
- Awake proning

KEY POINTS

- Italy was the first western country to face a large coronavirus disease 2019 (COVID-19) outbreak.
- COVID19 Lombardy Network responded to the surge of hospital admissions in Northern Italy; it organized a rapid increase in intensive care unit (ICU) beds and implemented measures for containment.
- Scientific evidence was provided by Italian centers to characterize the clinical history of COVID-19 associated respiratory failure.
- Relevant experience was collected in Italy during the pandemic about the use of noninvasive continuous positive airway pressure and awake proning, which were implemented to manage respiratory failure out of the ICU setting.
- Recommendations from national guidelines were structured to guide health care providers on resource allocation; promotion of awareness among Italian citizens within specific humanitarian and educational programs was implemented.

This article previously appeared in *Anesthesiology Clinics*, Volume 39, Issue 2, June 2021.
Funded by: CRUI2020.
[a] Department of Medicine and Surgery, University of Milano-Bicocca, Via Cadore, 48, Monza 20900, Italy; [b] Department of Emergency and Intensive Care, San Gerardo Hospital, Via G. B. Pergolesi, 33, Monza 20900, Italy; [c] Department of Pathophysiology and Transplantation, University of Milan, Via Francesco Sforza 35, Milano 20122, Italy; [d] Department of Anesthesia, Intensive Care and Emergency, Fondazione IRCCS Ca' Granda Ospedale Maggiore Policlinico, Via della Commenda, 10, Milano 20122, Italy
* Corresponding author. Department of Medicine and Surgery, University of Milano-Bicocca, Via Cadore 48, Monza (MB) 20900, Italy.
E-mail address: emanuele.rezoagli@unimib.it

Clinics Collections 12 (2022) 15–34
https://doi.org/10.1016/j.ccol.2021.12.002
2352-7986/22/© 2021 Elsevier Inc. All rights reserved.

INTRODUCTION

Italy was the first western country facing an outbreak of coronavirus disease 2019 (COVID-19).[1] The first Italian patient diagnosed with COVID-19 was admitted, on Feb. 20, 2020, to the intensive care unit (ICU) in Codogno Hospital (Lodi, Lombardy, Italy), and the number of reported positive cases increased to 36 in the next 24 hours, and then exponentially for 18 days. This triggered a prompt, coordinated response of the ICUs in the epicenter region of the outbreak that resulted in a massive surge in the ICU bed capacity.[2]

An Italian registry from 3 northern Italian regions (Lombardy, Emilia-Romagna and Veneto) showed that the rate of ICU admission was 12.6% of COVID-19 hospital admissions. Eight hundred and five patients were admitted and treated in the ICU among 6378 patients hospitalized for COVID-19 in the period between Feb. 24 through March 8, 2020.[3] The coordination of a critical care response in Italy happened in collaboration with out-of-hospital, and out-of-ICU management of patients with respiratory failure.

Furthermore, as part of the implementation of an organizational response to the SARS-CoV2 outbreak, many Italian research groups collected data and provided scientific evidence to understand how to better defeat coronavirus, and make this information quickly publicly available to help other countries that would have to face a similar challenge.

DEVELOPMENT OF A CRITICAL CARE RESPONSE – CORONAVIRUS DISEASE 2019 LOMBARDY INTENSIVE CARE UNIT NETWORK ORGANIZATIONAL PERSPECTIVE

The critical care response to the COVID-19 pandemic started with the formation of an emergency task force on Feb. 21, created by the Lombardy region authorities and health care representatives: the COVID-19 Lombardy ICU Network (2). The aim of the COVID-19 Lombardy ICU Network was to manage the allocation of resources for all COVID-19 patients requiring ICU treatment in the region. The intensive care team of the Policlinico Maggiore Hospital in Milan led the clinical task force, which was active 24 hours per day, 7 days per week to manage bed request calls.

The 2 primary goals of the network in the initial response phase were to increase surge ICU capacity and to implement measures for containment.

Increase of Surge Intensive Care Unit Capacity

The precrisis ICU capacity was

- Lombardy: approximately 738 ICU beds (7.4 beds/100,000 people, equal to 2.9% of the total number of hospital beds)
- Italy: approximately 4682 ICU beds[4]

An exponential model for the prediction of ICU admission rate estimated a need of up to 2500 ICU beds in only 1 week for COVID-19 patients.[5] Using this model, the whole Italian National Health System would be saturated by mid-April. Drawing from the experience of the Venous-Venous ECMO Respiratory Failure Network,[6] one of the first initiatives of the network was to create 15 COVID-19 dedicated hub hospitals, with specific expertise in the management of patients with acute respiratory distress syndrome (ARDS) and infectious diseases.

Specific tasks of the hub hospitals were to:

1. Create dedicated ICU cohorts for COVID-19 patients
2. Create triage areas with the possibility to assist critical patients waiting for diagnostic test results for COVID-19

3. Establish local protocols for triage and rapid allocation of patients with respiratory symptoms
4. Ensure adequate personal protective equipment (PPE) availability and training of health care workers
5. Immediately notify the regional coordinating center of every confirmed case of critical COVID-19

Through a central coordination of the ICU Network, 130 ICU beds dedicated to COVID-19 patients were created in Lombardy in 48 hours. After the saturation of the designated hub hospitals, almost all hospitals of the region created dedicated ICUs, and on April 2, the ICU capacity reached 1750 beds. In addition, on March 31, 2020, the Milan Fair COVID-19 Intensive Care Hospital was inaugurated. The project, developed by Fondazione Fiera Milano in partnership with Lombardy Region consisted of a temporary hospital with up to 250 ICU beds developed in 20 days, and covering more than 25,000 square meters (**Fig. 1**). The hospital reorganization process, with the opening of newly dedicated ICUs, has been a multidisciplinary effort, with the involvement of health care providers, hospital managers, and political authorities.[7–9] The Italian government allocated 845 million euros to the National Health System to ensure a progressive increase of the number of ICU beds for invasive mechanical ventilation, up to 14% of the total hospital beds.[10]

Implementation of Measures for Containment

The government instituted extraordinary measures for containment: restrictions within lockdown areas (red zones) were implemented gradually, and then expanded to the entire country on March 9, 2020, until May 18, 2020. A second wave of infections is currently ongoing in several European countries, including Italy. Measures for containment and restrictions within Italian territory were instituted again from Oct. 26, 2020,

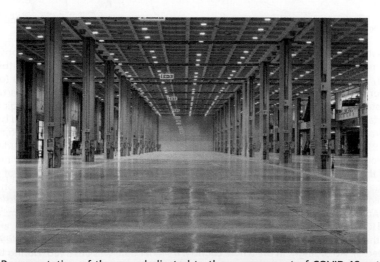

Fig. 1. Representation of the area dedicated to the management of COVID-19 patients at the Fair Milan Covid-19 Intensive Care Hospital covering more than 25,000 square meters of area Portello Pavilions 1 and 2 at Fieramilanocity, Milan, Italy. The image represents the empty space before Fair Milan Covid-19 Intensive Care Hospital was yet staged (permission obtained to reproduce the image by Fondazione Fiera – All Rights reserved – https://www.ospedalefieramilano.it/it/l-progetto.html).

based on the estimate of transmissibility within each region.[11] As of Dec. 13, 2020, the number of hospitalized patients in Lombardy and Italy was 5873 and 30,893, respectively; the number of ICU patients was 714 and 3,158, respectively. Overall, during the last 8 months, totals of 23,810 and 64,520 patients have died of SARS-CoV2 in Lombardy (**Fig. 2**A,B) and Italy (**Fig. 2**C,D), respectively.

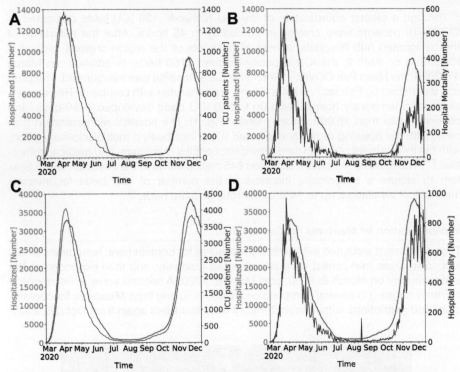

Fig. 2. Number of daily hospital versus ICU admissions (*A, C*) and hospital admissions versus hospital mortality (*B, D*) during the Italian first and second wave of SARS-CoV2 outbreak in Lombardy (top panels) and in Italy (bottom panels) from Feb. 24 to Dec. 13, 2020 (original data reports from the public source of "Presidenza del Consiglio dei Ministri - Dipartimento della Protezione Civile" https://github.com/pcm-dpc/COVID-19/blob/master/dati-regioni/dpc-covid19-ita-regioni.csv). (*D*) The peak of mortality reported on Aug. 15 was explained by internal verification of mortality data of Azienda Unità Sanitaria Locale of Parma (Emilia Romagna) that reported 154 deaths over March, April, and May that were not previously included. The distribution of hospitalized patients, ICU admissions, and deaths was different during the 2 peaks of the Italian SARS-CoV2 pandemic. In Lombardy, while the highest number of deaths during the first wave (ie, 546 deaths) was reported approximately 10 days before (ie, on March 20) the highest number of hospitalized patients (ie, 13,328 on April 4) and ICU admissions (ie, 1381 on April 3), during the second coronavirus peak, the highest capacitance in terms of hospital and ICU beds (ie, 9340 and 949, respectively) was reached earlier (ie, on Nov. 22), and contrary to the first wave, 10 days in advance compared with the highest number of deaths (ie, 347 on Dec. 3). Accordingly, in the whole country, a similar date was observed. During the first SARS-CoV2 wave, the highest number of deaths (ie, 969 deaths) was reported about 10 days before (ie, on March 26) compared with the highest request of hospital (ie, 33,004 on April 4) and ICU beds (ie, 4068 on April 3). In contrast, during the second peak of the pandemic, the highest numbers of hospital and ICU admissions (ie, 38,507 and 3848, respectively) were recorded on Nov. 23 and 25, respectively, about 10 days before the peak of COVID-19 deaths (ie, 993 on Dec. 3). (Visual courtesy of Francesco Casola.)

OUT-OF-HOSPITAL CORONAVIRUS DISEASE 2019 RESPONSE - AN ORGANIZATIONAL PERSPECTIVE
Organization of the Emergency Medical Service

The Emergency Medical Services (EMS) of the Lombardy region had to deal with an unprecedented increase in telephone calls to 112 (European emergency number) after the announcement of the first COVID-19 positive patient in Italy on Feb. 20, 2020. Call volumes registered a 264% increase compared with the 3 previous years on the 23rd of February in the metropolitan area of Milan (SOREU metropolitan).[12] Similar reports from other areas showed an increase in calls up to 440% compared with the pre-COVID-19 period.[13]

Several callers were just requesting information and guidance about COVID-19. Many others were suspected symptomatic patients deserving a prompt evaluation of respiratory symptoms, home isolation, and domicile SARS-CoV-2 testing or hospitalization. To cope with the escalation of calls, a COVID-19 response team was instituted by the EMS of the metropolitan area of Milan.[14] The team, composed of 10 health care professionals and 2 technicians, worked 24 hours per day 7 days per week in assessing the clinical condition of screened individuals to determine the need for hospital admission, or for home testing for SARS-CoV-2 and subsequent isolation. In essence, patients were screened for fever and any respiratory symptoms in order to

1. Organize ambulance
   dispatch and hospitalization in case of moderate or severe respiratory symptoms
2. Counsel, record, and isolate suspected or confirmed COVID-19 cases with mild symptoms

Despite efforts to maintain ordinary EMS activities through the creation of the COVID-19 response team, the reorganization of the 112 emergency response system, and the implementation of the staff, recent data showed that EMS arrival times were significantly higher compared with the same period in 2019 in Milan,[11] and in other provinces of Lombardy and Veneto, particularly for time-dependent conditions like out-of-hospital cardiac arrest.[15,16]

The Lombardy EMS coped with a dramatic increase in events caused by the outbreak in the region in an extremely short timeframe, and in a limited area, as occurred in the province of Bergamo. Data about the events managed by the dispatch center for the EMS of Brescia and Bergamo describe a devastating scenario. Fagoni and colleagues reported an increase of 50% in the number of events managed in March to April 2020, compared with the same period in 2019, with a tenfold increase in the number of the so-called respiratory or infective events. An alarming increase in the number of deaths was reported: +246% (odds ratio [OR] 1.7, *P*<.0001) in March to April 2020, compared with 2019.[17] This high mortality was in line with other reports from Italian cities severely affected by the COVID-19 pandemic in northern Italy.[18]

The Challenging Experience of Out-of-Hospital Cardiac Arrest During the Coronavirus Disease 2019 Outbreak

An almost 60% increase in out-of-hospital cardiac arrest (OHCA) incidence, coupled with a reduction in the short-term outcomes during the COVID-19 outbreak, was observed in Italy for the first time.[15] Specifically, during the first 40 days of the COVID-19 pandemic (Feb. 21 through March 31, 2020), the number of OHCAs occurring in the provinces of Lodi, Cremona, Pavia, and Mantua, increased up to 58% compared with the same period in 2019. An increase in the number of OHCA was seen in all 4 provinces, with a worrisome peak in the 2 most afflicted by COVID-19 infection: Lodi (+187%) and Cremona (+143%).

Among different etiologies, medical causes were more represented in OHCA during the COVID-19 pandemic. Age and sex of the patients were similar in the 2 study periods, but in 2020 home location and unwitnessed OHCA were more frequent compared with 2019. A decrease in bystander cardiopulmonary resuscitation rate of 15.6% was observed compared with the 2019 period. The median arrival time of emergency medical service was 3 minutes longer in 2020 than in 2019, and the incidence of out-of-hospital death was almost 15% higher in 2020 than in 2019. The cumulative incidence of out-of-hospital cardiac arrest in 2020 was strongly associated with the cumulative incidence of COVID-19. The authors then expanded the analysis to the following 60 days after the first COVID-19 patient was isolated, replicating the same results reported for the first 40 days.[19] On the contrary, a report from Padua in Veneto (northeast of Italy), did not highlight an increase in OHCA incidence and mortality.[16] However, in line with previous findings, the authors reported an increased EMS arrival time of 1.2 min in 2020 compared with 2019. Interestingly, when they broke the total arrival time into its main components (ie, call to dispatch, dispatch to departure, and departure to arrival), an increase in the time between the call and EMS departure was observed. The authors suggest that the longer call-to-departure time of the EMS could be due to the time spent to investigate COVID-19 status, while the delay in ambulance departure could be explained by PPE procedures and requirements.

IN-HOSPITAL CORONAVIRUS DISEASE 2019 RESPONSE - BUILDING SCIENTIFIC EVIDENCE

Intensive Care Unit Management of Coronavirus Disease 2019 Respiratory Failure

The COVID-19 Lombardy ICU Network was created to promptly respond to the SARS-CoV2 outbreak in Italy, and to manage the exponential surge of patients with respiratory failure, needing respiratory support in ICU. Fondazione IRCCS Ca' Granda Ospedale Maggiore Policlinico in Milan was the coordinating center of COVID-19 Lombardy ICU Network, which connected all the ICUs in the Lombardy region. Dedicated staff in the coordinator center of this consortium performed at least 2 telephone calls every day to obtain real-time granular information on most clinical characteristics and outcomes of patients admitted to the ICU.[20–22]

Despite the massive clinical and logistical efforts, COVID-19 Lombardy ICU Network was able to collect and provide scientific evidence about clinical characteristics, risk factors, pathophysiology, and prognosis of patients with SARS-CoV2 induced lung injury. Data collection was not limited to the mentioned phone calls, but also by local granular data collection in a centralized eCRF.

One of the aims of the COVID-19 Lombardy ICU Network was to deliver knowledge as rapidly as possible on a disease still poorly described, ultimately to help other countries facing a similarly dramatic health care experience.[23] Essentially, the research commitment of Ospedale Maggiore Policlinico was twofold in its objectives:

1. To build a registry that included all epidemiologic, clinical, and prognostic information of adult patients admitted to the hospital from the onset of the pandemic.
2. To create a biobank of samples to perform translational studies.

Data from this registry for national and international researchers will benefit patient care worldwide.[24] The authors summarized in **Table 1** the main scientific evidence reported by the COVID-19 Lombardy ICU Network, together with other Italian investigators, during the pandemic outbreak.

Table 1

Scientific evidence provided by the COVID-19 Lombardy ICU Network together with other Italian investigators during the pandemic outbreak to characterize the clinical history of critically ill COVID-19 patients

Areas of Research	Group of Research	Patient Population	Time of Inclusion	Main Findings
Clinical characteristics of COVID-19 ICU patients	COVID-19 Lombardy ICU Network[20]	1591 critically ill COVID-19 patients	Feb. 20 to March 8, 2020	• Median age of 63 (IQR 56–70) • Male-to-female ratio 4:1 • Hypertension was the most common comorbidity (49% of cases) • Of 1300 patients with ventilator data, 88% on mechanical ventilation, 11% on noninvasive ventilation • Median PEEP = 14 cmH$_2$O (IQR 12–16) -median Pao$_2$/Fio$_2$ = 160 (114–220) • Median Fio$_2$ = 70 (IQR 50–80) • Prone positioning was used in 27% of 875 patients • Patients with hypertension – compared to patients without hypertension – were older, with a more severe ARDS, requiring higher levels of PEEP and showing a higher ICU mortality (38 vs 22%, overall mortality 26%) • Short-term follow-up and half of patients with complete data at follow-up (March 25, 2020) were still in ICU

(continued on next page)

Table 1
(continued)

Areas of Research	Group of Research	Patient Population	Time of Inclusion	Main Findings
Risk factors of mortality in COVID-19 ICU patients	COVID-19 Lombardy ICU Network[21]	3988 critically ill COVID-19 patients	Feb. 20 to April 22	• Mortality was higher in males; in patients with at least 1 comorbidity; and in older patients (56 years old was the cut off – follow-up until May 30) • A higher severity of lung injury (ie, patients with a lower Pao_2, a higher Fio_2, and higher PEEP levels [$\geq$13 cmH$_2$O]) and a shorter duration of mechanical ventilation and hospital length of stay were correlated with a higher mortality rate • Among independent predictors of mortality – adjusted for time effect – 1. Older age and male sex (ie, baseline characteristics); 2. Hypercholesterolemia, type 2 diabetes, and chronic obstructive pulmonary disease (COPD) (ie, comorbidities); 3. A higher PEEP, a higher Fio_2 and a lower Pao_2/Fio_2 at admission (severity of lung injury): and 4. A trend to the use of any mechanical respiratory support (either noninvasive or invasive) was associated with a higher mortality rate

Pathophysiology of COVID-19 ARDS patients	Grasselli et al,[22] 2020	301 critically ill COVID-19 patients	March 9 -22	• Prospective multicenter observational study conducted in different regions from north to south of Italy
				• Median respiratory system compliance was 9 mL/cmH$_2$O higher in COVID-19 associated ARDS compared to patients with ARDS unrelated to COVID-19
				• Lung injury associated to COVID-19 appeared not only to be characterized by a parenchymal damage but included also an endothelial injury
				• The study reported a strong association between D-dimer concentration and areas of pulmonary hypoperfusion that was assessed by computed tomography (CT)-pulmonary angiography in a subgroup of patients
				• The role of different combination of levels of respiratory system compliance and D-dimer on outcome was investigated - in a multivariate model adjusted for sex, age, and severity of ARDS using Pao$_2$/Fio$_2$ the group of patients at the higher risk of mortality was the one with the worse epithelial and endothelial lung injury, as suggested by the combination of high D-dimer concentration and low compliance of the respiratory system

(continued on next page)

Table 1
(continued)

Areas of Research	Group of Research	Patient Population	Time of Inclusion	Main Findings
Hematological characteristics of COVID-19 patients	• Angelo Bianchi Bonomi Hemophilia and Thrombosis Center in Milan (COHERENT project)[25] • Angelo Bianchi Bonomi Hemophilia and Thrombosis Center in Milan[26]	• 62 COVID-19 patients – with low, intermediate or high intensity of care • 24 critically ill COVID-19 patients	First peak of the Italian COVID-19 outbreak	Both studies – according to the analyses of laboratory biomarkers of pro and anticoagulation, together with data regarding the viscoelastic properties of blood of COVID-19 patients by the use of thromboelastography – do not support hematological characteristics of disseminated intravascular coagulation – in contrast they demonstrated the presence of a prothrombotic phenotype that leads to a procoagulant imbalance that originates from a complex interplay between the inflammatory insult, hemostasis, and endothelial cells perturbation

Double patient ventilation with a single ventilator – feasible and ethical?
During a pandemic, there may be an imbalance between the numbers of critically ill patients requiring invasive ventilation, and the numbers of mechanical ventilators that are available. An interesting option that was proposed almost 15 years ago by Neyman and Irvin is to connect multiple patients to a single ventilator in order to compensate for the equipment shortage.[27] Researchers from Milano and Bologna in Italy successfully tested the feasibility of using a single turbine ventilator to provide ventilation in 2 simulated patients with different respiratory mechanic characteristics.[28] Beitler and colleagues took this experience to the next level and provided evidence of feasibility in COVID-19 patients with ARDS who shared ventilators for at least 2 days, under rigorous protocols, and experienced no adverse events.[29] This strategy still remains experimental. Critical points still need to be addressed such as the matching of respiratory mechanic characteristics of patients ventilated with a single ventilator – in order to avoid harm in one of them - and the safety of prolonged ventilator sharing.

Out of Intensive Care Unit Management of Coronavirus Disease 2019 Respiratory Failure

Noninvasive ventilation – state-of-the-art and guidelines
As stated, the massive burden of SARS-CoV2 on the Italian health care system quickly saturated the availability of ICU beds and mechanical ventilators. Among several, one of the challenges for health care providers was to manage and contain severe intrahospital respiratory failure outside the critical care environment. Noninvasive ventilation allowed physicians to stabilize patients, avoiding the progression to severe hypoxemia and muscle exhaustion that would eventually require invasive mechanical ventilation. Noninvasive positive pressure oxygenation strategies have been recently confirmed to be associated with a lower mortality risk compared to standard oxygen therapy.[30]

Noninvasive positive pressure ventilation (NIPPV) has played a key role in the management of COVID-19 patients out of the ICU during the Italian crisis surge. The rapid guidelines of the European Society of Intensive Care Medicine suggested on 1 side high-flow nasal cannula (HFNC) and NIPPV as strategies to reduce the need for intubation and overcome shortages of mechanical ventilators; on the other side, NIPPV was suggested for invasive ventilation as a last option in a scenario of a shortage of standard full-featured ventilators.[31] The worldwide guidelines on the management of critically ill COVID-19 patients confirmed the suggestion of the implementation of HFNC and NIPPV in acute hypoxemic respiratory failure (AHRF) and recommended early intubation in a controlled setting if worsening occurred.[32] The potential increase of virus aerosolization with NIPPV remains a significant concern regarding transmission of infection to health care providers.[33]

The Italian helmet continuous positive airway pressure experience during the coronavirus disease pandemic
The Italian approach to noninvasive ventilator management of COVID-19 AHRF was characterized in northern Italy by the use of helmet continuous positive airway pressure (c-PAP), because of the large Italian experience in the management of AHRF with this interface.[34]

The helmet is an interface of utmost utility in a pandemic scenario, in order to avoid the risk of aerosolization when helmet NIPPV is delivered through a ventilator, as suggested by Cabrini and colleagues[35] However, the use of helmet c-PAP has an excellent performance simply with a free-flow generator and a positive end-expiratory pressure (PEEP) valve at the helmet outlet, combined with a high-efficiency particulate air (HEPA) filter at the helmet outlet to reduce the risk of environmental contamination.[31,36] Furthermore, the helmet c-PAP bundle was proposed to optimize patient comfort using

1. A heat and moisture exchanger (HME) filter to decrease incoming noise
2. Counterweight fixing systems to stabilize the helmet position
3. Heated wire tubing with active humidification[37]

Early consensus management of non-ICU patients with SARS-CoV2 in Italy suggested the use of helmet c-PAP without humidification as the first choice.[38] Three Italian studies have reported data on the use of helmet c-PAP and NIPPV out of a critical care environment in COVID-19 patients.[39–41]

1. In a multicenter observational prospective study, Aliberti and colleagues described the characteristics and the outcome of patients undergoing c-PAP treatment in 3 high-dependency units in 2 Italian hospitals in Milan during the first pandemic wave. Out of 157 patients, helmet c-PAP successfully improved oxygenation from a $Pao_2/Fio_2 = 143$ to 206. However, intubation or death was higher compared to non-COVID-19 patients with the same severity of AHRF (45% vs 23%). Interestingly, patients with c-PAP failure showed higher inflammation (eg, high interleukin [IL]-6 levels) and activation of the coagulation cascade (eg, high D-Dimer levels) compared with patients who did not fail helmet c-PAP.[39]

2. In the emergency department of Papa Giovanni XXIII hospital (HPG23) from Bergamo (a city overly affected by the surge), Duca and colleagues described patient characteristics and the ventilator management. In a time frame of 10 days, the authors reported that out of 611 patients admitted to the emergency department with suspected COVID-19, 99 received ventilator support (12% invasive and 88% noninvasive) in the emergency department, and 85 of them were confirmed positive to SARS-CoV2 (median age 70 years, median Pao_2/Fio_2 ratio $= 128$). Given the resource limitation in the ICU setting at the outbreak onset, the internal hospital protocol in the emergency department of HPG23 adopted the use of helmet c-PAP or NIPPV in the presence of hypoxemia (SpO2<90%) or RR greater than 30/min during the administration of oxygen therapy by non-rebreather mask with an oxygen flow of 15 L/min. Patients were admitted to the ward until availability of an ICU bed. The follow-up mortality 2 months later was 77%, which was potentially explained by the severity of hypoxemia of patients admitted to the emergency department with standard oxygen therapy already maximized.[40]

3. The results from the largest data set that described the prevalence and the clinical characteristics of patients with COVID-19 treated with NIV outside the ICU, and that explored the factors associated with NIV failure (defined as need of intubation or death) were reported by Bellani and colleagues in a prospective single-day prevalence study (WARd-COVID). In 31 centers within the COVID-19 Lombardy ICU Network 8753 COVID-19 patients were present, accounting for an average of 62% of the overall hospital beds. Of these, 909 subjects (10.4%) received NIV out of the ICU. The use of the helmet or face-mask was used in a ratio of 3:1. NIV failed in 300 patients (37.6%). A higher c-reactive protein and lower Pao_2/Fio_2 and platelet counts were independent predictors of NIV failure. Mortality rate was 25% at 60-day follow-up. Although with a large sample size and the multicentric design of the study, the lower rates of NIV failure and mortality in the WARd-COVID – compared with previous reported studies[39,40] - may be explained by the different timing of patient enrollment and data collection (ie, 1 month later that the Italian SARS-CoV2 outbreak). At that time, the organizational optimization

of the ICU resources was already implemented by the COVID-19 Lombardy ICU Network. This consisted of an exponential increase of the number of ICU beds that might have allowed to treat patients with a less severe acute hypercapnic respiratory failure (AHRF) on the ward at the moment of patient enrollment (average $Pao_2/Fio_2 = 168$).[41] An exemplary image representing the use of helmet c-PAP in prone positioning – as performed in the authors' Institutions in Monza and Milano – is provided in **Fig. 3**.

The Italian experience with prone-positioning in spontaneously breathing patients
As with ARDS from other causes,[42] COVID-19 guidelines propose cycles of 12 to 16 hours of prone positioning in patients with moderate-severe ARDS and undergoing mechanical ventilation,[33] based on strong physiologic rationale.[43,44] No information was provided on the use of proning in awake, non-intubated patients in the recent guidelines where the knowledge of the benefits is limited. Nonsystematic differences have been reported in prone positioning compared to supine positioning in healthy volunteers, with the presence of a more homogeneous perfusion in selected subjects that might improve ventilation/perfusion matching.[45] The use of PEEP has been described to increase the ventilation/perfusion ratio in the dorsal areas of healthy subjects.[46] However, little is known in terms of the physiologic effects of PEEP in patients undergoing prone positioning with a severe impairment of gas exchange, as in the case with COVID-19 related ARDS.

Italy pioneered the use of prone positioning in awake COVID-19 patients spontaneously breathing and explored the role of noninvasive ventilation during protonation outside the ICU.

1. In a prospective study, Coppo and colleagues explored the feasibility and physiologic effects of prone positioning in 56 patients - on supplemental oxygen therapy only (21%) or with helmet c-PAP (79%). Prone positioning was feasible in 84% of patients. Oxygenation was significantly improved in the prone position (average Pao_2/Fio_2, 286 vs 181, $P<.0001$), and the oxygenation gain was maintained in 50% of the patient population after resupination. Among other factors, prone positioning seemed more effective if applied early after hospital admission.[47]
2. Data from a retrospective study by Ramirez and colleagues reported that pronation was feasible outside the ICU. Furthermore, patient mobilization, which included prone positioning, was effective in reducing failure rates of c-PAP in COVID-19 patients.[48]

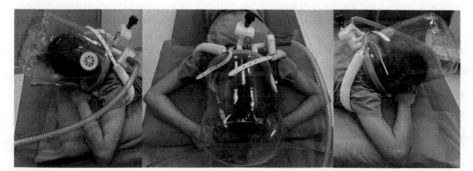

Fig. 3. Exemplary image of continuous positive pressure ventilation delivered by a helmet c-PAP during prone positioning in a healthy volunteer as per the authors' practice at San Gerardo Hospital, Monza and Policlinico Maggiore Hospital, Milano.

3. Bastoni and colleagues reported a series of 10 patients who met criteria for proning. In 6 patients, with a median Pao_2/Fio_2 of 68 mm Hg, prone positioning was effective at increasing oxygenation to a median Pao_2/Fio_2 of 97 mm Hg 1 hour after.[49]

4. The use of both prone and lateral positioning for 1 hour has been tested in 26 COVID-19 patients during helmet c-PAP admitted to the high-dependency unit of Policlinico Hospital in Milan. Retucci and colleagues observed that the success rate (ie, oxygenation improvement) of proning was higher compared with the use of lateral positioning. However, the short duration of patient positioning may have contributed to the loss of the beneficial improvement of oxygenation when patients returned to the semiseated position.[50]

In-hospital interplay and differences in the use of critical care resources between critical and noncritical care environments

Three regions in northern Italy joined together in a common effort to build a large network that included different experiences from the part of Italy that was severely hit by the outbreak. This led to the development of the COVID-19 Northern Italian ICU Network, which strived to report scientific evidence on the management and patient characteristics from different Italian areas.

In an interesting analysis from the COVID-19 Northern Italian ICU Network, the investigators reported differences among patients managed in and out of the ICU during the first 14 days of the pandemic outbreak (Feb. 24 to March 8, 2020). In the ICU, bed capacity rapidly increased from 1545 to 1989 beds (28.7%). In data obtained in 802 patients within 14 days, the percentage of patients who received respiratory support increased from 0.6% to 37% out of the ICU. Patients were located in the infectious disease ward, pneumology ward, emergency medicine, and intermediate care unit, with a proportion of 47%, 31%, 15%, and 7%, respectively. The proportion of patients admitted to ICU decreased from 20.3% to 15.2%. Patients located out of the ICU, compared to within the ICU, had more comorbidities, received more oxygen therapy and NIV, (with the exception of c-PAP that did not differ between the 2 groups), had higher Pao_2/Fio_2 and pH, and lower respiratory rate, $Paco_2$, and base excess.[3]

A useful score to predict clinical deterioration (defined as escalation of care to the ICU or death) in COVID-19 patients was proposed by Cecconi and colleagues. Higher levels of C-reactive protein (CRP) and creatinine, together with the presence of coronary artery disease, higher degree of hypoxemia, and a respiratory rate above or equal to 20 breaths per minute were used to build a prognostic index with a high predictive accuracy (85%) and easy implementation at bedside.[51] The findings obtained by Cecconi and coworkers were confirmed by the CORIST study – including almost 4000 patients from 30 clinical centers from northern, central and southern Italy – in which elevated CRP, impaired renal function, and advanced age predicted in-hospital mortality.[52]

SURGICAL PROCEDURES – CORONAVIRUS DISEASE 2019 POSITIVE AND NEGATIVE PATIENTS

The hospital overload of COVID-19 patients led to a sudden and unplanned interruption of elective surgical activities that led to the difficult process of balancing between the risk of delaying a cancer diagnosis and treatment, versus suffering a potential COVID-19 exposure, An individualized approach, based on a case-by case evaluation, is suggested.[53] Furthermore, in COVID-19-positive patients, precise, well-established plans and protocols must be implemented to perform emergent and nondeferrable surgical procedures.[54]

NATIONAL GUIDELINES ON RESOURCE ALLOCATION DURING CORONAVIRUS DISEASE 2019 – THE RESPONSE OF THE ITALIAN SOCIETY OF ANESTHESIA, ANALGESIA, RESUSCITATION, AND INTENSIVE CARE

The Italian Society of Anesthesia, Analgesia, Resuscitation, and Intensive Care (SIAARTI) provided documents and recommendations to manage the SARS-CoV2 outbreak at different levels, including both clinical practice[55] and ethical considerations.[56,57]

From an ethical perspective, SIAARTI elaborated recommendations in a scenario in which the surge of critical patients admitted to the hospital created an "imbalance between the real clinical needs of the population and the effective availability of intensive resources." The society highlighted 3 principles that should guide the decision-making process for appropriate allocation of limited health care resources:

1. Clinical appropriateness
2. Proportionality of care
3. Distributive justice

The SIAARTI guidelines aimed to help the clinicians in managing the potential emotional burden associated with resource allocation and make explicit the criteria for resource allocation. Although individual judgment must be considered part of the clinical decision, the presence of national recommendations served as a guide for clinicians to avoid frank disparities in the judgment and an arbitrary perspective in the presence of dramatic choices.

Scarce resources should be evaluated and considered in the presence of a higher probability of survival and of saved years of life – evaluating patient age, comorbidities, and the functional status before the event – and aiming to achieve a better outcome for the highest number of people.[56,57] Ethical and legal nuances of the national recommendations have been provided by the SIAARTI.[58,59]

SIAARTI, with the collaboration of Società Italiana di Infermieri di Terapia Intensiva (ANIARTI), Società Italiana di Medicina di Emergenza e Urgenza (SIMEU), Società Italiana di Cure Palliative (SICP), also provided guidance to health care workers for the management of communication on patient clinical conditions to the families that were completely isolated during the lockdown, and could not have any visual or physical interaction with their relative admitted to the hospital. The document, shared by these 4 societies, had 3 components, including a statement on communication with families, the key points used to develop the statements, and a checklist with instructions for how to make appropriate phone calls.[60]

Communication of clinical information to patient families was made difficult not only by the severity and acuity of such a novel disease, but also by the fear of the disease in non–health care workers, which created situations where health care professionals were praised while they were at work, but experienced discrimination when outside of the hospital setting.[61] This may have contributed to a psychological effect in the frontline personnel of the SARS-CoV2 pandemic.[62]

To promote awareness among people about the clinical condition of patients, and the daily working conditions of the health care workers during the COVID outbreak in Italy, Hope Onlus was created in collaboration with the Ospedale Maggiore Policlinico in Milan, and promoted the project "#Covid-19 con Hope" #Covid-19@storiedisperanza (www.hopeonlus.org). This important project has an educational and cultural mandate to explain the impact of COVID-19 on the society to Italian citizens within a humanitarian program of Hope Onlus, at both national and international levels. This project is composed of photo exhibitions, including images of the real-life conditions in the hospitals, together with stories of the health care workers in action (**Fig. 4**). The

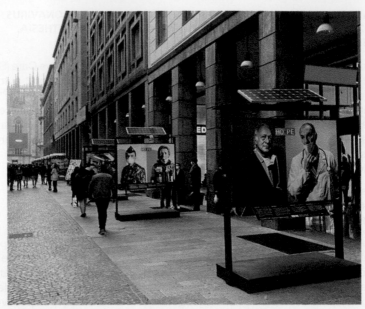

Fig. 4. Humanitarian Program Hope Onlus "#Covid-19 con Hope" #Covid-19@storiedisper-anza. On the first stand, Prof. Antonio Pesenti, on the left, and Prof. Giacomo Grasselli, on the right – Clinical Director and Clinical Lead of the Intensive Care Unit of Policlinico Maggiore Hospital, Milano – the 2 main actors who led the Lombardy Crisis Unit and coordinated the COVID-19 Lombardy ICU network.

authors' university is also participating in the FLOWS project, led by the National University of Ireland in Galway, which aims to identify the needs and development of best practice guidance for the psychological support of frontline health care workers during and after COVID-19.[63]

In conclusion, the Italian critical care experience during the first wave of the COVID-19 pandemic was a pioneer example of an organizational and clinical response to the outbreak. At the same time, a continuous effort was made to provide scientific evidence to understand how to better defeat coronavirus, and make this information available to help other countries worldwide.

CLINICS CARE POINTS

- Italy was the first western country to face a large COVID-19 outbreak.
- COVID19 Lombardy Network responded to the surge of hospital admissions in the Northern Italy; it organized a rapid increase in ICU beds and implemented measures for containment.
- Scientific evidence was provided by Italian centers to characterize the clinical history of COVID-19 associated respiratory failure
- Relevant experience was collected in Italy during the pandemic about the use of noninvasive continuous positive airway pressure and awake proning, which were remarkably implemented to manage respiratory failure out of the ICU setting.
- Recommendations from national guidelines were structured to guide health care providers on resource allocation; promotion of awareness among Italian citizens within specific humanitarian and educational programs was implemented

ACKNOWLEDGMENTS

The authors thank Francesco Casola, PhD, for his help with the visual of **Fig. 2.**

DISCLOSURE

The authors have nothing to disclose.

REFERENCES

1. WHO Director-General's opening remarks at the media briefing on COVID-19: 11 March 2020. 2020. Available at: https://covid19.who.int/?gclid=Cj0KCQiA-OeBBhDiARIsADyBcE4_O7cTc98_eNV7hXefnM_DNAfVfCmwKaXlmvzHipvRpqTF mrIaGBsaAq0VEALw_wcB.
2. Grasselli G, Pesenti A, Cecconi M. Critical care utilization for the COVID-19 outbreak in Lombardy, Italy: early experience and forecast during an emergency response. JAMA 2020;323(16):1545–6.
3. Tonetti T, Grasselli G, Zanella A, et al. Use of critical care resources during the first 2 weeks (February 24-March 8, 2020) of the Covid-19 outbreak in Italy. Ann Intensive Care 2020;10(1):133.
4. Pecoraro F, Clemente F, Luzi D. The efficiency in the ordinary hospital bed management in Italy: An in-depth analysis of intensive care unit in the areas affected by COVID-19 before the outbreak. PLoS One 2020;15(9):e0239249.
5. Remuzzi A, Remuzzi G. COVID-19 and Italy: what next? Lancet 2020;395(10231): 1225–8.
6. Patroniti N, Zangrillo A, Pappalardo F, et al. The Italian ECMO network experience during the 2009 influenza A(H1N1) pandemic: preparation for severe respiratory emergency outbreaks. Intensive Care Med 2011;37(9):1447–57.
7. Fagiuoli S, Lorini FL, Remuzzi G, et al. Adaptations and Lessons in the Province of Bergamo. N Engl J Med 2020;382(21):e71.
8. Carenzo L, Costantini E, Greco M, et al. Hospital surge capacity in a tertiary emergency referral centre during the COVID-19 outbreak in Italy. Anaesthesia 2020;75(7):928–34.
9. Buoro S, Di Marco F, Rizzi M, et al. Papa Giovanni XXIII Bergamo Hospital at the time of the COVID-19 outbreak: Letter from the warfront. Int J Lab Hematol 2020; 42(Suppl 1):8–10.
10. Available at: https://www.gazzettaufficiale.it/eli/id/2020/03/09/20G00030/sg. Accessed December 13, 2020.
11. Cori A, Ferguson NM, Fraser C, et al. A new framework and software to estimate time-varying reproduction numbers during epidemics. Am J Epidemiol 2013; 178(9):1505–12.
12. Marrazzo F, Spina S, Pepe PE, et al. Rapid reorganization of the Milan metropolitan public safety answering point operations during the initial phase of the COVID-19 outbreak in Italy. J Am Coll Emerg Physicians Open 2020;1(6):1240–9.
13. Perlini S, Canevari F, Cortesi S, et al. Emergency department and out-of-hospital emergency system (112-AREU 118) integrated response to coronavirus disease 2019 in a northern Italy centre. Intern Emerg Med 2020;15(5):825–33.
14. Spina S, Marrazzo F, Migliari M, et al. The response of Milan's emergency medical system to the COVID-19 outbreak in Italy. Lancet 2020;395(10227):e49–50.
15. Baldi E, Sechi GM, Mare C, et al. Out-of-hospital cardiac arrest during the covid-19 outbreak in Italy. N Engl J Med 2020;383(5):496–8.

16. Paoli A, Brischigliaro L, Squizzato T, et al. Out-of-hospital cardiac arrest during the COVID-19 pandemic in the Province of Padua, Northeast Italy. Resuscitation 2020;154:47–9.
17. Fagoni N, Perone G, Villa GF, et al. The Lombardy emergency medical system faced with COVID-19: the impact of out-of-hospital outbreak. Prehosp Emerg Care 2020;25:1–7.
18. Piccininni M, Rohmann JL, Foresti L, et al. Use of all cause mortality to quantify the consequences of covid-19 in Nembro, Lombardy: descriptive study. BMJ 2020;369:m1835.
19. Baldi E, Sechi GM, Mare C, et al. COVID-19 kills at home: the close relationship between the epidemic and the increase of out-of-hospital cardiac arrests. Eur Heart J 2020;41(32):3045–54.
20. Grasselli G, Zangrillo A, Zanella A, et al. Baseline characteristics and outcomes of 1591 patients infected with SARS-CoV-2 Admitted to ICUs of the lombardy region, Italy. JAMA 2020;323(16):1574–81.
21. Grasselli G, Greco M, Zanella A, et al. Risk factors associated with mortality among patients with COVID-19 in intensive care units in Lombardy, Italy. JAMA Intern Med 2020;180(10):1–11.
22. Grasselli G, Tonetti T, Protti A, et al. Pathophysiology of COVID-19-associated acute respiratory distress syndrome: a multicentre prospective observational study. Lancet Respir Med 2020;8(12):1201–8.
23. Cook DJ, Marshall JC, Fowler RA. Critical illness in patients with COVID-19: mounting an effective clinical and research response. JAMA 2020;323(16): 1559–60.
24. Bandera A, Aliberti S, Gualtierotti R, et al. Response of an Italian reference institute to research challenges regarding a new pandemic: COVID-19 network. Clin Microbiol Infect 2020;S1198-743X(20):30374–8.
25. Peyvandi F, Artoni A, Novembrino C, et al. Hemostatic alterations in COVID-19. Haematologica 2020. https://doi.org/10.3324/haematol.2020.262634.
26. Panigada M, Bottino N, Tagliabue P, et al. Hypercoagulability of COVID-19 patients in intensive care unit: a report of thromboelastography findings and other parameters of hemostasis. J Thromb Haemost 2020;18(7):1738–42.
27. Neyman G, Irvin CB. A single ventilator for multiple simulated patients to meet disaster surge. Acad Emerg Med 2006;13:1246–9.
28. Tonetti T, Zanella A, Pizzilli G, et al. One ventilator for two patients: feasibility and considerations of a last resort solution in case of equipment shortage. Thorax 2020;75(6):517–9.
29. Beitler JR, Mittel AM, Kallet R, et al. Ventilator sharing during an acute shortage caused by the COVID-19 pandemic. Am J Respir Crit Care Med 2020;202(4): 600–4.
30. Ferreyro BL, Angriman F, Munshi L, et al. Association of noninvasive oxygenation strategies with all-cause mortality in adults with acute hypoxemic respiratory failure: a systematic review and meta-analysis. JAMA 2020;324(1):57–67.
31. Aziz S, Arabi YM, Alhazzani W, et al. Managing ICU surge during the COVID-19 crisis: rapid guidelines. Intensive Care Med 2020;46(7):1303–25.
32. Alhazzani W, Møller MH, Arabi YM, et al. Surviving sepsis campaign: guidelines on the management of critically ill adults with coronavirus disease 2019 (COVID-19). Intensive Care Med 2020;46(5):854–87.
33. Hui DS, Chow BK, Ng SS, et al. Exhaled air dispersion distances during noninvasive ventilation via different Respironics face masks. Chest 2009;136:998–1005.

34. Bellani G, Patroniti N, Greco M, et al. The use of helmets to deliver non-invasive continuous positive airway pressure in hypoxemic acute respiratory failure. Minerva Anestesiol 2008;74(11):651–6.

35. Cabrini L, Landoni G, Zangrillo A. Minimise nosocomial spread of 2019-nCoV when treating acute respiratory failure. Lancet 2020;395(10225):685.

36. Lucchini A, Giani M, Winterton D, et al. Procedures to minimize viral diffusion in the intensive care unit during the COVID-19 pandemic. Intensive Crit Care Nurs 2020;60:102894.

37. Lucchini A, Giani M, Isgrò S, et al. The "helmet bundle" in COVID-19 patients undergoing non invasive ventilation. Intensive Crit Care Nurs 2020;58:102859.

38. Vitacca M, Nava S, Santus P, et al. Early consensus management for non-ICU ARF SARS-CoV-2 emergency in Italy: from ward to trenches. Eur Respir J 2020;55(5):2000632.

39. Aliberti S, Radovanovic D, Billi F, et al. Helmet CPAP treatment in patients with COVID-19 pneumonia: a multicenter, cohort study. Eur Respir J 2020;56(4):2001935.

40. Duca A, Memaj I, Zanardi F, et al. Severity of respiratory failure and outcome of patients needing a ventilatory support in the Emergency Department during Italian novel coronavirus SARS-CoV2 outbreak: preliminary data on the role of Helmet CPAP and non-invasive positive pressure ventilation. EClinicalMedicine 2020;24:100419.

41. Bellani G, Grasselli G, Cecconi M, et al. Noninvasive ventilatory support of COVID-19 patients outside the Intensive Care Units (WARd-COVID). Ann Am Thorac Soc 2021. https://doi.org/10.1513/AnnalsATS.202008-1080OC.

42. Fan E, Del Sorbo L, Goligher EC, et al. An Official American Thoracic Society/European Society of Intensive Care Medicine/Society of Critical Care Medicine clinical practice guideline: mechanical ventilation in adult patients with acute respiratory distress syndrome. Am J Respir Crit Care Med 2017;195(9):1253–63.

43. Gattinoni L, Taccone P, Carlesso E, et al. Prone position in acute respiratory distress syndrome. Rationale, indications, and limits. Am J Respir Crit Care Med 2013;188(11):1286–93.

44. Guerin C, Baboi L, Richard JC. Mechanisms of the effects of prone positioning in acute respiratory distress syndrome. Intensive Care Med 2014;40(11):1634–42.

45. Musch G, Layfield JDH, Harris RS, et al. Topographical distribution of pulmonary perfusion and ventilation, assessed by PET in supine and prone humans. J Appl Physiol (1985) 2002;93(5):1841–51.

46. Mure M, Nyrén S, Jacobsson H, et al. High continuous positive airway pressure level induces ventilation/perfusion mismatch in the prone position. Crit Care Med 2001;29(5):959–64.

47. Coppo A, Bellani G, Winterton D, et al. Feasibility and physiological effects of prone positioning in non-intubated patients with acute respiratory failure due to COVID-19 (PRON-COVID): a prospective cohort study. Lancet Respir Med 2020;8(8):765–74.

48. Ramirez GA, Bozzolo EP, Castelli E, et al. Continuous positive airway pressure and pronation outside the intensive care unit in COVID 19 ARDS. Minerva Med 2020. https://doi.org/10.23736/S0026-4806.20.06952-9.

49. Bastoni D, Poggiali E, Vercelli A, et al. Prone positioning in patients treated with non-invasive ventilation for COVID-19 pneumonia in an Italian emergency department. Emerg Med J 2020;37(9):565–6.

50. Retucci M, Aliberti S, Ceruti C, et al. Prone and lateral positioning in spontaneously breathing patients with COVID-19 pneumonia undergoing noninvasive helmet CPAP Treatment. Chest 2020;158(6):2431–5.
51. Cecconi M, Piovani D, Brunetta E, et al. Early predictors of clinical deterioration in a cohort of 239 patients hospitalized for COVID-19 infection in Lombardy, Italy. J Clin Med 2020;9(5):1548.
52. Di Castelnuovo A, Bonaccio M, Costanzo S, et al. Common cardiovascular risk factors and in-hospital mortality in 3,894 patients with COVID-19: survival analysis and machine learning-based findings from the multicentre Italian CORIST Study. Nutr Metab Cardiovasc Dis 2020;30(11):1899–913.
53. Moletta L, Sefora Pierobon E, Capovilla G, et al. International guidelines and recommendations for surgery during COVID-19 pandemic: a systematic review. Int J Surg 2020;79:180–8.
54. Coccolini F, Perrone G, Chiarugi M, et al. Surgery in COVID-19 patients: operational directives. World J Emerg Surg 2020;15(1):25.
55. Sorbello M, El-Boghdadly K, Di Giacinto I, et al. The Italian coronavirus disease 2019 outbreak: recommendations from clinical practice. Anaesthesia 2020; 75(6):724–32.
56. Vergano M, Bertolini G, Giannini A, et al. SIAARTI recommendations for the allocation of intensive care treatments in exceptional, resource-limited circumstances. Minerva Anestesiol 2020;86(5):469–72.
57. Vergano M, Bertolini G, Giannini A, et al. Clinical ethics recommendations for the allocation of intensive care treatments in exceptional, resource-limited circumstances: The Italian perspective during the COVID-19 epidemic. Crit Care 2020;24:165.
58. Piccinni M, Aprile A, Benciolini P, et al. [Ethical, deontologic and legal considerations about SIAARTI document "clinical ethics recommendations for the allocation of intensive care treatments, in exceptional, resource-limited circumstances." Recenti Prog Med 2020;111(4):212–22.
59. Sulmasy DP. Principled decisions and virtuous care: an ethical assessment of the SIAARTI Guidelines for allocating intensive care resources. Minerva Anestesiol 2020;86(8):872–6.
60. Multidisciplinary Working Group. ComuniCovid." Italian Society of Anesthesia and Intensive Care (SIAARTI), Italian Association of Critical Care Nurses (Aniarti), ItalianSociety of Emergency Medicine (SIMEU), and Italian SocietyPalliative Care (SICP). How to communicate with families of patients in complete isolation during SARS-CoV-2 pandemic multidisciplinary working group "ComuniCoViD. Recenti Prog Med 2020;111(6):357–67.
61. Cabrini L, Grasselli G, Cecconi M, et al. Yesterday heroes, today plague doctors: the dark side of celebration. Intensive Care Med 2020;46(9):1790–1.
62. Azoulay E, De Waele J, Ferrer R, et al. Symptoms of burnout in intensive care unit specialists facing the COVID-19 outbreak. Ann Intensive Care 2020;10(1):110.
63. Available at: https://hrbopenresearch.org/articles/3-54. Accessed December 13, 2020.

Severe Acute Respiratory Syndrome Coronavirus 2 Serology Testing – A Laboratory Primer

Patricia R. Slev, PhD, D(ABCC)[a,b,*]

KEYWORDS

- SARS-CoV-2 serology • COVID-19 • Antibody laboratory testing

KEY POINTS

- There are dozens of EUA serology assays,for SARS-CoV-2 that differ in methodology, antibody class detected, antigenic target, and performance characteristics. Although there are recommendations against using IgM as a standalone and IgA, there are no other specific recommendations with regard to antigenic target or antibody class.
- The vast majority of antibody assays are qualitative and detect binding antibodies which include neutralizing antibodies. There is one EUA serology assay that specifically detects neutralizing antibodies. Multiple studies have demonstrated a positive correlation between binding and neutralizing antibody assays.
- Antibody testing should not be used for diagnosing SARS-CoV-2 infection and utility is currently limited to seroprevalence studies, as an aid in supporting a multisystem inflammatory syndrome in children (MIS-C) diagnosis, or diagnosis in adults presenting late in the disease course, and identifying eligible donors for COVID-19 convalescent plasma (CCP).
- As of May 2021, there are no recommendations from any of the professional societies (IDSA, CDC, AACC) for antibody testing to qualify for vaccine administration postnatural infection or for assessing adequate immune response due to vaccination.

INTRODUCTION

In 2019, a new coronavirus virus, SARS-CoV-2, emerged that would lead to a worldwide pandemic and highlight the importance of laboratory medicine in infectious disease management.[1] In 2021, SARS-CoV-2 remains a priority for laboratory testing. Although diagnostic testing to determine who was infected with the virus was at the forefront of the pandemic, as serology testing became available, public interest in

This article previously appeared in *Clinics in Laboratory Medicine*, Volume 42, Issue 1, March 2022.

[a] Immunology Division, ARUP Laboratories, 500 Chipeta Way, Salt Lake City, UT 80108, USA;
[b] Department of Pathology, University of Utah School of Medicine, Salt Lake City, UT, USA
* ARUP Laboratories, 500 Chipeta Way, Salt Lake City, UT 80108, USA
E-mail address: Patricia.slev@aruplab.com

2352-7986/22/© 2021 Elsevier Inc. All rights reserved.

testing quickly rose and demanded that laboratories offer serology testing, even though antibody testing utility was limited. In the early days of the pandemic, March and April 2020, serology testing was not recommended for clinical purposes and was deemed of limited clinical value.[2,3] Therefore, the FDA did not see a need for strict regulations for antibody testing. This led to a proliferation of SARS-CoV-2 antibody tests, dominated early on by lateral flow assays (LFA) imported from various parts of the world. At the time, the FDA only required that the manufacturer notify the FDA of their intent to bring an antibody assay to market without any data requirements to support the performance characteristics of the assay. The consequence was a rapid and unprecedented proliferation of unvalidated, expensive assays quickly made available to anyone who wanted access. In addition, many were confused about rapid tests and incorrectly assumed that because of the ease of use that these rapid tests could be used in any setting, such as physicians' offices, without laboratory oversight or validation. The combination of public curiosity as to whether they had been infected with the virus and the lack of validated antibody tests used indiscriminately in any setting was accompanied by a considerable amount of bad press because many of the assays were inaccurate. This situation quickly escalated and highlighted the need for quality serology tests, FDA oversight, and the importance of the laboratory in validating serology assays. In early May 2020, the FDA issued new guidance for Emergency Use Authorization (EUA) claims for serology assays, that stated that, although manufacturers could notify the FDA of their intent to bring a serology assay to market as a first step to obtaining EUA, the manufacturer also had to provide supporting data to the FDA within 10 days of the notification. In addition, the FDA instituted an umbrella protocol that allowed for serology assays to be independently evaluated through NIH by agencies such as the National Cancer Institute (NCI), CDC, and Biomedical Advanced Research and Development Authority (BARDA). The FDA has also published templates for test manufacturers with recommendations for the number of samples that should be evaluated to determine performance characteristics and threshold requirements for performance characteristics (please refer to the section on serology assay evaluation).

The pandemic and serology testing have rapidly evolved and today we have a plethora of EUA serology assays available, and the list is still growing every day. There have been 21 new serology assays approved just since January 1, 2021. The good news is that many advances have been made and there are many high-quality assays but there is now increased confusion about test choice, test utility, and test result interpretation. The SARS-CoV-2 EUA serology testing landscape has been recently reviewed by Ravi and colleagues.[4] Confusion is driven not just by a large number of assay options but also by the rapidly evolving science about antibody kinetics, antibody durability, and protective immunity in the context of SARS-CoV-2 infection and now, vaccination.

SEVERE ACUTE RESPIRATORY SYNDROME CORONAVIRUS 2 HUMORAL RESPONSE
Not All Antibodies Are Created Equal

One concept that is not typically highlighted for other infectious diseases as far as the choice of serologic assay that has become critical to our understanding of SARS-CoV-2 infection is the different categories of antibodies and their role in the adaptive immune response. All antibodies bind to an antigen and serve a role in clearing infection. However, binding antibodies consist of both nonneutralizing and neutralizing antibodies (Nabs). Non-Nabs typically develop before Nabs and may function in viral clearance but do not extinguish infective virus. In contrast, there is a category of binding antibodies that are referred to as Nabs that can be of various antibody classes and have the unique ability to prevent cellular infection, potentially limiting initial infection and disease severity, as well as possibly preventing reinfection. For example, in the case of SARS-CoV-2 infection, Nabs develop that bind to the receptor-binding domain (RBD) region of the virus, thereby interfering with the virus's ability to interact with the angiotensin-converting enzyme 2 (ACE2) cellular receptor on the cell surface and thereby preventing cellular infection.[5-10] The typical laboratory antibody assays measure binding antibodies, without distinguishing between neutralizing and non-Nabs. Although Nab assays provide a functional indication of the immune system and may correlate with protective immunity, it is not established what concentration of Nabs confers protective immunity due to natural infection or vaccination.

Due to the role of Nabs, many studies have investigated a correlation between commercial serology assays that measure binding antibodies and neutralization assay results. There is a general qualitative agreement and a positive correlation between binding and Nab assays. Studies also show that not surprisingly, there is a higher degree of correlation between Nab assays and binding antibody assays that use the spike protein as a target.[11-13] Nab concentrations provide important information about levels of functional antibody and have been used in vaccine development; however, there are currently no recommendations for the clinical use of neutralization assays to specifically assess vaccine response, determine infection risk or predict disease severity.[14-16]

Antibody Kinetics and Durability

Although we continue to learn about the fine details of the humoral response against SARS-CoV-2 as the pandemic unfolds, we do have a basic understanding of the antibody response in SARS-CoV-2 infection. The majority of studies indicate that infected individuals mount a SARS-CoV-2 specific antibody response in the acute stage of the disease and over 90% of infected individuals have detectable antibodies 3-weeks postsymptom onset. For IgM, the time to seroconversion ranges from 4 to 14 days.[17] Mean time to seroconversion for IgG is 12 to 15 days, and generally detectable 7 to 14-days postsymptom onset. For IgA, most studies suggest seroconversion within 4-days postsymptom onset. IgM and IgG develop almost simultaneously without a significant delay between detectable IgM and IgG.[18] The majority of studies demonstrate that IgM peaks 2 to 5-weeks postsymptom onset, and rapidly declines thereafter. IgA is less well studied but also seems to decline within a few weeks postinfection.

Early studies suggested that IgG antibody responses waned rapidly during the convalescent stage[18] and that IgG may not be durable, particularly in individuals who experienced mild forms of COVID-19.[19] More recent studies suggest that the IgG antibody response postnatural infection is detectable during the convalescent stage, and although IgG levels decline over time and may vary with disease severity, an IgG response can remain detectable up to several months, with at least one study reporting detection of RBD-spike IgG seropositivity in 88% of individuals at 8-months postinfection.[17,20-22] Studies also indicate that 4% to 10% of infected individuals may have undetectable or a delayed antibody response following SARS-CoV-2 infection.[22]

Nab titers have been shown to correlate with disease severity, and individuals with a more severe form of disease had higher titers of Nabs.[17,23-25] Most studies demonstrated that Nabs are detectable between 7 and 15-days postsymptom onset and most individuals were positive by 21-days postdisease onset.[26] Although asymptomatic individuals had lower antibody titers, Nab titers varied considerably between individuals.[24] Furthermore, although disease severity affected the magnitude of the Nab response, some studies suggest that the kinetics of the response were not impacted.[27] For example, in one study, individuals with more severe disease had higher Nab titers than individuals with milder forms of disease but the number of days to peak neutralization titers did not differ based on disease severity.[27] Although Nab titers plateau within a few weeks, Nab titers may be detectable for months.[20] The humoral response in the context of SARS-CoV-2 has been reviewed by multiple groups[5,8,17,28]

Antibody durability has also been studied in response to vaccination. Although there was a slight decline over time, both binding and Nabs were detectable and remained elevated at least 6-months postvaccination with the Moderna vaccine.[29] Postvaccine studies for the Pfizer vaccine yielded similar results, demonstrating sustained antibody durability at least in response to mRNA vaccines. Studies are ongoing to determine when antibodies wane to levels that may warrant a booster dose of these vaccines.

In conclusion, individuals who are infected with SARS-CoV-2 and are symptomatic develop SARS-CoV-2 specific antibodies. IgM rises quickly and peaks 2 to 5-weeks postsymptom onset and then rapidly declines to undetectable levels within another 3 to 5 weeks. In contrast, IgG peaks 3 to 7-week postdisease onset, then plateaus and moderately declines for the next few weeks but can persist and be detected for several months postinfection.[20,22] Because there is no significant delay between IgM and IgG seroconversion, serology should not be used to diagnose SARS-CoV-2 infection, and there is no substantial benefit for using IgM standalone assays. In addition, for assessing exposure weeks after symptom onset IgG is useful as it is more durable. Vaccine-induced antibodies are detectable at least 6-months postvaccine administration of either of the 2 mRNA vaccines, Moderna and Pfizer.[14,30] Ongoing studies will further refine these findings.

SEVERE ACUTE RESPIRATORY SYNDROME CORONAVIRUS 2 SEROLOGY TESTING LANDSCAPE

As of April 2021, the FDA site lists 75 serology assays that have received EUA in the United States. Currently available commercial serology assays vary in methodology, antibody class detection, and antigen targets. There are 3 general types of methodologies: ELISA, LFA that provide rapid results and chemiluminescent immunoassays (CIA) Often, an individual major manufacturer may have multiple assays that have received EUA. For example, a single manufacturer may have an IgG, an IgM, and a total antibody assay. In addition, some vendors also have the same antibody class for a different target, such as a nucleocapsid IgG assay and a spike IgG assay. A few assays detect antibodies to more than one viral protein target. The vast majority of the assays are approved for use in high and moderate complexity settings. Only 5 of the many rapid, LFA are CLIA-waived. Sample types include plasma and serum, fingerstick whole blood, and the most recent addition, dried blood spot for home collection. Only a handful of the assays are semiquantitative, and one has EUA claim for specifically detecting Nabs. The following link (https://www.fda.gov/medical-devices/coronavirus-disease-2019-covid-19-emergency-use-authorizations-medical-devices/in-vitro-diagnostics-euas-serology-and-other-adaptive-immune-response-tests-sars-cov-2) to the FDA site is a helpful reference as it lists the current EUA serology assays available and general overview of the assay. Another useful link is: https://www.fda.gov/medical-devices/coronavirus-disease-2019-covid-19-emergency-use-authorizations-medical-devices/eua-authorized-serology-test-performance. At this site, one can not only read the instructions for use (IFU), instructions for health care providers and test recipients for each assay but can also quickly ascertain the performance characteristics of a serology assay based on the data the manufacturer provided and additional findings if the assay was independently evaluated by NCI, CDC, or BARDA. Needless to say, the sheer number of serology assay options for a single infectious agent is not only unprecedented but makes navigating the testing landscape increasingly difficult.

SEVERE ACUTE RESPIRATORY SYNDROME CORONAVIRUS 2 SEROLOGY ASSAY DESIGNS
Binding Antibody Assays

The vast majority of commercial assays are geared toward detecting the IgG isotype, but there are several total antibody assays, IgM & IgG combination (particularly for LFA), and a few IgM standalone assays that have received EUA. Although IgA assays have been developed, they are not in use in the United States, as studies have shown that they lack specificity. Professional guidelines do not recommend IgA assays or the use of a standalone IgM assay but do not otherwise express a preference for assays based on antibody class(es) detected.[15,16,31] IgG and total antibody assays have become the most commonly used assays because antibody testing is not recommended for diagnosis. Therefore, assays that detect IgG or total antibodies can be used to determine exposure and are the most widely used.

Antibody isotype is just one of the SARS-CoV-2 serology assay attributes that a laboratory must consider when choosing which SARS-CoV-2 assay to implement. Another important consideration is the viral target of the assay. SARS-CoV-2 consists of a single-stranded positive-sense RNA genome which encodes for nonstructural and 4 structural proteins, including the spike (S) and the nucleocapsid (N) proteins. The spike glycoprotein, S1 subunit is a surface protein present on the virion that contains the RBD which binds the angiotensin-converting enzyme 2 (ACE2) receptor and mediates entry into the host cell. The RBD and spike protein are the primary targets for Nabs in SARS-CoV-2 infection. Nabs prevent viral infection of the cell by interfering with the ability of the virus to interact with the ACE2 cell surface receptor.[32,33] Assays may contain different spike regions as targets, including S1 & S2, S1 only, or RBD only. The N protein is the most abundantly expressed viral protein and encapsulates viral RNA. It is well established that antibody responses against the nucleocapsid and spike proteins of the SARS-CoV-2 virus are readily detected in individuals who have been infected with SARS-CoV-2 and have also become the favored targets for serology assays.[25] There are some assays that use both the S and N proteins as antigenic targets.[4,34,35] Although both of these targets have been used extensively in developing serology assays for determining exposure to SARS-CoV-2, recent attention has turned to IgG antibody assays against the spike protein, as a possible tool for assessing immune response due to vaccination.

Severe Acute Respiratory Syndrome Coronavirus 2 Nab Assays

Although Nabs play a crucial role in SARS-CoV-2 infection, there is only one assay that has received EUA that specifically detects Nabs. This is in part because developing a Nab assay that can be adapted to a clinical laboratory is difficult to achieve. The gold standard for measuring Nabs is the plaque reduction neutralization test (PRNT). A classic PRNT assay determines the serum dilution that inhibits viral growth (50% or 90% inhibition) in cell culture and can therefore provide a titer. However, these assays require expertise in cell culture, are labor-intensive and require live virus, which in the case of SARS-CoV-2 would necessitate a biosafety level 3 (BSL3) facility. Another methodology is the pseudovirus-based live cell neutralization assay. This methodology uses a pseudoviral vector to express the protein target of interest, such as the spike for SARS-CoV-2, therefore eliminating the need for live SARS-CoV-2 virus and a BSL3 facility. However, this method still requires viral and cell culture expertise and is not amenable to high throughput settings and rapid turnaround time (TAT), as needed for implementation in a clinical laboratory. These classical methods that use live or pseudotyped virus and determine the serum dilution that inhibits virus growth maybe the gold standard for measuring Nab concentrations but are really only suited for research.[24,36–38] More recently, surrogate viral neutralization tests (sVNT) have been developed. sVNT have a percent inhibition cut-off that allows for a qualitative determination of presence or absence of Nabs.[39] The Nab assay that has received EUA uses the spike protein as a target because the primary target of Nabs is the spike protein. The assay does not detect a particular antibody class. The role of Nab assays in the clinical laboratory remains to be determined.

EVALUATION OF SEVERE ACUTE RESPIRATORY SYNDROME CORONAVIRUS 2 SEROLOGY ASSAYS

As mentioned above, the FDA now requires that manufacturers of SARS-CoV-2 antibody assays submit supporting data to FDA within 10 days of notifying the FDA of the intent to bring an antibody assay to market and has published specific templates with sample size and performance threshold recommendations for EUA submission for serology assays. Although there are many caveats in the template depending on whether the assay is designed to detect individual or combined SARS-CoV-2 antibody classes, there are some general rules. Evaluation of at least 75 unique samples, preferably collected from subjects before December 2020, is recommended for specificity studies. Furthermore, if the 75 samples were tested from a population that has a high prevalence of vaccination against, and/or infection with common viruses and the observed percent positive agreement (PPA) is greater than 95% then specific cross-reactivity studies are not required. Evaluation of sensitivity requires a minimum of 30 unique samples collected from individuals with RT-PCR confirmed SARS-CoV-2 infection. Clinical performance data for sensitivity is stratified by days postsymptom onset and the typical timeframes suggested are 0 to 7 days, 8 to 14 days, and $\geq$ 15 days. For IgG and total antibody assays, 30 samples collected at day 15 or later postsymptom onset, are recommended. Therefore, for SARS-CoV-2 serology assays, generally, the minimum PPA required is 90% and the minimum negative percent agreement is 95%.[40]

SEVERE ACUTE RESPIRATORY SYNDROME CORONAVIRUS 2 SEROLOGY TESTING RECOMMENDATIONS

SARS-CoV-2 serology testing is recommended by a number of professional societies for the following applications: (1) seroprevalence and epidemiologic studies, (2) as an aid in diagnosing multisystem inflammatory syndrome in children (MIS-C), (3) support a diagnosis in individuals with symptoms consistent with SARS-CoV-2 infection who repeatedly test negative by NAAT, and (4) identifying eligible COVID-19 convalescent plasma (CCP) donors.

Serology assays have been used extensively for seroprevalence studies.[41] Given that a large proportion of adults have now been immunized in the United States, serology-based seroprevalence studies are more difficult to interpret. Careful consideration must be given to the choice of the assay and respective antigenic target used for this type of investigation (please see below).

Serologic testing can also be helpful clinically for the diagnosis of both MIS-C and adults who present late in the disease course. MIS-C develops in some children infected with SARS-CoV-2, often after the viral infection is no longer detectable by NAAT.[42] Serology testing for MIS-C is now a criterion included in the case definition..[31] For adults who have symptoms consistent with SARS-CoV-2 infection or have been exposed to SARS-CoV-2 infection but are repeatedly NAAT negative, antibody testing can also be used as the confirmation of SARS-CoV-2 infection. Generally, the use of either an IgG or a total antibody assay at 3 to 4 weeks (no sooner than 14 days) post-symptom onset for optimal accuracy, when using serology assays as an adjunct for the confirmation of SARS-CoV-2 infection is recommended.[15,31,34]

The use of convalescent plasma to treat patients with COVID-19 was implemented early during the pandemic. Passive antibody transfer as a therapy has been used for a number of infectious diseases in the past, including influenza.[43] Initially, only one commercial assay was approved for the selection of individuals considered to have "high SARS-CoV-2 antibody titers" and who were eligible for COVID-19 convalescent donations. However, in recent months, the FDA has updated the guidelines and has now established individual manufacturer-dependent cut-offs for several commercial assays that measure binding antibodies that can be used for the qualification of high antibody titer samples that can be used for CCP donations.

One serology testing application that has been used in the research setting but has yet to be used clinically, is to monitor vaccine response. As of May 2021, there are no recommendations for determining who should qualify for vaccination or what is considered an appropriate or protective immune response postvaccine administration based on serology results.[16] This is due to both the way vaccine efficacy was assessed during the vaccine clinical trials and the lack of standardization for both binding and Nab assays. Vaccine trials evaluated vaccine efficacy by comparing how many individuals became infected with SARS-CoV-2 in the control and vaccinated groups during the course of the clinical trials. And although various binding and Nab assays were used to determine if individuals mounted an immune response there was no cut-off on any assay that was evaluated for protective immunity.[14] In fact, 100% of vaccinated individuals developed robust levels of binding and Nabs in response to vaccination with the Moderna mRNA vaccine.[14] Although currently there are no recommendations for monitoring or assessing appropriate immune response due to vaccination using serology testing, many individuals who have been vaccinated have sought serology testing postvaccination. And although a detectable immune response postvaccination indicates that the individual has mounted an immune response to the vaccination, it is imperative to emphasize that there is no threshold antibody level associated with protective immunity on any platform, including Nab assays.

SEVERE ACUTE RESPIRATORY SYNDROME CORONAVIRUS 2 SEROLOGY TEST REPORTING AND INTERPRETATION

SARS-CoV-2 antibody test result interpretation is complex. Although in its simplest form, a negative antibody result indicates no SARS-CoV-2 exposure or vaccination, and a positive antibody result suggests exposure or possibly vaccination, all results must be interpreted in context. Variables that impact interpretation include: timing of the sample collection, patient clinical history, antigen target, and performance characteristics of the assay used.

Timing of sample collection in serology testing is crucial for appropriate test interpretation. Most notably, suboptimal timing due to the early collection of sample postsymptom onset can result in a false-negative result. A false-negative result in someone who was exposed to SARS-CoV-2 is also possible in patients who are immunocompromised or individuals who had asymptomatic infection.[44]

Antigenic targets further complicate the interpretation. Due to the mass vaccination success in the United States, the antigen target has become a recent conundrum. Clinicians and epidemiologists may want to determine who has been exposed to infection and who has been vaccinated. Because the spike protein is the target of the vaccines that have been approved to date in the United States, it is reasonable to think that one can distinguish between these 2 scenarios by testing for spike and nucleocapsid antibodies. For example, individuals who are positive by nucleocapsid assays must have had a natural infection because the vaccines do not use nucleocapsid as the antigen for antibody stimulation. Indeed most recent updates from the CDC reflect this approach and test interpretation.[16] However, caution must be taken because, in the absence of clinical history, this approach is predicated on the assumption that the nucleocapsid and spike assays used in a laboratory have the same sensitivity and specificity which is not likely. There have been reports of known, confirmed SARS-COV-2 cases that subsequently tested positive by a spike assay but negative by a nucleocapsid assay.[45,46] Clinical history is crucial to correct test result interpretation, otherwise, test results could translate in misclassifying an individual's status. Seroprevalence studies and reference laboratories may be particularly challenged by the lack of clinical history to assist in test interpretation. The merits of using nucleocapsid and spike assays to distinguish between vaccinated and previously infected individuals is an active area of research and publications are forthcoming.[47]

In addition, assay performance characteristics not only vary between assays, but even small differences in specificity and sensitivity between assays can translate to substantial differences in positive predictive value (PPV) and negative predictive value (NPV) depending on disease prevalence. For example, an assay that has 98.1% sensitivity and 99.6% specificity that translates into 99.9% NPV and only 92% PPV when disease prevalence is 5.0%. If the disease prevalence is 10% the NPV only drops to 99.8% but the PPV increases to 96.1%. It is understandable that PPV was of particular concern during the early days of the pandemic, when disease prevalence was low. Therefore, the CDC made the following recommendation to increase PPV: (1) test only individuals who have a high likelihood of exposure to SARS-CoV-2, (2) test with an assay that has greater than 99.5% specificity, and (3) if not possible to test with an assay that has greater than 99.5% specificity then implement an orthogonal approach to testing.[16]

The orthogonal approach to testing is based on testing with one serology assay and if the sample is positive by the first assay, then the sample is tested by a second assay. Ideally, the assay with the highest specificity should be used first to minimize discrepant results between the 2 assays used in an orthogonal testing approach. Otherwise, the assays used in this type of algorithm can be the same antigenic target but different method (ELISA spike and CIA spike), or the same method but different antigenic targets (CIA nucleocapsid, CIA spike). If both test results are positive, then the PPV is very high, assuring that the result is a true positive. However, if the second test is negative interpretation is less clear. Although at first glance this would suggest a false-positive result with the first assay, it may be that the discrepant results are due to differences in sensitivity between the assays and not a reflection of the accuracy of the first test. Discrepant results must be interpreted with caution and considered in the context of the patient's clinical history. Orthogonal testing has also been applied for seroprevalence studies.[41] Today, the prevalence of disease has increased across the country and assays with greater than 99.5% specificity are more readily available;

therefore, the need for orthogonal testing to increase PPV is no longer a priority for most laboratories.

In summary, many variables, including patient history, have an impact on the accuracy of the test result and interpretation. Both the FDA and best practices require that clinical serology results must be accompanied by clear footnotes on the patient chart that state the limitations of serology testing. Most, importantly, serology testing should not be used for diagnosing SARS-CoV-2 infection. Other important limitations include that a negative SARS-CoV-2 antibody result does not rule out current or past infection and a positive SARS-CoV-2 antibody test can be due to cross-reaction with other commonly circulating human coronaviruses. The clearer and more comprehensive yet concise information a laboratory can provide in the test order recommendations and/or chart comments regarding the details of the assay used (such as the antigenic target, antibody class detected) and specific limitations, the more helpful it is for clients, clinicians, and patients.

SEVERE ACUTE RESPIRATORY SYNDROME CORONAVIRUS 2 ANTIBODY TESTING PERSPECTIVE

Although many studies have been conducted to address immunity postinfection and postvaccination, some aspects of humoral immunity in response to SARS-CoV-2 infection are still being defined. Studies have often yielded conflicting results about various aspects of SARS-CoV-2 infection humoral response. It is important to note that many of the studies, particularly early in the pandemic, were limited in patient numbers, patient demographics, and temporal follow-up. More recent studies have had access to larger and more diverse cohorts and extended study duration. Another complicating factor that can affect the result of studies attempting to address the fundamental serology questions in the context of SARS-CoV-2 infection is that the assay used for these studies may also have an impact on the findings. Fundamentally, it is still not known what constitutes a protective immune response when assessing antibody response, in the context of natural infection or vaccination.

Another challenge to making a meaningful interpretation for SARS-CoV-2 antibody test results is the lack of standardization for both binding and Nab assays. Substantial test performance variation and therefore choice of assay can have a significant impact on the overall conclusion of a study or clinical test interpretation.

The lack of standardization between any of the EUA serology assays, neutralizing, and binding antibody assays makes it difficult to interpret results obtained with different serology assays. This is the case for both clinical interpretation and a confounding factor in research studies. Semiquantitative assay results have no commutability and cannot be used interchangeably between assays, even if the assays are semiquantitative. Although the need for standardization is undeniable, the first step is to determine what constitutes humoral protective immunity. Antibodies as a correlate of protective immunity and accompanying standard threshold have been developed for other infectious diseases such as hepatitis B, whereby hepatitis B surface antibody levels more than 10 mIU/mL indicate protective immunity.[43] It is, therefore, possible that someday there will be SARS-CoV-2 antibody manufacturer-specific cut-offs, as has been established for SARS-CoV-2 antibody assays in the context of CCP, or a standard that can be used to firmly establish what constitutes a protective antibody response in the context of SARS-CoV-2.

In summary, the SARS-CoV-2 pandemic continues to dominate the world and US health care. Laboratory testing, including serology testing, remains at the forefront of the public health response. Current antibody testing is not limited by technology or supply chain issues, but important limitations do exist. The limitations consist of rapidly changing understanding of the immune response to natural infection with SARS-CoV-2, evolving knowledge regarding vaccine response to a new form of vaccine technology, and the lack of standardization for serology assays. Although antibody tests are widely available, there is a need for standardization to increase the clinical utility of antibody testing in the future.

The laboratory must remain vigilant in staying current with advancing knowledge, rapid developments in testing methods, and updated recommendations. The laboratory remains critical to ensuring a quality result by validating/verifying the test and implementing appropriate quality control measures.[15] Finally, the laboratory is crucial to educating clinicians, patients, and the public alike about the complexity and limitations of SARS-CoV-2 antibody testing.

CLINICS CARE POINTS

- SARS CoV-2 serology assays are not standardized.

- Clinical utility remains limited.

- If a serology assay is used as an adjunct to nucleic acid amplification tests (NAATs) for supporting a clinical diagnosis in MIS-C or in adults with suspicion of SARS-CoV-2 who are NAAT negative, IgG, and total antibody assays should be used 3 to 4 weeks postsympom onset for optimal accuracy.

DISCLOSURE

The author has nothing to disclose.

REFERENCES

1. Wu F, Zhao S, Yu B, et al. A new coronavirus associated with human respiratory disease in China. Nature 2020;579(7798):265–9.
2. Theel ES, Slev P, Wheeler S, et al. The role of antibody testing for SARS-CoV-2: is there one? J Clin Microbiol 2020;58(8). e00797-20.
3. Farnsworth CW, Anderson NW. SARS-CoV-2 serology: much hype, little data. Clin Chem 2020;66(7):875–7.
4. Ravi N, Cortade DL, Ng E, et al. Diagnostics for SARS-CoV-2 detection: a comprehensive review of the FDA-EUA COVID-19 testing landscape. Biosens Bioelectron 2020;165:112454.
5. Carrillo J, Izquierdo-Useros N, Avila-Nieto C, et al. Humoral immune responses and neutralizing antibodies against SARS-CoV-2; implications in pathogenesis and protective immunity. Biochem Biophys Res Commun 2021;538:187–91.
6. Zhao J, Yuan Q, Wang H, et al. Antibody responses to SARS-CoV-2 in patients with novel coronavirus disease 2019. Clin Infect Dis 2020;71(16):2027–34.
7. Chi X, Yan R, Zhang J, et al. A neutralizing human antibody binds to the N-terminal domain of the Spike protein of SARS-CoV-2. Science 2020;369(6504):650–5.
8. Hueston L, Kok J, Guibone, et al. The antibody response to SARS-CoV-2 infection. Infectious Diseases Society of merica; 2020. p. 1–8. https://doi.org/10.1093/ofid/ofaa387.
9. Ju B, Zhang Q, Ge J, et al. Human neutralizing antibodies elicited by SARS-CoV-2 infection. Nature 2020;584(7819):115–9.

10. Liu L, Wang P, Nair MS, et al. Potent neutralizing antibodies against multiple epitopes on SARS-CoV-2 spike. Nature 2020;584(7821):450–6.

11. Suhandynata RT, Bevins NJ, Tran JT, et al. SARS-CoV-2 serology status detected by commercialized platforms distinguishes previous infection and vaccination adaptive immune responses. medRxiv : the preprint server for health sciences. medRxiv 2021. https://doi.org/10.1101/2021.03.10.21253299.

12. Liu W, Liu L, Kou G, et al. Evaluation of nucleocapsid and spike protein-based enzyme-linked immunosorbent assays for detecting antibodies against SARS-CoV-2. J Clin Microbiol 2020;58(6). e00461-20.

13. Rychert J, Couturier MR, Elgort M, et al. Evaluation of 3 SARS-CoV-2 IgG antibody assays and correlation with neutralizing antibodies. J Appl Lab Med 2021;6(3):614–24.

14. Jackson LA, Anderson EJ, Rouphael NG, et al. An mRNA vaccine against SARS-CoV-2 - preliminary report. N Engl J Med 2020;383(20):1920–31.

15. Zhang YV, Wiencek J, Meng QH, et al. AACC practical recommendations for implementing and interpreting SARS-CoV-2 EUA and LDT Serologic Testing in Clinical Laboratories. Clin Chem 2021;67(9):1188–200.

16. CDC. Interim guidelines for COVID-19 antibody testing. Available at: https://www.cdc.gov/coronavirus/2019-ncov/lab/resources/antibody-tests-guidelines.html. Accessed May 20, 2021.

17. Post N, Eddy D, Huntley C, et al. Antibody response to SARS-CoV-2 infection in humans: a systematic review. PLoS One 2020;15(12):e0244126.

18. Long QX, Liu BZ, Deng HJ, et al. Antibody responses to SARS-CoV-2 in patients with COVID-19. Nat Med 2020;26(6):845–8.

19. Long QX, Tang XJ, Shi QL, et al. Clinical and immunological assessment of asymptomatic SARS-CoV-2 infections. Nat Med 2020;26(8):1200–4.

20. Wajnberg A, Amanat F, Firpo A, et al. Robust neutralizing antibodies to SARS-CoV-2 infection persist for months. Science 2020;370(6521):1227–30.

21. Dan JM, Mateus J, Kato Y, et al. Immunological memory to SARS-CoV-2 assessed for up to 8 months after infection. Science 2021;371(6529). eabf4063.

22. Gudbjartsson DF, Norddahl GL, Melsted P, et al. Humoral immune response to SARS-CoV-2 in Iceland. N Engl J Med 2020;383(18):1724–34.

23. Wang P, Liu L, Nair MS, et al. SARS-CoV-2 neutralizing antibody responses are more robust in patients with severe disease. Emerg Microbes Infect 2020;9(1):2091–3.

24. Wu F, Liu M, Wang A, et al. Evaluating the association of clinical characteristics with neutralizing antibody levels in patients who have recovered from mild COVID-19 in shanghai, China. JAMA Intern Med 2020;180(10):1356–62.

25. Shrock E, Fujimura E, Kula T, et al. Viral epitope profiling of COVID-19 patients reveals cross-reactivity and correlates of severity. Science 2020;370(6520). eabd4250.

26. Wang K, Long QX, Deng HJ, et al. Longitudinal dynamics of the neutralizing antibody response to SARS-CoV-2 infection. Clin Infect Dis 2021 Aug 2;73(3):e531–9.

27. Seow J, Graham C, Merrick B, et al. Longitudinal observation and decline of neutralizing antibody responses in the three months following SARS-CoV-2 infection in humans. Nat Microbiol. 2020 Dec;12(5):1598–607.

28. Vabret N, Britton GJ, Gruber C, et al. Immunology of COVID-19: current state of the science. Immunity 2020;52(6):910–41.

29. Doria-Rose N, Suthar MS, Makowski M, et al. Antibody persistence through 6 Months after the second dose of mRNA-1273 vaccine for covid-19. N Engl J Med 2021;384(23):2259–61.
30. pfizer. PFIZER AND BIONTECH CONFIRM HIGH EFFICACY AND NO SERIOUS SAFETY CONCERNS THROUGH UP TO SIX MONTHS FOLLOWING SECOND DOSE IN UPDATED TOPLINE ANALYSIS OF LANDMARK COVID-19 VACCINE STUDY. 2021. Available at: https://www.pfizer.com/news/press-release/press-release-detail/pfizer-and-biontech-confirm-high-efficacy-and-no-serious#:%7E:text=19%20Vaccine%20Study-,PFIZER%20AND%20BIONTECH%20CONFIRM%20HIGH%20EFFICACY%20AND%20NO%20SERIOUS%20SAFETY%20CONCERNS%20THROUGH%20UP%20. Accessed May 20, 2021.
31. Hanson KE, Caliendo AM, Arias CA, et al. Infectious diseases society of America guidelines on the diagnosis of COVID-19:serologic testing. Clin Infect Dis 2020. https://doi.org/10.1093/cid/ciaa1343.
32. Walls AC, Park YJ, Tortorici MA, et al. Structure, function, and Antigenicity of the SARS-CoV-2 spike glycoprotein. Cell 2020;181(2):281–92.e6.
33. Wu Y, Wang F, Shen C, et al. A noncompeting pair of human neutralizing antibodies block COVID-19 virus binding to its receptor ACE2. Science 2020; 368(6496):1274–8.
34. Deeks JJ, Dinnes J, Takwoingi Y, et al. Antibody tests for identification of current and past infection with SARS-CoV-2. Cochrane Database Syst Rev 2020;6: CD013652.
35. Lisboa Bastos M, Tavaziva G, Abidi SK, et al. Diagnostic accuracy of serological tests for covid-19: systematic review and meta-analysis. Bmj 2020;370:m2516.
36. Zheng Y, Larragoite ET, Lama J, et al. Neutralization assay with SARS-CoV-1 and SARS-CoV-2 spike pseudotyped murine leukemia virions. bioRxiv 2020. https://doi.org/10.1101/2020.07.17.207563.
37. Amanat F, Stadlbauer D, Strohmeier S, et al. A serological assay to detect SARS-CoV-2 seroconversion in humans. Nat Med 2020;26(7):1033–6.
38. Okba NMA, Müller MA, Li W, et al. Severe acute respiratory syndrome coronavirus 2-specific antibody responses in coronavirus disease patients. Emerg Infect Dis 2020;26(7):1478–88.
39. Tan CW, Chia WN, Qin X, et al. A SARS-CoV-2 surrogate virus neutralization test based on antibody-mediated blockage of ACE2-spike protein-protein interaction. Nat Biotechnol 2020;38(9):1073–8.
40. (FDA) UFaDA. Serology template for test developers. Available at: https://www.fda.gov/medical-devices/coronavirus-disease-2019-covid-19-emergency-use-authorizations-medical-devices/in-vitro-diagnostics-euas. Accessed May 20, 2021.
41. Ripperger TJ, Uhrlaub JL, Watanabe M, et al. Orthogonal SARS-CoV-2 serological assays enable surveillance of low-prevalence communities and reveal durable humoral immunity. Immunity 2020;53(5):925–33.e4.
42. Whittaker E, Bamford A, Kenny J, et al. Clinical characteristics of 58 children with a pediatric inflammatory multisystem syndrome temporally associated with SARS-CoV-2. JAMA 2020;324(3):259–69.
43. Plotkin SA. Updates on immunologic correlates of vaccine-induced protection. Vaccine 2020;38(9):2250–7.
44. Ye X, Xiao X, Li B, et al. Low humoral immune response and ineffective clearance of SARS-cov-2 in a COVID-19 patient with CLL during a 69-day follow-up. Front Oncol 2020;10:1272.

45. Wang H, Wiredja D, Yang L, et al. Case-control study of individuals with discrepant nucleocapsid and spike protein SARS-CoV-2 IgG results. Clin Chem 2021;67(7):977–86.
46. Röltgen K, Powell AE, Wirz OF, et al. Defining the features and duration of antibody responses to SARS-CoV-2 infection associated with disease severity and outcome. Sci Immunol 2020;5(54). eabe0240.
47. Demmer RT, Baumgartner B, Wiggen TD, et al. Identification of natural SARS-CoV-2 infection in seroprevalence studies among vaccinated populations. medRxiv 2021. https://doi.org/10.1101/2021.04.12.21255330.

Vaccine-Induced Severe Acute Respiratory Syndrome Coronavirus 2 Antibody Response and the Path to Accelerating Development (Determining a Correlate of Protection)

Amy C. Sherman, MD[a,b,1,*], Michaël Desjardins, MD[a,b,c,1], Lindsey R. Baden, MD[a,b]

KEYWORDS

- SARS-CoV-2 • Vaccines • Serologic diagnostics

KEY POINTS

- A marker of immunity that describes clinical efficacy for SARS-CoV-2 vaccines would be a valuable clinical and epidemiological tool.
- A "correlate" or "surrogate" of SARS-CoV-2 vaccine-induced protection needs to be well-defined, including clear endpoints (e.g., hospitalization, severe disease, transmission).
- Different statistical models and methodologies can be used to determine a correlate or surrogate of protection.
- Many factors including host characteristics, vaccine platform, and immunologic parameters may impact the correlate or surrogate of protection.

INTRODUCTION

Less than 18 months after the identification of severe acute respiratory syndrome coronavirus 2 (SARS-CoV-2) and its genome, 13 authorized or approved COVID-19 vaccines are being deployed around the world,[1] and many more candidates are

This article previously appeared in *Clinics in Laboratory Medicine*, Volume 42, Issue 1, March 2022.

[a] Division of Infectious Diseases, Brigham and Women's Hospital, 75 Francis Street, Boston, MA 02115, USA; [b] Harvard Medical School, Boston, MA 02115, USA; [c] Division of Infectious Diseases, Centre Hospitalier de l'Université de Montréal, 1000 Rue Saint-Denis, Bureau F06.1102b, Montreal, Quebec H2X 0C1, Canada

[1] Co-first authors.

* Corresponding author. Division of Infectious Diseases, Brigham and Women's Hospital, 75 Francis Street, Boston, MA 02115, USA

E-mail address: acsherman@bwh.harvard.edu

https://doi.org/10.1016/j.ccol.2021.12.004
2352-7986/22/© 2021 Elsevier Inc. All rights reserved.

currently undergoing evaluation in clinical trials. In the United States, 3 vaccines have been granted an Emergency Use Authorization (EUA) by the Food and Drug Administration: BNT162b2 (Pfizer/BioNTech), mRNA-1273 (Moderna), and Ad26.CoV2.S (Janssen Biotech, Inc). Although the phase 3 clinical trials have demonstrated clinical efficacy in preventing moderate to severe COVID-19 disease, the underlying immune mechanisms that confer protection are still not known. Furthermore, determining protection against SARS-CoV-2 infection in vaccinated people using laboratory markers would be extremely useful. Efficacy studies, such as randomized controlled trials (RCTs), depend on large and expensive clinical trials, whereas large population studies during vaccine rollout often have confounding variables. Using a "surrogate" or "correlate" of protection allows for easier monitoring and surveillance of a particular vaccine's effectiveness, which can aid in both vaccine development and licensure.[2] Markers of immune responses can also be applied to determine a population response for new variants or strains of a virus, across unique characteristics of a population (eg, elderly, immunocompromised), and across different manufacturing or lots. Furthermore, COVID-19 vaccine boosters may be necessary, and a correlate of protection (CoP) would allow for efficient measurement of persistent protection. To date, there is no accepted CoP for COVID-19 vaccine-induced immunity.

The current knowledge regarding antibody-induced responses to SARS-CoV-2 vaccines, the definition of a CoP, proposed CoP for SARS-CoV-2, and special considerations for defining an SARS-CoV-2 vaccine-induced CoP are discussed.

SEVERE ACUTE RESPIRATORY SYNDROME CORONAVIRUS 2 VACCINES AND ANTIBODY RESPONSES

The varied COVID-19 vaccines that have been approved for emergency use or are still undergoing clinical evaluation use different technologies, administration schedules, and antigen targets (**Table 1**), which may result in different cellular and humoral responses following immunization. The available data on the dynamics, duration, and magnitude of the antibody responses following COVID-19 immunization are discussed in relation to different vaccine platforms.

Antibody responses to COVID-19 vaccines are commonly reported using 2 different assays: immunoassays to detect binding antibodies (bAb) and neutralization assays to detect neutralizing antibodies (nAb).[3] Immunoassays, such as enzyme-linked immunosorbent assays (ELISA), detect and quantify antibodies that have the capacity to bind a specific antigen in vitro. Except for inactivated vaccines, all available COVID-19 vaccines target the SARS-CoV-2 spike protein or one of its components (eg, receptor binding domain or RBD, S1, S2). Thus, it is expected that these vaccines will lead to the production of bAb against the spike protein, but not against the nucleocapsid protein. This antibody response signature is different from what is seen after natural infection or vaccination with inactivated vaccines, where detection of both spike and other antigens (such as nucleocapsid) bAb is expected. Neutralization assays are used to quantify functional antibodies that have the capacity to inhibit the replication of SARS-CoV-2 in vitro. Alternatively, a pseudovirus expressing SARS-CoV-2 spike protein can be used instead of wild-type SARS-CoV-2, providing significant safety and versatility advantages. In most phase 1/2 trials, a strong correlation was seen between bAb and nAb elicited postvaccination.[4–7]

Dynamics of Antibody Responses Postvaccination

In participants without previous SARS-CoV-2 infection, bAb, such as immunoglobulin G (IgG) against the full spike, S1, S2, or RBD, are usually detectable 14 days after the

Table 1
Vaccine platforms, dose and schedule, and antigen targets

Vaccine Platform	Vaccine Name	Approved/ Authorized	Vaccine Dose and Schedule	Antigen Target
mRNA-based vaccines	BNT162b2 (Pfizer/BioNTech)	≥85 countries US EUA 12/11/2020	30 µg, 2 doses, 21 d apart[9]	Prefusion-stabilized full-length S protein
	mRNA-1273 (Moderna)	≥46 countries US EUA 12/18/2020	100 µg, 2 doses, 28 d apart[5,11,85]	Prefusion-stabilized full-length S protein
Vector vaccines	AZD1222 (Astra-Zeneca) Vector: ChAdeno	≥139 countries Not in the US	5×10^{10} VP, 2 doses, 4–12 wk apart[8,86]	Full-length S protein
	Ad26.CoV2.S (Janssen) Vector: Ad26	≥41 countries USA EUA 2/27/2021	5×10^{10} VP, 1 dose[4]	Prefusion-stabilized full-length S protein
	Sputnik V (Gamaleya Center) Vector: rAd26/rAd5	≥65 countries Not in the US	10^{11} VP, 2 doses 21 d apart[6]	Full-length S protein
	Convidicea (CanSino) Vector: rAd5	≥5 countries Not in the US	5×10^{10} VP, 1 dose[7]	Full-length S protein
Inactivated vaccines	CoronaVac (Sinovac)	≥24 countries Not in the US	3 µg, 2 doses 14–28 d apart[10,87]	Inactivated SARS-CoV-2 (CN02 strain)
	BBIBP-CorV (Sinopharm)	≥40 countries Not in the US	4 µg, 2 doses 21–28 d apart[63]	Inactivated SARS-CoV-2 (HB02 strain)
	Covaxin (Bharat Biotech)	≥9 countries Not in the US	6 µg, 2 doses 28 d apart[15,88]	Inactivated SARS-CoV-2 (NIV-2020-770 strain)
	WIBP-CorV (Sinopharm)	2 countries Not in the US	5 µg, 2 doses 21 d apart[89]	Inactivated SARS-CoV-2 (WIV04 strain)
	CoviVac (Chumakov Center)	1 country Not in the US	N/A, 2 doses, 14 d apart	Inactivated SARS-CoV-2 (strain N/A)
Subunit vaccine	EpiVacCorona (Vector Institute)	2 countries Not in the US	N/A, 2 doses 21–28 d apart (NCT04780035)	Synthesized peptide antigens of SARS-CoV-2
	ZF2001 (Anhui Zhifei Longcom Biopharmaceutical)	2 countries Not in the US	25 µg, 3 doses, 0–30–60 d[16]	Receptor-binding domain

initial dose and tend to further increase on days 21 to 28, when the second dose is administered.[5,8] All the 2-dose schedule vaccines show a *prime-boost* effect, with further significant increase of bAb peaking around 7 to 14 days after the second dose.[5,9,10]

In general, nAb are detected at a low level starting at day 14 and significantly increase after the second dose.[5,6,8] nAb tend to increase at a rate slower than bAb, however, like bAb, tend to peak 7 to 14 days postdosing schedule. The single-dose vaccines Ad26.CoV2.S (Janssen Biotech, Inc), a nonreplicating adenovirus serotype 26 (Ad26) vector vaccine, and Convidicea (CanSino), a nonreplicating adenovirus serotype 5 vector vaccine, produce bAb and nAb by day 28, that tend to further increase by day 56 for Ad26.CoV2.S.[4,7]

Limited data are available regarding the duration of antibody responses post-COVID-19 vaccines. Data generated from the phase 1 and phase 3 clinical trials are critical to better understand the duration of protection, as participants in these trials were vaccinated as early as March 2020 and July 2020, respectively. This prolonged follow-up period provides early understanding of the kinetics of antibody response and vaccine efficacy over time and may guide the need for future booster dose. In the mRNA-173 phase 1 study, in which 33 participants received 2 doses of vaccine 28 days apart, bAb and nAb titers decreased but persisted through 6 months after the second dose as assessed by 3 different assays.[11] There is also growing evidence from the phase 3 trials that vaccination with messenger RNA (mRNA) vaccines remains clinically effective to prevent confirmed symptomatic cases of COVID-19 for at least 6 months.[12,13]

Magnitude of Antibody Responses

The magnitude of postvaccination bAb and nAb published to date is difficult to compare between COVID-19 vaccine types, because researchers use different assays and methods to quantitate antibody levels. Furthermore, for bAb, assays target different antigens, such as the full spike protein or one of its fragments (S1, S2, RBD).[14] For this reason, some groups have included a panel of control convalescent serum specimen from individuals with prior COVID-19 to compare the vaccine-induced responses with the natural infection. mRNA and vector vaccines were shown to induce bAb and nAb titers similar to or higher than what is detected in convalescent sera.[4,5,8,9] For inactivated vaccines, only CoronaVac and Covaxin trials reported comparison with convalescent sera and showed respectively lower or similar nAb titers in sera from vaccinated participants compared with convalescents sera.[15] The recombinant vaccine ZF2001 showed significantly higher nAb titers in vaccinated participants than in convalescent sera.[16] However, these data must be cautiously interpreted because the serum panels differ among the different studies. Antibody titers after natural infection can vary significantly in convalescent individuals, based on host's characteristics, severity of disease, and timing from symptom onset.[3,17]

Impact of Previous Infection on Antibody Responses to Vaccines

In individuals with previous SARS-CoV-2 infection, postvaccination humoral responses differ significantly in terms of dynamics and magnitude. In those who received BNT162b2 (Pfizer, Inc) or mRNA-1273 (ModernaTx, Inc), a rapid increase of bAb is seen after the first dose, starting as early as 5 to 8 days.[18] The titers quickly peak at high levels between days 9 and 12 and do not significantly increase after the second dose. In comparison with those without preexisting immunity, the titers were 10 to 45 times higher after the first dose and remained 6 times higher after the second dose. Another study showed that 2 doses of BNT162b2 (Pfizer, Inc) in previously uninfected individuals induced lower nAb titers than a single dose in those with previous infection.

COVID-19 Vaccines Humoral Responses and Variants

In the early phase 1/2 COVID-19 vaccine trials, vaccine-induced neutralizing activity was assessed by neutralization assays using pseudovirus expressing the wild-type Spike protein or using wild-type SARS-CoV-2. However, since January 2021, many different genetic variants of SARS-CoV-2 have emerged around the world. These variants have various substitutions, insertions, and/or deletions in the spike protein gene that may lead to increased transmissibility or disease severity, and may also reduce vaccine-induced protection.[19] Current variants of concern according to the Centers for Disease Control and Prevention include B.1.1.7 (first identified in United Kingdom), P1 (first identified in Brazil), B1.351 (first identified in South Africa), and B.1.427 and B.1.429 (first identified in California, USA). Emerging data have shown reduced, but variable neutralizing activity of postvaccination sera on these variants, with a small to moderate reduction in activity on the B.1.1.7, P1, B.1.427, and B.1.429,[20,21] and more significant reduction of neutralization was shown on the B1.351 variant, particularly with AZD1222, where complete virus escape has been described.[22] In patients with previous SARS-CoV-2 infection, a single dose of BNT162b2 substantially increased the serum neutralizing activity against B.1.1.7, P1, and B.1.351, with similar titers across patients for each variant.[23]

DEFINITION AND HISTORICAL EXAMPLES OF CORRELATES OF PROTECTION AND RISKS

There are several definitions of the terms "correlate of protection" and "correlates of risk." Plotkin and Plotkin[24] define a CoP as "a specific immune response to a vaccine that is closely related to protection against infection, disease, or other defined end point." A CoP is typically a measurable immune marker, and preferably one that is relatively easy to obtain by standard laboratory techniques, for facile scalability and reproducibility. Importantly, Plotkin and Plotkin argue that the correlate itself confers protection, which they distinguish from a "surrogate," which is not itself protective but is an appropriate substitute for a different immune response that does offer protection. When defining a CoP, it is equally important to define the endpoint being described. For example, does the immunologic parameter provide protection against infection, transmission, hospitalization, or death? Depending on the outcome measure, the threshold value of a CoP may vary. The term "correlates of risk" was described by Qin and colleagues[25,26] as the statistical assessment of a CoP in the context of a clinical trial. In this assessment, the clinical endpoint is the outcome measure of efficacy as predetermined in the clinical trial.

The humoral immune response is an essential feature of protection for many vaccine-preventable diseases. Antibodies have been described as good correlates of protection for several different types of pathogens, including tetanus, pneumococcus, hepatitis A, hepatitis B, diphtheria, and *Haemophilus influenzae* b.[27–29] Passive immunity from transfer of antibodies can be shown to be protective. For example, antibodies transferred from maternal transmission to the fetus or antibodies provided clinically by injection can confer protection, which demonstrates a direct protective effect of the immune marker in question. Often, a discrete and quantitative antibody threshold value for protection can be described. However, it should be noted that antibody quality rather than quantity may also be important, and thus, a potential limitation in identifying a simplistic quantity of antibody as being protective for a given pathogen.

The immune system is complex and redundant. Thus, some have proposed that a CoP for a given vaccine is not reflective in a single immune marker, but rather could be a series of immune markers in an immune cascade, or numerous independent immune markers. For example, a clear correlate for measles protection has been identified, with an antibody level of plaque reduction neutralization greater than 120 mIU/mL, as demonstrated by successful protection with maternal-fetal transmission of antibodies.[30] However, individuals who are unable to produce antibodies because of humoral deficiencies can clear measles infection, demonstrating an alternative pathway of T-cell–induced immunity that confers protection.[31,32] Therefore, multiple immune pathways may be important for generating protection depending on the pathogen and characteristics of the host, with several unique correlates of protection.

Methods to Evaluate Immune Correlates

Much controversy exists in the literature regarding the meaning and utilization of immune-based correlates. A vaccine can be shown to induce a specific immune response; however, this does not necessarily translate to clinical efficacy. A vaccine may also have an immune response that is statistically associated with an assessment of efficacy; however, this value does not directly translate into a causal relationship between the immune marker and protection. To further refine how correlates should be described and thereby applied, several investigators have suggested validation models using a combination of statistical and clinical data.

Prentice[33] developed 4 criteria to evaluate endpoints for RCTs. These criteria have been adapted in the context of vaccine trials, as listed below[34]:

1. Protection against the clinical endpoint is significantly related to having received the vaccine.
2. The substitute endpoint is significantly related to the vaccination status.
3. The substitute endpoint is significantly related to protection against the clinical endpoint.
4. The full effect of the vaccine on the frequency of the clinical endpoint is explained by the substitute endpoint, as it lies on the sole causal pathway.

Although described specifically for RCTs, others have demonstrated that the Prentice criteria can also be applied for observational studies, although this was elucidated in relation to cancer research and not vaccinology research.[35]

Qin and colleagues[25] proposed a framework to statistically describe 3 different levels of correlates of protection and defined the data requirements needed to systematically validate the immune marker for each level. The 3 levels are defined as follows: (1) "correlate of risk," which is most closely associated with protection against a clinical outcome as determined in a clinical trial; followed by (2) "level 1 specific surrogate of protection" (further split between statistical and principal surrogates); and (3) "level 2 general surrogate of protection." Although "correlate of risk" was initially described in the context of a clinical trial, Qin's methods have been adapted for use in the setting of outbreak investigations, as with Ebola vaccinations in the Democratic Republic of the Congo.[36] Qin's "level 1" statistical category must adhere to the Prentice criteria, and "level 2" can be determined only through a large-scale phase 3 trial or large postlicensure studies that have the statistical power to calculate vaccine efficacy across populations.

The threshold method has also been described, in which a specific level of the immune marker is identified. Individuals who have values above the threshold are considered protected against the clinical endpoint, whereas those with levels below the threshold are susceptible.[29,37] Different statistical tests can estimate the threshold by either (1) comparing preexposure immune marker levels to disease incidence immune marker levels in observational/cohort studies or (2) examining the proportion of vaccinated and unvaccinated individuals below the threshold and calculating the immune marker-derived vaccine efficacy.[38,39] The threshold method and variations have been used to describe specific antibody-associated levels of protection for several vaccines, including the pneumococcal conjugate vaccine,[29] meningococcal C conjugate vaccine,[40] and rubella vaccine.[39]

Although the methodologies described by Prentice, Qin, and others can be valuable to statistically validate a CoP, the foundation rests on the measurement of the immunologic marker. Assays that have a wide degree of variability and measurement error will impact the subsequent statistical calculations used in these models. Measurement errors should be carefully considered for the SARS-CoV-2 antibody assays, which have shown varying degrees of sensitivity and specificity, with no gold standard, and with various types of assays used for different COVID-19 vaccine trials and post-EUA analyses.[41,42]

THE PATH TO DEFINING CORRELATE OF PROTECTION FOR SEVERE ACUTE RESPIRATORY SYNDROME CORONAVIRUS 2 VACCINES

Determining a CoP for SARS-CoV-2 is essential to determine both individual and population level immunity, and to describe protection both after natural infection and after vaccination. Furthermore, as new variants emerge and current vaccines are adapted, a defined CoP will be useful to efficiently generate and implement vaccination programs and identify novel vaccines for use in specific populations. As described above, an important factor in describing a CoP is defining and harmonizing the clinical or efficacy endpoint. A uniform endpoint for SARS-CoV-2 has not been clearly defined, with heterogeneous outcome measures described across clinical trials and other COVID-19 studies.[43] The current literature describes the insights gained from passive immunization of monoclonal antibodies in humans as well as possible correlates of protection as shown in animal models and cohort studies (summarized in **Table 2**). RCTs, large population observational studies, and challenge trials may also aid in identifying CoPs for SARS-CoV-2. Furthermore, as new SARS-CoV-2 variants emerge, sieve analyses may be used to better understand the mechanism behind vaccine protection by using genetic and statistical approaches to measure dissimilarity between virus strains in vaccinated individuals as compared with virus strains in placebo recipients.[44] Similar approaches have been used in the field of HIV-1 vaccines and prevention.[45]

Passive Immunity

described earlier, a true CoP is an immune component that is responsible for protection against a disease endpoint and can be demonstrated by passive transfer from an immune individual to a naïve individual. For SARS-CoV-2, monoclonal antibodies (mAb) have been developed that validate the role of neutralization antibodies as a mechanism of protection against disease.[46] A double-blind, phase 1 to 3 trial investigated the use of an antibody cocktail (REGN-COV2) in nonhospitalized, symptomatic patients.[47] The cocktail is composed of 2 neutralizing human IgG1 antibodies that target the RBD of SARS-CoV-2. The interim analysis demonstrated reduction of the SARS-CoV-2 viral load in participants who received the REGN-COV2 antibody

Table 2
Proposed correlates of protection

Study Design	Authors	Natural Infection or Postimmunization	Endpoint	Correlates of Protection Identified
Passive immunity	Weinreich et al,[47] 2021 Chen et al,[48] 2021	Passive antibody transfer	SARS-CoV-2 viral load	nAb, no specific threshold determined
Animal model	McMahan et al,[50] 2021	Natural infection	SARS-CoV-2 PCR detection in BAL	50 for pseudovirus nAb titers; 100 for RBD ELISA titers; 400 for S ELISA titers
Animal model	Corbett et al,[52] 2020	Postimmunization	SARS-CoV-2 PCR detection in BAL	nAb, no specific threshold determined
Animal model	Mercado et al,[51] 2020	Postimmunization	SARS-CoV-2 PCR detection in BAL	nAb 100–250
Cohort study	Addetia et al,[58] 2020	Natural infection	SARS-CoV-2 PCR (nasopharyngeal) and clinical symptoms	nAb were protective in 3 crew members with levels of 1:174, 1:161, and 1:3082

cocktail, with a more pronounced effect in individuals who had not yet produced endogenous antibody. Another randomized, placebo-controlled phase 2 study (BLAZE-1) evaluated the role of LY-CoV555, an anti-spike neutralizing mAb that binds with high affinity to the RBD region of SARS-CoV-2 in patients with mild to moderate COVID-19 disease in the outpatient setting.[48] For one of the 3 dose levels tested, there was a significant decline in viral load by day 11 as compared with the placebo group as well as a trend toward fewer hospitalizations and lower symptom burden in patients who received LY-CoV555. These data suggest a direct beneficial role of nAb in COVID-19. Studies are ongoing to better understand if mAb would also be beneficial in preventing SARS-CoV-2 infection in close contacts of infected individuals (eg, NCT04452318), which would provide additional insight into the role of humoral immunity in protection.

Animal Models

An animal model with rhesus macaques was developed and demonstrated SARS-CoV-2 infection and replication in pneumocytes and bronchial epithelial cells.[49] All macaques produced SARS-CoV-2 anti-spike bAb and nAb responses as well as SARS-CoV-2–specific cellular immune responses. After 35 days from the initial viral infection, the macaques were rechallenged with the same dose of SARS-CoV-2. Limited levels to no levels of viral RNA were detected from bronchoalveolar lavage (BAL) or nasal swabs in the rechallenged animals, which exhibited asymptomatic or mild clinical disease. These data suggest immunologic control upon rechallenge. However, because of the small sample size and near complete protection of the animals after rechallenge, no immune correlates of protection were identified. Given the positive responses of bAb, nAb, and cellular immune activation, the relative dominance of any one of these immune markers could not be determined.

The investigators next investigated the use of IgG transfer from convalescent macaque sera to naïve macaques who were subsequently challenged with SARS-CoV-2 as well as depletion of CD8+ T cells in convalescent macaques to identify a CoP.[50] The macaques who received the purified IgG were protected against the challenge infection in a dose-dependent manner. Using logistic regression models, antibody thresholds greater than 50 for pseudovirus nAb titers, 100 for RBD ELISA titers, and 400 for S ELISA titers were demonstrated to be protective. In the CD8+ T-cell–depleted group, some breakthrough infections occurred, suggesting that protection is not independently related to T-cell function, but that cellular immunity likely plays a role, especially in the setting of low antibody titers.

The same macaque model was then used to assess for vaccine-induced protection with DNA vaccine candidates and Ad26 vector vaccines.[51] Viral replication in BAL fluid and nasal secretions was measured for the endpoint analyses. Because of variability in the outcomes based on the different vaccine constructs administered, the investigators were able to evaluate for immune CoPs. An inverse correlation was described between nAb (both pseudovirus and live virus nAb titers) and RNA levels from BAL and nasal secretions, suggesting nAb as an immune CoP, with nAb titers between 100 and 250 offering complete protection.

Nonhuman primate challenge models have also been used to evaluate immune responses and determine CoP after vaccination. To evaluate CoP in the context of mRNA-1273 administration, nonhuman primates were challenged with intratracheal and intranasal SARS-CoV-2 four weeks after the second vaccination with mRNA-1273.[52] The endpoint assessment was quantification of SARS-CoV-2 RNA in BAL fluid and nasal secretions. mRNA-1273–induced serum neutralization activity was then correlated with RNA from BAL and nasal secretions and was found to be negatively correlated. Given this finding, in combination with the rapid reduction in viral replication 24 to 48 hours after challenge, the investigators speculated that antibodies do serve as the primary mechanism of protection. However, a specific threshold could not be determined, because the vaccine-induced immune response offered high protection with limited variation in viral replication.

A limitation of animal models is the inability to entirely recapitulate human pathogenesis and disease. The concentration and inoculation of virus for the challenge in animals may not reflect true transmission dynamics in humans.

Cohort and Observational Studies

Cohort and observational studies can provide information about CoP through epidemiologic analyses. Several cohort studies have examined rates of reinfection within distinct populations, which can also provide clues regarding CoP.[53–55] For example, a large, prospective cohort study in the United Kingdom, the SIREN (SARS-CoV-2 Immunity and Reinfection Evaluation) study, enrolled more than 30,000 health care workers and documented SARS-CoV-2 polymerase chain reaction (PCR) and antibody testing every 2 to 4 weeks.[56] The investigators describe that the seropositive participants (those with a prior history of SARS-CoV-2 infection) had an 84% lower risk of reinfection (adjusted incidence rate ratio 0.159; 95% CI 0.13–0.19). The data provide evidence that antibodies are protective against reinfection, although the investigators did not correlate specific antibody thresholds with protection.[57]

The outbreak that occurred on a fishery boat departing from Seattle was essential in determining that nAb were protective against SARS-CoV-2. One hundred three out of 117 individuals were seronegative before departure and were subsequently infected. Three members of the crew were seropositive with high nAb (1:174, 1:161, and 1:3082) before departure and did not develop infection as evidenced by negative SARS-CoV-2 PCR from nasopharyngeal swabs and lack of clinical symptoms.[58] Thus, high nAb were associated with protection, but no exact threshold could be determined from this observational study.

Challenge Studies

Human challenge studies involve the direct and controlled infection of healthy human volunteers and have been used to investigate novel vaccine candidates. Unlike RCTs or large population-based studies, controlled human challenge studies are faster and require fewer participants to measure efficacy and immune responses. These designs have been used to study other respiratory viral pathogens like influenza[59] and HCoV-229E and have been proposed to evaluate SARS-CoV-2.[60,61] Challenge models are attractive designs to determine immune CoP, because the exact timing of natural infection and/or immunization and dose can be tightly controlled, allowing for high-resolution assessment of correlations between immune markers and efficacy endpoints.

COVID-19 human challenge studies have begun in the United Kingdom.[62] The trials are currently ongoing; no data have been released yet regarding early findings. Later stages may offer insight to discerning CoP.

Randomized Controlled Trials

RCTs are well suited to define CoP, because clear clinical endpoints are established and measures of both vaccine efficacy and immune markers are documented at defined intervals. Using the threshold method and other statistical calculations, the vaccine efficacy can be correlated with an immune marker level to determine a CoP. Current evaluation of the phase 3 data is ongoing to determine a CoP, which may vary for different vaccine constructs.

OTHER CONSIDERATIONS RELATING TO CORRELATES OF PROTECTION

Based on correlates of protection for other infectious diseases, other important factors must be considered when defining immunologic markers of protection after COVID-19 vaccination. This section reviews some of these considerations, such as host factors, the vaccine platform and target antigen, and other important immunologic aspects of the immune response to vaccination.

Host Factors

Host factors, such as age, chronic medical conditions, and the use of immunosuppressive therapies, have been shown to impact the antibody responses to COVID-19 vaccines. These factors may also impact definitions of COVID-19 postvaccination correlates or surrogates of protection.

Age is an important factor influencing humoral vaccine responses. Most of the COVID-19 vaccine phase 1/2 trials showed that the magnitude of the vaccine-induced antibody responses in older individuals is generally lower than the antibody magnitude produced by younger individuals. For example, mRNA vaccines were shown to produce lower titers of bAb and lower or similar titers of nAb in participants older than 55 to 65 years of age.[5,9] The same tendency was shown with vector vaccines, except for AZD1222, which showed similar bAb and nAb titers in all age groups.[4,8,10] BBIP-CorV, an inactivated vaccine, led to lower nAb production in those aged 60 and older.[63]

The components of the immune response postvaccination that best correlate with protection may differ quantitively and qualitatively because of immunosenescence.[64] For example, in adults up to 50 years old, serum influenza hemagglutination inhibition levels of about 1:40 correlate well with protection.[24] However, higher postvaccination titers $\geq$1:40 are common among older individuals who develop influenza, suggesting that this threshold is not protective for older individuals.[65] In older individuals, T-cell responses may be a better correlate of vaccine protection against influenza.[66]

The effect of age on COVID-19 vaccine immune correlates is currently unknown. The correlation of bAb and nAb titers after Ad26.CoV2.S was stronger in younger individuals than in those 65 years and older.[4] This suggests a variation in the immune response phenotype in older individuals, which could influence the definition of immune correlates in this population.

Data are emerging regarding other host factors that are associated with lower humoral responses to COVID-19 vaccines, such as chronic comorbidities and immunocompromised states. For example, patients undergoing maintenance hemodialysis showed significant lower bAb than controls after 2 doses of BNT162b2.[67] Individuals with chronic inflammatory disease treated with immunosuppressive therapies, in particular those receiving B-cell depletion therapy of corticosteroids, exhibit significantly lower bAb and nAb titers after mRNA vaccines.[68] Solid organ transplant recipients were shown to have poor humoral responses after mRNA vaccines,[69,70] with older individuals and those receiving antimetabolite therapy having some of the poorest humoral responses.

Immunocompromised individuals have a significantly reduced humoral response to COVID-19 vaccines. CoP in this population may be different than in the general population. For example, patients treated with B-cell depletion therapy (anti-CD20) are usually unable to mount strong humoral immune responses to COVID-19 vaccines or SARS-CoV-2 infection.[71,72] However, infected individuals on such therapy still have the ability to clear the virus, which suggest that the cellular immune response or other arms of the immune system may have an important role.

Socioeconomic status, usually closely related to other factors, such as nutritional status, risk, and frequency of exposure, has been shown to impact immune correlates for other diseases. For example, the antibody titers associated with protection against pneumococcal infection has been shown to be higher among infants who live in low-resource settings.[29,73] The impact of socioeconomic status of environmental factors on correlates of protection from SARS-CoV-2 vaccination is unknown. However, because lower socioeconomic status has been already recognized as a risk factor for disease incidence and mortality,[74,75] it may be an important factor to consider as well when defining immune correlates after vaccination.

Vaccine Platform and Vaccine Antigens

Vaccines using different technological platforms and antigen targets may induce different qualitative and quantitative antibodies, which is another important factor to consider when establishing immune correlates for COVID-19 vaccines. This concept has been well described with other vaccines, such as those against *H influenzae* type b (polysaccharide vs conjugated vaccine) and *Bordetella pertussis* (whole cell vs acellular vaccine),[76,77] where different platforms were shown to yield different immune repertoire. COVID-19 vaccines use different technologies (mRNA, vector, subunit, inactivated) and different antigen targets (full spike, prefusion stabilized spike protein, RBD, inactivated virus), which may lead to different immune response quality and repertoire. Inactivated vaccines have the unique characteristic of presenting the whole virus to the immune system, which leads to the production of antibodies other than anti-spike, such as antinucleocapsid.[15] Even if the main target of nAb against SARS-CoV-2 appears to be the spike protein,[78] the antibody repertoire and diversity produced by inactivated vaccines may have immunologic significance against SARS-CoV-2 and the circulating variants that possess critical spike protein mutations.[79,80]

Immunologic Factors

The immune mechanisms leading to protection are complex and usually involve a combination of both humoral and cellular responses.[81] The impact of the relative importance of these 2 branches of the adaptive immune system for protection against SARS-CoV-2 is still unknown. Many studies have shown that antibodies are associated with protection against reinfection,[56] but few have evaluated the implication of cellular immune response on reinfection. COVID-19 vaccines have been shown to induce strong humoral immunity, but T-cell responses were also elicited after vaccination.[4,5] In a nonhumate primate study using an adenovirus-based vaccine (Ad26-S.PP), T-cell responses did not seem to correlate with protection.[51] It is still unknown if the cellular response contributes to protection in humans; however, there are clues that cellular responses are important. For example, the clinical protection from BNT162 against COVID-19 may start as soon as 12 days after the first dose.[82] However, nAb titers within the first 21 days after vaccination are low or undetectable.[9] Researchers showed that 3 weeks after the first BNT162b2 dose, nAb were not detected, but strong responses of RBD and spike antibodies with Fc-mediated effector functions and cellular responses largely by CD4+ T-cell responses were seen.[83]

Mucosal immunity is another possible key component of COVID-19 protection, as SARS-CoV-2 initially infects the respiratory mucosal surfaces.[84] However, the mucosal immunity that results from COVID-19 natural infection and vaccination and its implication in defining COVID-19 correlates of protection remain largely unknown.

SUMMARY

The vaccine-induced CoP for SARS-CoV-2 has yet to be defined. When establishing a CoP, it will be essential not only to identify the appropriate immune marker but also to properly define the endpoint measure (eg, clinical disease, especially severe illness; transmission, SARS-CoV-2 PCR positivity) and understand the nuances of CoP in terms of host and antigen characteristics. Furthermore, standardized assays for the chosen immune marker or markers must be established in order to ensure comparability between disparate vaccine platforms and conditions of use. Ideally, these assays should be a test that is relatively easy to perform and does not require specialized equipment or reagents to promote easy scalability across the globe. Much of the focus has been to determine a humoral CoP, in part because of the ease of collection and evaluation, although cellular responses are also likely to be important.

As new public health challenges relating to COVID-19 emerge, such as variant strains, waning vaccine efficacy over time, and decreased vaccine efficacy for special populations (such as immunocompromised hosts), it is important to determine a CoP to allow accurate bridging studies for special populations and against variants of concern. In the context of a global pandemic with dynamic threats to public health, large-scale phase 3 clinical trials are inefficient to rapidly assess novel vaccine candidates for variant strains or for special populations, because these trials are slow and costly. Defining a practical CoP will aid in efficiently conducting future assessments to further describe protection for individuals and on a population level for surveillance.

CLINICS CARE POINTS

- The clinical utility of a correlate or surrogate of vaccine-induced immunity would be useful to assess individual and population-level protection, and allow for new vaccine candidates to be tested without costly and large efficacy trials.
- Further standardization of laboratory SARS-CoV-2 serologic tests are an equally important step to be able to use a correlate of protection in clinical practice.
- Clinicians and laboratorians must acknowledge that different vaccine platforms, circulating variants, and host factors may impact the correlate of the protection, and that a single marker of immunity may not be able specifically predict protection for all scenarios.

REFERENCES

1. COVID-19 vaccine tracker. Available at: https://www.raps.org/news-and-articles/news-articles/2020/3/covid-19-vaccine-tracker. Accessed April 25, 2021.
2. Plotkin SA. Immunologic correlates of protection induced by vaccination. Pediatr Infect Dis J 2001;20:63–75.
3. Immunogenicity of clinically relevant SARS-CoV-2 vaccines in nonhuman primates and humans | Science Advances. Available at: https://advances.sciencemag.org/content/7/12/eabe8065. Accessed April 25, 2021.
4. Sadoff J, Le Gars M, Shukarev G, et al. Interim results of a phase 1–2a trial of Ad26.COV2.S Covid-19 vaccine. New Engl J Med 2021;0. https://doi.org/10.1056/NEJMoa2034201.
5. Jackson LA, Anderson EJ, Rouphael NG, et al. An mRNA vaccine against SARS-CoV-2 — preliminary report. New Engl J Med 2020;0. https://doi.org/10.1056/NEJMoa2022483.

6. Logunov DY, Dolzhikova IV, Zubkova OV, et al. Safety and immunogenicity of an rAd26 and rAd5 vector-based heterologous prime-boost COVID-19 vaccine in two formulations: two open, non-randomised phase 1/2 studies from Russia. Lancet 2020;396:887–97.

7. Zhu F-C, Guan X-H, Li Y-H, et al. Immunogenicity and safety of a recombinant adenovirus type-5-vectored COVID-19 vaccine in healthy adults aged 18 years or older: a randomised, double-blind, placebo-controlled, phase 2 trial. Lancet 2020;396:479–88.

8. Folegatti PM, Ewer KJ, Aley PK. Safety and immunogenicity of the ChAdOx1 nCoV-19 vaccine against SARS-CoV-2: a preliminary report of a phase 1/2, single-blind, randomised controlled trial. Lancet 2020;396:467–78.

9. Walsh EE, Frenck RW, Falsey AR, et al. Safety and immunogenicity of two RNA-based Covid-19 vaccine candidates. New Engl J Med 2020;383:2439–50.

10. Zhang Y, Zeng G, Pan H, et al. Safety, tolerability, and immunogenicity of an in-activated SARS-CoV-2 vaccine in healthy adults aged 18–59 years: a rando-mised, double-blind, placebo-controlled, phase 1/2 clinical trial. Lancet Infect Dis 2021;21:181–92.

11. Doria-Rose N, Suthar MS, Makowski M, et al. Antibody persistence through 6 months after the second dose of mRNA-1273 vaccine for Covid-19. New En-gland Journal of Medicine 2021. https://doi.org/10.1056/NEJMc2103916.

12. Pfizer and BioNTech confirm high efficacy and no serious safety concerns through up to six months following second dose in updated topline analysis of landmark COVID-19 vaccine study. 2021. Available at: https://www.businesswire.com/news/home/20210401005365/en/Pfizer-and-BioNTech-Confirm-High-Efficacy-and-No-Serious-Safety-Concerns-Through-Up-to-Six-Months-Following-Second-Dose-in-Updated-Topline-Analysis-of-Landmark-COVID-19-Vaccine-Study. Accessed May 3, 2021.

13. Moderna provides clinical and supply updates on COVID-19 vaccine program ahead of 2nd annual vaccines day | Moderna, Inc., (n.d.). Available at: https://investors.modernatx.com/news-releases/news-release-details/moderna-provides-clinical-and-supply-updates-covid-19-vaccine/. Accessed May 20, 2021.

14. Klasse PJ, Nixon DF, Moore JP. Immunogenicity of clinically relevant SARS-CoV-2 vaccines in nonhuman primates and humans. Sci Adv 2021;7:eabe8065.

15. Ella R, Reddy S, Jogdand H, et al. Safety and immunogenicity of an inactivated SARS-CoV-2 vaccine, BBV152: interim results from a double-blind, randomised, multicentre, phase 2 trial, and 3-month follow-up of a double-blind, randomised phase 1 trial. Lancet Infect Dis 2021. https://doi.org/10.1016/S1473-3099(21)00070-0.

16. Yang S, Li Y, Dai L, et al. Safety and immunogenicity of a recombinant tandem-repeat dimeric RBD-based protein subunit vaccine (ZF2001) against COVID-19 in adults: two randomised, double-blind, placebo-controlled, phase 1 and 2 trials. Lancet Infect Dis 2021. https://doi.org/10.1016/S1473-3099(21)00127-4.

17. Seow J, Graham C, Merrick B, et al. Longitudinal observation and decline of neutralizing antibody responses in the three months following SARS-CoV-2 infec-tion in humans. Nat Microbiol 2020;5:1598–607.

18. Krammer F, Srivastava K, Alshammary H, et al. Antibody responses in seroposi-tive persons after a single dose of SARS-CoV-2 mRNA vaccine. New Engl J Med 2021;384:1372–4.

19. CDC. Cases, Data, and surveillance. Centers for Disease Control and Prevention; 2020. Available at: https://www.cdc.gov/coronavirus/2019-ncov/cases-updates/variant-surveillance/variant-info.html. Accessed April 30, 2021.

20. Shen X, Tang H, Pajon R, et al. Neutralization of SARS-CoV-2 variants B.1.429 and B.1.351. New Engl J Med 2021;0. https://doi.org/10.1056/NEJMc2103740.

21. Wu K, Werner AP, Koch M, et al. Serum neutralizing activity elicited by mRNA-1273 vaccine. New Engl J Med 2021;384:1468–70.

22. Madhi SA, Baillie V, Cutland CL, et al. Efficacy of the ChAdOx1 nCoV-19 Covid-19 vaccine against the B.1.351 variant. New Engl J Med 2021;0. https://doi.org/10.1056/NEJMoa2102214.

23. Lustig Y, Nemet I, Kliker L, et al. Neutralizing response against variants after SARS-CoV-2 infection and one dose of BNT162b2. New Engl J Med 2021;0. https://doi.org/10.1056/NEJMc2104036.

24. Plotkin SA, Plotkin SA. Correlates of vaccine-induced immunity. Clin Infect Dis 2008;47:401–9. https://doi.org/10.1086/589862.

25. Qin L, Gilbert PB, Corey L, et al. A framework for assessing immunological correlates of protection in vaccine trials. J Infect Dis 2007;196:1304–12.

26. Plotkin SA, Gilbert PB. Nomenclature for immune correlates of protection after vaccination. Clin Infect Dis 2012;54:1615–7.

27. Denoël PA, Goldblatt D, de Vleeschauwer I, et al. Quality of the Haemophilus influenzae type b (Hib) antibody response induced by diphtheria-tetanus-acellular pertussis/Hib combination vaccines. Clin Vaccin Immunol 2007;14:1362–9.

28. Jack AD, Hall AJ, Maine N, et al. What level of hepatitis B antibody is protective? J Infect Dis 1999;179:489–92.

29. Siber GR, Chang I, Baker S, et al. Estimating the protective concentration of anti-pneumococcal capsular polysaccharide antibodies. Vaccine 2007;25:3816–26.

30. Chen RT, Markowitz LE, Albrecht P, et al. Measles antibody: reevaluation of protective titers. J Infect Dis 1990;162:1036–42.

31. Plebani A, Fischer MB, Meini A, et al. T cell activity and cytokine production in X-linked agammaglobulinemia: implications for vaccination strategies. Int Arch Allergy Immunol 1997;114:90–3.

32. Gans HA. Deficiency of the humoral immune response to measles vaccine in infants immunized at age 6 Months. JAMA 1998;280:527.

33. Prentice RL. Surrogate endpoints in clinical trials: definition and operational criteria. Stat Med 1989;8:431–40.

34. World Health Organization. Correlates of vaccine-induced protection: methods and implications. 2013. Available at: https://apps.who.int/iris/bitstream/handle/10665/84288/WHO_IVB_13.01_eng.pdf. Accessed April 13, 2021.

35. Schatzkin A, Freedman LS, Dorgan J, et al. Using and interpreting surrogate endpoints in cancer research. IARC Sci Publ.; 1997. p. 265–71.

36. Halloran ME, Longini IM, Gilbert PB. Designing a study of correlates of risk for Ebola vaccination. Am J Epidemiol 2020;189:747–54.

37. Chen X, Bailleux F, Desai K, et al. A threshold method for immunological correlates of protection. BMC Med Res Methodol 2013;13:29.

38. Siber GR. Methods for estimating serological correlates of protection. Dev Biol Stand 1997;89:283–96.

39. Skendzel LP. Rubella immunity. Defining the level of protective antibody. Am J Clin Pathol 1996;106:170–4.

40. Validation of serological correlate of protection for meningococcal C conjugate vaccine by using efficacy estimates from postlicensure surveillance in England, (n.d.). Available at: https://www.ncbi.nlm.nih.gov/pmc/articles/PMC193909/. Accessed April 15, 2021.

41. Galipeau Y, Greig M, Liu G, et al. Humoral responses and serological assays in SARS-CoV-2 infections. Front Immunol 2020;11. https://doi.org/10.3389/fimmu.2020.610688.
42. Whitman JD, Hiatt J, Mowery CT, et al. Evaluation of SARS-CoV-2 serology assays reveals a range of test performance. Nat Biotechnol 2020;38:1174–83.
43. Mehrotra DV, Janes HE, Fleming TR, et al. Clinical endpoints for evaluating efficacy in COVID-19 vaccine trials. Ann Intern Med 2020;174:221–8.
44. Rolland M, Gilbert PB. Sieve analysis to understand how SARS-CoV-2 diversity can impact vaccine protection. PLOS Pathog 2021;17:e1009406.
45. Corey L, Gilbert PB, Juraska M, et al. Two randomized trials of neutralizing antibodies to prevent HIV-1 acquisition. New Engl J Med 2021;384:1003–14.
46. Taylor PC, Adams AC, Hufford MM, et al. Neutralizing monoclonal antibodies for treatment of COVID-19. Nat Rev Immunol 2021;1–12.
47. Weinreich DM, Sivapalasingam S, Norton T, et al. REGN-COV2, a neutralizing antibody cocktail, in outpatients with Covid-19. New Engl J Med 2021;384:238–51.
48. Chen P, Nirula A, Heller B, et al. SARS-CoV-2 neutralizing antibody LY-CoV555 in outpatients with Covid-19. New Engl J Med 2021;384:229–37.
49. Chandrashekar A, Liu J, Martinot AJ, et al. SARS-CoV-2 infection protects against rechallenge in rhesus macaques. Science 2020;369:812–7.
50. McMahan K, Yu J, Mercado NB, et al. Correlates of protection against SARS-CoV-2 in rhesus macaques. Nature 2021;590:630–4.
51. Mercado NB, Zahn R, Wegmann F, et al. Single-shot Ad26 vaccine protects against SARS-CoV-2 in rhesus macaques. Nature 2020;586:583–8.
52. Corbett KS, Flynn B, Foulds KE, et al. Evaluation of the mRNA-1273 vaccine against SARS-CoV-2 in nonhuman primates. New Engl J Med 2020;383:1544–55.
53. Lumley SF, O'Donnell D, Stoesser NE, et al. Antibody status and incidence of SARS-CoV-2 infection in health care workers. New Engl J Med 2021;384:533–40.
54. Hansen CH, Michlmayr D, Gubbels SM, et al. Assessment of protection against reinfection with SARS-CoV-2 among 4 million PCR-tested individuals in Denmark in 2020: a population-level observational study. The Lancet 2021;397:1204–12.
55. Harvey RA, Rassen JA, Kabelac CA, et al. Association of SARS-CoV-2 seropositive antibody test with risk of future infection. JAMA Intern Med 2021. https://doi.org/10.1001/jamainternmed.2021.0366.
56. Hall VJ, Foulkes S, Charlett A, et al. SARS-CoV-2 infection rates of antibody-positive compared with antibody-negative health-care workers in England: a large, multicentre, prospective cohort study (SIREN). Lancet 2021;397:1459–69.
57. Krammer F. Correlates of protection from SARS-CoV-2 infection. Lancet 2021;397:1421–3.
58. Addetia A, Crawford KHD, Dingens A, et al. Neutralizing antibodies correlate with protection from SARS-CoV-2 in humans during a fishery vessel outbreak with a high attack rate. J Clin Microbiol 2020;58. https://doi.org/10.1128/JCM.02107-20.
59. Sherman AC, Mehta A, Dickert NW, et al. The future of flu: a review of the human challenge model and systems biology for advancement of influenza vaccinology. Front Cell. Infect. Microbiol. 2019;9. https://doi.org/10.3389/fcimb.2019.00107. Available at:.
60. Deming ME, Michael NL, Robb M, et al. Accelerating development of SARS-CoV-2 vaccines — the role for controlled human infection models. New Engl J Med 2020;383:e63.
61. Callow KA, Parry HF, Sergeant M, et al. The time course of the immune response to experimental coronavirus infection of man. Epidemiol Infect 1990;105:435–46.

62. Kirby T. COVID-19 human challenge studies in the UK. Lancet Respir Med 2020; 8:e96.

63. Xia S, Zhang Y, Wang Y, et al. Safety and immunogenicity of an inactivated SARS-CoV-2 vaccine, BBIBP-CorV: a randomised, double-blind, placebo-controlled, phase 1/2 trial. The Lancet Infect Dis 2021;21:39–51.

64. Grubeck-Loebenstein B, Della Bella S, Iorio AM, et al. Immunosenescence and vaccine failure in the elderly. Aging Clin Exp Res 2009;21:201–9.

65. Gravenstein S, Drinka P, Duthie EH, et al. Efficacy of an influenza hemagglutinin-diphtheria toxoid conjugate vaccine in elderly nursing home subjects during an influenza outbreak. J Am Geriatr Soc 1994;42:245–51.

66. McElhaney JE, Xie D, Hager WD, et al. T cell responses are better correlates of vaccine protection in the elderly. J Immunol 2006;176:6333–9.

67. Grupper A, Sharon N, Finn T, et al. Humoral response to the Pfizer BNT162b2 vaccine in patients undergoing maintenance hemodialysis,. CJASN 2021. https://doi.org/10.2215/CJN.03500321.

68. Glucocorticoids and B Cell depleting agents substantially impair immunogenicity of mRNA vaccines to SARS-CoV-2 | medRxiv. Available at: https://www.medrxiv.org/content/10.1101/2021.04.05.21254656v2. Accessed April 30, 2021.

69. A. Grupper, L. Rabinowich, D. Schwartz, et al, Reduced humoral response to mRNA SARS-Cov-2 BNT162b2 vaccine in kidney transplant recipients without prior exposure to the virus, Am J Transplant. Available at: 10.1111/ajt.16615.

70. Boyarsky BJ, Werbel WA, Avery RK, et al. Immunogenicity of a single dose of SARS-CoV-2 messenger RNA vaccine in solid organ transplant recipients. JAMA 2021. https://doi.org/10.1001/jama.2021.4385.

71. Fallet B, Kyburz D, Walker UA. Mild course of COVID-19 and spontaneous virus clearance in a patient with depleted peripheral blood b cells due to rituximab treatment. Arthritis Rheumatol 2020;72:1581–2.

72. Herishanu Y, Avivi I, Aharon A, et al. Efficacy of the BNT162b2 mRNA COVID-19 vaccine in patients with chronic lymphocytic leukemia. Blood 2021. https://doi.org/10.1182/blood.2021011568.

73. Jódar L, Butler J, Carlone G, et al. Serological criteria for evaluation and licensure of new pneumococcal conjugate vaccine formulations for use in infants. Vaccine 2003;21:3265–72.

74. Karmakar M, Lantz PM, Tipirneni R. Association of social and demographic factors with COVID-19 incidence and death rates in the US. JAMA Netw Open 2021; 4:e2036462.

75. Clouston SAP, Natale G, Link BG. Socioeconomic inequalities in the spread of coronavirus-19 in the United States: a examination of the emergence of social inequalities. Soc Sci Med 2021;268:113554.

76. Edwards KM, Meade BD, Decker MD, et al. Comparison of 13 acellular pertussis vaccines: overview and serologic response. Pediatrics 1995;96:548–57.

77. Jelonek MT, Chang SJ, Chiu CY, et al. Comparison of naturally acquired and vaccine-induced antibodies to Haemophilus influenzae type b capsular polysaccharide. Infect Immun 1993;61:5345–50.

78. Barnes CO, Jette CA, Abernathy ME, et al. SARS-CoV-2 neutralizing antibody structures inform therapeutic strategies. Nature 2020;588:682–7.

79. Huang B, Dai L, Wang H, et al. Serum sample neutralisation of BBIBP-CorV and ZF2001 vaccines to SARS-CoV-2 501Y.V2. Lancet Microbe 2021;0. https://doi.org/10.1016/S2666-5247(21)00082-3.

80. Abdool Karim SS, de Oliveira T. New SARS-CoV-2 variants — clinical, public health, and vaccine implications. New Engl J Med 2021;0. https://doi.org/10.1056/NEJMc2100362.
81. Amanna IJ, Slifka MK. Contributions of humoral and cellular immunity to vaccine-induced protection in humans. Virology 2011;411:206–15.
82. Polack FP, Thomas SJ, Kitchin N, et al. Safety and efficacy of the BNT162b2 mRNA Covid-19 vaccine. New Engl J Med 2020;383:2603–15.
83. Tauzin A, Nayrac M, Benlarbi M, et al. A single BNT162b2 mRNA dose elicits antibodies with Fc-mediated effector functions and boost pre-existing humoral and T cell responses. BioRxiv 2021;2021. https://doi.org/10.1101/2021.03.18.435972.
84. Russell MW, Moldoveanu Z, Ogra PL, et al. Mucosal immunity in COVID-19: a neglected but critical aspect of SARS-CoV-2 infection. Front Immunol 2020;11. https://doi.org/10.3389/fimmu.2020.611337.
85. Anderson EJ, Rouphael NG, Widge AT, et al. Safety and immunogenicity of SARS-CoV-2 mRNA-1273 vaccine in older adults. New Engl J Med 2020. https://doi.org/10.1056/NEJMoa2028436.
86. Ramasamy MN, Minassian AM, Ewer KJ, et al. Safety and immunogenicity of ChAdOx1 nCoV-19 vaccine administered in a prime-boost regimen in young and old adults (COV002): a single-blind, randomised, controlled, phase 2/3 trial. Lancet 2020;396:1979–93.
87. Wu Z, Hu Y, Xu M, et al. Safety, tolerability, and immunogenicity of an inactivated SARS-CoV-2 vaccine (CoronaVac) in healthy adults aged 60 years and older: a randomised, double-blind, placebo-controlled, phase 1/2 clinical trial. Lancet Infect Dis 2021;0. https://doi.org/10.1016/S1473-3099(20)30987-7.
88. Safety and immunogenicity clinical trial of an inactivated SARS-CoV-2 vaccine, BBV152 (a phase 2, double-blind, randomised controlled trial) and the persistence of immune responses from a phase 1 follow-up report | medRxiv. Available at: https://www.medrxiv.org/content/10.1101/2020.12.21.20248643v1. Accessed April 30, 2021.
89. Xia S, Duan K, Zhang Y, et al. Effect of an inactivated vaccine against SARS-CoV-2 on safety and immunogenicity outcomes: interim analysis of 2 randomized clinical trials. JAMA 2020;324:951.

Role of Digital Health During Coronavirus Disease 2019 Pandemic and Future Perspectives

Adnan Ahmed, MD[a], Rishi Charate, MD[a],
Naga Venkata K. Pothineni, MD[a], Surya Kiran Aedma, MD[b],
Rakesh Gopinathannair, MD[a], Dhanunjaya Lakkireddy, MD[a],*

KEYWORDS

- Digital health • Artificial intelligence (AI) • Machine learning (ML) • Deep learning (DL)
- COVID-19 pandemic • Telemedicine • Remote monitoring

KEY POINTS

- COVID-19 pandemic brought a significant paradigm shift in mode of health care delivery.
- Adoption of digital health served as a necessary tool to ensure safety of patients and health care professionals.
- Telemedicine, a concept that existed pre-COVID, was used to deliver care in outpatient as well as inpatient care settings to restrict exposure and conserve PPE.
- Barriers to wide-scale availability of digital health are related to lack of infrastructure, digital literacy, and patients belonging to underserved and underrepresented population with socioeconomic constraints.
- Economics of digital medical care and insurance reimbursements will continue to be a matter of debate in the near future.

INTRODUCTION

The coronavirus disease 19 (COVID-19) pandemic has yielded an unparalleled global challenge in the delivery of health care. From nationally mandated quarantines and mass vaccination efforts to ushering in a new era of virtual communication, it has necessitated a new perspective on health care moving forward. Specifically, it has led to institutionalized changes to health care systems, hospitals, medical professionals, ancillary staff, training programs, and health care polices. Aims to both safely

This article previously appeared in *Cardiac Electrophysiology Clinics*, Volume 14, Issue 1, March 2022.
[a] Kansas City Heart Rhythm Institute, 5100 W, 110th Street, Suite 200 Overland Park, KS 66211, USA; [b] Carle Foundation Hospital, 611 West Park Street, Urbana, IL 61801, USA
* Corresponding author. Kansas City Heart Rhythm Institute, 5100 W, 110th Street, Suite 200, Overland Park, KS 66211, USA.
E-mail address: dhanunjaya.lakkireddy@hcahealthcare.com

preserve the best qualities of face-to-face traditional patient care as well as integrate technology and virtual care have been at the forefront of each specialty. Digital health care has been a revolution in this effort in effective management of patients with complex conditions. This paradigm shift has called for our advocacy to improve upon and incorporate even newer emerging digital health solutions as well as alleviate previous barriers to digital health care. Cardiac electrophysiology (EP) has been uniquely poised as a specialty that has been accustomed to using digital health techniques such as remote monitoring and artificial intelligence (AI) supplementary tools even in the prepandemic period.[1] In this article, we explain the obstacles encountered with in-person care during the pandemic, review currently available digital health platforms specifically in relation to cardiac EP, and explore further avenues for advancing digital and in-person care delivery in the future.

TRADITIONAL CARE DURING THE PANDEMIC

The COVID-19 pandemic has abruptly ushered in a foundational change to the traditional practice of medicine. Despite clinical research and advancements continually evolving and reshaping the field of medicine, the practice of face-to-face patient encounters had previously remained stable. Although face-to-face care was accepted as the norm for centuries, the pandemic forced us to revisit this idea as a community. This pandemic was the catalyst for not only a sudden but also a widespread paradigm shift in patient care, with nearly 80% of the US population indicating that they have used one form of digital health.[2,3] The pandemic has also enabled health care providers and administrators to revisit the intricacies of in-person care delivery and improve overall efficiency. In-person care depends on a variety of supporting frameworks that include providers, administrative personnel, patients, caregivers, and family members and is very time and resource intensive. Testing for COVID-19 and limiting physical contact between personnel for in-person care made for a more complex, time-consuming, and inefficient process. One study advocated for creating a safe workplace by universal testing for COVID-19 in asymptomatic patients and health care workers. Out of 1670 subjects, 758 were patients and 912 were caregivers, Emergency Medical Service, and EP laboratory personnel. The study found 3.8% positivity rates in the asymptomatic population.[4] While hospitals began cancellation of elective clinic and procedural visits in efforts to allocate health care resources toward tackling the pandemic, a steep decline in patient comfort levels in attending in-person visits was also noted. Several reports have indicated patient hesitancy to attend for in-person care even for concerning anginal symptoms. In fact, there was a reduction in patients presenting to the emergency room with acute myocardial infarction during the peak of the pandemic, and those that presented had higher mechanical complications due to late presentations.[5] These data highlight the hesitancy and overt concern that patients may have to seek medical care in this current global crisis, which can sometimes be life threatening. Cardiac EP has also seen a decline in in-person visits across the globe during the pandemic. However, EP has an advantage of decision making being driven by abstract data such as rhythm monitors, electrocardiograms, and device interrogations, which enabled a smoother transition to virtual care.

DIGITAL HEALTH IN ELECTROPHYSIOLOGY DURING CORONAVIRUS DISEASE 2019
Remote Monitoring

Cardiac EP has been a leader in digital health care. Over the years multitude of devices have been developed and implemented in clinical practice, and these services were increasingly used during the pandemic in addition to development of some novel tools. Remote cardiac monitoring can be classified into 3 broad categories:[1]

- Medical-grade wearable monitors such as Holter monitor and external and internal loop recorder.
- Consumer-grade wearable monitors such as smartwatches.
- Cardiac implantable electronic devices (CIEDs) such as pacemakers and defibrillators.

These diverse range of devices generate different types of data. Holter and loop recorders only function as data collectors, whereas CIEDs can recognize critical findings and intervene based on programming. As a result, remote monitoring bears a prognostic value and helps in reducing worse outcomes. CIEDs received a class I recommendation for remote monitoring in 2015.[6] However, in the prepandemic times remote monitoring was underused due to patient- and system-based issues. The pandemic made remote monitoring an important tool to help identify critical and noncritical issues and address them accordingly.[7] Enrollment of existing patients in device clinics in remote monitoring was an important initiative undertaken by various EP programs in response to the pandemic.[8] One Italian study reported an experience of 332 patients introduced to remote monitoring during the lockdown. Patients were categorized based on modality, divided between remote monitoring at home versus office. Study findings reported high patient satisfaction, and providers were better able to provide continuous health care coverage in eligible CIED patients.[9]

Remote monitoring enables informed triage of patients needing urgent procedures, clinical decision making and diagnosis, and implementation of appropriate therapeutic interventions while bypassing an in-person visit. Similarly, patients adopting digital health tools like pulse oximeters, automated blood pressure equipment, glucose monitors, and single-lead electrocardiography (ECG) recorders were able to provide their respective physicians with important data without risking exposure.

One important aspect of remote monitoring is the burden of data received and the challenge of trained personnel being available to accurately review and act upon the data. Development of novel AI tools that can incorporate machine learning (ML) can help stratify the findings, so that appropriate measures can be taken.[1]

The concept of drive-through pacing clinics fills the gap for the subset of patients who may not be suitable for remote monitoring. This familiar concept involved patients driving up parallel to a kiosk occupied by a health care worker. A study by Akhtar and colleagues[10] evaluated 316 patients of which 66.8% had pacemakers, 21.8% had cardiac resynchronization therapy (CRT) devices, and 4.1% had implantable cardioverter-defibrillators. A total of 50 wound inspections were performed, and 2 were diagnosed and treated for superficial infections. Seven were diagnosed with new-onset atrial fibrillation (AF) and were referred for anticoagulation. Device settings were adjusted in 16.1% of cases, and only 22 patients were referred to a physician for a variety of symptoms. Most patients (57.1%) preferred this drive-through format over the conventional methods.[10]

Telemedicine

The concept of telemedicine existed in the pre-COVID era, but it was limited and often complicated with reimbursement issues for physicians. The COVID-19 crisis led to rapid adoptions of virtual medical care. At present telemedicine is provided by telephones, secure messaging, and audio-video conference calls via commercial applications. The Office for Civil Right expressed willingness to forego penalties for Health

Insurance Portability and Accountability Act noncompliance among providers enacting in good faith measures for telemedicine during the pandemic.[11]

In an attempt to conserve personal protective equipment (PPE), avoid exposure for patients and clinicians, and limit both hospitalizations for non-COVID reasons and outpatient office visits, an array of tele-health care was provided to patients in inpatient and outpatient settings. The Heart Rhythm Society (HRS)/American college of cardiology (ACC)/American Heart Association (AHA) provided an early guidance for electrophysiologists on how to practice during the pandemic. The guidance advocated for virtual visits, emphasizing social distancing, conservation of PPE, and minimizing face-to-face encounters when possible; it also clearly addressed nonurgent/nonemergent procedures, protocols for performing procedures on patients with COVID-19.[12]

Berman and colleagues[13] shared their experience of managing 29 inpatient EP consultations at the heart of the pandemic in New York. The investigators were able to manage 55% of patients remotely and were able to provide guideline- and evidence-based recommendations.[13] Similar reports came from other specialties like OB/GYN in which they were able to provide telehealth to 1352 patients for prenatal care, of which 61.5% were maternal-fetal medicine visits.[14] Another pilot study was reported by Renner and colleagues[15] from Helsinki University Hospital in Finland. The investigators performed 25 tele-rounds in 15 patients in the pulmonary ward; they concluded that tele-rounding is feasible in select patients with COVID-19 and can improve health care workers' safety and conserve PPE.[15]

Whether the current exponential growth in telemedicine will continue to grow after the pandemic is over is yet to be seen. However, with mass-scale vaccinations being delivered globally and humanity seeking a return to normalcy, we do believe the unexpected outcome of COVID-19 is reliance upon digital health, which can be seen in forms like physical fitness, adherence to therapies, ordering medications, and disease screening tools as part of smartphone/tablet apps.

We hypothesize that these adoptions may improve patient satisfaction, avoid long wait times in offices, avoid travel, and discuss medical care at the comfort of their homes. A study by Han and colleagues[3] reported that 60% of patients and 70% of clinicians would prefer to continue with virtual telehealth visits in future. This concept will also aid busy specialist physicians who tend to cover multiple hospitals to make recommendations via digital visits, improve recommendation times, and eventually improve hospital length of stay.

Artificial Intelligence Tools

AI has been incorporated into medicine for some decades now, but its incorporation to modern day clinical practice is reaching new horizons with the start of the COVID 19 pandemic. AI refers to machine-based processing of data that typically requires human cognitive function. ML is a subgroup of AI that uses algorithms to learn patterns empirically from data; it identifies nonlinear relationships and higher-order interactions between multiple variables, which are often difficult to obtain via traditional statistics. Deep learning (DL) is a powerful ML approach that analyzes large complex data sets and enables efficient decisions. AI tools have brought about significant change in cardiac EP and cardiovascular imaging as well. AI has shown promise in assisting in diagnosis, disease prediction models, and response to treatment and prognosis.[16]

The concept of AI is not new in cardiac EP with automated ECG interpretations existing since the 1970s.[17] However, interpretation of ECGs relies on expert opinion and requires training and expertise. Algorithms for the computerized automated diagnosis of 12-lead ECGs in prehospital setting can really aid emergency medical personnel or nonspecialist physicians to identify a condition and timely start treatment in high-risk patients. However, current automated ECG diagnosis algorithms lack accuracy and result in misdiagnosis if not reviewed carefully. There has been substantial progress in these areas where ECG-based deep neural networks (DNNs) have been tested to identify arrhythmias, classify supraventricular tachycardias, and predict left ventricular hypertrophy. A study by Attia and colleagues,[18] which included 180,922 patients, in which AI-enabled ECG during normal sinus rhythm was able to identify AF with almost 80% accuracy. Another good example is the study by Ko and colleagues in which they used a trained and validated convolutional neural network using 12-lead ECG and were able to detect hypertrophic cardiomyopathy with a sensitivity up to 95%. We do believe that these DNN models require more refinement and validation but in future are likely to aid specialists and nonspecialists with improved ECG diagnosis and perhaps as screening tools.[19–22]

Other dimensions related to ECGs are the use of implantable devices, smartwatches, and smartphone-based apps, which can generate large amounts of data sets that are not amenable for manual evaluation. Arrhythmia detection algorithms on DNNs on large sets of ambulatory patients with single-lead plethysmography have shown similar diagnostic performance as cardiologists and implantable loop recorders. Continuous monitoring provides the opportunity to pick up asymptomatic cardiac arrhythmias and overcome serious adverse events in future.[21]

Electroanatomic mapping in complex invasive EP procedures provides another opportunity. By combining data from diagnostic tools like MRI and fluoroscopy, previous electroanatomical mapping can help identify arrhythmogenic substrates and decrease the invasive catheter ablation times. There has been development in integrating fluoroscopy and electroanatomical mapping with MRI with ML.[23,24]

The above-mentioned examples provide a framework of tools in AI, but their widescale validation and translation into clinical practice may not be that far away.

Electrophysiology-Specific Innovations

Some examples of EP-specific innovations are described in the following sections.

Tele-atrial fibrillation project

AF is the most common cardiac arrhythmia; its traditional management requires face-to-face evaluations with cardiologist and primary care doctors and checking heart rate (HR) and rhythm control with ECG. With lockdowns and health facilities under pressure, telehealth visits became the backbone for providing care. However, effective management is limited in patients with AF because it did not allow for measurements of HR or checking the rhythm during the telehealth visit. To overcome this and make a unified structure all over Europe, The Cardiology Department of the Maastricht University Medical Center+ (MUMC+) in Maastricht, the Netherlands, innovated a standard operating procedure document describing the TeleCheck-AF approach. This approach involved teleconsultation coupled with remote photoplethysmography-based HR and heart rhythm monitoring (FibriCheckVR) to allow the treating clinicians to manage their patients comprehensively. FibriCheckVR currently enrolls 2492 patients in about 40 clinical centers around Europe. Patients once enrolled are requested to check their HR and heart rhythm via the application twice a day for at least 7 days before doctor's visit. The physician evaluates the rhythms in real time and reports it in a user-friendly dashboard. Further changes in clinical management will be addressed by physicians via teleconsultations.

This is a great example in which varying infrastructure in different countries were able to set up the concept of mobile health (mHealth) in a short duration of time.

FibriCheckVR was easy to use and install by patients. Further prospective trials are underway to assess if mHealth is noninferior to current standard care guided by face-to-face consultations.[2,25]

Smartphone electrocardiographic surveillance

Another great example in this association is the use of smartphone for ECG surveillance to preserve hospital capacity during the pandemic. The idea was to empower primary care physicians and patients with appropriate tools to identify patients with concerns for clinical deterioration with stable COVID-19 infection. The study involved 21 primary care physicians who enrolled 521 patients. The physicians were equipped with 8/12-lead hospital-grade smartphone-operated ECG device (D-Heart). First ECG was done under the supervision of the physician, and they were instructed to record at least one ECG at day 4 of infection or whenever cardiac symptoms were present during the first 10 days of infection. ECG was evaluated 24/7 within 15 minutes of arrival via telecardiology platform by cardiologists. This is reported to be the first study of its kind and enabled primary care physicians for early detection and avoiding a worse clinical outcome. The study concluded that the smartphone-controlled ECG devices are ideal for simple arrhythmia assessments but may not be adequate for complex ECG evaluation.[26] Certainly, this methodology lays a nice platform for multiparametric telemonitoring for patients in the future with improvement and acceptability of telehealth.

Home antiarrhythmic drug loading with smartphone tracings

Outpatient loading of antiarrhythmic drugs (AAD) like sotalol and dofetilide has been a matter of debate. Although outpatient initiation of sotalol is approved in certain cases, clinicians prefer to admit patients and monitor them closely for QT interval prolongation and development of ventricular arrhythmias. As COVID-19 stretched the health care systems all over the world, it led to delays in hospitalization for initiation of AAD and elective ablation procedures to help ensure maintenance of sinus rhythm versus rate control strategy. These circumstances led to the initiative of starting these medications in outpatient setting with patients who had CIEDs. Two separate studies by Mascarenhas and colleagues[27,28] for dofetilide (n = 30 patients) and sotalol (105 patients) demonstrated that they were able to successfully initiate these medications in the outpatient setting with careful telemonitoring. In both studies Permanent Pace makers and Intra-cardiac defibrillators were programmed to provide a lower rate of pacing at 70 bpm and Implantable loop recorders were programmed to detect an HR greater than 150 to 160 bpm depending on the device used. A mandatory 2-hour manual transmission was obtained after initiation of medication. Patients were seen in office for the first 3 days of initiation of medication.[27,28]

Although larger cohorts may be needed to validate these findings, these studies do lay a good foundation and direction for future studies. This outpatient initiative not only decreases the risk of nosocomial infections, including COVID-19, but also helps to decrease the cost burden by avoiding hospitalization of 3 days.

Heart logic

CRT devices have now been incorporated in multiple studies with ML to predict end points like heart failure or death after CRT by using multitude of baseline variables. Heart Logic is a good example of a personalized, remote heart failure diagnostic and monitoring solution and has been validated to provide weeks of advance notice for early signs of worsening heart failure.[29]

The ML models have outperformed current guidelines in predicting response and improved event-free survivals, although these findings are modest at this time. In other reports ML has been able to predict mortality better than preexisting clinical risk scores.[30,31]

BARRIERS TO DIGITAL HEALTH DELIVERY

Virtual care and digital health were instrumental in care delivery during the pandemic. Cancellation of elective procedures and visits was the immediate response, whereas creation of alternative digital solutions such as virtual telemedicine visits and remote patient monitoring measures represented a long-term viable strategy.[7] However, this transition was far from seamless and posed significant difficulties during its immediate implementation. First, the resource burden from the COVID-19 pandemic required a prioritization of essential procedures, and with this in mind a return to full force in the postpandemic period can place additional strain on digital health care delivery given that it continues to be evolving in terms of familiarity and efficiency.[32] Furthermore, the sheer volume of data inflow that can be expected with CIEDs, both medical- and consumer-grade wearable monitors, and incorporated AI tools can be overwhelming. This burden of increased data can present challenges to incorporation into clinical practice and can be overwhelming once in-person care returns to full volumes. Additional quality control parameters are needed because the accuracy of some of these devices is still precocious.[1] Along with this data influx, an efficient and accurate triaging system must be in place, and AI tools, although improving, still lack this ability reliably.[1] In a comparative prepandemic and peripandemic survey regarding the changes in the digital health landscape among cardiac EP professionals, the most common barrier cited was a lack of infrastructure, which despite showing an improvement between the 2 surveys still remained a prominent problem even after reassessment and highlights the lag of a supportive framework despite advancements in digital health.[3] This fact must be taken into consideration with the reintegration of face-to-face encounters, and with the progression of digital health moving forward. Our familiarity with digital health and its limits is still expanding, although more specifically this puts us as providers in the impactful role to ensure digital literacy to our patients.[33] Although smartphone applications, digital wearable devices, and virtual telemedicine appointments have served to further patient care, this comes with a learning curve for the user itself and makes providers the fulcrum of digital literacy education and patient advocacy in this area. Furthermore, these digital health solutions also serve both themselves as social barriers to health and can further highlight already present health care disparities.[3] Digital health usually requires access to Wi-Fi, Bluetooth, and/or smartphones, which may not be routinely available to all patients. Patients in underserved or underrepresented populations and with socioeconomic barriers are experiencing a compounded gap in care.[34] Specifically, a multivariate analysis consisting of 148,402 patients who had either completed or missed telemedicine appointments revealed that age greater than 55 years, Asian ethnicity, Medicaid insurance care, and non-English-speaking patients were most vulnerable to the digital divergence in care.[35] African American and Latinx communities with household incomes of less than $50,000 had lower rates of video telemedicine visits compared with telephone visits, which could limit some of the offered video conference benefits such as medication reconciliations or virtual physical examinations.[35] The demand, therefore, for more applications of digital health must also be met with equal support for digital health equity, an equally vital social disparity in the current state of medicine.[34] Finally, a virtual move to collective educational platforms such as national and global health conferences has remained a topic of discussion, with some claiming its potential to reach a wider audience yet others highlighting the inability to provide

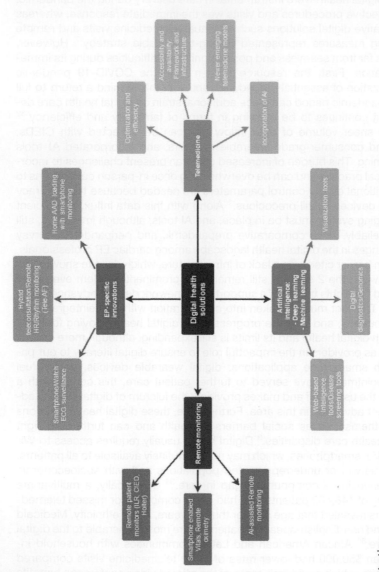

Fig. 1. Central illustration.

hands-on experience, and interdisciplinary learning.[32] As vaccination efforts continue to curb the impact of the pandemic, and in-person patient care has been slowly reintegrating, resurgences can halt this process, and the supplementary role of digital health must be continually reevaluated. Finding a steady state in which overreliance is not placed upon digital health while still using these resources to extract as much patient data to complement face-to-face interactions is paramount.

Fig. 1 summarizes the flow of digital health in clinical cardiac EP.

DIGITAL HEALTH IN THE POSTPANDEMIC PERIOD

Two main overarching factors will outline the future of digital health: digital health infrastructure and government policies for reimbursement.[3] Economics remains a fundamental driver for impacting changes in medical care. The Centers for Medicare and Medicaid have responded with base billing code implementation and addition for telemedicine to encompass a wide spectrum and acuity of patient encounters, and it remains to be seen if other insurance carriers will follow this pathway, as well as if this continues to be fostered and expanded in the future.[1,32]

Other improvements have come in the form of applicability and accessibility. The utilization of learning models such as Project ECHO (Extension of Community Healthcare Outcomes) is a collaborative multispecialty videoconferencing program that aims to promote peer-to-peer, multidisciplinary learning to health care providers, as well as make them comfortable as a technology provider in the digital health landscape.[36] Furthermore, the advocacy seen from organizations such as Telehealth for Seniors, Inc, a Florida-based nonprofit organization aiding in provision of digital health devices and education for seniors, has emerged during the pandemic, as well as increases in telehealth platform funding from the Coronavirus Aid, Relief, and Economic Security (CARES) Act[3,37]; these have contributed to the increase in accessibility to digital health, although these gaps in digital health disparity have not been bridged and advocacy for digital health equity must remain pressured.[34] Successful continued advocacy and resultant expansion of digital health can hope to present new telemedicine models to more remote areas and reach a wider spectrum of patients.

A further application of digital health in the future postpandemic period will hope to focus on the impact of digital health on clinical research and, namely, its recruitment. Predating the COVID-19 pandemic, efforts such as the MyHeart Counts and Heart eHealth studies used app-based recruitment and wearable monitoring devices to create larger cohorts and easier, prolonged periods of study.[38] Pairing this with the advancements necessitated in digital health, there is an optimistic outlook on the contribution of digital health tools in patient recruitment and ease of monitoring to contribute to higher cohorts in clinical research.

EP serves as a fertile foundation for the incorporation of AI, and the ideal role it plays in the future is still budding. The hope for AI to assist in triaging and risk stratification in various cardiac diseases provides for an enticing outlook, and it can be hoped that these advancements will continue to be cultivated, as their application currently remains limited.

SUMMARY

New digital health innovations and an accommodating digital health landscape have shown promise during this pandemic, and we find ourselves as a field faced with the challenge of continuing to cultivate and incorporate this aspect of medicine. Consumer-grade wearable monitors, AI triaging and diagnostic supplementary tools, and improved accessibility to technology mark some of the foreseen changes to the field of cardiac EP. This knowledge will allow us to focus on restructuring the comprehensive and traditional albeit resource-intensive in-person model of patient care, and we hope to transition to a more efficient, patient-centered, and communicative framework both incorporating digital health and reincorporating in-person care moving forward.

REFERENCES

1. Slotwiner DJ, Al-Khatib SM. Digital health in electrophysiology and the COVID-19 global pandemic. Heart Rhythm O2 2020;1(5):385–9.

2. Gawalko M, Duncker D, Manninger M, et al. The European TeleCheck-AF project on remote app-based management of atrial fibrillation during the COVID-19 pandemic: centre and patient experiences. Europace 2021;23(7):1003–15.

3. Han JK, Al-Khatib SM, Albert CM. Changes in the digital health landscape in cardiac electrophysiology: a pre-and peri-pandemic COVID-19 era survey. Cardiovasc Digit Health J 2021;2(1):55–62.

4. Mohanty S, Lakkireddy D, Trivedi C, et al. Creating a safe workplace by universal testing of SARS-CoV-2 infection in asymptomatic patients and healthcare workers in the electrophysiology units: a multi-center experience. J Interv Card Electrophysiol 2020;62(1):171–6.

5. Primessnig U, Pieske BM, Sherif M. Increased mortality and worse cardiac outcome of acute myocardial infarction during the early COVID-19 pandemic. ESC Heart Fail 2021;8(1):333–43.

6. Slotwiner D, Varma N, Akar JG, et al. HRS Expert Consensus Statement on remote interrogation and monitoring for cardiovascular implantable electronic devices. Heart Rhythm 2015;12(7):e69–100.

7. Lakkireddy DR, Chung MK, Deering TF, et al. Guidance for rebooting electrophysiology through the COVID-19 pandemic from the Heart Rhythm Society and the American Heart Association Electrocardiography and Arrhythmias Committee of the Council on Clinical Cardiology: Endorsed by the American College of Cardiology. Circ Arrhythm Electrophysiol 2020;13(7):e008999.

8. Pothineni NVK, Santangeli P, Deo R, et al. COVID-19 and electrophysiology procedures-review, reset, reboot!!! J Interv Card Electrophysiol 2020;59(2):303–5.

9. Piro A, Magnocavallo M, Della Rocca DG, et al. Management of cardiac implantable electronic device follow-up in COVID-19 pandemic: lessons learned during Italian lockdown. J Cardiovasc Electrophysiol 2020;31(11):2814–23.

10. Akhtar Z, Montalbano N, Leung LWM, et al. Drive-Through Pacing Clinic: A Popular Response to the COVID-19 Pandemic. JACC Clin Electrophysiol 2021;7(1):128–30.

11. enforcement, U.S.D.o.H.H.S.H.g.N.o., et al., U.S. Department of Health & Human Services. HHS.gov. Notification of enforcement for discretion for telehealth remote communications during the COVID-19 nationwide public health emergency. March 30, 2020. Available at: https://www.hhs.gov/hipaa/for-professionals/special-topics/emergency-preparedness/notification-enforcement-discretion-telehealth/index.html.

12. Lakkireddy DR, Chung MK, Gopinathannair R, et al. Guidance for cardiac electrophysiology during the COVID-19 pandemic from the Heart Rhythm Society COVID-19 task force; Electrophysiology Section of the American College of Cardiology; and the Electrocardiography and Arrhythmias Committee of the Council

on Clinical Cardiology, American Heart Association. Heart Rhythm 2020;17(9): e233–41.

13. Berman JP, Abrams MP, Kushnir A, et al. Cardiac electrophysiology consultative experience at the epicenter of the COVID-19 pandemic in the United States. Indian Pacing Electrophysiol J 2020;20(6):250–6.

14. Madden N, Emeruwa UN, Friedman AM, et al. Telehealth uptake into prenatal care and provider attitudes during the COVID-19 pandemic in New York City: a quantitative and qualitative analysis. Am J Perinatol 2020;37(10):1005–14.

15. Renner A, Paajanen J, Reijula J. Tele-rounding in a university hospital pulmonary ward during the COVID-19 pandemic: a pilot study. Infect Dis (Lond) 2020;52(9): 669–70.

16. Feeny AK, Chung MK, Madabhushi A, et al. Artificial intelligence and machine learning in arrhythmias and cardiac electrophysiology. Circ Arrhythm Electrophysiol 2020;13(8):e007952.

17. Nygårds ME, Hulting J. An automated system for ECG monitoring. Comput Biomed Res 1979;12(2):181–202.

18. Attia ZI, Noseworthy PA, Lopez-Jimenez F, et al. An artificial intelligence-enabled ECG algorithm for the identification of patients with atrial fibrillation during sinus rhythm: a retrospective analysis of outcome prediction. Lancet 2019;394(10201): 861–7.

19. Hannun AY, Rajpurkar P, Haghpanahi M, et al. Cardiologist-level arrhythmia detection and classification in ambulatory electrocardiograms using a deep neural network. Nat Med 2019;25(1):65–9.

20. Perlman O, Katz A, Amit G, et al. Supraventricular tachycardia classification in the 12-lead ECG using atrial waves detection and a clinically based tree scheme. IEEE J Biomed Health Inform 2016;20(6):1513–20.

21. van de Leur RR, Boonstra MJ, Bagheri A, et al. Big data and artificial intelligence: opportunities and threats in electrophysiology. Arrhythm Electrophysiol Rev 2020; 9(3):146–54.

22. Ko WY, Siontis KC, Attia ZI, et al. Detection of hypertrophic cardiomyopathy using a convolutional neural network-enabled electrocardiogram. J Am Coll Cardiol 2020;75(7):722–33.

23. van Es R, van den Broek HT, van der Naald M, et al. Validation of a novel stand-alone software tool for image guided cardiac catheter therapy. Int J Cardiovasc Imaging 2019;35(2):225–35.

24. van den Broek HT, Wenker S, van de Leur R, et al. 3D Myocardial Scar Prediction Model Derived from Multimodality Analysis of Electromechanical Mapping and Magnetic Resonance Imaging. J Cardiovasc Transl Res 2019;12(6):517–27.

25. Pluymaekers NAHA, Hermans ANL, van der Velden RMJ, et al. On-demand app-based rate and rhythm monitoring to manage atrial fibrillation through teleconsultations during COVID-19. Int J Cardiol Heart Vasc 2020;28:100533.

26. Maurizi N., Fumagalli C., Cecchi F., et al. 2021;ztab009. Published 2021 Jan 29. Use of Smartphone-operated ECG for home ECG surveillance in COVID-19 patients. 2021. https://doi.org/10.1093/ehjdh/ztab009.

27. Mascarenhas DAN, Mudumbi PC, Kantharia BK. Outpatient initiation of dofetilide: insights from the complexities of atrial fibrillation management during the COVID-19 lockdown. J Interv Card Electrophysiol 2021;1–8. https://doi.org/10.1007/s10840-021-00942-y.

28. Mascarenhas DAN, Mudumbi PC, Kantharia BK. Outpatient initiation of sotalol in patients with atrial fibrillation: utility of cardiac implantable electronic devices for

therapy monitoring. Am J Cardiovasc Drugs 2021;1–8. https://doi.org/10.1007/s40256-021-00493-7.

29. Gardner RS, Singh JP, Stancak B, et al. HeartLogic Multisensor Algorithm Identifies Patients During Periods of Significantly Increased Risk of Heart Failure Events: Results From the MultiSENSE Study. Circ Heart Fail 2018;11(7):e004669.

30. Feeny AK, Rickard J, Patel D, et al. Machine learning prediction of response to cardiac resynchronization therapy: improvement versus current guidelines. Circ Arrhythm Electrophysiol 2019;12(7):e007316.

31. Hu SY, Santus E, Forsyth AW, et al. Can machine learning improve patient selection for cardiac resynchronization therapy? PLoS One 2019;14(10):e0222397.

32. Alkhouli M, Coylewright M, Holmes DR. Will the COVID-19 Epidemic reshape cardiology? Eur Heart J Qual Care Clin Outcomes 2020;6(3):217–20.

33. Cowie MR, Lam CSP. Remote monitoring and digital health tools in CVD management. Nat Rev Cardiol 2021;18(7):457–8.

34. Crawford A, Serhal E. Digital health equity and COVID-19: The innovation curve cannot reinforce the social gradient of health. J Med Internet Res 2020;22(6):e19361.

35. Eberly LA, Kallan MJ, Julien HM, et al. Patient characteristics associated with telemedicine access for primary and specialty ambulatory care during the COVID-19 pandemic for primary and specialty ambulatory care during the COVID-19 pandemic. JAMA Netw Open 2020;3(12):e2031640.

36. Hunt RC, Struminger BB, Redd JT, et al. Virtual peer-to-peer learning to enhance and accelerate the health system response to COVID-19: The HHS ASPR Project ECHO COVID-19 Clinical Rounds Initiative. Ann Emerg Med 2021;78(2):223–8.

37. Verma A. 2020. Available at: https://www.telehealthforseniors.org/contact. Accessed July 30, 2021; TeleHealth Access for Seniors, Inc.

38. Sharma A, Harrington RA, McClellan MB, et al. Using digital health technology to better generate evidence and deliver evidence-based care. J Am Coll Cardiol 2018;71(23):2680–90.

Mental Health Effects of the COVID-19 Pandemic on Children and Adolescents

A Review of the Current Research

Jill Meade, PhD

KEYWORDS

- COVID-19 • Child • Adolescent • Mental health • Psychological • Anxiety
- Depression

KEY POINTS

- Research is ongoing regarding mental health effects of the coronavirus disease 2019 pandemic on children and adolescents.
- Early studies show children and adolescents experiencing increased anxiety and depression.
- Isolation, loneliness, lack of physical activity, family stress, and racism may contribute to the effects of the coronavirus disease 2019 pandemic on child and adolescent mental health.

BACKGROUND

Coronavirus disease 2019 (COVID-19) has created unimaginable challenges for children, adolescents, and their families around the world. This virus, which was first identified in Wuhan, China, in December 2019,[1] has led to 23,440,774 cases of COVID-19 in the United States (as of January 16, 2021) and has caused more than 390,938 total US deaths.[2] Pandemic-related school and business closings and community lockdowns have had significant effects on families. The earliest world-wide lockdowns that started in China around January 23, 2020,[3] included restrictions on schools and gatherings, and resulted in children being transitioned to online school. In the United States, many school districts began transitioning to online school in March 2020 in conjunction with community closures.[4] Since then, individual communities and states within the United States have continued to impose and lift restrictions in

This article previously appeared in *Pediatric Clinics*, Volume 68, Issue 5, October 2021.
Children's Hospital of Michigan, Department of Psychiatry/Psychology, Box 137, 3901 Beaubien Boulevard, Detroit, MI 48201, USA
E-mail address: jmeade@med.wayne.edu

Clinics Collections 12 (2022) 79–93
https://doi.org/10.1016/j.ccol.2021.12.006
2352-7986/22/© 2021 Elsevier Inc. All rights reserved.

response to COVID-19 outbreaks. This situation has been and continues to be a constantly changing situation, with new stressors occurring constantly.

COVID-19–RELATED SOURCES OF STRESS FOR CHILDREN AND ADOLESCENTS

Everyday life for children and adolescents has been significantly disrupted by the COVID-19 pandemic. Potential stressors for children and adolescents during this challenging time could include:

- Increased social isolation
- Heightened concerns over safety and health
- Increased stress of parents and caregivers owing to work, financial, or other impacts
- Increased family conflict, parent–child conflict, and/or child abuse
- Placements with friends or relatives owing to parent work situation
- Loss of prosocial activities (school, sports, social activities, hobbies)
- Adjustment to online schooling processes and demands
- Increased screen time and sedentary behaviors
- Decreased access to medical and mental health care, including exacerbated health disparities

ADDED EFFECTS OF SOCIOPOLITICAL EVENTS

In addition to the pandemic-related changes discussed, co-occurring sociopolitical stressors during this time also likely impact the mental health of children and adolescents. Given that the first cases of COVID-19 were identified China,[1] some American politicians began referring to it as the "Wuhan virus" or the "Chinese virus," which led to reports of a racism pandemic against Asian Americans in the United States.[5] Early research on this topic demonstrated that nearly one-half of Chinese American parents and their children ages 10 to 18 who were surveyed reported being targeted by or witnessing COVID-19 racial discrimination.[6]

Additional racial-based stressors occurred in the United States beginning May 25 with the death of George Floyd at the hands of the police.[7] Through media coverage and a video of his death, many children were exposed to examples of violence and/or racism. Outrage over police violence focused the country on issues of racial justice and resulted in months of protests and demonstrations, peaking in June 2020.[8] It is difficult to disentangle the effects of the COVID-19 pandemic stressors from these sociopolitical events in the United States.

EARLY REVIEWS ON COVID-19 AND CHILD MENTAL HEALTH

The earliest identified reviews of original research looking at COVID-19 effects on child and adolescent mental health identified concerns about increasing levels of depression and anxiety[9] as well as post-traumatic symptoms.[10] A review by Fong and Iarocci[11] published in November 2020 combined past pandemic research with newly available COVID-19 findings and concluded that pandemic-related social isolation and quarantining is resulting in significant anxiety, post-traumatic stress disorder (PTSD), and fears in children and adolescents. The authors emphasized the importance of reducing barriers to mental health services for children and families.

CURRENT STUDIES

The purpose of this article is to provide an updated review of the current body of research findings to date on the specific impacts of COVID-19 on the mental health functioning of children and adolescents. Original data studies examining mental health outcomes in the general population of children and adolescents during COVID-19 were identified through search engines and publications. **Table 1** provides a summary of studies reviewed, including authors, country of origin, month(s) of data collection, number and ages of subjects, and major findings with regards to child and adolescent mental health. These studies present a snapshot in time, and it will be important that research be ongoing in order to understand the short- and long-term effects of the pandemic on children and adolescents.

Changes in Mental Health Owing to COVID-19

To investigate changes in child/adolescent mental health functioning in relation to the pandemic, studies have examined parent and youth retrospective symptoms reports and have compared current data to that from previous years. Longitudinal data analyses would be ideal, but are not yet available.

Parent and child report of changes

The worsening of child mental health during the pandemic has been reported by parents and children. A US study of 1000 parents with at least 1 child under age 18 years found that 14.3% of parents reported observing worsening in child's behavioral health after March, with little difference in racial, ethnic, income, or education groups.[23] Reported declines in parent and child mental health for these families were linked to having younger children, loss of child care, and reported increased food insecurity. Canadian researchers collected data from both clinical and community samples of youth ages 14 to 28 approximately 1 month after pandemic onset. Both groups reported significant declines in mental health compared with prepandemic functioning, with the community sample reporting the greatest decline. Interestingly, this primarily college-aged sample reported decreased substance use from before to after the onset of the pandemic, possibly owing to a return to parents' homes.

Suicide statistics across times periods

Studies examining large health-related datasets have been able to compare changes in suicide-related behaviors from year to year. Hill and colleagues[17] examined the outcomes of routine screening for suicide in 18,247 youth ages 11 to 21 years in a large US city hospital emergency department (ED), comparing percentage of youth seen reporting recent suicidal ideation and recent attempts from March through July 2020 with the same months in 2019. They found higher rates of both suicidal ideation in March and July 2020 (compared with 2019), and higher rates of recent suicide attempts in February through April and July 2020 (compared with 2019), suggesting that events in 2020 were leading to these increases. In contrast, in Japan researchers used public data to compare rates of completed suicides in youth under age 20 years for March through May of 2019 and the same months in 2020.[18] Although they found that youth suicide in Japan did increase from March to May each year, rates were not worse in 2020. Researchers hypothesized that youth remaining at home with family (owing to COVID-19 restrictions) may have been a protective factor.

Table 1
Research examining mental health impacts of COVID-19 on children and adolescents

Author	Country (Data Collection Dates)	Participants	Findings Regarding Child and Adolescent Mental Health
Cheah et al,[6] 2020	United States (March 14 to May 31, 2020)	543 parents in the United States who identify as Chinese and 320 of their children, ages 10–18 y	Majority of parents and children reported directly experiencing or witnessing racial discrimination against Chinese or Asian Americans owing to COVID-19. Both parent report of poorer child well-being and child report of anxiety linked to experiences of racial discrimination.
Chen et al,[12] 2020	Guiyang, China (April 2020)	1036 children, ages 6–15 y	11.78% rate of depression, 18.92% rate of anxiety, and 6.56% rate of both. Factors linked with depression: being female, being older teen, lower parent education, no companion on weekdays, and less physical exercise. Factors linked with anxiety: being female, no companion on weekdays, and less physical exercise. Some belief physical exercise serves a protective factor.
Duan et al,[13] 2020	20 provinces in mainland China (article submitted in April 2020)	3613 children ages 7–18 y	22.28% of sample reported depressive symptoms above clinical threshold. Anxiety in children was 23.87% and 29.27% in adolescents. Increased anxiety linked to being aged 13–18, female, living in urban area, emotion-focused coping style. Increased depression linked to smartphone addiction, Internet addiction. Problem-focused coping and fewer hours on the Internet before pandemic related to decreased depressive symptoms.

Study	Country (Dates)	Sample	Findings
Fitzpatrick et al,[14] 2020	United States (April to July 2020)	133 caregivers of at least 1 child aged 1–19 y	Parents reported top mental health problems in their most challenging child; Results grouped by age: 1–5 y: misbehavior, social isolation, boredom, needing attention, anxiety 6–12 y: academics, misbehavior, anxiety, social isolation, depression 13–19 y: depression, anxiety, misbehavior, social isolation, inattention or impulsivity
Gassman-Pines et al,[15] 2020	United States (Feb to April 2020)	645 parents of children 5–7 y	In children of hourly service-industry workers, more COVID-related hardships (job loss, loss of income, caregiver burden) resulted in increased children's uncooperative and worry behaviors.
Hawke et al,[16] 2020	Canada (April 2020)	Clinical sample of 276 youth, and community sample of 346 youth, majority Caucasian, ages 14–28 y.	Significant mental health decline reported by participants across groups. Internalizing disorder: 68.4% of clinical sample and 39.9% youth in the community sample had high likelihood of meeting criteria. Externalizing disorders: 40.2% of clinical and 16.9% of community sample had high likelihood.
Hill et al,[17] 2020	United States (February to July 2020)	11- to 21-year-old youth seen at a city emergency department	City ED screened youth for reported recent suicidal ideation and suicide attempts; rates were higher in several months of February to July 2020 compared with same period in 2019

(continued on next page)

Table 1
(continued)

Author	Country (Data Collection Dates)	Participants	Findings Regarding Child and Adolescent Mental Health
Isumi et al,[18] 2020	Japan (March to May, 2018, 2019, 2020)	Nationwide suicides among youth <20 y	Concluded pandemic did not have significant effect on suicide rates compared with previous years or pre–post school closure. Discussed possible positive connections, cohesion, and social support for children.
Jiao et al,[19] 2020	Shaanxi Province, China (February 2020)	320 parents of children and adolescents, ages 3–18 y	Younger children (3–6 y) had more clinginess and fear about safety of family members from COVID (compared with older children). Older children (6–18 y) had more inattention and "obsessive request of updates." Most common symptoms in entire sample were clinging, inattention, and irritability.
Leeb et al,[20] 2020	United States (January to October, 2019 and 2020)	Examined data from the CDC's National Syndromic Surveillance Program regarding ED visits among children <18 y	Children had fewer total mental health ED visits after lockdown, but percentage of visits that were for mental health-related increased in late March and continued through October. Percentage of mental health-related visits in late March through October was significantly higher than during same months in 2019. Ages 5–11 y: 24% increase in percentage. Ages 12–17 y 31% increase in percentage.

Reference	Location (date)	Sample	Findings
Liu et al,[21] 2020	China (February to March 2020)	Grades 5–6 (estimated ages 10–11 y) and college students (estimated ages 17–22y)]	In primary school children, concerns regarding threat to life and health (endorsed by 39.7%) was related to somatic symptoms and anxiety but not depression. Overall rates were low, however.
Liu et al,[22] 2021	Wuhan and Huangshi, China (February to March 2020)	1264 children ages 7–12 y and their parents.	Higher inattention-hyperactivity and problems with prosocial behaviors when children did little or no physical exercise. Children in Wuhan at higher risk for peer problems and overall behavior difficulties vs Huangshi.
Patrick et al,[23] 2020	United States (June 2020)	1000 parents with $\geq$1 child <18 y	14.3% reported worsening in child's behavioral health with little difference in racial, ethnic, income, or education groups. Worsening of mental health in parent and child linked to having younger children, loss of child care, and reported increased food insecurity.
Tang et al,[24] 2021	China (March 2020)	4342 Primary and secondary school students, ages 6–17 y	Higher reported depression, anxiety, and stress among senior secondary students, those who saw quarantine having more problems vs benefits, and those whose parents had not discussed COVID with them.

(continued on next page)

Table 1
(continued)

Author	Country (Data Collection Dates)	Participants	Findings Regarding Child and Adolescent Mental Health
Xie et al,[3] 2020	Wuhan and Huangshi, China (February to March 2020)	1784 children, Chinese grades 2–6 (approx. ages: 7–12 y)	Rates of anxiety and depression higher than previous population studies in China. Higher depression scores found in children from Wuhan vs Huangshi, those who rated themselves as "quite worried" about being affected by COVID-19, or those who rated themselves as "not optimistic about the epidemic."
Yeasmin et al,[25] 2020	Bangladesh (April to May 2020)	384 parents of children ages 5–15 y	Severity of depressive, anxiety, and sleep symptoms was higher for children in urban area, who had more COVID + family/neighbors, and whose parents had higher education, needed to go to workplace, who smoked, or were at risk of losing job.
Yue et al,[26] 2020	China (February 2020)	1360 children and parents; average child age 10.56 y (SD = 1.79)	Anxiety and PTSD symptoms in children related to spending more time on COVID media reports.
Zhou et al,[27] 2020	China (March 2020)	8079 teens ages 12–18 y	Found higher depressive and anxious symptoms in females, in rural areas, and in higher grades. Protective factors included: knowing more about COVID, taking safety precautions, and being optimistic about pandemic

Abbreviations: CDC, Centers for Disease Control and Prevention; ED, emergency department.

Mental health emergency visit rates

Hospital emergency departments are often the site for crisis mental health evaluations of children and adolescents. Using data from the Centers for Disease Control and Prevention reporting general mental health-related visits for children less than 18 years of age at hospital emergency departments across 47 US states, Leeb and colleagues[20] examined rates of visits for the period of January through October in 2019 and 2020. When examining proportion of mental health-related visits per 100,000 emergency department visits, sharp increases were found after March 2020, and these increases continued through October. Additionally, the proportion of mental health-related visits in late March through October was significantly higher than during same months in 2019. More specifically, the proportion of such visits for ages 5 to 11 demonstrated a 24% increase from 2019 to 2020 (from 783 per 100,000 visits to 972 per 100,000), and the proportion of adolescents aged 12 to 17 years presenting for mental health-related visits increased 31% (from 3098 per 100,000 emergency department visits to 4051 per 100,000). These increases may well reflect increased distress among children and adolescents owing to pandemic-related stressors. Additionally, the authors raised the possibility that these increases are related to the public's difficulties accessing mental health services in the community.[20]

Predominant COVID-19–Related Mental Health Concerns by Age

Across studies reviewed, rates of mental health symptoms during COVID-19 have varied by age. Findings here are grouped for younger children, school-aged children, and adolescents.

Younger children

Studies examining the most significant mental health concerns in younger children (eg, <7 years of age) during the pandemic have found reports of more clinginess and fear about safety,[19] increased uncooperative and worry behaviors,[15] and misbehavior, boredom, needing attention, and anxiety.[14] Young children of hourly service workers who experienced significant COVID-related stressors displayed increased uncooperative and worry behaviors.[15]

School-aged children

Children of elementary school age (approximately 7–13 years) have been reported to display rates of anxiety and depression that are higher than normal during the COVID-19 pandemic.[3] Rates of significant depressive symptoms in studies of children during this time have ranged from 2.2%[26] to 11.78%.[12] Rates of significant anxiety symptoms have ranged from 1.8%[26] to 18.92%[12] to 23.87%.[13] The rate of PTSD was reported as 3.16%.[26] The most problematic behaviors have been reported to be increased inattention and need for reassurance,[19] as well as difficulties with academics, misbehavior, anxiety, social isolation, and depression.[14]

Adolescents

Parents have reported that the most significant behavioral concerns in adolescents during the pandemic have included depression, anxiety, misbehavior, social isolation, (poor) attention, and impulsivity.[14] Self-report rates of significant anxiety symptoms have been found to range from 10.4%[27] to 29.27%.[13] Rates of significant depressive symptoms have been reported to range from 17.3%[27] to 22.28%[13] and were found to be higher in female adolescents compared with males.[12,13,27] Several studies indicated that high school seniors (as compared with younger children) demonstrated the highest ratings for depression,[27] anxiety, and stress.[24] Mental health-related emergency department visits were more common in ages 12 to 17 during the postpandemic months (March to October, 2020) with females having the higher proportion of visits.[20] In a community sample of primarily college-aged youth, 39.9% reported symptoms of an internalizing disorder (eg, depression or anxiety), and 16.9% reported symptoms of an externalizing disorder (eg, aggression, oppositionality).[16] Another study of college age youth indicated high rates of somatic symptoms (34.85%), particularly when worried about necessities of daily life.[21]

Factors Found to Contribute to Mental Health Symptoms

Research on mental health and psychosocial functioning has identified multiple factors that seem to affect rates of mental health symptoms in children and adolescents.

Social isolation

Research has shown that social isolation and loneliness increase the risk of depression and possibly anxiety, with duration of loneliness having the biggest impact on child mental health.[28] The COVID-19 studies reviewed here did indeed link social isolation to increased depression and anxiety, including children who were unhappy with home quarantine,[24] those whose parents went to work while children stayed at home,[25] and children who had no companion on weekdays.[12] Sexual minority youth may be particularly vulnerable to the mental health effects of social isolation. A study by Fish and colleagues[29] with lesbian, gay, bisexual, transgender, and youth questioning sexual orientation (LGBTQ) youth identified the challenges of youth being homebound with unsupportive families, as well as loss of in-person support and socialization. Researchers stressed the importance of assisting LGBTQ youth in maintaining social supports and mental health through electronic connections.

Screen time

The use of phones and the Internet have become integral parts of coping with the COVID-19 pandemic. Although some parents reported successfully using media entertainment to soothe children during the initial weeks of the pandemic,[19] a large study of children and adolescents linked smartphone and Internet addiction (defined as excessive use) to increased depression.[13]

Lack of physical activity

Children engaging in regular physical activity during the pandemic seemed to fare better, demonstrating less hyperactive–inattentive behavior and more prosocial behaviors.[22] Conversely, a lack of physical exercise during COVID-19 has been linked to higher levels of depression and anxiety, and investigators suggest that physical activity may serve as a protective factor.[12] Mittal and colleagues[30] raised concerns about significant negative effects of sedentary behavior on children's mental health, noting that children's play is crucial to meet developmental milestones. They emphasized the importance of alternatives such as zoom to continue physical activity, as well as community and academic partnerships to ensure that children remain active.

Perceived COVID-19 risk

Child and adolescent mental health has been found to vary directly with perceived risks of COVID-19. Two studies examined negative effects of living near high rates of COVID-19 (ie, City of Wuhan compared with other areas in China). Children living near Wuhan displayed higher levels of depression,[3] more peer problems, and overall behavior difficulties.[31] Consistent with this finding, primary school children were found to have increased somatic symptoms and anxiety when experiencing higher concerns regarding threats to their life and health.[21] Yeasmin and colleagues[25] found that children with a greater severity of sleep problems had more COVID-positive family members or neighbors. Fitzpatrick and colleagues[14] examined the effects of community COVID-19 rates and restrictions, finding that number of COVID-19 cases in a family's geographic region was significantly associated with child and adolescent internalizing problems. More leniency in community restrictions was associated with greater child and adolescent internalizing, as well as externalizing problems, suggesting that children felt safer and had better mental health outcomes when community restrictions were in place.

Exposure to COVID-19 information

Some evidence has been found that exposure to COVID-related information can affect mental health. In a large study 1 month after quarantine, grade school children who reported spending more time on COVID-19 media reports also reported higher levels of anxiety and PTSD symptoms. In the same study, the amount of attention paid to such reports was related to PTSD symptoms only.[26] In contrast, a separate study found that children seemed to benefit from discussions about COVID-19 with parents; those whose parents did not discuss COVID-19 with them reported higher levels of depression, anxiety, and stress.[24] A large study of adolescents found that those reporting greater knowledge about COVID-19, more optimism about it, and engaging in more safety steps reported lower levels of depressive and anxious symptoms.

Parenting stress

It is difficult to separate child and parent well-being from each other. Studies examining parent well-being during the COVID-19 pandemic found that it was directly related to hardships such as decreases in work, incomes and increased caregiving burden.[15] In a US study of 1000 parents, 26.9% reported worsening of their own mental health since onset of the pandemic, especially in mothers, unmarried parents, and families with younger children.[23] Such stressors can lead to increased risks of domestic violence and child abuse.[32] Studies during COVID-19 have found that parental depression, job loss, and previous maltreatment predicted higher rates of maltreatment for children ages 4 to 10 years of age.[33] A study examining parenting of a wider range of children (<18 years) found that greater received support and perception of control resulted in parents being less likely to maltreat.[34] Rodriguez and colleagues noted that the pandemic serves as a perfect storm, given the economic hardships, effects on parental mental health, and the increased time families are spending together during the COVID-19 restrictions.[35] The authors call for investment in primary prevention, rather than a reactive approach, to support and educate families and communities to protect children.

DISCUSSION

Experts have cautioned that the high number of deaths, continued experience of grief and loss, and exacerbation of current mental health disorders mean that a "second wave" of mental health consequences from this pandemic is "imminent."[36] Consequently, the need for effective social supports and mental health interventions is crucial.

Kaslow and colleagues[37] proposed a behavioral health response continuum to "flatten the emotional distress curve," which was inspired by the Centers for Disease Control and Prevention's pandemic intervals framework. Through strategic planning, behavioral health experts can mobilize and provide large-scale interventions such as education on coping strategies, social connectedness, and other behavioral health education. Continued data gathering and research would then help to identify continued needs and provide information on program effectiveness. Using a public health model to address the mental health needs of a population is a promising approach.

Going forward, the need for accessible mental health services for children and families has never been greater. Decreasing financial and insurance barriers to access will be essential, including continued development of parity for mental health care. The increase in telehealth mental health services in the United States has been dramatic[38] and offers one way to expand access to families with distance, safety, or transportation barriers. The disproportionate effect of COVID-19 on communities of Black, Latino, and Native American families requires collaborative behavioral health care in which experts build capacity around the needs of these communities.[39]

Medical settings are often the front line with regard to identifying mental health needs. Professionals in these settings will want to assess for depression and anxiety in children and adolescents during this continued pandemic. Standardized, empirically based mental health screening measures can quickly identify those in need of further assessment and/or referrals for mental health services. The American Academy of Pediatrics provides recommended screening measures (Mental Health Tools) within their Mental Health Initiatives website, which can be found here: https://www.aap.org/en-us/advocacy-and-policy/aap-health-initiatives/Mental-Health/Pages/Primary-Care-Tools.aspx.[40] The site provides information on the measures, as well as information on obtaining them. Integrating mental health professionals within medical care can be ideal for assessing and treating overall psychosocial functioning of patients.

As we approach the 1-year anniversary of COVID-19 pandemic, continued research will be critical to understand ongoing impacts to child and adolescent mental health. There is a need for more research within communities disproportionally affected by COVID-19 such as the Black, Latino, and Native American populations. There is also a need for further research of COVID-19 impacts on children and adolescents with disabilities. There is a need to identify effective prevention strategies and treatment interventions.

SUMMARY

Research on the mental health effects of the COVID-19 pandemic on children and adolescents confirms the presence of significant anxiety and depression, as well as increases in these symptoms compared with prepandemic levels. Research reviewed suggests that teenagers, especially females and high school seniors, may suffer the most. There is evidence that social isolation and sedentary behaviors contribute to these mental health problems. Children who feel unsafe with regard to COVID-19 may be more likely to experience somatic symptoms, depression, and anxiety. Exposure to excessive information about COVID without parental communication on the topic may lead to higher anxiety and PTSD symptoms.

Many parents are experiencing significant economic and personal stress along with increasing mental health symptoms, especially single parents and parents of young children. It is clear that parental stress and mental health problems directly affect their children, and some children may be at increased risk for child maltreatment owing to pandemic-related stressors and situations.

Increasing access to mental health services for children and families will be vital. Integrating mental health care into medical settings would be ideal to provide frontline and comprehensive care. Research on the continuing effects of COVID-19 will be necessary as the situation continues to change, and studies of effective prevention and treatments strategies are also needed.

CLINICS CARE POINTS

- Professionals are just beginning to understand how the ongoing COVID-19 pandemic has significantly impacted the lives and mental health of children and adolescents.
- Current research shows children are displaying increased anxiety and depression, and that social isolation and a lack of physical activity may worsen these factors.
- Racial minority children and adolescents may be at even greater risk, given the additive effects of racism on health.
- Health care professionals should screen patients routinely for unmet mental health needs and provide links to care when indicated. Increasing access to mental health care is crucial.

DISCLOSURE

The author has nothing to disclose.

REFERENCES

1. CDC. About COVID-19. CDC: Centers for Disease Control and Prevention. 2020. Available at: https://www.cdc.gov/coronavirus/2019-ncov/cdcresponse/about-COVID-19.html. Accessed January 16, 2021.
2. CDC. COVID Data Tracker: United States COVID-19 Cases and Deaths by State. Centers for Disease Control and Prevention (CDC). 2021. Available at: https://covid.cdc.gov/covid-data-tracker/#cases_casesper100klast7days. Accessed January 16, 2021.
3. Xie X, Xue Q, Zhou Y, et al. Mental Health Status Among Children in Home Confinement During the Coronavirus Disease 2019 Outbreak in Hubei Province, China. JAMA Pediatr 2020;174(9):898–900.
4. Taylor DB. A Timeline of the Coronavirus Pandemic. New York Times. 2021. Available at: https://www.nytimes.com/article/coronavirus-timeline.html. Accessed January 16, 2021.
5. Gee GC, Ro MJ, Rimoin AW. Seven Reasons to Care About Racism and COVID-19 and Seven Things to Do to Stop It. Am J Public Health 2020;110(7):954–5.
6. Cheah CSL, Wang C, Ren H, et al. COVID-19 racism and mental health in Chinese American families. Pediatrics 2020;146(5). https://doi.org/10.1542/peds.2020-021816.
7. Taylor DB. George Floyd protests: a timeline. New York Times. Available at: https://www.nytimes.com/article/george-floyd-protests-timeline.html. Accessed January 16, 2021.
8. Buchanan L, Bui Q, Patel JK. Black Lives Matter May Be the Largest Movement in U.S. History. New York Times. 2020. Available at: https://www.nytimes.com/interactive/2020/07/03/us/george-floyd-protests-crowd-size.html. Accessed January 16, 2020.
9. Racine N, Cooke JE, Eirich R, et al. Child and adolescent mental illness during COVID-19: a rapid review. Psychiatry Res 2020;292:113307.
10. Marques de Miranda D, da Silva Athanasio B, Sena Oliveira AC, et al. How is COVID-19 pandemic impacting mental health of children and adolescents? Int J Disaster Risk Reduction 2020;51:101845.
11. Fong VC, Iarocci G. Child and family outcomes following pandemics: a systematic review and recommendations on COVID-19 policies. J Pediatr Psychol 2020;45(10):1124–43.

12. Chen F, Zheng D, Liu J, et al. Depression and anxiety among adolescents during COVID-19: a cross-sectional study [Letter to the Editor]. Brain Behav Immun 2020;88:36–8.

13. Duan L, Shao X, Wang Y, et al. An investigation of mental health status of children and adolescents in China during the outbreak of COVID-19. J Affect Disord 2020; 275:112–8.

14. Fitzpatrick O, Carson A, Weisz JR. Using mixed methods to identify the primary mental health problems and needs of children, adolescents, and their caregivers during the coronavirus (covid-19) pandemic. Child Psychiatry Hum Dev 2020. https://doi.org/10.1007/s10578-020-01089-z.

15. Gassman-Pines A, Ananat EO, Fitz-Henley J II. COVID-19 and parent-child psychological well-being. Pediatrics 2020;146(4). https://doi.org/10.1542/peds.2020-007294.

16. Hawke LD, Barbic SP, Voineskos A, et al. Impacts of COVID-19 on youth mental health, substance use, and well-being: a rapid survey of clinical and community samples: Répercussions de la COVID-19 sur la santé mentale, l'utilisation de substances et le bien-être des adolescents : un sondage rapide d'échantillons cliniques et communautaires. Can J Psychiatry 2020;65(10):701–9.

17. Hill RM, Rufino K, Kurian S, et al. Suicide ideation and attempts in a pediatric emergency department before and during CoViD-19. Pediatrics 2020;147(3). e2020029280.

18. Isumi A, Doi S, Yamaoka Y, et al. Do suicide rates in children and adolescents change during school closure in Japan? The acute effect of the first wave of COVID-19 pandemic on child and adolescent mental health. Child Abuse Neglect 2020;110(Part 2). https://doi.org/10.1016/j.chiabu.2020.104680.

19. Jiao WY, Wang LN, Liu J, et al. Behavioral and Emotional Disorders in Children during the COVID-19 Epidemic. J Pediatr 2020;221:264–6.e1.

20. Leeb RT, Bitsko RH, Radhakrishnan L, et al. Mental Health-Related Emergency Department Visits Among Children Aged <18 Years During the COVID-19 Pandemic - United States, January 1-October 17, 2020. MMWR Morb Mortal Wkly Rep 2020;69(45):1675–80.

21. Liu S, Liu Y, Liu Y. Somatic symptoms and concern regarding COVID-19 among Chinese college and primary school students: a cross-sectional survey. Psychiatry Res 2020;289:113070.

22. Liu Q, Zhou Y, Xie X, et al. The prevalence of behavioral problems among school-aged children in home quarantine during the COVID-19 pandemic in China. J Affect Disord 2021;279:412–6.

23. Patrick SW, Henkhaus LE, Zickafoose JS, et al. Well-being of parents and children during the COVID-19 pandemic: a national survey. Pediatrics 2020;146(4). https://doi.org/10.1542/peds.2020-016824.

24. Tang S, Xiang M, Cheung T, et al. Mental health and its correlates among children and adolescents during COVID-19 school closure: the importance of parent-child discussion. J Affect Disord 2021;279:353–60.

25. Yeasmin S, Banik R, Hossain S, et al. Impact of COVID-19 pandemic on the mental health of children in Bangladesh: a cross-sectional study. Child Youth Serv Rev 2020;117:105277.

26. Yue J, Zang X, Le Y, et al. Anxiety, depression and PTSD among children and their parent during 2019 novel coronavirus disease (covid-19) outbreak in China. Curr Psychol 2020. https://doi.org/10.1007/s12144-020-01191-4.

27. Zhou S-J, Zhang L-G, Wang L-L, et al. Prevalence and socio-demographic correlates of psychological health problems in Chinese adolescents during the

outbreak of covid-19. Eur Child Adolesc Psychiatry 2020. https://doi.org/10.1007/s00787-020-01541-4.

28. Loades ME, Chatburn E, Higson-Sweeney N, et al. Rapid systematic review: the impact of social isolation and loneliness on the mental health of children and adolescents in the context of COVID-19. J Am Acad Child Adolesc Psychiatry 2020; 59(11):1218–39.

29. Fish JN, McInroy LB, Paceley MS, et al. 'I'm kinda stuck at home with unsupportive parents right now': LGBTQ youths' experiences with COVID-19 and the importance of online support. J Adolesc Health 2020;67(3):450 2.

30. Mittal VA, Firth J, Kimhy D. Combating the dangers of sedentary activity on child and adolescent mental health during the time of COVID-19. J Am Acad Child Adolesc Psychiatry 2020;59(11):1197–8.

31. Liu D, Baumeister RF, Zhou Y. Mental health outcomes of coronavirus infection survivors: a rapid meta-analysis. J Psychiatr Res 2020. https://doi.org/10.1016/j.jpsychires.2020.10.015.

32. Fegert JM, Vitiello B, Plener PL, et al. Challenges and burden of the Coronavirus 2019 (COVID-19) pandemic for child and adolescent mental health: a narrative review to highlight clinical and research needs in the acute phase and the long return to normality. Child Adolesc Psychiatry Ment Health 2020;14:20.

33. Lawson M, Piel MH, Simon M. Child maltreatment during the COVID-19 pandemic: consequences of parental job loss on psychological and physical abuse towards children. Child Abuse Neglect 2020;110(Part 2). https://doi.org/10.1016/j.chiabu.2020.104709.

34. Brown SM, Doom JR, Lechuga-Peña S, et al. Stress and parenting during the global COVID-19 pandemic. Child Abuse Neglect 2020;110(Part 2). https://doi.org/10.1016/j.chiabu.2020.104699.

35. Rodriguez CM, Lee SJ, Ward KP, et al. The perfect storm: hidden risk of child maltreatment during the Covid-19 pandemic. Child Maltreat 2020. https://doi.org/10.1177/1077559520982066. 1077559520982066.

36. Simon NM, Saxe GN, Marmar CR. Mental health disorders related to COVID-19–Related Deaths. JAMA 2020;324(15):1493–4.

37. Kaslow NJ, Friis-Healy EA, Cattie JE, et al. Flattening the emotional distress curve: a behavioral health pandemic response strategy for COVID-19. Am Psychol 2020;75(7):875–86.

38. Patients with Depression and Anxiety Surge as Psychologists Respond to the Coronavirus Pandemic. November 2020, 2020.

39. Fortuna LR, Tolou-Shams M, Robles-Ramamurthy B, et al. Inequity and the disproportionate impact of COVID-19 on communities of color in the United States: the need for a trauma-informed social justice response. Psychol Trauma Theor Res Pract Policy 2020;12(5):443–5.

40. Pediatrics AAo. Mental health initiatives: primary care tools. Available at: https://www.aap.org/en-us/advocacy-and-policy/aap-health-initiatives/Mental-Health/Pages/Primary-Care-Tools.aspx. Accessed January 16, 2021.

Health Disparities and Their Effects on Children and Their Caregivers During the Coronavirus Disease 2019 Pandemic

Lynn C. Smitherman, MD[a],*, William Christopher Golden, MD[b],
Jennifer R. Walton, MD, MPH[c]

KEYWORDS

- COVID-19 pandemic • Health disparities in children • Systemic racism

KEY POINTS

- COVID-19 disproportionately affects children of color, and children considered vulnerable due to their living situations or underlying health conditions.
- Children of color have higher rates of hospitalization and more serious disease from COVID-19 than white children, mirroring the demographics of adult patients with COVID-19.
- Health disparities of children uncovered during the COVID-19 pandemic are due to structural racism, underlying medical problems, limited access to care, the occupations/employment of their caregivers, and the limited ability to minimize exposure/transmission in their home environments.
- To reduce health disparities among vulnerable populations of children during this pandemic and in the future, an intensified effort must be initiated and sustained to dismantle the social determinants of health, particularly measures to provide economic stability for families and access to health care and community infrastructure to support technology needed for education and telemedicine to achieve health equity.

This article previously appeared in *Pediatric Clinics*, Volume 68, Issue 5, October 2021.
[a] Department of Pediatrics, Wayne State University School of Medicine, 400 Mack Avenue, Suite 1 East, Detroit, MI 48201, USA; [b] Eudowood Neonatal Pulmonary Division, Department of Pediatrics, Johns Hopkins University School of Medicine, 1800 Orleans Street, Bloomberg 8523, Baltimore, MD 21287, USA; [c] Division of Developmental Behavioral Pediatrics, Department of Pediatrics, Nationwide Children's Hospital, The Ohio State University College of Medicine, 700 Children's Drive, Columbus, OH 43205, USA
* Corresponding author.
E-mail address: lsmither@med.wayne.edu

Clinics Collections 12 (2022) 95–107
https://doi.org/10.1016/j.ccol.2021.12.007
2352-7986/22/© 2021 Elsevier Inc. All rights reserved.

INTRODUCTION

As of the end of January 2021, there have been more than 26,000,000 infections and more than 435,000 deaths attributable to COVID-19.[1] Unfortunately, racial and ethnic minorities have been affected most significantly by this pandemic, particularly African Americans, Latinx Americans, and Indigenous Americans.[2] For example, African Americans compose 13.4% of the US population but represent 15.5% of COVID-19-related deaths.[1] In addition, although severe acute respiratory syndrome coronavirus 2 (SARS-CoV-2) affects children to a lesser extent than adults, non-Hispanic black and Hispanic children are hospitalized at a higher rate than white children and have more serious disease.[3,4] Finally, children with underlying health conditions, including obesity, chronic lung disease, and prematurity are hospitalized with COVID-19 at a higher rate than those without chronic medical conditions.[3] This disproportionate impact of COVID-19 in minoritized communities has been linked to preexisting health disparities.[5–7]

Health disparities are defined as differences among specific populations in the ability to achieve full health potential (as measured by differences in incidence, prevalence, mortality, burden of disease, and other adverse health conditions).[5] Among children, multiple factors contribute to these disparities, including economic stability, and access to health care. According to the Annie E. Casey Foundation, before the current pandemic, 12 million children in the United States were living in poverty in 2019, including one-third of African American and Native American children and 25% of Latinx children.[8] During the same period, of the 4.4 million children without health insurance, 14% were Native American, 9% were of Hispanic descent, and 18% were immigrants.[8] At present, owing to the impact of the pandemic on job security, more than 50% of African American, Latinx, and multiethnic adults are now without medical insurance, directly affecting the health security of their children.[8] With the onset of the pandemic and the social and political upheaval felt by many disenfranchised communities, these well-documented disparities (and the importance of addressing them) have again been brought to the attention of the medical community.[2–8]

This overview will examine the effects of these health disparities in various populations of children in this country. We will first examine the historical context of health disparities, how they developed, and why they still exist. We will then examine how specifically the COVID-19 pandemic impacted these disparities among children and adolescents, both directly and indirectly. Finally, we hope to provide some recommendations to reduce these disparities.

Historical Review of Health Care Disparities

Health care disparities have been described in the medical literature over the decades. Unequal distribution of resources along with the social determinants of health (economic stability, education, social and community context, health and health care and neighborhood) all contribute to the overall health and well-being of individuals in our society.[9]

A well-established reason for inequitable distribution of resources is systemic racism (racial bias across institutions and society), which has operated over centuries and has impacted generations of citizens in this country. This form of racism is more subtle than interpersonal racism and is unattributable to a particular individual or group of individuals. Examples include "red-lining" (restricting financial services, including loans and mortgages, to persons living in certain neighborhoods based on race), denying land ownership to ethnic/racial minorities, and minimizing access to resources such as healthy foods and transportation in communities where racial/ethnic minorities tend to live. Systemic racism has also contributed to decreased property values in communities of color, reducing federal, state, and local services (such as school funding and community resources) to impoverished communities. These policies have become embedded into the fabric of our society, and over time have become the status quo.[9,10]

Systemic racism has resulted in devastating effects on communities of color. Over centuries, policies endorsed and supported by systemic racism have limited opportunities where racial/ethnic minorities live, work, and obtain an education.[9] A longstanding history of the denial of basic rights and resources has burdened African Americans with lower socioeconomic status relative to whites, along with underresourced communities, which over time has contributed to comorbid conditions leading to vulnerability to poor health outcomes.[11] In addition, migrants from certain countries were not automatically granted citizenship, resulting in diminished opportunities to improve their economic status. Citizens of Hispanic descent, particularly those whose families emigrated from Mexico and Central America, have been denied home ownership and have lived under the scrutiny of immigration laws and policies.[12] Indigenous Americans have suffered forced migration and forced assimilation under racist laws and policies. Therefore, based on the policies, laws, and social structure of the United States, structural racism was successful in preventing communities of color to thrive. Structural racism also significantly accounts for the differences in health and well-being among ethnic and racial minorities in this country.[13,14] In effect, centuries of discrimination and racial trauma have negatively impacted the overall health of people of color.[11-14]

While racism has played a major role in health disparities, poorer health outcomes also have been demonstrated in patients with other medical and social constraints. Homelessness,[15] physical disability and/or special care needs,[16-19] and geography[20] all have been implicated in disparate health outcomes among adults and children. Recent work has suggested that vulnerable populations warrant close attention to ensure receipt of appropriate health care during the current COVID-19 pandemic.[21]

Health Disparities and Pandemics, Including Coronavirus Disease 2019

Historically, communities that are most impacted by new epidemics are often facing other threats to health and overall well-being.[7] Looking back at the Spanish flu in 1918 and the AIDS epidemic in the 1980s to the 1990s, marginalized communities were hit the hardest.[7]

Evidence demonstrates that although whites may have higher cases of COVID-19 based on raw numbers, blacks and Hispanics have higher rates and mortality based on percentage of the population.[1] There are many reasons for these discrepancies, most of which surround social determinants of health. Access to health care, immigration status, and language barriers all contribute to health inequity among Hispanics. For example, currently, Hispanics have the lowest rates of medical insurance coverage of all racial/ethnic groups in the United States (19.8% compared with 5.4% non-Hispanic whites). Compounding this statistic is that immigration status might impede eligibility to access health care, and almost 30% of this population is not fluent in English, thus posing additional barriers.[12] In addition, underfunding of the American Indian health system along with the additional burden of chronic disease predisposes this population to poorer outcomes secondary to COVID-19.[14]

Historically, blacks and Hispanics have higher disease burdens in the case of chronic lung disease, heart disease, diabetes, and obesity, conditions that also are risk factors of higher risk of mortality due to COVID-19.[11,12] These disparities extend to children as well. For children hospitalized with COVID-19-related illnesses, 45.7% of Hispanic children and 29.8% of black children had an underlying medical condition (obesity, chronic lung disease, or prematurity) compared with 14.9% of white children.[3] However, when social determinants of health, including neighborhood conditions, employment, and access to healthy foods are superimposed on these biological risks, the reasons for the higher case load and mortality become clear.[7] Many African Americans, Hispanic Americans, and Indigenous Americans live in dense housing (often in multigenerational families) and therefore are unable to socially distance. Strategies to minimize risk, such as facial coverings and frequent handwashing, may not always be attainable if someone in the household tests positive for COVID-19, making appropriately quarantining/isolation impossible.[6,11–14] In addition, essential workers typically tend to be people of color, who, despite the pandemic, must interact daily with the public (as opposed to telecommuting), increasing their risk of exposure.[6]

Impact of Health Disparities and Coronavirus Disease 2019 on Specific Pediatric Populations

Newborns

Amid this pandemic, important attention must be directed to the medical outcomes of neonates. The effects of SARS-CoV-2 extend across the antenatal to neonatal continuum, particularly affecting communities that traditionally have been marginalized. Studies of pregnant and parturient women in major US cities have demonstrated increased SARS-CoV-2 infection and/or seroprevalence among ethnic/racial minorities, and national data indicate an increased risk of death among infected Hispanic and non-Hispanic black women.[22–25] Additionally, pregnant women infected with SARS-CoV-2 have an increased risk of preterm delivery,[26,27] which may exacerbate the known disparity in such deliveries among African American women in the United States.[28,29] Finally, Niles and colleagues[30] argue that care and non–evidence-based policies implemented during the outbreak, including early inductions and elective cesarean deliveries (to manage hospital volumes) and limiting care partners during labor and delivery, disproportionately affect outcomes among women of color. These factors may reduce or eliminate opportunities for establishment of the maternal-neonatal dyad.

Data indicate rates of neonatal acquisition of SARS-CoV-2 at approximately 2% to 7%, with newborns presenting predominately with respiratory symptoms and being more significantly ill than older children.[31,32] Intrauterine and postnatal acquisition of SARS-CoV-2 infection in newborns has been described, although the mechanisms and risk factors for neonatal infection are not completely clear.[31,33–35] Additionally, specific data on racial disparities among SARS-CoV-2-infected newborns still are being investigated.

Further challenges remain in hospital-based newborn care during the pandemic, which may directly impact minoritized communities. In April, 2020, the American Academy of Pediatrics (AAP) recommended temporary separation of SARS-CoV-2-positive mothers from their newborns after birth to minimize the risk of neonatal infection.[36] Subsequent data demonstrated decreased rates of immediate and long-term breastfeeding among separated maternal-neonatal dyads.[37] These results, along with data showing no increased risk of neonatal infection with rooming-in, led the AAP in July 2020 to endorse room sharing (with appropriate infection control practices) for healthy babies with their nonacutely ill mothers.[36] However, the previous restrictions may have impaired nursing practices among African American mothers, who are less likely to initiate and continue breastfeeding through infancy.[38]

Additional stressors may occur at home and in outpatient settings. Newborn care (and provision of discharge instructions) to nonmaternal caregivers may be required, especially if an ill mother remains hospitalized. However, as a disproportionate number of cases of SARS-CoV-2 occur in racial/ethnic minorities,[39] these additional caretakers may place the baby at risk for postnatal viral acquisition and illness. Furthermore, hand hygiene and mask wearing (with breastfeeding and other components of neonatal care) still are recommended for mothers and family members convalescing from SARS-CoV-2 illness,[36] which may represent an additional expense for families. Finally, routine newborn appointments (for state newborn screening, hyperbilirubinemia monitoring, and weight/feeding assessment) may be delayed due to limitations in physical space (for isolating infected or at-risk patients) and personal protective equipment (for providers) in primary care offices. Telemedicine and home health nursing visits, evolving alternatives to traditional office appointments, seem to be attractive models for pediatric primary care in the midst of the pandemic. However, minoritized communities, many with limited financial resources and technology access, residua of racial residential segregation, and existent language barriers, may be unable to use these opportunities, possibly worsening disparities in short-term neonatal outcomes.

School-aged children and adolescents

Almost 60 million students have been significantly affected from school closures due to COVID-19.[40] Evidence has grown about the adverse effects on the physical, developmental, socioemotional, and environmental health of children before the COVID-19 pandemic by various social determinants of health, including poverty and racism. The impact has exponentially increased since the pandemic's arrival.

One example of these effects on children is the growth of the nation's digital divide. Before the pandemic, underserved and marginalized populations already had difficulty accessing stable telephone and Internet connections. Per the Pew Research Center, in 2019, 79% of white households had home broadband connection, compared with 66% of black households and 61% of Hispanic households.[41] Financial disparities also impact this divide; 92% of those who make $75,000 or more had home broadband compared with 87% who make $50,000 to $74,999, 72% who make $30,000 to $49,999, and 56% who make $30,000 or less.[41] The pandemic has intensified this inequity, and as health care systems nationwide converted to telehealth options to continue to provide care, so did the amplification of the digital divide. Social determinants of health fostered this negative impact, in mechanisms ranging from limited or lack of Internet access, patients' level of literacy on use of technology, building rapport and trust with patients, and cost.[42] This divide leads to families trying to access the Internet in not ideal ways via public spaces, such as parking lots.[43] Those individuals who come from a lower socioeconomic status, elderly, racial/ethnic minority, and/or with disabilities, need to be considered as the digital divide is addressed.[44] Cities (such as Baltimore, Philadelphia, and San Antonio) and organizations have become creative in delivering secure Internet connections to underserved communities. The need for continued advocacy nationwide on this effort is imperative.[43]

The COVID-19 pandemic may also have impacted childhood obesity. One study using a microsimulation model of students followed from kindergarten through fifth grade showed that mean body mass indices and childhood obesity prevalence increased as the time of the school closure increased (based on different scenarios of school closures due to COVID-19).[45] A 0.640% change in childhood obesity was noted from a 2-month closure alone for kindergarten students (closed April and May 2020), and a 2.373% change was noted from closures and decreased activity from April 2020 through December 2020.[45] More of an impact on childhood obesity was noted in male, non-

Hispanic black and Hispanic children.[45] Another study demonstrated that decreased physical activity and increased sedentary behavior were noted in children in the United States, early in the COVID-19 pandemic, and specifically more among children aged 9 to 13 years compared with children aged 5 to 8 years.[46] There is guidance from the AAP on identifying children at risk for obesity, acknowledging and addressing the inequities in accessing opportunities and obesity rates, and supporting families on the importance of healthy eating and physical activity during the COVID-19 pandemic.[47]

Unique childhood populations

During the 2018 to 2019 academic year, more than 7 million children in the nation received special education services in school, with the highest percentage for American Indian/Alaska Native students at 18%.[48] It was reported that 16% of Black students, 14% of white students, 14% of students of 2 or more races, and 13% of Hispanic students were reported to have disabilities requiring special education services.[48] Jeste and colleagues,[49] in evaluating how access to educational and health care services have changed since the pandemic, noted that 74% of parents of children with disabilities reported their children lost at least one therapy or educational service, 56% reported their children received "at least some" services, and 36% reported losing access to a health care provider. These data indicate that the pandemic has adversely affected daily functioning and routine of children with special needs. Depending on the type of disability (for example, autism spectrum disorder), this decrease in support may lead to an increase in challenging behaviors by frequency and/or intensity.[50] Guidance to support children with disabilities and their families receiving their educational services exist at federal and state levels, including virtual options. Although some virtual options have shown success for some students with disabilities, addressing the barriers to access and education (as previously discussed) to those options are vital for true equitable academic success for students from all backgrounds.

Before the pandemic, cases of pediatric mental illness and suicide trends have been on the rise and are concerning, as children as young as 5 years have been identified with mental health problems.[51] COVID-19 has gravely affected pediatric mental health, both directly and indirectly. This pandemic is traumatizing, leading to children becoming fearful of having COVID-19 or a family member becoming ill or dying. In addition, children realize this pandemic has affected their ability to interact with peers, celebrate birthdays (or other holidays), and attend school. Parents and caregivers are also enduring this trauma and the difficulties navigating employment, providing for their families, and keeping everyone healthy. These stressors have led to missed appointments with health care providers, and for some families, worsening housing and food insecurity, significantly increasing adverse childhood experiences.

Researchers reviewed the mental health effects in children impacted by the pandemic and noted abuse, neglect, and a variety of psychiatric disorders, including suicidal ideations.[52] Leeb and colleagues[53] found that starting in April 2020, pediatric mental health-related emergency department visits increased 24% in children aged 5 to 11 years, and increased 31% in children aged 12 to 17 years, when compared with 2019 data. Additionally, given the importance of schools as an option for health care delivery (specifically for mental health treatment), closures significantly disrupted these services, particularly for racial and ethnic minority students.[54] Leff and colleagues[55] further noted that black children were more than 50% less likely to come to the emergency department (ED) with a mental health condition compared with before the pandemic, possibly for a few reasons, such as unequal access to care (especially with school closures) and COVID-19 disproportionately affecting black communities and delaying seeking care.[55]

Children with medical complexity are at risk of reduced health care access during the pandemic due to decreased care from home health aides and school closures, where medical care was provided during the day.[56] Because of the increased vulnerability of these children, parents were at risk for unemployment if they were not able to work from home and at risk for mental/emotional stress without respite and in-home support[56]; this further increases the isolation of these families and increases the vulnerability of children with medical complexity. Medical visits may be reduced as parents/caregivers fear exposure to COVID-19.[8,56]

During this time of the pandemic, children are at a higher risk for maltreatment.[56,57] With school closures the number of mandatory reporters that see children on a regular basis is significantly reduced. The more than 400,000 children in the foster care system during the pandemic are particularly vulnerable because of the shelter-in-place and social distancing executive orders that were placed to decrease the transmission of COVID-19.[56,57] Many children in foster care have experienced adversity and trauma, which led to their initial placement.[56–58] Compounding this is that social distancing in many areas meant that these children were not able to have face-to-face visits with their birth families, which may contribute to their emotional stress.[56] In some states, case workers have been either furloughed or unable to make home visits with children in care for routine safety checks, delaying the potential for reunification with birth families. In addition, delays in court proceedings delay adoptions for children in care.[56] Furthermore, children who age out of the system during the pandemic are left in a more vulnerable state as they try to navigate life as adults during a public health and economic crisis.[56]

Homeless families with children do not have the privilege of adhering to the public health recommendations to decrease the spread of COVID-19.[56] Sheltering in place, access to hygiene supplies, and practicing social distancing are not always possible or practical for families with housing insecurity.[55] Of those families, approximately 75% are "doubling up," that is, living with another family; approximately 14% live in shelters, 7% live in hotels or motels, and approximately 3% are unsheltered.[56,57] During the pandemic, 78% of families experiencing homelessness are Hispanic, again in line with the health disparities seen during the pandemic.[56] Unaccompanied youth who are homeless are more likely to be African American; identify as lesbian, gay, bisexual, transgender, and gender or sexual orientation questioning (LGBTQ), or have less than a high school education.[57] According to the Annie E. Casey Foundation, 18% of families are concerned that they will not be able to pay for their rent on time during the pandemic, with higher proportions of African American families (31%) and Hispanic families (26%) compared with white families (12%).[8] Families who are doubling up are frequently under the threat of being asked to leave due to financial or safety reasons.[56] Those living in shelters use communal bathrooms and kitchens, again making social distancing and hygiene difficult.[56] In general, contact tracing, prevention, and treatment are more difficult for families that are homeless.[56]

Impact of Coronavirus Disease 2019 on Caregivers

Children depend on their parents, guardians, and/or caregivers for basic needs (food, shelter, clothing) as well as transportation, education, and health care access (ie, insurance). Any condition that impacts the caregivers' ability to provide these needs negatively impacts the overall well-being of the child. For example, a caregiver employed as an essential worker during this pandemic might be unable to provide supervision of children at home as they attend school virtually. Caregivers may be at a greater risk of exposure to COVID-19 depending on his or her employment status and might not adequately be able to quarantine upon exposure, thus increasing the risk of infection to the entire family.[6] In addition, many frontline jobs do not compensate workers who have to stay home due to illness, placing workers at risk of losing their source of income.[6,8] Furthermore, many of these workers have inadequate health insurance coverage and may delay care once symptomatic, risking their own health and the health of their family and community.[6,8]

Although the percentage of whites working essential jobs was only slightly lower than nonwhites (Hispanics, blacks, and Asians), job characteristics of essential workers varies with race/ethnicity.[6] Approximately 12% of Whites and 17% of Asians are essential workers able to work from home, compared with 10% blacks and 9% Hispanics.[6,8] A higher proportion of blacks tend to work in health care (eg, nursing assistants, home health care aides, ambulance drivers, housekeeping) and public safety (eg, police officers, firefighters, security guards, corrections officers, postal employees, public transportation workers, and those who work in funeral homes and crematoriums).[6,59] Hispanics are overrepresented in the foodservice industry.[6,60] These occupations increase the exposure risk to COVID-19 among minorities.

Impact of Coronavirus Disease 2019 on Physicians and Other Health Care Workers of Color

The COVID-19 pandemic has also had a significant effect on physician and skilled health workers of color. Of the 18.6 million health care workers in the United States, 40% are people of color (16% blacks, 13% Hispanic, and 7% Asian).[60,61] At present, African Americans, Hispanics, and Native American constitute 5%, 5.8%, and 0.4% of practicing physicians, respectively.[60,61] These discrepancies in themselves have led to some of the health disparities seen in minority communities, and one of the interventions to counteract this is to increase the pipeline to include more physicians of color into the profession.[61] However, this pandemic has caused a disparate toll on these physicians of color. Many disproportionately practice in communities with higher rates of COVID-19 and thus are at a higher risk of exposure.[60,61] In addition, these physicians are more likely to have chronic health conditions, placing them at higher risk for severe morbidity and mortality from COVID-19.[60,61] Also, those physicians in private practice have witnessed the economic impact of the pandemic on their livelihood, and those who serve their communities in safety net health care institutions have had to deal with understaffed and underresourced personnel.[61] Furthermore, when African Americans enter the health care system as patients, they are at a higher risk of receiving lower-quality care, particularly if they are treated using diagnostic criteria and clinical pathways embedded with racial bias.[61] Finally, physicians of color in general are at a greater risk of developing mental health problems including anxiety, depression, posttraumatic stress disorder, imposter syndrome, and survivor guilt.[12,61]

SUMMARY
Steps to Minimize Health Disparities and Their Impact on Children, Caregivers, and Health Care Workers During the Coronavirus Disease 2019 Pandemic and Beyond

COVID-19 has illuminated the areas of needed improvement in the delivery of equitable child health and education. Several agencies and organizations are providing guidelines on how to support families, schools, and health care systems in this effort. The Economic Policy Institute has highlighted the lessons learned and suggested a plan through "relief, recovery, and rebuilding,"[62] where this nation critically reviews its resources and interest in child development. The Centers for Disease Control and Prevention created a resource kit to support child behavioral and mental health, categorized by age groups.[63] Pediatric providers must continue to check in with their families and keep open communication. A resource to assist providers is the Roadmap to Resilience, Emotional, and Mental Health from the American Board of Pediatrics.[64]

For parents and caregivers who are unable to secure economic stability and health care through employment, there must be mechanisms available to assist with access to safety net resources easily and without the threat of legal action or deportation.[12–14,56–60]

For children of unique populations, steps to minimize the impact of COVID-19 include:

- Providing access to telehealth visits
- Endorsing caregiver support groups
- Ensuring respite care for children with complex medical conditions and their families
- Heightening awareness among other mandatory reporters
- Providing paid leave and economic assistance to foster families
- Enhancing technical support and connectivity for parents for telemedicine visits and resource acquisition
- Increasing state funding for family preservation services for children in foster care
- Offering emergency rental assistance and upholding a moratorium on evictions and foreclosures for homeless children[55–58]

Whatever obstacle may come, be it COVID-19 or another global disaster, steps must be taken to ensure the resilience of children and adolescents and their families. In addition to those efforts, we must also ensure that our health care system has the resources and personnel needed to ensure the equitable delivery of health care services to everyone. Policies to promote the overall health and well-being of children, adolescents, and their families, including the promotion and sustaining of safety net resources, access to health care, safe living environments, and economic security, should continue to be this nation's top priority.

CLINICS CARE POINTS

- Compared with the general population, non-Hispanic blacks, indigenous Americans/Alaskan Natives, and Hispanics have higher rates of COVID-19 infection and deaths, because of several factors including:
  - Timely access to medical care
  - Poverty
  - Occupation
  - Systemic racism
- Although children in general have lower rates of COVID-19 infection and hospitalization, non-Hispanic black and Hispanic children have higher rates of hospitalization due to COVID-19 infection.
- In addition to people of color, unique populations of children at higher risk of medical complications of COVID-19 due to health disparities include:
  - Children who are immigrants
  - Children who are obese
  - Children with chronic illnesses and/or disabilities
  - Children who are homeless
  - Children who are impoverished
  - Children who are in foster care
- Health disparities during the COVID-19 pandemic have also been demonstrated in education, safety net programs, and mental health support services.

- Recommendations to decrease these disparities include addressing social determinants of health:
  - Education: providing schools and families with appropriate resources to stabilize and enhance virtual learning, offering individualized instruction for students falling behind, and redesigning the educational system to focus on the whole child
  - Health and health care: monitoring and addressing the physical and mental health of patients and families during the pandemic, advocating for the elimination of barriers to COVID-19 testing and vaccines, and recommending appropriate compensation for telemedicine care
  - Economic stability: providing personal protective equipment (PPE) for all essential workers, supporting fair housing practices (rental assistance, eviction moratoria) during the pandemic, and promoting affordable/free PPE supplies to families with high-risk household members.

DISCLOSURE

The authors have nothing to disclose.

REFERENCES

1. Center for Disease Control. Available at: https://covid.cdc.gov/covid-data-tracker/#cases_casesper100klast7days. Accessed January 17, 2021.
2. Abedi v. Olulana O, Avula V, Chaudhary D, Khan A, Shahjouei S, Li J, and Zand R. Racial, Economic and Health Inequality and COVID-19 Infection in the United States. J Racial Ethn Health Disparities 2020;1–11.
3. Kim L, Whitaker M, O'Halloran A, et al. Hospitalization Rates and Characteristics of Children Aged <18 Years Hospitalized with Laboratory-Confirmed COVID-19- COVID-NET, 14 States, March 1-25, 2020. MMWR Morb Mortal Wkly Rep 2020; 69:1081–8.
4. Lee EH, Kepler KL, Geevarughese A, Paneth-Pollak R, Dorsinville MS, Ngai S, Reilly KH. Race/Ethnicity Amoung Children with COVID-19-Associated Multi-system Inflammatory Syndrome. JAMA Netw Open 2020;3(11):e20302800.
5. Baciu A, Negussie Y, Geller A, et al, editors. The state of health disparities in the United States in communities in action: pathways to health equity. National Academies of Sciences, Engineering, and medicine; health and medicine Division; board on population health and public health practice; Committee on community-based Solutions to promote health equity in the United States. Washington (DC): National Academies Press; 2017.
6. Selden TM, Berdahl TA. COVID-19 and Racial/Ethnic Disparities in Health Risk, Employment, and Household Composition. Health Aff 2020;39(9):1624–32.
7. Gravlee C. Systemic racism, chronic health inequities, and COVID-19: A syndemic in the making? Am J Hum Biol 2020;e23482.
8. Kids, Families and COVID-19: Pandemic Pain Points and the Urgent Need to Respond. Annie E. Casey Foundation. December 2020;14.
9. Jones CP. Confronting Institutional Racism. Phylon 2002;50(1–2):7–22, 1960.
10. Johnson T. Intersection of Bias, Structural Racism and Social Determinants with Health Care Inequities. Pediatrics 2020;146(2). e2020003657.
11. Yancy CW. COVID-19 and African Americans. JAMA 2020;323(19):1891–2.
12. Gil R, Marcelin JR. Zuniga-Blanco, Marquez C, Mathew T, Piggott D. COVID-19 Pandemic: Disparate Health Impact on the Hispanic/Latinx Population in the United States. J Infect Dis 2020;222(10):1592–5.

13. Fingling MG, Casey LS, Fryberg SA, Hafner S, Blendon RJ, Benson JM, Sayde JM, Miller C. Discrimination in the US: Experiences of Native Americans. Health Serv Res 2019;54:1431–41.
14. Hatcher SM, Agnew-Brune C, Anderson M, et al. COVID-19 Among American Indian and Alaska Native Persons-23 States, January 31-July 3, 2020. MMWR Morb Mortal Wkly Rep 2020;69:1166–9.
15. Oppenheimer SC, Nurius PS, Green S. Homelessness history impacts on health outcomes and economic and risk behavior intermediaries: new insights from population data. Fam Soc 2016;97(3):230–42.
16. Na L, Singh S. Disparities in mental health, social support and coping among individuals with mobility impairment. Disabil Health J 2021;14(2):101047.
17. Minnaert J, Kenney MK, Ghandour R, et al. CSHCN with hearing difficulties: Disparities in access and quality of care. Disabil Health J 2020;13(1):100798.
18. Jolles MP, Thomas KC. Disparities in self-reported access to patient-centered medical home care for children with special health care needs. Med Care 2018;56(10):840–6.
19. Acharya K, Meza R, Msall ME. Disparities in life course outcomes for transition-aged youth with disabilities. Pediatr Ann 2017;46(10):e371–6.
20. Morales DA, Barksdale CL, Beckel-Mitchener A. A call to action to address rural mental health disparities. J Clin Transl Sci 2020;4(5):463–7.
21. Verduzco-Gutierrez M, Lara AM, Annaswamy TM. When Disparities and Disabilities Collide: Inequities during the COVID-19 Pandemic. PM&R 2021;13(4):412–4.
22. Emeruwa UN, Spiegelman J, Ona S, et al. Influence of race and ethnicity on severe acute respiratory syndrome coronavirus 2 (SARS-CoV-2) infection rates and clinical outcomes in pregnancy. Obstet Gynecol 2020;136(5):1040–3.
23. Sakowicz A, Ayala AE, Ukeje CC, et al. Risk factors for severe acute respiratory syndrome coronavirus 2 infection in pregnant women. Am J Obstet Gynecol MFM 2020;2(4):100198.
24. Flannery DD, Gouma S, Dhudasia MB, et al. SARS-CoV-2 seroprevalence among parturient women in Philadelphia. Sci Immunol 2020;5(49):eabd5709.
25. Zambrano LD, Ellington S, Strid P, et al. Update: characteristics of symptomatic women of reproductive age with laboratory-confirmed SARS-CoV-2 infection by pregnancy status - United States, January 22-October 3, 2020. MMWR Morb Mortal Wkly Rep 2020;69(44):1641–7.
26. Marín Gabriel MA, Vergeli MR, Carbonero SC, et al. Maternal, perinatal and neonatal outcomes with COVID-19: a multicenter study of 242 pregnancies and their 248 infant newborns during their first month of life. Pediatr Infect Dis J 2020;39(12):e393–7.
27. Allotey J, Stallings E, Bonet M, et al. Clinical manifestations, risk factors, and maternal and perinatal outcomes of coronavirus disease 2019 in pregnancy: living systematic review and meta-analysis. BMJ 2020;370:m3320.
28. Johnson JD, Green CA, Vladutiu CJ, et al. Racial disparities in prematurity persist among women of high socioeconomic status. Am J Obstet Gynecol MFM 2020;2(3):100104.
29. Kistka ZA, Palomar L, Lee KA, et al. Racial disparity in the frequency of recurrence of preterm birth. Am J Obstet Gynecol 2007;196(2):131.e131–6.
30. Niles PM, Asiodu IV, Crear-Perry J, et al. Reflecting on equity in perinatal care during a pandemic. Health Equity 2020;4(1):330–3.
31. Barrero-Castillero A, Beam KS, Bernardini LB, et al. COVID-19: neonatal-perinatal perspectives. J Perinatol 2021;41(5):940–51.

32. Liguoro I, Pilotto C, Bonanni M, et al. SARS-COV-2 infection in children and newborns: a systematic review. Eur J Pediatr 2020;179(7):1029–46.
33. Naz S, Rahat T, Memon FN. Vertical transmission of SARS-CoV-2 from COVID-19 infected pregnant women: a review on intrauterine transmission. Fetal Pediatr Pathol 2021;40(1):80–92.
34. Wang W, Xu Y, Gao R, et al. Detection of SARS-CoV-2 in different types of clinical specimens. JAMA 2020;323(18):1843–4.
35. Kimberlin DW, Stagno S. Can SARS-CoV-2 Infection be acquired in utero?: More definitive evidence is needed. JAMA 2020;323(18):1788–9.
36. American Academy of Pediatrics. FAQ: Management of Infants Born to Mothers with Suspected or Confirmed COVID-19. Available at: https://services.aap.org/en/pages/2019-novel-coronavirus-covid-19-infections/clinical-guidance/faqs-management-of-infants-born-to-covid-19-mothers/. Accessed January 18, 2020.
37. Popofsky S, Noor A, Jill Leavens-Maurer J, et al. Impact of maternal severe acute respiratory syndrome coronavirus 2 detection on breastfeeding due to infant separation at birth. J Pediatr 2020;226:64–70.
38. Beauregard JL, Hamner HC, Chen J, et al. Racial disparities in breastfeeding initiation and duration among U.S. infants born in 2015. MMWR Morb Mortal Wkly Rep 2019;68(34):745–8.
39. COVID-19 Racial and Ethnic Health Disparities. Available at: www.cdc.gov/coronavirus/2019-ncov/community/health-equity/racial-ethnic-disparities/increased-risk-illness.html. Accessed January 18, 2021.
40. Masonbrink AR, Hurley E. Advocating for Children During the COVID-19 School Closures. Pediatrics 2020;146(3):e20201440.
41. Internet Broadband Fact Sheet. Pew Research Center Internet & Technology. 2019. Available at: https://www.pewresearch.org/internet/fact-sheet/internet-broadband/#who-has-home-broadband. Accessed January 17, 2021.
42. Ramsetty A, Adams C. Impact of the digital divide in the age of COVID-19. J Am Med Inform Assoc 2020;27(7):1147–8.
43. Flaherty C, Wood SM, Chen K. Broadband Internet Access, Education & Child Health: From Differences to Disparities, Part 1. PolicyLab Blog post September 2020 Notes. Available at: https://policylab.chop.edu/blog/broadband-internet-access-education-child-health-differences-disparities-part-1. Accessed January 17, 2021.
44. Gray DM, Joseph JJ, Olayiwola JN. Strategies for Digital Care of Vulnerable Patients in a COVID-19 World—Keeping in Touch. JAMA Health Forum Published Online 2020. https://doi.org/10.1001/jamahealthforum.2020.0734.
45. An R. Projecting the impact of the coronavirus disease-2019 pandemic on childhood obesity in the United States: A microsimulation model. J Sport Health Sci 2020;9:302–12.
46. Dunton GF, Do B, Wang SD. Early effects of the COVID-19 pandemic on physical activity and sedentary behavior in children living in the U.S. BMC Public Health 2020;20:1351.
47. Supporting Healthy Nutrition and Physical Activity During the COVID-19 Pandemic. American Academy of Pediatrics; 2020. Available at: https://services.aap.org/en/pages/2019-novel-coronavirus-covid-19-infections/clinical-guidance/supporting-healthy-nutrition-and-physical-activity-during-the-covid-19-pandemic/. Accessed January 27, 2021.
48. The Condition of Education: Students with Disabilities. National Center for Education Statistics, May 2020. Available at: https://nces.ed.gov/programs/coe/indicator_cgg.asp. Accessed January 17, 2021.

49. Jeste S, Hyde C, Distefano C, Halladay A, Ray S, Porath M, Wilson RB, Thurm A. Changes in access to educational and healthcare services for individuals with intellectual and developmental disabilities during COVID-19 restrictions. J Intellect Disabil Res 2020;64:825–33.

50. Eshraghi AA, Li C, Alessandri M, Messinger DS, Eshraghi RS, Mittal R, Armstrong FD. COVID-19: overcoming the challenges faced by individuals with autism and their families. The Lancet Psychiatry 2020;7(6):481–3.

51. Bridge JA, Asti L, Horowitz LM, et al. Suicide Trends Among Elementary School–Aged Children in the United States From 1993 to 2012. JAMA Pediatr 2015;169(7):673–7.

52. de Figueiredo CS, Sandre PC, Portugal LCL, et al. COVID-19 pandemic impact on children and adolescents' mental health: Biological, environmental, and social factors. Prog Neuro-psychopharmacology Biol Psychiatry 2021;106:110171.

53. Leeb RT, Bitsko RH, Radhakrishnan L, Martinez P, Njai R, Holland KM. Mental Health–Related Emergency Department Visits Among Children Aged <18 Years During the COVID-19 Pandemic — United States, January 1–October 17, 2020. MMWR Morb Mortal Wkly Rep 2020;69:1675–80.

54. Golberstein E, Wen H, Miller BF. Coronavirus Disease 2019 (COVID-19) and Mental Health for Children and Adolescents. JAMA Pediatr 2020;174(9):819–20.

55. Leff RA, Setzer E, Cicero MX, Auerbach M. Changes in pediatric emergency department visits for mental health during the COVID-19 pandemic: A cross-sectional study. Clin Child Psychol Psychiatry 2021;26(1):33–8.

56. Wong CA, Ming D, Maslow G, Gifford EJ. Mitigating the Impacts of the COVID-19 Pandemic Response on At-Risk Children. Pediatrics 2020;146(1):e20200973.

57. Annie E. Casey Foundation. Foster Care. Available at: https://www.aecf.org/topics/foster-care/?gclid=Cj0KCQiAmL-ABhDFARIsAKywVafrrw_UzGo3vVK7-wiDLkeYCl7xnGDkenDz4LX4Ge3Lli8kfNx5SCUaAgc_EALw_wcB. Accessed January 26, 2021.

58. Hilavinka E, Firth S. CCOVID-19 Strips Safety Net for Foster Youth "Aging Out' During Pandemic. Medpage Today 12/8/20. Available at: https://www.medpagetoday.com/special-reports/exclusives/90072?vpass=1. Accessed January 24, 2021.

59. Beharry MS, Christensen R. Homelessnes in pediatric populations: strategies for prevention, assistance and advocacy. Pediatr Clin North Am 2020;67(2):357–72.

60. Artiga S, Rae M, Pham O, Hamel L, Munan C. COVID-19 Risks and Impacts Among Health Care Workers by Race and Ethnicity. 2020. Available at: https://www.kff.org/racial-equity-and-health-policy/issue-brief/covid-19-risks-impacts-health-care-workers-race-ethnicity/. Accessed January 17, 2021.

61. Filut A, Carnes M. Will Losing Black Physicians be a Consequence of the COVID-19 Pandemic? Acad Med 2020;95(12):1796–8.

62. Garcia E, Weiss E. COVID-19 and student performance, equity, and U.S. education policy. Economic Policy Institute. 2020. Available at: https://www.epi.org/publication/the-consequences-of-the-covid-19-pandemic-for-education-performance-and-equity-in-the-united-states-what-can-we-learn-from-pre-pandemic-research-to-inform-relief-recovery-and-rebuilding/. Accessed January 17, 2021.

63. COVID-19 Parental Resources Kit. Center for Disease Control and Prevention. 2020. Available at: https://www.cdc.gov/coronavirus/2019-ncov/daily-life-coping/parental-resource-kit/index.html. Accessed January 17, 2021.

64. Roadmap to Resilience. Emotional, and Mental Health. The American Board of Pediatrics. 2020. Available at: https://www.abp.org/foundation/roadmap. Accessed January 17, 2021.

The Effect of COVID-19 on Education

Jacob Hoofman, MS2[a], Elizabeth Secord, MD[b],*

KEYWORDS

- COVID-19 • Education • Virtual learning • Special education
- Medical school education

KEY POINTS

- Virtual learning has become a norm during COVID-19.
- Children requiring special learning services, those living in poverty, and those speaking English as a second language have lost more from the pandemic educational changes.
- For children with attention deficit disorder and no comorbidities, virtual learning has sometimes been advantageous.
- Math learning scores are more likely to be affected than language arts scores by pandemic changes.
- School meals, access to friends, and organized activities have also been lost with the closing of in-person school.

BACKGROUND

The transition to an online education during the coronavirus disease 2019 (COVID-19) pandemic may bring about adverse educational changes and adverse health consequences for children and young adult learners in grade school, middle school, high school, college, and professional schools. The effects may differ by age, maturity, and socioeconomic class. At this time, we have few data on outcomes, but many oversight organizations have tried to establish guidelines, expressed concerns, and extrapolated from previous experiences.

GENERAL EDUCATIONAL LOSSES AND DISPARITIES

Many researchers are examining how the new environment affects learners' mental, physical, and social health to help compensate for any losses incurred by this pandemic and to better prepare for future pandemics. There is a paucity of data at

This article previously appeared in *Pediatric Clinics*, Volume 68, Issue 5, October 2021.
[a] Wayne State University School of Medicine, 540 East Canfield, Detroit, MI 48201, USA;
[b] Department of Pediatrics, Wayne Pediatrics, School of Medicine, Pediatrics Wayne State University, 400 Mack Avenue, Detroit, MI 48201, USA
* Corresponding author.
E-mail address: esecord@med.wayne.edu

Clinics Collections 12 (2022) 109–117
https://doi.org/10.1016/j.ccol.2021.12.008
2352-7986/22/© 2021 Elsevier Inc. All rights reserved.

this juncture, but some investigators have extrapolated from earlier school shutdowns owing to hurricanes and other natural disasters.[1]

Inclement weather closures are estimated in some studies to lower middle school math grades by 0.013 to 0.039 standard deviations and natural disaster closures by up to 0.10 standard deviation decreases in overall achievement scores.[2] The data from inclement weather closures did show a more significant decrease for children dependent on school meals, but generally the data were not stratified by socioeconomic differences.[3,4] Math scores are impacted overall more negatively by school absences than English language scores for all school closures.[4,5]

The Northwest Evaluation Association is a global nonprofit organization that provides research-based assessments and professional development for educators. A team of researchers at Stanford University evaluated Northwest Evaluation Association test scores for students in 17 states and the District of Columbia in the Fall of 2020 and estimated that the average student had lost one-third of a year to a full year's worth of learning in reading, and about three-quarters of a year to more than 1 year in math since schools closed in March 2020.[5]

With school shifted from traditional attendance at a school building to attendance via the Internet, families have come under new stressors. It is increasingly clear that families depended on schools for much more than math and reading. Shelter, food, health care, and social well-being are all part of what children and adolescents, as well as their parents or guardians, depend on schools to provide.[5,6]

Many families have been impacted negatively by the loss of wages, leading to food insecurity and housing insecurity; some of loss this is a consequence of the need for parents to be at home with young children who cannot attend in-person school.[6] There is evidence that this economic instability is leading to an increase in depression and anxiety.[7] In 1 survey, 34.71% of parents reported behavioral problems in their children that they attributed to the pandemic and virtual schooling.[8]

Children have been infected with and affected by coronavirus. In the United States, 93,605 students tested positive for COVID-19, and it was reported that 42% were Hispanic/Latino, 32% were non-Hispanic White, and 17% were non-Hispanic Black, emphasizing a disproportionate effect for children of color.[9] COVID infection itself is not the only issue that affects children's health during the pandemic. School-based health care and school-based meals are lost when school goes virtual and children of lower socioeconomic class are more severely affected by these losses. Although some districts were able to deliver school meals, school-based health care is a primary source of health care for many children and has left some chronic conditions unchecked during the pandemic.[10]

Many families report that the stress of the pandemic has led to a poorer diet in children with an increase in the consumption of sweet and fried foods.[11,12] Shelter at home orders and online education have led to fewer exercise opportunities. Research carried out by Ammar and colleagues[12] found that daily sitting had increased from 5 to 8 hours a day and binge eating, snacking, and the number of meals were all significantly increased owing to lockdown conditions and stay-at-home initiatives. There is growing evidence in both animal and human models that diets high in sugar and fat can play a detrimental role in cognition and should be of increased concern in light of the pandemic.[13]

The family stress elicited by the COVID-19 shutdown is a particular concern because of compiled evidence that adverse life experiences at an early age are associated with an increased likelihood of mental health issues as an adult.[14] There is early evidence that children ages 6 to 18 years of age experienced a significant increase in their expression of "clinginess, irritability, and fear" during the early pandemic school shutdowns.[15] These emotions associated with anxiety may have a negative impact on the family unit, which was already stressed owing to the pandemic.

Another major concern is the length of isolation many children have had to endure since the pandemic began and what effects it might have on their ability to socialize. The school, for many children, is the agent for forming their social connections as well as where early social development occurs.[16] Noting that academic performance is also declining the pandemic may be creating a snowball effect, setting back children without access to resources from which they may never recover, even into adulthood.

Predictions from data analysis of school absenteeism, summer breaks, and natural disaster occurrences are imperfect for the current situation, but all indications are that we should not expect all children and adolescents to be affected equally.[4,5] Although some children and adolescents will likely suffer no long-term consequences, COVID-19 is expected to widen the already existing educational gap from socioeconomic differences, and children with learning differences are expected to suffer more losses than neurotypical children.[4,5]

SPECIAL EDUCATION AND THE COVID-19 PANDEMIC

Although COVID-19 has affected all levels of education reception and delivery, children with special needs have been more profoundly impacted. Children in the United States who have special needs have legal protection for appropriate education by the Individuals with Disabilities Education Act and Section 504 of the Rehabilitation Act of 1973.[17,18] Collectively, this legislation is meant to allow for appropriate accommodations, services, modifications, and specialized academic instruction to ensure that "every child receives a free appropriate public education . . . in the least restrictive environment."[17]

Children with autism usually have applied behavioral analysis (ABA) as part of their individualized educational plan. ABA therapists for autism use a technique of discrete trial training that shapes and rewards incremental changes toward new behaviors.[19] Discrete trial training involves breaking behaviors into small steps and repetition of rewards for small advances in the steps toward those behaviors. It is an intensive one-on-one therapy that puts a child and therapist in close contact for many hours at a time, often 20 to 40 hours a week. This therapy works best when initiated at a young age in children with autism and is often initiated in the home.[19]

Because ABA workers were considered essential workers from the early days of the pandemic, organizations providing this service had the responsibility and the freedom to develop safety protocols for delivery of this necessary service and did so in conjunction with certifying boards.[20]

Early in the pandemic, there were interruptions in ABA followed by virtual visits, and finally by in-home therapy with COVID-19 isolation precautions.[21] Although the efficacy of virtual visits for ABA therapy would empirically seem to be inferior, there are few outcomes data available. The balance of safety versus efficacy quite early turned to in-home services with interruptions owing to illness and decreased therapist availability owing to the pandemic.[21] An overarching concern for children with autism is the possible loss of a window of opportunity to intervene early. Families of children and adolescents with autism spectrum disorder report increased stress compared with families of children with other disabilities before the pandemic, and during the pandemic this burden has increased with the added responsibility of monitoring in-home schooling.[20]

Early data on virtual schooling children with attention deficit disorder (ADD) and attention deficit with hyperactivity (ADHD) shows that adolescents with ADD/ADHD found the switch to virtual learning more anxiety producing and more challenging than their peers.[22] However, according to a study in Ireland, younger children with ADD/ADHD and no other neurologic or psychiatric diagnoses who were stable on medication tended to report less anxiety with at-home schooling and their parents and caregivers reported improved behavior during the pandemic.[23] An unexpected benefit of shelter in home versus shelter in place may be to identify these stressors in face-to-face school for children with ADD/ADHD. If children with ADD/ADHD had an additional diagnosis of autism or depression, they reported increased anxiety with the school shutdown.[23,24]

Much of the available literature is anticipatory guidance for in-home schooling of children with disabilities rather than data about schooling during the pandemic. The American Academy of Pediatrics published guidance advising that, because 70% of students with ADHD have other conditions, such as learning differences, oppositional defiant disorder, or depression, they may have very different responses to in home schooling which are a result of the non-ADHD diagnosis, for example, refusal to attempt work for children with oppositional defiant disorder, severe anxiety for those with depression and or anxiety disorders, and anxiety and perseveration for children with autism.[25] Children and families already stressed with learning differences have had substantial challenges during the COVID-19 school closures.

HIGH SCHOOL, DEPRESSION, AND COVID-19

High schoolers have lost a great deal during this pandemic. What should have been a time of establishing more independence has been hampered by shelter-in-place recommendations. Graduations, proms, athletic events, college visits, and many other social and educational events have been altered or lost and cannot be recaptured.

Adolescents reported higher rates of depression and anxiety associated with the pandemic, and in 1 study 14.4% of teenagers report post-traumatic stress disorder, whereas 40.4% report having depression and anxiety.[26] In another survey adolescent boys reported a significant decrease in life satisfaction from 92% before COVID to 72% during lockdown conditions. For adolescent girls, the decrease in life satisfaction was from 81% before COVID to 62% during the pandemic, with the oldest teenage girls reporting the lowest life satisfaction values during COVID-19 restrictions.[27] During the school shutdown for COVID-19, 21% of boys and 27% of girls reported an increase in family arguments.[26] Combine all of these reports with decreasing access to mental health services owing to pandemic restrictions and it becomes a complicated matter for parents to address their children's mental health needs as well as their educational needs.[28]

A study conducted in Norway measured aspects of socialization and mood changes in adolescents during the pandemic. The opportunity for prosocial action was rated on a scale of 1 (not at all) to 6 (very much) based on how well certain phrases applied to them, for example, "I comforted a friend yesterday," "Yesterday I did my best to care for a friend," and "Yesterday I sent a message to a friend." They also ranked mood by rating items on a scale of 1 (not at all) to 5 (very well) as items reflected their mood.[29] They found that adolescents showed an overall decrease in empathic concern and opportunity for prosocial actions, as well as a decrease in mood ratings during the pandemic.[29]

A survey of 24,155 residents of Michigan projected an escalation of suicide risk for lesbian, gay, bisexual, transgender youth as well as those youth questioning their sexual orientation (LGBTQ) associated with increased social isolation. There was also a 66% increase in domestic violence for LGBTQ youth during shelter in place.[30] LGBTQ youth are yet another example of those already at increased risk having disproportionate effects of the pandemic.

Increased social media use during COVID-19, along with traditional forms of education moving to digital platforms, has led to the majority of adolescents spending significantly more time in front of screens. Excessive screen time is well-known to be associated with poor sleep, sedentary habits, mental health problems, and physical health issues.[31] With decreased access to physical activity, especially in crowded inner-city areas, and increased dependence on screen time for schooling, it is more difficult to craft easy solutions to the screen time issue.

During these times, it is more important than ever for pediatricians to check in on the mental health of patients with queries about how school is going, how patients are keeping contact with peers, and how are they processing social issues related to violence. Queries to families about the need for assistance with food insecurity, housing insecurity, and access to mental health services are necessary during this time of public emergency.

MEDICAL SCHOOL AND COVID-19

Although medical school is an adult schooling experience, it affects not only the medical profession and our junior colleagues, but, by extrapolation, all education that requires hands-on experience or interning, and has been included for those reasons.

In the new COVID-19 era, medical schools have been forced to make drastic and quick changes to multiple levels of their curriculum to ensure both student and patient safety during the pandemic. Students entering their clinical rotations have had the most drastic alteration to their experience.

COVID-19 has led to some of the same changes high schools and colleges have adopted, specifically, replacement of large in-person lectures with small group activities small group discussion and virtual lectures.[32] The transition to an online format for medical education has been rapid and impacted both students and faculty.[33,34] In a survey by Singh and colleagues,[33] of the 192 students reporting 43.9% found online lectures to be poorer than physical classrooms during the pandemic. In another report by Shahrvini and colleagues,[35] of 104 students surveyed, 74.5% students felt disconnected from their medical school and their peers and 43.3% felt that they were unprepared for their clerkships. Although there are no pre-COVID-19 data for comparison, it is expected that the COVID-19 changes will lead to increased insecurity and feelings of poor preparation for clinical work.

Gross anatomy is a well-established tradition within the medical school curriculum and one that is conducted almost entirely in person and in close quarters around a cadaver. Harmon and colleagues[36] surveyed 67 gross anatomy educators and found that 8% were still holding in-person sessions and 34 ± 43% transitioned to using cadaver images and dissecting videos that could be accessed through the Internet.

Many third- and fourth-year medical students have seen periods of cancellation for clinical rotations and supplementation with online learning, telemedicine, or virtual rounds owing to the COVID-19 pandemic.[37] A study from Shahrvini and colleagues[38] found that an unofficial document from Reddit (a widely used social network platform with a subgroup for medical students and residents) reported that 75% of medical schools had canceled clinical activities for third- and fourth-year students for some part of 2020. In another survey by Harries and colleagues,[39] of the 741 students who responded, 93.7% were not involved in clinical rotations with in-person patient contact. The reactions of students varied, with 75.8% admitting to agreeing with the decision, 34.7% feeling guilty, and 27.0% feeling relieved.[39] In the same survey, 74.7% of students felt that their medical education had been disrupted, 84.1% said they felt increased anxiety, and 83.4% would accept the risk of COVID-19 infection if they were able to return to the clinical setting.[39]

Since the start of the pandemic, medical schools have had to find new and innovative ways to continue teaching and exposing students to clinical settings. The use of electronic conferencing services has been critical to continuing education. One approach has been to turn to online applications like Google Hangouts, which come at no cost and offer a wide variety of tools to form an integrative learning environment.[32,37,40] Schools have also adopted a hybrid model of teaching where lectures can be prerecorded then viewed by the student asynchronously on their own time followed by live virtual lectures where faculty can offer question-and-answer sessions related to the material. By offering this new format, students have been given more flexibility in terms of creating a schedule that suits their needs and may decrease stress.[37]

Although these changes can be a hurdle to students and faculty, it might prove to be beneficial for the future of medical training in some ways. Telemedicine is a growing field, and the American Medical Association and other programs have endorsed its value.[41] Telemedicine visits can still be used to take a history, conduct a basic visual physical examination, and build rapport, as well as performing other aspects of the clinical examination during a pandemic, and will continue to be useful for patients unable to attend regular visits at remote locations. Learning effectively now how to communicate professionally and carry out telemedicine visits may better prepare students for a future where telemedicine is an expectation and allow students to learn the limitations as well as the advantages of this modality.[41]

Pandemic changes have strongly impacted the process of college applications, medical school applications, and residency applications.[32] For US medical residencies, 72% of applicants will, if the pattern from 2016 to 2019 continues, move between states or countries.[42] This level of movement is increasingly dangerous given the spread of COVID-19 and the lack of currently accepted procedures to carry out such a mass migration safely. The same follows for medical schools and universities.

We need to accept and prepare for the fact that medial students as well as other learners who require in-person training may lack some skills when they enter their profession. These skills will have to be acquired during a later phase of training. We may have less skilled entry-level resident physicians and nurses in our hospitals and in other clinical professions as well.

SUMMARY

The COVID-19 pandemic has affected and will continue to affect the delivery of knowledge and skills at all levels of education. Although many children and adult learners will likely compensate for this interruption of traditional educational services and adapt to new modalities, some will struggle. The widening of the gap for those whose families cannot absorb the teaching and supervision of education required for in-home education because they lack the time and skills necessary are not addressed currently. The gap for those already at a disadvantage because of socioeconomic class, language, and special needs are most severely affected by the COVID-19 pandemic school closures and will have the hardest time compensating. As pediatricians, it is critical that we continue to check in with our young patients about how they are coping and what assistance we can guide them toward in our communities.

CLINICS CARE POINTS

- Learners and educators at all levels of education have been affected by COVID-19 restrictions with rapid adaptations to virtual learning platforms.

- The impact of COVID-19 on learners is not evenly distributed and children of racial minorities, those who live in poverty, those requiring special education, and children who speak English as a second language are more negatively affected by the need for remote learning.

- Math scores are more impacted than language arts scores by previous school closures and thus far by these shutdowns for COVID-19.

- Anxiety and depression have increased in children and particularly in adolescents as a result of COVID-19 itself and as a consequence of school changes.

- Pediatricians should regularly screen for unmet needs in their patients during the pandemic, such as food insecurity with the loss of school meals, an inability to adapt to remote learning and increased computer time, and heightened anxiety and depression as results of school changes.

DISCLOSURE

The authors have nothing to disclose.

REFERENCES

1. Harris D, Larsen M. The Effects of the New Orleans Post-Katrina Market-based School Reforms on Medium Term Student Outcomes. Education Research Alliance for New Orleans. New Orleans (LA): Tulane University; 2019. p. 160215. Available at: http://educationresearchalliancenola.org/files/publications/Harris-Larsen-Reform-Effects-2019-08-01.

2. Hansen D, Larden M. School year length and student performance: quasi experimental evidence. Social Sci Res Netw Paper 2011. https://doi.org/10.2139/ssrn.2269846.

3. Marcotte DE, Helmelt SW. Unscheduled school closings and student performance. Educ Finance Policy 2008;3(3):316–38.

4. Kuhfeld M, Soland J, Tarasawa B, et al. Projecting the potential impact of COVID-19 school closures on academic achievement. Educ Res 2020;49(8):549–65.

5. Kuhfeld M, Tarasawa B. The COVID-19 slide: what summer learning loss can tell us about the potential impact of school closures on student academic achievement. NWEA; 2020. ED609141.NWEA. Available at: eric.ed.gov/?id.

6. Wolfson JA, Leung CW. Food insecurity and COVID-19: disparities in early effects for US Adults. Nutrients 2020;12(6):1648.

7. Fegert JM, Vitiello B, Plener PL, et al. Challenges and burden of the coronavirus 2019 (COVID-19) pandemic for child and adolescent mental health: a narrative review to highlight clinical and research needs in the acute phase and the long return to normality. Child Adolesc Psychiatry Ment Health 2020;14:20.

8. Bobo E, Lin L, Acquaviva E, et al. How do children and adolescents with attention deficit hyperactivity disorder (ADHD) experience during the COVID-19 outbreak? Encephale 2020;46(3S).

9. Leeb RT, Price S, Sliwa S, et al. COVID-19 trends among school-aged children - United States, March 1-September 19, 2020. MMWR Morb Mortal Wkly Rep 2020; 69(39):1410–5.

10. Anderson S, Haeder S, Caseman K, et al. When adolescents are in school during COVID-19, coordination between school-based health centers and education is key. J Adolesc Health 2020;67(6):745–6.

11. Ruiz-Roso MB, de Carvalho Padilha P, Mantilla-Escalante DC, et al. Covid-19 confinement and changes of adolescent's dietary trends in Italy, Spain, Chile, Colombia and Brazil. Nutrients 2020;12(6):1807.

12. Ammar A, Brach M, Trabelsi K, et al. Effects of COVID-19 home confinement on eating behaviour and physical activity: results of the ECLB-COVID19 international online survey. Nutrients 2020;12(6):1583.

13. Yeomans M. Adverse effects of consuming high fat–sugar diets on cognition: Implications for understanding obesity. Proc Nutr Soc 2017;76(4):455–65.

14. Merrick MT, Ports KA, Ford DC, et al. Unpacking the impact of adverse childhood experiences on adult mental health. Child Abuse Negl 2017;69:10–9.

15. Singh S, Roy D, Sinha K, et al. Impact of COVID-19 and lockdown on mental health of children and adolescents: a narrative review with recommendations. Psychiatry Res 2020;293:113429.

16. Elkin F, Handel G. The child and society: the process of socialization. New York: Random House; 1972. The Child and Society: The Process of Socialization - Frederick Elkin, Gerald Handel - Google Books.

17. Keogh B. Celebrating PL 94-142: the education of All Handicapped Children Act of 1975. Issues Teach Educ Fall 2007;16(2):65–9.

18. United States Department of Education, Office of Special Education and Rehabilitative Services. History: twenty-five years of progress in educating children with disabilities through IDEA. Available at: http://www.ed.gov/policy/speced/leg/idea/history.pdf.

19. Spreat S. Chapter 10: behavioral treatments for children with ASDs. In: Reber M, editor. The autism Spectrum: Scientific Foundations and Treatment. Cambridge University Press; 2012. p. 239–57.

20. Cox DJ, Plavnick JB, Brodhead MT. A proposed process for risk mitigation during OID-19 pandemic. Behav Anal Pract 2020;13(2):299–305 (Behavior Analyst Certification Board.(2020) Ethics guidelines for ABA providers during COVID-19 pandemic. Available at: http://www.back.com/ethics-guidelines-for-aba-providers-during-covid-19-pandemic-2/.

21. Nicolson AC, Lazo-Pearson JF, Shandy J. ABA finding its heart during a pandemic: an exploration in social validity. Behav Anal Pract 2020;13:757–66.

22. Becker SP, Breaux R, Cusick C, et al. Remote learning during COVID-19: examining school practices, service continuation, and difficulties for adolescents with and without attention deficit hyperactivity disorder. J Adolesc Health 2020;67(6):769–77.

23. McGrath J. ADHD and COVID-19: current roadblocks and future opportunities. Ir J Psychol Med 2020;21:1–8.

24. Cortese S, Asherson P, Sonuga-Barke E, et al. ADHD management during the COVID-19 pandemic: guidance from the European ADHD Guidelines Group. Lancet Child Adolesc Health 2020;4(6):412–4.

25. Spinks-Franklin A. Available at: https://www.healthychildren.org/English/health-issues/conditions/COVID-19/Pages/ADHD-and-Learning-During-COVID-19.aspx. Accessed: January 27, 2021.

26. Liang L, Ren H, Cao R, et al. The effect of COVID-19 on youth mental health. Psychiatr Q 2020;91:841–52.

27. Soest TV, Bakken A, Pedersen W, et al. Life satisfaction among adolescents before and during the COVID-19 pandemic. Tidsskr Nor Laegeforen 2020;(10):140.
28. Lee J. Mental health effects of school closures during COVID-19 [published correction appears in Lancet Child Adolesc Health. 2020 Apr 17]. Lancet Child Adolesc Health 2020;4(6):421.
29. Van de Groep S, Zanolie K, Green KH, et al. A daily diary study on adolescents' mood, empathy, and prosocial behavior during the COVID-19 pandemic. PLoS One 2020;(10):15.
30. Edwards E, Janney CA, Mancuso A, et al. Preparing for the behavioral health impact of COVID-19 in Michigan. Curr Psychiatry Rep 2020;22(12):88.
31. Nagata JM, Abdel Magid HS, Gabriel KP. Screen time for children and adolescents during the COVID-19 pandemic. Obesity (Silver Spring) 2020;28:1582–3.
32. Rose S. Medical student education in the time of COVID-19. JAMA 2020;323(21): 2131–2.
33. Singh K, Srivastav S, Bhardwaj A, et al. Medical education during the COVID-19 pandemic: a single institution experience. Indian Pediatr 2020;57(7):678–9.
34. Wilcha RJ. Effectiveness of virtual medical teaching during the COVID-19 crisis: systematic review. JMIR Med Educ 2020;6(2):e20963.
35. Shahrvini B, Baxter SL, Coffey CS, et al. Pre-clinical remote undergraduate medical education during the COVID-19 pandemic: a survey study. Preprint Res Sq 2020;rs.3:rs-33870.
36. Harmon DJ, Attardi SM, Barremkala M, et al. An analysis of anatomy education before and during Covid-19: May-August 2020. Anat Sci Educ 2021;2:132–47.
37. Sandhu P, de Wolf M. The impact of COVID-19 on the undergraduate medical curriculum. Med Educ Online 2020;25(1):1764740.
38. Shahrvini B, Baxter SL, Coffey CS, et al. Pre-clinical remote undergraduate medical education during the COVID-19 pandemic: a survey study. BMC Med Educ 2021;21:13.
39. Harries AJ, Lee C, Jones L, et al. Effects of the COVID-19 pandemic on medical students: a multicenter quantitative study. BMC Med Educ 2021;21(1):14.
40. Moszkowicz D, Duboc H, Dubertret C, et al. Daily medical education for confined students during coronavirus disease 2019 pandemic: a simple videoconference solution. Clin Anat 2020;33(6):927–8.
41. Iancu AM, Kemp MT, Alam HB. Unmuting medical students' education: utilizing telemedicine during the COVID-19 pandemic and beyond. J Med Internet Res 2020;22(7):e19667.
42. Byrne LM, Holmboe ES, Combes JR, et al. From medical school to residency: transitions during the COVID-19 pandemic. J Grad Med Educ 2020;12(4): 507–11.

Impact of COVID-19 on Resettled Refugees

Micah Brickhill-Atkinson, Fern R. Hauck, MD, MS, FAAFP*

KEYWORDS

- COVID-19 • Refugees • Vulnerable populations • Health care access

KEY POINTS

- Refugees experience unique challenges during the COVID-19 pandemic, including suspension of resettlement.
- Other harms of COVID-19 that affect the population at large have intensified effects on refugees, such as economic and disease vulnerability, mental illness exacerbations, communication challenges, and educational disruption.
- The Society of Refugee Healthcare Providers published guidelines for assessing refugees' barriers to following COVID-19 preventive recommendations.
- Recent reports from refugee health care providers offer suggestions for mitigating pandemic-related harm, including communication, case management, and advocacy.

INTRODUCTION

The novel coronavirus SARS-CoV-2 (COVID-19) has infected nearly 13 million people and has caused more than 570,000 deaths globally.[1] As the pandemic creates new challenges for worldwide communities, the refugee crisis remains another of humanity's grave tragedies. Refugees displaced due to war, violence, and oppression number 21.3 million worldwide.[2] As of April 4, 2020, thirty-four countries with substantial refugee resettlement reported local COVID-19 transmission.[3] Statistical data about the impact of COVID-19 on this population is scarce,[4] but a growing body of literature reveals that bureaucracy, poverty, and discrimination have threatened the well-being of refugees during the pandemic.[2] COVID-19 has additionally highlighted barriers to accessing health care for refugees,[5] who stand foremost among the world's most vulnerable people. The United Nations 2030 Agenda for Sustainable Development contains a promise to ensure no one is left behind,[3] and COVID-19 will only be controlled when all populations are included in the response.[5] Current literature

This article previously appeared in *Primary Care: Clinics in Office Practice*, Volume 48, Issue 1, March 2021.
Department of Family Medicine, University of Virginia, PO Box 800729, Charlottesville, VA 22908-0729, USA
* Corresponding author.
E-mail address: frh8e@virginia.edu

2352-7986/22/© 2021 Elsevier Inc. All rights reserved.

highlights 6 themes of the refugee pandemic experience (**Table 1**) and elucidates techniques for assessing barriers and alleviating harms.

SUSPENSION OF RESETTLEMENT AND RELATED SERVICES

Case 1: A.N. is a 30-year-old man from Afghanistan. He arrived in the United States 1 year ago. Soon after, his marriage to an Afghan woman was finalized, and he was assured that his wife would follow him to the United States. Now, he reports significant anxiety after his wife's migration was delayed due to COVID-19. The couple was informed that reunification would be deferred for at least 6 months.

Kathleen Newland of the Migration Policy Institute aptly pronounces, "COVID-19 has been the greatest disruption to human movement since World War II."[6] On March 10, 2020, the International Organization for Migration and the United Nations High Commissioner for Refugees (UNHCR) suspended refugee resettlement in the wake of worldwide travel restrictions.[7] The hold was lifted on June 18, 2020, after 10,000 refugee migrations were deferred. Some travel restrictions remain in place and continue to delay life-saving departures for persecuted people.[8] In addition, downstream effects such as expiration of security checks and overseas health examinations postpone travel for months after the resumption of resettlement.[9] Displaced persons are at risk of persecution in their countries of origin, and families face prolonged separation. Precedents from Ebola and SARS show that travel bans additionally incite stigma for migrant communities already in host countries.[10] Suspensions tend to harm refugees without benefiting host countries because many migrants would travel from an unaffected country to a nation with already high case counts. According to a World Health Organization report in 2018, refugees are at a low risk of transferring communicable disease to the host population in general.[7]

Table 1
Impacts of COVID-19 on resettled and accepted refugees

Suspension of Resettlement and Related Services	• Prolonged persecution • Delayed reunification • Expiration of security and health checks • Modified resettlement assistance after arrival
Economic Hardship	• Disproportionate job loss • Difficulty accessing relief • Reduced support for overseas family members
Disease Vulnerability	• Overcrowded living conditions • Comorbidities • High risk occupations • Delayed care and public health measures
Mental Illness Exacerbations	• Higher need • Memories of forced isolation and hiding • Modified and reduced mental health services
Communication Challenges	• Need for linguistically appropriate information • Barriers to virtual communication
Pediatric Impacts	• Boredom and loss of daily structure • School closings

Newly arrived refugees also face reduced volunteer and public services during the pandemic.[7] Volunteers and staff may be quarantined or restricted by government mandates, which disturbs provision of resettlement resources.[2] For example, the International Rescue Committee (IRC) in Charlottesville, Virginia typically provides an orientation for refugees attending their first medical appointment. Staff members transport clients to the family medicine clinic and show them how to find the waiting room and register. COVID-19 restrictions do not allow such transportation or accompaniment, and refugees must navigate the unfamiliar health system alone (E. Uhlmann, MPH, personal communication, July 16, 2020).

ECONOMIC HARDSHIP

Case 2: M.K. is a 35-year-old single mother of four. She and her daughters arrived in the United States 2 years ago, and she began working as a hotel housekeeper. She lost her job during COVID-19 and has not found new employment. Her landlord comes to the apartment for rent, evoking tremendous anxiety. The family fears eviction as funds become scarce.

For resettled refugees, the impact of COVID-19 manifests in part through economic hardship. Migrant groups tend to fill difficult, low-paying occupations in their host countries.[4] In a study of 8 nations that house more than one-third of the world's refugee population, refugees were 60% more likely to lose jobs or income due to COVID-19 than the local population. About 60% worked in the most affected occupations, such as food services and retail, compared with 37% of the host population.[11] Low-income households have less ability to work remotely, which creates increased susceptibility to job loss amid the pandemic.[12] Refugees often carry the additional burden of sending money to family in their country of origin, so pandemic-related economic hardship reaches even further than those immediately affected by job loss.[6] Refugees also face barriers in accessing public services and safety nets. The Kovler Center Child Trauma Program (KCCTP), which serves refugee families in Chicago, recently noted that families frequently experienced job loss and struggled to access unemployment benefits.[13]

DISEASE VULNERABILITY

Case 3: N.D., her husband, and 5 children are refugees living in an apartment with 1 bathroom. Even prepandemic, sharing a bathroom caused problems such as constipation in one of the children due to withholding bowel movements. COVID-19 measures seem nearly impossible to the family in light of their crowded home.

COVID-19's disease burden is higher in low-income settings such as resettled refugee populations due to living conditions, comorbidities, high-risk jobs, and delayed care and public health measures. The London School of Hygiene and Tropical Medicine reports that large and multigenerational households are a major reason for the disproportionate impact.[12] Overcrowded housing confers an increased risk of contracting disease,[7] and refugees often live in conditions that make hygiene and distancing impossible.[5] Management of chronic illnesses, such as diabetes mellitus and human immunodeficiency virus (HIV), is especially challenging among refugee populations during the pandemic.[14] Patients may be afraid to leave the house and may not be able to access prescriptions or appointments.

Endale and colleagues[13] propose that refugees are disproportionately affected by COVID-19 due to the frequency of high-risk jobs. For example, a high proportion of African refugees in the United States fill nursing home caretaker roles, which places them in one of the most vulnerable settings.[15] Low-income families are disincentivized from infection control measures, such as staying home from work, because their livelihoods are stretched too far.[12]

Refugees are vulnerable to stigma about disease transmission, which may make them fearful to disclose symptoms.[15] They may also delay seeking care due to fears of contagion or loss of legal protection.[10] In addition, widespread testing and contact tracing are less feasible in low-income settings; therefore, the current extent of disease is likely underestimated.[12]

MENTAL ILLNESS EXACERBATIONS

Case 4: S.A. is a 25-year-old female refugee with depression, anxiety, and posttraumatic stress disorder (PTSD) who presents to clinic with a chief concern of "stomach pain." During the interview, she becomes tearful as she describes increased nightmares and feeling hopeless when she thinks of her family members still in her country of exit. She fears leaving her apartment and contracting COVID-19, which evokes memories of forced hiding in her childhood.

Mental health is a chief concern among refugees during both pre- and post-pandemic circumstances. Systematic reviews estimate prevalences of up to 44% for anxiety, 44% for depression, and 36% for PTSD.[2] Migrants are more vulnerable to mental health risks in pandemics than the host population.[13] A 2020 literature review of international journals examined factors that worsen refugee mental health and found substantial commonality with risk factors for COVID-19.[2] Overlapping themes included overcrowding; disrupted sewage disposal; lower standards of hygiene; poor nutrition; reduced sanitation; and lack of shelter, health care, public services, and safety.[2] Boredom, isolation, inadequate supplies, lack of information, financial concerns, and disease-related stigma exacerbate the psychosocial effects of pandemics and quarantine.[13] Isolation and lack of control, prominent conditions in the COVID-19 setting, are known to exacerbate PTSD. Memories of forced hiding may be evoked by lockdowns and empty streets, and the pandemic may be reminiscent of Ebola and cholera for African migrants.[15]

Host countries face overloaded mental health care at baseline, making them ill equipped to adequately care for the pandemic-induced exacerbations among refugees.[2] Community-based mental health resources have moved to remote operations, making access even more difficult.[13] Baseline shortages combined with the exacerbating factors of a pandemic set up an environment for crisis among refugee mental health patients.

COMMUNICATION CHALLENGES

Case 5: D.N. is a 30-year-old female refugee from Afghanistan who recently arrived to the United States. She has a history of domestic abuse and fled her husband's family with her 3 children. In the few months since her arrival, she presented to clinic four times with vague somatic concerns, anxiety, and depressed mood. She was offered telephone therapy, as the clinic had paused in-person counseling sessions due to the health system's COVID-19 precautions. However, she is reluctant to share her traumatic experiences over the phone and reports little benefit from these sessions. She asks if she can instead participate in in-person therapy, where she would feel more comfortable discussing her trauma history.

Communication is a particular challenge for refugee patients in the pandemic setting. Lau and colleagues remind providers that communication is especially important for displaced populations who distrust authorities because of past experiences.[10] One challenge arises in accessible information sharing. Refugees struggle to find culturally and linguistically appropriate data about COVID-19.[7] Obstacles also present in the arena of telecommunication. The KCCTP noted the following barriers to refugee telemedicine: computer and Internet access; technological proficiency; attention span; decreased speed of interpretation; and privacy concerns.[13] Shared living conditions and unstable housing make private virtual communication difficult for many families. Providers at the Boston Center for Refugee Health and Human Rights (BCRHHR) noted that patients were sometimes unwilling to share trauma or torture histories over phone or video.[15] Although the host population may rely on virtual information sharing, refugees face added barriers in accessing these alterative communication modalities.

PEDIATRIC IMPACTS

Case 6: C.K. and M.K. are 7-year-old twins who arrived to the United States 1 year ago. In clinic, it is noted that they speak and understand little English. Their mother relates that they cannot read in any language. They do not speak English at home, and they did not attend school the past 4 months due to closings.

Pediatric refugees' daily functioning has suffered during COVID-19, attributable to boredom, isolation, and loss of daily structure.[13] IRC Medical Case Manager Erica Uhlmann in Charlottesville, Virginia notes a pattern of refugee parents overprotecting their children and prohibiting them from going outside. The IRC and partnering medical providers are educating families that time outside is safe and healthy as long as social distance is maintained (E. Uhlmann, MPH, personal communication, July 16, 2020).

School closings detrimentally affect refugee children. A systematic review of factors influencing pediatric refugee mental health found that schooling is essential for their adaptation and positive mental health. A sense of belonging at school is associated with lower PTSD and higher self-esteem, whereas lack of school attendance correlates with externalizing behavior. Poor connectedness with a school increases risk of depression, anxiety, and somatic stress.[16] Schools also provide a vital role in language acquisition for recently resettled children. Refugee students of all ages learn academic English in 4 to 7 years under ideal circumstances, but the interval increases to 10 years with interruptions to formal education. Schools maintain an indispensable role for educating migrant students and reducing achievement disparities.[17] Although distance learning may be accessible for some students, limited technological proficiency among refugee families poses a barrier to remote schooling.[13] The isolating conditions created by COVID-19 may have devastating impacts on pediatric refugee health and development.

TECHNIQUES TO ASSESS BARRIERS

The Society of Refugee Healthcare Providers issued guidelines to assess resettled refugees' barriers to following COVID-19 preventive behaviors. These include questions about fear of stigma or discrimination (eg, How have others in your community acted toward those who have become sick?); disease understanding (eg, Can you tell me about the symptoms of COVID-19?); how the patient communicates with providers and accesses information (eg, Before the pandemic, how did you normally communicate with your health care provider?); difficulties with prevention recommendations (eg, Do you have face masks, soap, hand sanitizer, etc.?); barriers to health care (eg, Do you know where to go for COVID-19 testing?); and social support (eg, Is there someone you can call if you need assistance with groceries, medications, or other essential needs if you become sick?).[18] The full assessment is available in **Box 1**.

TECHNIQUES TO MITIGATE HARMS

Refugee providers have published recommendations for reducing the harms of COVID-19. The BCRHHR issued the following suggestions: provide weekly email blasts about available community resources; watch for PTSD reemerging out of remission; remain mindful of patients' tolerance and attention span in telehealth sessions and consider shorter sessions if needed; maintain flexibility with in-person visits if patients are uncomfortable over the phone, especially patients who dissociate; and know the area's concrete food bank, unemployment, and shelter resources.[15]

The KCCTP offered the following resources to migrant families: exercise videos; guided relaxation and meditation; educational activities; caregiver guides; peer group video calls; virtual storybook readings; and cognitive behavioral therapy. The organization also initiated a response termed "Psychological First Aid." The approach started with information dissemination, dedicating attention to language accessibility. Next, providers turned their focus to active outreach, extensive case management, and telemedicine services.[13] The University of Virginia International Family Medicine Clinic similarly prioritized information dissemination and mailed handouts from the Centers for Disease Control and Prevention (CDC) to families in their first languages (Fern R. Hauck, MD, MS, personal communication, July 21, 2020). Multilingual print resources from the CDC can be found at the following Web address: https://wwwn.cdc.gov/pubs/other-languages. The UNHCR found that digital communication techniques are also useful for sharing information with refugees.[2]

Fawad and colleagues discuss the unique challenges of refugee chronic disease management in a pandemic.[14] The 2009 H1N1 influenza outbreak demonstrated the need for contingency planning in chronic disease management; deaths from stroke, myocardial infarction, and acute heart failure increased in this epidemic setting. Providers may consider extended medication supplies, especially for heart disease, HIV, tuberculosis, and contraception.[10]

Policy-level mitigation can also help alleviate harms for refugees during COVID-19. For example, public health leaders in the United Kingdom call for temporary citizenship rights for all migrant groups.[4] The UNHCR recommends full health care service access for refugees, reminding leaders that protecting all members ultimately shields the community at large.[10] The Center for Global Development advocates for fast-track credentialing of refugees who could contribute to the nation's health response or assist with personal protective equipment manufacturing, contact tracing, and delivery services. Allocating COVID-19 relief money to local nongovernmental organizations is another strategy to meet refugee needs. Currently, only 0.07% of US COVID-19 relief funds reach these nonprofit agencies that have a record of effective local community service.[11]

Local and national leaders, providers, and neighbors can also mitigate harm by maintaining a posture of openness and trust. Lessons from Ebola and SARS offer reminders that engaging communities and building trust contribute to the achievement of public health measures, whereas stigmatization opposes success. Transparency, trust, and community partnership are essential for disease control.[10]

Box 1
Society of Refugee Healthcare Providers Guide to Assessing Barriers to Following COVID-19 Prevention Guidance Among Resettled Refugees

Patient Communication
1. Before the COVID-19 pandemic, how did you normally communicate with your health care provider?
2. Did you use an interpreter to communicate with your health care provider?
3. What is your preferred method of communication with health care providers? (eg, email, telephone, text messaging, mailed letter, direct provider interaction)
   a. *If text message, mail, email, or telephone:* do you have anyone who can interpret (verbal) or translate (nonverbal, ie, documents) for you if needed? If so, is it a professional interpreter, community member, friend, or family member?
   b. *If the interpreter was a community member, friend, or family:* have you felt fear or embarrassment when someone other than a professional interpreter was used to discuss health conditions?
4. How do you access information about COVID-19? (eg, Internet, television, newspaper, friends, social group, faith-based group, social media such as WhatsApp, TikTok)

Patient Understanding of COVID-19
1. Can you tell me about the symptoms of COVID-19?
2. Can you tell me about some health complications of COVID-19?
3. How do you protect yourself from getting sick with COVID-19?
4. How do you prevent family members and others from getting sick with COVID-19?
5. How would you normally treat *[list symptoms that are currently associated with COVID-19]*:
   a. Fever?
   b. Dry Cough?
   c. Fatigue?
   d. Headache?
   e. Aches and pains?
   f. Sore throat?
   g. Chest pain?
   h. Difficulty breathing or shortness of breath?

Fear of Stigma or Discrimination
1. Do you know anyone in your community who has either become sick with COVID-19 or tested positive for COVID-19?
2. How have others in your community acted toward those who have become sick?
3. Would you communicate with someone who was diagnosed with COVID-19? If so, how? When would you resume meeting the person face-to-face?

Barriers to Following COVID-19 Prevention Recommendations
1. Is there any person in your home who can help with household responsibilities if you were to become sick? *[this is primarily asked to persons living with others, such as adults and children]*.
2. If someone in your house was to get sick with COVID-19, do you have a way to keep a six feet distance from other household members within your house?
3. Are you or anyone else in your household currently working?
   a. If yes:
      i. where are you/they working?
      ii. what information has your/their employer provided?
      iii. what steps have your/their employer taken to keep you and your family safe?
      iv. If you or someone in your household were to become sick with COVID-19, do you think you would be able to miss work until you or your family member feel better and a medical professional said it was safe for you to go back to work?
   b. If no one in the household is currently working, what support are you receiving financially?
4. Do you have access to:
   a. Face masks and gloves?
   b. Soap and/or hand sanitizer?

    c. Household cleaners and disinfectants?
    d. Enough dishware, eating utensils, clothes, towels, and bedding for sick and healthy family members?
    e. Essential needs such as a food, medications, and basic amenities (eg, electricity)?

Barriers to Health Care Access
1. Do you know where to go to receive testing for COVID-19? If yes, how did you find out about the testing site?
2. Do you know where to go to receive health care for COVID-19?
3. How would you get to a health care facility if you were sick and needed to see a health care provider?
4. Can you describe when you would feel you need to call 911? Are you comfortable calling 911?
5. Do you have health insurance that can help support your health care needs if you get sick?
6. Is there any reason that would prevent you from seeking care if you become sick?

Available Social Support
1. Is there someone you can call to support you (and/or your family) if you become sick? If you need to go to the emergency room?
2. Do you think this person can continue to assist you if you were diagnosed with COVID-19?
3. Is there someone you can call if you need assistance with groceries, medications, laundry and/or other essential needs while you are sick?
4. Do you think this person can continue to assist you if you were diagnosed with COVID-19?

From Guide to Assessing Barriers to Following COVID-19 Prevention Guidance Among Resettled Refugees. New York: Society of Refugee Healthcare Providers; 2020. License: CC BY-NC-SA 4.0.; with permission.

SUMMARY

The novel coronavirus SARS-CoV-2 poses singular challenges to the world's resettled refugee population. Suspension of resettlement prolongs suffering for refugees accepted but not yet relocated and delays family reunification, and modified resettlement agency operations create challenges for new arrivals. Refugees are particularly vulnerable to both economic hardship and severe disease in the wake of the pandemic. Mental illnesses, prevalent among this population at baseline, are exacerbated by isolative and uncertain conditions. Communication challenges make the virtual world less accessible to resettled refugees, and children suffer the consequences of boredom and loss of school resources. Refugee providers can mitigate harms by comprehensively assessing barriers faced by their patients, providing accessible information, and advocating for policies that include vulnerable populations and promote trust.

CLINICS CARE POINTS

- Implement questions from the Society for Refugee Healthcare Providers Guide to assess refugee patients' needs during the pandemic.
- Watch for PTSD reemergence and other mental illness exacerbations.
- Review local resources to enable concrete recommendations for refugees and all patients in need during the challenging pandemic conditions.
- Offer linguistically appropriate information about COVID-19 and preventive measures.

ACKNOWLEDGMENTS

Special thanks to Erica Uhlmann, International Rescue Committee Charlottesville Medical Case Manager.

DISCLOSURE

The authors have nothing to disclose.

REFERENCES

1. World Health Organization. Coronavirus disease (COVID-19) Situation Report – 176. 2020. Available at: https://www.who.int/docs/default-source/coronaviruse/situation-reports/20200714-covid-19-sitrep-176.pdf. Accessed July 14, 2020.
2. Júnior JG, Sales JPD, Moreira MM, et al. A crisis within the crisis: The mental health situation of refugees in the world during the 2019 coronavirus (2019-nCoV) outbreak. Psychiatry Res 2020;288:113000. Available at: https://www.ncbi.nlm.nih.gov/pmc/articles/PMC7156944/. Accessed July 16, 2020.
3. The Lancet. COVID-19 will not leave behind refugees and migrants. Lancet 2020; 395(10230):1090.
4. Bhopal RS. COVID-19: Immense necessity and challenges in meeting the needs of minorities, especially asylum seekers and undocumented migrants. Public Health 2020;182:161–2.
5. Orcutt M, Patel P, Burns R, et al. Global call to action for inclusion of migrants and refugees in the COVID-19 response. Lancet 2020;395(10235):1482–3.
6. Newland K. Lost in transition. Science 2020;368(6489):343.
7. Kluge HHP, Jakab Z, Bartovic J, et al. Refugee and migrant health in the COVID-19 response. Lancet 2020;395(10232):1237–9.
8. Joint Statement: UN refugee chief Grandi and IOM's Vitorino announce resumption of resettlement travel for refugees. United Nations High Commissioner for Refugees website. 2020. Available at: https://www.unhcr.org/en-us/news/press/2020/6/5eeb85be4/joint-statement-un-refugee-chief-grandi-ioms-vitorino-announce-resumption.html. Accessed July 16, 2020.
9. Bhattacharya CB, Fisher B. Refugee Assistance During a Global Pandemic. *Sustaining Sustainability.* 2020. Available at: https://soundcloud.com/user-148611772/episode-12-refugee-assistance-during-a-global-pandemic-with-betsy-fisher. Accessed July 14, 2020.
10. Lau LS, Sarmari G, Moresky RT, et al. COVID-19 in humanitarian settings and lessons learned from past epidemics. Nat Med 2020;26:647–8.
11. Dempster H, Ginn T, Graham J, et al. Locked Down and Left Behind: The Impact of COVID-19 on Refugees' Economic Inclusion. Center for Global Development, Refugees International, and International Rescue Committee. 2020. Available at: https://www.refugeesinternational.org/reports/2020/7/6/locked-down-and-left-behind-the-impact-of-covid-19-on-refugees-economic-inclusion. Accessed July 16, 2020.
12. Dahab M, van Zandvoort K, Flasche S, et al. COVID-19 control in low-income settings and displaced populations: what can realistically be done? London School of Hygiene and Tropical Medicine website. 2020. Available at: https://www.lshtm.ac.uk/newsevents/news/2020/covid-19-control-low-income-settings-and-displaced-populations-what-can. Accessed July 16, 2020.
13. Endale T, Jean NS, Birman D. COVID-19 and refugee and immigrant youth: A community-based mental health perspective. Psychol Trauma 2020;12(S1):

S225–7. Available at: https://europepmc.org/article/med/32478552. Accessed July 16, 2020.

14. Fawad M, Rawashdeh F, Parmar PK, et al. Simple ideas to mitigate the impacts of the COVID-19 epidemic on refugees with chronic diseases. Confl Health 2020;14: 23. Available at: https://www.ncbi.nlm.nih.gov/pmc/articles/PMC7201387/. Accessed July 16, 2020.

15. Mattar S, Piwowarczyk LA. COVID-19 and U.S.-based refugee populations: Commentary. Psychol Trauma 2020;12(S1):S228–9. Available at: https://europepmc.org/article/med/32538665. Accessed July 16, 2020.

16. Fazel M, Reed RV, Panter-Brick C, et al. Mental health of displaced and refugee children resettled in high-income countries: risk and protective factors. Lancet 2012;379:266–82.

17. McNeely CA, Morland L, Doty SB, et al. How schools can promote healthy development for newly arrived immigrant and refugee adolescents: Research priorities. J Sch Health 2017;87(2):121–32.

18. Society of Refugee Healthcare Providers. Guide to Assessing Barriers to Following COVID-19 Prevention Guidance Among Resettled Refugees. 2020. Available at: http://refugeesociety.org/wp-content/uploads/2020/04/Guide-Assessing-Barriers-COVID-19-SRHP-June2020.pdf. Accessed July 16, 2020.

Delivering Holistic Transgender and Nonbinary Care in the Age of Telemedicine and COVID-19

Reflections and Implications for Best Practices

Henry Ng, MD, MPH[a,b,]*, Lyndsay Zimmerman, BSN[a],
Bailey Ferguson, MBA[a], Elizabeth Dimmock, MSN[a,c],
Richard Harlan, MD[a,d], James Hekman, MD[a,e], Hiba Obeid, MD[a,e]

KEYWORDS

- Transgender • Nonbinary • Primary care • Care navigation • Telehealth
- Gender affirmation care • Social determinants of health

KEY POINTS

- Describe the authors' process for providing affirming health care for transgender and nonbinary people.
- Describe the authors' experiences with telehealth to help facilitate care delivery for transgender and nonbinary people.
- Review some best practices and resources in delivering care for transgender and nonbinary people.

INTRODUCTION

Transgender people have a gender identity that does not align with the sex they were assigned at birth. The number of transgender people in the United States is not exactly known because many vital statistics and official records, including the United States Census, do not record gender identity. Studies estimate the number of transgender people in the United States to be between 1 million and 1.4 million adult Americans.[1,2] Younger adults are more likely to identify as transgender or nonbinary and approximately 2% of high school students self-identify as transgender in a 2017 national

This article previously appeared in *Primary Care: Clinics in Office Practice*, Volume 48, Issue 2, June 2021.

[a] Center for LGBTQ+ Health, Cleveland Clinic Foundation, 14601 Detroit Avenue, Lakewood, OH 44107, USA; [b] Internal Medicine & Geriatrics, Primary Care Pediatrics, Cleveland Clinic Community Care, Cleveland, Ohio, USA; [c] Internal Medicine, Cleveland Clinic Community Care, Cleveland, Ohio, USA; [d] Obstetrics, Gynecology & Women's Health Institute, Cleveland Clinic Foundation, Cleveland, Ohio, USA; [e] Internal Medicine & Geriatrics, Cleveland Clinic Community Care, Cleveland, Ohio, USA
* Corresponding author.
E-mail addresses: henry.ng.md@gmail.com; ngh@ccf.org

2352-7986/22/© 2021 Elsevier Inc. All rights reserved.

survey.[3] For primary care health professionals, changing patient demographics necessitate both clinical competence and cultural fluency in working with transgender and nonbinary (TGNB) patients. To better serve diverse patients and communities, health professionals need to be aware of the health concerns and challenges facing TGNB people, familiarize themselves with best practices and models of care in serving TGNB patients, and have awareness of the environmental factors that can affect health outcomes for TGNB people. In this article, the authors discuss health concerns facing TGNB communities, address clinical and environmental factors that have an impact on TGNB care, examine best practices that promote optimal health outcomes for TGNB people, and share their experiences in developing tools to provide affirming and respective care for TGNB people.

HEALTH CONCERNS, DISPARITIES, AND BARRIERS TO CARE FOR TRANSGENDER AND NONBINARY PEOPLE

In 2011, the Institute of Medicine published "The Health of Lesbian, Gay, Bisexual, and Transgender People: Building a Foundation for Better Understanding." This report was among the first to comprehensively assess the health needs and gaps for sexual and gender minority people in the United States.[4] Poor health outcomes and health care discrimination experienced by TGNB people have been documented in the 2015 US Transgender Survey, where respondents reported that in the 12 months before the survey nearly 1 in 4 respondents had problems with health insurance coverage because they were transgender, 55% of respondents were denied coverage for transition-related surgery, 33% of respondents had a negative experience with a health care provider/system, and 23% of survey respondents avoided seeing a doctor when needed due to fear of being mistreated for being transgender.[5]

In the United States and globally, health concerns and disparities affecting transgender people have focused on mental health, sexual and reproductive health, substance use, violence and victimization, stigma/discrimination, and a variety of general health topics (eg, mortality, hormone use, metabolic syndrome, diabetes, and cancer).[6] A 2016 systematic review of preventive health services for transgender patients found that a majority of studies discussed human immunodeficiency virus (HIV) rates or risk behaviors, whereas few studies mentioned tobacco abuse, cholesterol screening or cardiovascular health, or pelvic examinations. No studies reported addressed mammography or chest/breast tissue examinations, colorectal cancer screening, or vaccination against influenza.[7]

In addition to stigma and experiences of discrimination, TGNB people face barriers to accessing care for general health as well as gender affirmation care, with a lack of providers with expertise contributing the most to restricting health care access.[8] Some health professionals, however, have indicated a desire to improve their ability to care for and treat transgender patients and address knowledge gaps.[9,10] Although education and training in transgender health are outside the scope of this article, tools and resources have been developed in conjunction with models of care that can help health professionals augment their clinical knowledge and hone skills to better care for TGNB patients.

CARE GUIDELINES FOR TRANSGENDER AND NONBINARY PEOPLE

Several guidelines, frameworks, and recommendations[11–17] have been developed that address various aspects of TGNB care. These guidelines are summarized in **Table 1**. Guidelines vary in their scope and content but address health concerns in primary care, gender-affirming hormonal therapy (GAHT), reproductive health and

Table 1
Organizational gender affirmation care guidelines and recommendations

Organization	Year	Title (Citation)	Description (from Web Page/Abstract)
World Professional Association for Transgender Health	2011	Standards of Care, Version 7[11]	Standards of Care, Version 7, provides clinical guidance for health professionals to assist transsexual, transgender, and gender nonconforming people.
Endocrine Society	2017	Endocrine Treatment of Gender-Dysphoric/ Gender-Incongruent Persons: An Endocrine Society Clinical Practice Guideline[12]	The 2017 guideline on endocrine treatment of gender dysphoric/gender incongruent persons
University of California, San Francisco Transgender Care	2016	Guidelines for the Primary and Gender affirmation care of Transgender and Gender Nonbinary People[13]	Guidelines were developed to complement the existing World Professional Association for Transgender Health Standards of Care and the Endocrine Society guidelines in that they are specifically designed for implementation in everyday evidence-based primary care, including settings with limited resources.
The Fenway Institute, Fenway Health	2015	Comprehensive transgender healthcare: the gender affirming clinical and public health model of Fenway Health[14]	This report describes the evolution of a Boston community health center's multidisciplinary model of transgender health care, research, education, and dissemination of best practices.
American College of Obstetricians and Gynecologists	2011	Health Care for Transgender Individuals. Committee Opinion No. 512[15]	This committee opinion provides guidance and recommendations for the health care of transgender individuals.
American College of Obstetricians and Gynecologists	2017	Care for Transgender Adolescents. Committee Opinion No. 685[16]	This committee opinion reflects recommendations for care of transgender adolescents based on the emerging clinical and scientific advances in transgender health.

(continued on next page)

			Description (from Web
Organization	Year	Title (Citation)	Page/Abstract)
TransLine	2019	TransLine Gender Affirming Hormone Therapy Prescriber Guidelines[17]	National standardized guideline of best practices in hormonal therapy provision as a reference to achieve uniformity for the Transgender Medical Consultation Service.

Table 1
(continued)

fertility, contraception, sexual health and HIV prevention, mental health, aging, and adolescent health.

Additionally, recent books and articles on TGNB health describe not only how to deliver comprehensive primary and gender affirmation care to TGNB people[18–22] but also the importance of including cancer surveillance,[23–26] the fertility concerns of transgender patients,[27] pregnancy in transgender men,[28–30] mental health,[31,32] recognizing the effects of self-prescribed gender affirmation care[33–35] as well as HIV care[36] and social determinants of health.[37,38] These resources are presented in **Table 2**. A full discussion of the role of patient-centered communication,[39] Lesbian, Gay, Bisexual, Transgender, Queer/Questioning (LGBTQ)-affirming clinical environments,[40] legal resources for name changes,[41] and sexual orientation and gender identity (SOGI) data in electronic health records (EHRs)[42] falls outside the framework for this article, but the importance of each of these elements is recognized in establishing and maintaining relationships of trust with TGNB patients, especially at their initial point of contact.

DELIVERING TRANSGENDER AND NONBINARY–AFFIRMING PRIMARY CARE AND HORMONAL CARE: THE AUTHORS' EXPERIENCES

In March 2020, the authors' updated the patient intake process for TGNB people with a goal of "meeting patients where they are" amid the COVID-19 pandemic for safe, inclusive, and streamlined care. As patients call to schedule their initial visit for gender-affirming care, a scheduler administers a scheduling questionnaire in the EHR, prompting the call to be transferred to the Center for LGBTQ+ Care clinic coordinator. The coordinator identifies what services the patient is requesting and connects them to the appropriate service accordingly. If medical gender affirmation care is requested, the patient's information is routed to the medical team patient navigator (PN) in the EHR.

The PN contacts the patient to complete registration and demographic information in the EHR, including the "name the patient goes by" (a term the authors' group feels is more affirming than using "preferred name") and their pronouns, assists with activating an EHR patient portal account, and sends a code of conduct electronically for the patient to review and agree to. If a patient lacks health insurance coverage or has out-of-network insurance, the PN assists in linking the patient to a patient financial advocate to identify potential assistance program resources. Once completed, the PN schedules an in-person or telehealth visit with a provider based on the patient's preference. Additionally, the PN assures each patient has transportation to the appointment and offers to arrange through the patient's insurance or local agencies if needed.

Table 2
Selected clinical articles and resources

Care Domain	Title (Citation)	Authors	Year	Description
General/primary care	Comprehensive Care of the Transgender Patient, 1st Edition[18]	Ferrando CA	2020	A multidisciplinary resource on transgender health care and surgery covering many aspects of transgender health care, including epidemiology and history, mental health services, endocrine and hormone therapy treatment, and surgical options
	Care of the Transgender Patient[19]	Safer JD et al.	2019	Guide published by the American College of Physicians to assist primary care and family medicine physicians in caring for transgender patients
	Caring for Transgender and Gender-Diverse Persons: What Clinicians Should Know[20]	Klein DA et al.	2018	The article describes key information clinicians should know when caring for transgender and gender-diverse persons.
	Best Practices in LGBT Care: A Guide for Primary Care Physicians[21]	McNamara M and Ng H	2016	This article reviews some best practices for health screening and care for LGBT people.
	Trans Bodies, Trans Selves[22]	Erickson-Schroth L (editor)	2014	Comprehensive guide and resource for TGNB people, written by TGNB people

(continued on next page)

Table 2
(continued)

Care Domain	Title (Citation)	Authors	Year	Description
Cancer surveillance	Female-to-male patients have high prevalence of unsatisfactory Paps compared to non-transgender females: implications for cervical cancer screening.[23]	Peitzmeier SM et al.	2014	Research article examining Pap tests results at an urban community health center demonstrating female-to-male patients had more unsatisfactory examinations
	Cancer in Transgender People: Evidence and Methodological Considerations[24]	Braun H et al.	2017	Comprehensive review of cancer epidemiology in TGNB people
	Breast cancer risk in transgender people receiving hormone treatment: nationwide cohort study in the Netherlands[25]	de Blok Christel JM et al.	2019	Retrospective cohort study on breast cancer incidence and characteristics among transgender people in the Netherlands
	Cancer Screening for Transgender and Gender Diverse Patients[26]	Grimstad F et al.	2020	Review of sex-trait related cancer risks and screening guidelines in transgender and gender-diverse populations

Category	Title	Author	Year	Description
Reproductive/sexual health and fertility	From Erasure to Opportunity: A Qualitative Study of the Experiences of Transgender Men Around Pregnancy and Recommendations for Providers[28]	Hoffkling A et al.	2017	Exploratory qualitative study on the experiences of transgender men around pregnancy
	Fertility Concerns of the Transgender Patient[27]	Cheng PJ et al.	2019	Review article describing the fertility issues and concerns transgender people face
	Transgender men and Pregnancy[29]	Obedin-Maliver J and Makadon H	2016	Commentary providing guidance to clinicians caring for transgender men or gender nonconforming people who are contemplating, carrying or have completed a pregnancy
	Family Planning and Contraception Use in Transgender men[30]	Light A et al.	2018	Exploratory study describing current contraceptive practices and fertility desires of transgender men during and after transitioning
Mental health	Transgender Mental Health[31]	Erickson-Schroth L and Carmel T	2016	Guest editorial for a special issue of Psychiatric Annals addressing mental health concerns for transgender people
	Gender Dysphoria in Adults: An Overview and Primer for Psychiatrists[32]	Byne W et al.	2018	White paper describing the diagnostic nosology, epidemiology, gender development, mental health assessment, differential diagnosis, treatment and referral for gender-affirming somatic treatments in adults with gender dysphoria

(continued on next page)

Table 2
(continued)

Care Domain	Title (Citation)	Authors	Year	Description
Gender-affirming hormonal therapy self-care	Structural Inequities and Social Networks Impact Hormone Use and Misuse Among Transgender Women in Los Angeles County[33]	Clark K et al.	2018	Quantitative study examining associations between medically monitored hormone use, hormone misuse, structural inequities and social dynamics in a cohort of transgender women
	Nonprescribed Hormone Use and Self-Performed Surgeries: "Do-It-Yourself" Transitions in Transgender Communities in Ontario, Canada[34]	Rotondi NK et al.	2013	Case series describing nonprescribed hormone use and self-performed surgeries among a cohort of transgender adults
	Tranitioning Bodies: The Case of Self-Prescribing Sexual Hormones in Gender Affirmation in Individuals Attending Psychiatric Services[35]	Metatasio A et al.	2018	Case series describing transgender and gender nonconforming individuals self-prescribing and self-administration of hormones without medical; consultation
Social determinants of care	Barriers and Facilitators to Engagement and Retention in Care Among Transgender Women Living With Human Immunodeficiency Virus[36]	Sevelius JM et al.	2014	Qualitative study examining culturally unique barriers and facilitators to engagement and retention in HIV care among transgender women
	A Preliminary Assessment of Selected Social Determinants of Health in a Sample of Transgender and Gender Nonconforming Individuals in Puerto Rico[37]	Martinez-Velez JJ et al.	2019	Survey study using a community-based participatory research approach exploring social determinants of health affecting a cohort of transgender and gender nonconforming adults
	Social Determinants of Discrimination and Access to Health Care Among Transgender Women in Oregon[38]	Garcia J and Crosby RA	2020	Qualitative study exploring social determinants affecting patients' access to gender affirmation care

An intake form then is sent via the patient's EHR portal to complete the collection of SOGI data, health history, and specifically the patient's experience of gender, goals of care, and thoughts around fertility, contraception, and creating families. The form is presented in Appendix 1. The authors' electronic questionnaire is used with the philosophy of respectful inquiry when inquiring about potentially sensitive topics, such as sexuality and gender identity. If the intake is not completed, the patient is reminded that this helps tailor their plan of care to the patient's goals while maintaining safety. Once the intake by the PN is completed, patients are contacted by a support resource nurse (SRN) to complete a clinical intake, including determination of specific clinical care needs, clarify and set expectations for the upcoming appointment, and assess the need for laboratory testing and referrals. Patients also are provided the opportunity for referrals at that time for routine gynecologic care and cancer prevention as well as counseling for fertility preservation and referral of fertility services, according to recommendations by the American College of Obstetricians and Gynecologists.[15,16]

Patients are seen by caregivers, who are nurse practitioners, physician assistants, and physicians with formal training and years of clinical experience with gender affirmation care. Other learners and trainees also may participate in the patient's care with their permission. Initial visits often are performed via telehealth with video or Zoom-supported calls or telephone calls, where the provider reviews the patient's goals for the visit and ongoing clinical care, their existing care team, their health and anatomic inventory, their gender experience and gender care goals, and family planning, fertility, and reproductive health needs. The authors' patients, like many, have performed many hours of their own review of available online resources about transgender care. These resources range from care paths described by academic centers and health centers focused on TGNB care to subreddit forum posts and YouTube videos of TGNB people sharing their experiences with their gender affirmation care. Due to many barriers to care, TGNB communities often turn to social media as self-serve resource for medical knowledge.[43] The caregivers recognize the importance of affirming patients' use of e-health, a concept of using technology to improve the quality of health care, to explore gender on their road to self-discovery.[44] As described by Eysenbach,[44] the authors' team strives to address several of the "10 e's in "e-health"' including empowering TGNB patients' understanding of their care through an exchange of ideas around evidence-based interventions and shared decision making.

Informed consent for initiation or continuation of gender affirmation care is reviewed with patients and referrals to health services, such as mental health support and fertility preservation specialists, are made as appropriate. Hormonal care is initiated after patients have completed a physical examination and laboratory testing and have had a thorough discussion of the nuances of gender affirmation care, including microdosing (the use of hormonal treatments at doses lower than that of typical standard starting doses), medication administration, and insurance coverage in addition to reviewing the partially and completely irreversible effects of hormonal medications. The authors offer hormonal treatments like those described by TransLine Gender Affirming Hormone Therapy Guidelines.[17]

Sometimes, patients presenting for gender affirmation care may have unclear goals of care, medical, psychological, or other factors that may have an impact on their successful gender care and transition. In those instances, the authors review those patients in a multidisciplinary and interprofessional team meeting to determine the next steps of care to address a patient's gender care needs while promoting their well-being and safety. **Fig. 1** summarizes the care navigation process and steps employed to provide patients affirming care at the authors' center.

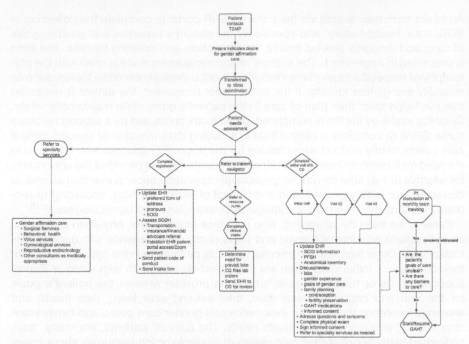

Fig. 1. Patient care navigation for gender affirmation care. CG, caregiver—doctor of medicine/doctor of osteopathic medicine/nurse practitioner/physician assistant; EHR, electronic health record; GAHT, gender affirmation hormonal therapy; PFSH, past medical history, family history, and social history; Pt, patient; SODH, social determinants of health; SOGI, sexual orientation & gender identity; TSMP, transgender surgery and medicine program.

The authors' caregivers serve as gender specialists and/or the primary care providers for TGNB patients who come to the authors' program. As patients progress through their gender affirmation care, they are offered referrals to subspecialty care in the hospital system, including behavioral health, medical specialty, surgical specialty, and gender-confirming surgical care. An interprofessional team is used to help patients achieve their care goals. For example, if patients are prescribed injectable hormonal therapies, they can meet with the SRN for education on injection technique and can contact her for follow-up questions or concerns, including medication coverage assistance. Another example of interprofessional teamwork is collaboration with clinical pharmacy. The caregivers work closely with a dedicated clinical pharmacist with prescribing authority for tobacco cessation treatment who assists with tobacco cessation medication management. Tobacco cessation is important not only for patients' cardiovascular and pulmonary health but also for those who seek eventual gender-affirming surgeries for optimal postsurgical healing. Finally, the navigation process utilizes the EHR to assess social determinants of health for each patient (insurance status, resource limitations, and so forth) and to identify and remove barriers to care.

DISCUSSION

Since implementing revised intake process, 166 patients have had contact with the authors' PN and SRN. Feedback on the process has been positive with patients who have shared that the act of asking them for the name they go by and their pronouns can have a profound effect on their experience. Many patients the authors have encountered shared that this was the first medical office to ask them these questions and expressed gratitude toward acts of inclusion. Additional feedback from patients has expressed that having a common caregiver, such as the SRN at primary care, and specialty visits, such as gynecology, have aided in providing them a sense of security and shared rapport in the team-based approach. The authors currently are exploring further opportunities to involve clinical pharmacy beyond tobacco cessation in the care of transgender patients. Pharmacists can have roles in TGNB care, including HIV prevention and treatment as well as helping patients and their families understand the medications used in gender affirmation care to anticipate and manage side effects.[45]

The SARS-CoV-2 pandemic has laid bare the disparities that TGNB people face in preserving and promoting their health. With limited personal and financial resources combined with the effects of institutional racism and transphobia, many TGNB patients continue to struggle to overcome structural barriers and microaggressions in their daily health care encounters. For optimal clinical outcomes, patient engagement, and trust-building, clinicians need to be aware of intersectional identities and how discrimination, real and perceived, negatively affects their patients, especially transgender people of color.[46] In addition to streamlining and creating affirming care navigation and using evidence-based care guidelines, telehealth has become an important tool to reach and better care for TGNB people. In 2020, the Centers for Medicare & Medicaid temporarily expanded coverage for telehealth services, which included reimbursement for diagnoses other than those related to COVID-19 infection, waiving or reducing cost-sharing for telehealth visits, lifting geographic restrictions that patients must be located in a rural area, and allowing providers licensed in one state to see patients in another state. Like many other health organizations, the authors' center has embraced telehealth to connect patients to health care professionals for all kinds of care, including GAHT services. Telehealth has become a vital part of the authors' approach to reduce and eliminate barriers to care for TGNB people, and future research is planned to measure the impact of these methods in improving health outcomes and care experiences for TGNB patients.

CLINICS CARE POINTS

- When working with TGNB patients, addressing patients by the name they go by and their pronouns helps create a welcoming clinical environment.

- Health care providers caring for TGNB patients should utilize evidence-based recommendations for transgender-inclusive primary care and gender affirmation care.

- Telehealth can be used to help reduce the anxiety and burden faced by TGNB patients who seek gender affirmation care, especially for those who reside away from urban centers.

- TGNB people face multiple barriers to care at the interpersonal, institutional, and policy levels. Health organizations serving TGNB people should help their patients navigate health care systems and barriers related to social determinants of health.

- Interprofessional and multidisciplinary approaches to gender affirmation care can promote patient satisfaction and help patients achieve their individual care goals.

ACKNOWLEDGMENTS

This scholarly work could not have been done without the leadership and efforts of our program's progenitor, Dr Cecile Ferrando, the Medical Director for the Transgender

Surgery & Medicine Program at the Cleveland Clinic. Additionally, we are grateful for the technical expertise offered by Richard Dimmock who helped with refining the figures shared in this article.

DISCLOSURE

The authors have no commercial or financial conflicts of interest to disclose. There are no funding sources to disclose.

SUPPLEMENTARY DATA

Supplementary data related to this article can be found online at https://doi.org/10.1016/j.ccol.2021.12.010.

REFERENCES

1. Meerwijk EL, Sevelius JM. Transgender population size in the united states: a meta-regression of population-based probability samples. Am J Public Health 2017;107(2):e1–8.
2. Flores AR, Herman JL, Gates GJ, et al. How many adults identify as transgender in the United States? Los Angeles (CA): The Williams Institute; 2016.
3. Johns MM, Lowry R, Andrzejewski J, et al. Transgender identity and experiences of violence victimization, substance use, suicide risk, and sexual risk behaviors among high school students — 19 states and large urban school districts, 2017. MMWR Morb Mortal Wkly Rep 2019;68:67–71.
4. Institute of Medicine. The health of Lesbian, Gay, Bisexual, and transgender people: building a Foundation for better understanding. Washington, DC: The National Academies Press; 2011. https://doi.org/10.17226/13128.
5. James SE, Herman JL, Rankin S, et al. Executive summary of the report of the 2015 U.S. Transgender survey. Washington, DC: National Center for Transgender Equality; 2016.
6. Reisner SL, Poteat T, Keatley J, et al. Global health burden and needs of transgender populations: a review. Lancet 2016;388(10042):412–36.
7. Edmiston EK, Donald CA, Sattler AR, et al. Opportunities and gaps in primary care preventative health services for transgender patients: a systemic review. Transgend Health 2016;1(1):216–30.
8. Safer JD, Coleman E, Feldman J, et al. Barriers to healthcare for transgender individuals. Curr Opin Endocrinol Diabetes Obes 2016;23(2):168–71.
9. Shires DA, Stroumsa D, Jaffee KD, et al. Primary care clinicians' willingness to care for transgender patients. Ann Fam Med 2018;16(6):555–8.
10. Paradiso C, Lally RM. Nurse practitioner knowledge, attitudes, and beliefs when caring for transgender people. Transgend Health 2018;3(1):47–56.
11. Selvaggi G, Dhejne C, Landen M, et al. The 2011 WPATH standards of care and penile reconstruction in female-to-male transsexual individuals. Adv Urol 2012; 2012:581712.
12. Hembree WC, Cohen-Kettenis PT, Gooren L, et al. Endocrine treatment of gender-dysphoric/gender-incongruent persons: an endocrine society clinical practice guideline. J Clin Endocrinol Metab 2017;102(11):3869–903.
13. Deutsch MB, editor. UCSF Transgender Care, Department of Family and Community Medicine, University of California San Francisco. Guidelines for the Primary and Gender-Affirming Care of Transgender and Gender Nonbinary People. 2nd edition. Deutsch MB, ed; June 2016. Available at: transcare.ucsf.edu/guidelines.

14. Reisner SL, Bradford J, Hopwood R, et al. Comprehensive transgender health-care: the gender affirming clinical and public health model of Fenway Health. J Urban Health 2015;92(3):584–92.
15. Health care for transgender individuals. Committee Opinion No. 512. American College of Obstetricians and Gynecologists. Obstet Gynecol 2011;118:1454–8.
16. Care for transgender adolescents. Committee Opinion No. 685. American College of Obstetricians and Gynecologists. Obstet Gynecol 2017;129:e11–6.
17. Transline Gender Affirming Hormone Therapy Prescriber Guidelines. 2019. Available at: https://transline.zendesk.com/hc/en-us/articles/229373288-TransLine-Hormone-Therapy-Prescriber-Guidelines. Accessed August 27, 2020.
18. Ferrando CA. Comprehensive care of the transgender patient. Philadelphia, PA, USA: Elsevier; 2020. https://doi.org/10.1016/C2015-0-05870-1.
19. Safer JD, Tangpricha V. Care of the transgender patient. Ann Intern Med 2019; 171(1):ITC1–16.
20. Klein DA, Paradise SL, Goodwin ET. Caring for transgender and gender-diverse persons: what clinicians should know. Am Fam Physician 2018;98(11):645–53.
21. McNamara MC, Ng H. Best practices in LGBT care: A guide for primary care physicians. Cleve Clin J Med 2016;83(7):531–41.
22. Erickson-Schroth L, editor. Trans Bodies, Trans Selves: A Resource for the Transgender Community. New York, NY, USA: Oxford University Press; 2014.
23. Peitzmeier SM, Reisner SL, Harigopal P, et al. Female-to-male patients have high prevalence of unsatisfactory Paps compared to non-transgender females: implications for cervical cancer screening. J Gen Intern Med 2014;29(5):778–84.
24. Braun H, Nash R, Tangpricha V, et al. Cancer in Transgender People: Evidence and Methodological Considerations. Epidemiologic Rev 2017;39(1):93–107.
25. de Blok Christel JM, Wiepjes Chantal M, Nota Nienke M, et al. Breast cancer risk in transgender people receiving hormone treatment: nationwide cohort study in the Netherlands. BMJ 2019;365:l1652.
26. Grimstad F, Tulimat S, Stowell J. Cancer screening for transgender and gender diverse patients. Curr Obstet Gynecol Rep 2020;9:146–52.
27. Cheng PJ, Pastuszak AW, Myers JB, et al. Fertility concerns of the transgender patient. Transl Androl Urol 2019;8(3):209–18.
28. Hoffkling A, Obedin-Maliver J, Sevelius J. From erasure to opportunity: a qualitative study of the experiences of transgender men around pregnancy and recommendations for providers. BMC Pregnancy Childbirth 2017;17(Suppl 2):332.
29. Obedin-Maliver J, Makadon HJ. Transgender men and pregnancy. Obstet Med 2016;9(1):4–8.
30. Light A, Wang LF, Zeymo A, et al. Family planning and contraception use in transgender men. Contraception 2018;98(4):266–9.
31. Erickson-Schroth L, Carmel T. Transgender mental health. Psychiatr Ann 2016;46: 330–1.
32. Byne W, Karasic DH, Coleman E, et al. Gender dysphoria in adults: an overview and primer for psychiatrists. Transgend Health 2018;3(1):57–70.
33. Clark K, Fletcher JB, Holloway IW, et al. Structural inequities and social networks impact hormone use and misuse among transgender women in los angeles county. Arch Sex Behav 2018;47(4):953–62.
34. Rotondi NK, Bauer GR, Scanlon K, et al. Nonprescribed hormone use and self-performed surgeries: "do-it-yourself" transitions in transgender communities in Ontario, Canada [published correction appears in Am J Public Health. 2013 Nov;103(11):e11]. Am J Public Health 2013;103(10):1830–6.

35. Metastasio A, Negri A, Martinotti G, et al. Transitioning Bodies. The Case of Self-Prescribing Sexual Hormones in Gender Affirmation in Individuals Attending Psychiatric Services. Brain Sci 2018;8(5):88.
36. Sevelius JM, Patouhas E, Keatley JG, et al. Barriers and facilitators to engagement and retention in care among transgender women living with human immunodeficiency virus. Ann Behav Med 2014;47(1):5–16.
37. Martinez-Velez JJ, Melin K, Rodriguez-Diaz CE. A Preliminary Assessment of Selected Social Determinants of Health in a Sample of Transgender and Gender Nonconforming Individuals in Puerto Rico. Transgend Health 2019;4(1):9–17.
38. Garcia J, Crosby RA. Social Determinants of Discrimination and Access to Health Care Among Transgender Women in Oregon. Transgend Health 2020;225–33. https://doi.org/10.1089/trgh.2019.0090.
39. Ross KA, Castle Bell G. A Culture-Centered Approach to Improving Healthy Trans-Patient–Practitioner Communication: Recommendations for Practitioners Communicating with Trans Individuals. Health Commun 2017;32(6):730–40.
40. Keuroghlian AS, Ard KL, Makadon HJ. Advancing health equity for lesbian, gay, bisexual, and transgender (LGBT) people through sexual health education and LGBT-affirming health care environments. Sex Health 2017;14:119–22.
41. Hill BJ, Crosby R, Bouris A, et al. Exploring transgender legal name change as a potential structural intervention for mitigating social determinants of health among transgender women of color. Sex Res Social Policy 2018;15(1):25–33.
42. Burgess C, Kauth MR, Klemt C, et al. Evolving Sex and Gender in Electronic Health Records. Fed Pract 2019;36(6):271–7.
43. Blotner C, Rajunov M. Engaging transgender patients: using social media to inform medical practice and research in transgender health. Transgend Health 2018;3(1):225–8.
44. Eysenbach G. What is e-health? J Med Internet Res 2001;3(2):E20.
45. Redfern JS, Jann MW. The evolving role of pharmacists in transgender health care. Transgend Health 2019;118–30. https://doi.org/10.1089/trgh.2018.0038.
46. Howard SD, Lee KL, Nathan AG, et al. Healthcare experiences of transgender people of color. J Gen Intern Med 2019;34:2068–74.

Blood Banking and Transfusion Medicine Challenges During the COVID-19 Pandemic

Andy Ngo, MD, Debra Masel, MT, (ASCP) SBB, Christine Cahill, RN, MS, Neil Blumberg, MD, Majed A. Refaai, MD*

KEYWORDS

- COVID-19 • Blood banking • Transfusion medicine • Blood shortage
- Blood wastage • FDA donation policies • Convalescent plasma

KEY POINTS

- COVID-19 has had a negative impact on blood collection.
- The Centers for Disease Control, blood centers, and American Red Cross have developed new policies to protect donors and the blood supply.
- Blood management has become more important with decreasing supply as well as management of blood bank personnel.
- Convalescent plasma, although touted as a possible treatment, has limited literature on its efficacy.

INTRODUCTION

Within 3 months of the first diagnosed case, the outbreak of acute respiratory disease caused by the novel coronavirus (SARS-CoV-2), also known as COVID-19, rapidly grew into a global pandemic. The eruption of this virus, reportedly, may have been linked to a seafood and wildlife market in Wuhan, Hubei Province, China.[1,2] Person-to-person spread is thought to occur via respiratory droplet contact (≤6 feet), skin contacts, and even the transmission through air while speaking. Despite the extraordinary universal attempts to limit the spread of this virus, new cases are diagnosed on a daily basis throughout the world and have dramatically affected, among other health care disciplines, the blood bank and transfusion medicine. Because of the growing prevalence and highly infectious nature of COVID-19, new policies and guidelines

This article previously appeared in *Clinics in Laboratory Medicine*, Volume 40, Issue 4, December 2020.
Department of Pathology and Laboratory Medicine, Transfusion Medicine Unit, University of Rochester, Strong Memorial Hospital - Blood Bank, 601 Elmwood Avenue, Box 608, Rochester, NY 14642, USA
* Corresponding author.
E-mail address: Majed_Refaai@URMC.Rochester.edu

Clinics Collections 12 (2022) 143–157
https://doi.org/10.1016/j.ccol.2021.12.011
2352-7986/22/
© 2021 Elsevier Inc. All rights reserved.

have started to develop in transfusion medicine practices. In this article the authors address the myriad of ways that COVID-19 has affected blood banking and transfusion medicine, including the safety of both blood donors and blood product recipients, the management and distribution of blood products during a pandemic, and the use of blood product–derived therapeutics.

CLINICAL MANIFESTATIONS OF COVID-19

Common symptoms of COVID-19 infection, which typically appear within 2 to 14 days after exposure, include fever, sore throat, cough, shortness of breath, chills, muscle pain, headache, and sensory changes such as loss of smell or taste. Nausea, vomiting, diarrhea, skin rash, delirium, and dizziness have also been reported.[3,4] In advanced cases, mild-to-severe lower respiratory tract infection can be seen and may progress to critical status, as a result of the cytokine storm, requiring intubation and mechanical ventilation. Acute respiratory failure and a widespread thromboembolic disease are also common in these critical cases.[5,6] However, conservative estimates of 30% to as high as 96% of infected individuals may manifest mild to no symptoms, posing huge challenges in containing this pandemic crisis and protecting blood donors.[7]

In one of the earlier studies of COVID-19 patients, Guan and colleagues[8] reported that in addition to the usual viral route of respiratory droplets, the virus could be transmitted by saliva, urine, and stool.[9] Extracted data of 1099 patients with laboratory-confirmed COVID-19–related acute respiratory distress syndrome (ARDS) showed a predominant male gender (58%), median age of 47 years with most common symptoms of fever (88%) and cough (68%). The median incubation period was found to be 3 days with a range of 0 to 24 days. Only 1.2% of patients reported to have a direct contact with wildlife and 31% had been to Wuhan city, whereas the majority (72%) had contact with people from Wuhan city. At time of admission, ground-glass opacity was the typical (56.4%) radiological finding on chest computed tomography (CT). Interestingly, a significant number of severe cases were diagnosed by clinical symptoms and real-time reverse transcriptase polymerase chain reaction (RT-PCR) with normal radiological findings. Multivariate analysis revealed that severe pneumonia was an independent factor associated with either intensive care unit (ICU) admission, mechanical ventilation, or death (hazard ratio, 9.80; 95% confidence interval, 4.06–23.67).[8]

COVID-19 DIAGNOSIS

Ideally, testing every blood donor for COVID-19 would be the best practice; however, at least for the time being, this task cannot realistically be accomplished. To date, 7 recognized types of coronavirus strains that can infect humans have been identified, including *Alpha coronavirus* (229E and NL63) and *Beta coronavirus* (OC43 and HKU1). The rare but more severe types are called MERS-CoV, which lead to Middle East respiratory syndrome (MERS), and SARS-CoV, responsible for severe acute respiratory syndrome (SARS) endemic.[10]

Laboratory confirmation of COVID-19 infection is based on detection of unique sequences of viral RNA by RT-PCR. Sputum samples provide better detection than throat samples, whereas lower respiratory tract samples are superior to those from the upper respiratory tract.[11] The presence of SARS-CoV-2 RNA in the blood is a marker of severe illness based on 113 studies.[12] Additional laboratory findings in COVID-19 infection include lymphopenia (83%); neutrophilia; and elevated levels of serum alanine aminotransferase, aspartate aminotransferase, lactate dehydrogenase, C-reactive protein (CRP), ferritin, and D-dimer.[13] Substantial increase in CRP, ferritin, and D-dimer levels were found to be associated with severe infection.[14] In addition, significant association has been recognized between lymphopenia and high levels of D-dimer with mortality.[15,16]

Bilateral air-space consolidation is typically seen on chest radiograph; however, findings may be unremarkable early in the disease. Chest CT images usually demonstrate bilateral, peripheral ground glass opacities, which is nonspecific to COVID-19 infection.

MANAGEMENT OF COVID-19

An effective COVID-19 vaccine would be the ultimate solution for all of the concerns surrounding blood bank industry. However, currently there is no vaccine available to protect against SARS-CoV-2. Likewise, no prophylactic therapy has yet been proved to be effective in patients who have been exposed to SARS-CoV-2 nor a clearly successful treatment of those who develop the infection.[17] Patients who are confirmed positive for COVID-19 and present with mild symptoms are usually managed by self-isolation at home for up to 14 days, which is also the minimal deferral period recommended by many blood centers.[7-10] In advanced cases, hospitalization may be required for clinical observation and supportive management with fluid and oxygen resuscitations, anticoagulation, empirical antibiotics in case of a secondary infection, and nonsteroidal antiinflammatory agents in some cases. Critical cases may require ICU admission for possible intubation and mechanical ventilation. Corticosteroids and immunosuppressive agents are usually not recommended except when required for other indications or in a cytokine storm. Extracorporeal membrane oxygenation can be considered but is associated with a high mortality rate.

Complications of COVID-19 infection include pneumonia, respiratory failure, ARDS, sepsis and septic shock, cardiomyopathy and arrhythmia, acute kidney injury, bacterial infections, thromboembolism, gastrointestinal bleeding, polyneuropathy, and death.

The only means we have for reducing infection in the general population and protecting blood donors relies on recommended infection control. Measures, such as proper hand and environmental hygiene, and appropriate use of personal protective equipment along with maintaining the social distancing (at least 6 feet) are necessary to prevent COVID-19 spreading. Early detection, triage, and isolation of potentially infectious patients are also important considerations. A combination of these measures is the basis of current blood donation protocols, which will hopefully protect and maintain our blood supply.

BLOOD DONATION AND BLOOD PRODUCTS

There are multiple Federal Drug Administration (FDA) criteria a blood donor must meet before donating blood products. These parameters range from physical requirements, such as age, weight, temperature, blood pressure, and pulse, to a background check of the donor's sexual, medical, and travel history. Any discrepancies or issues that arise during the interview process and the physical examination could temporarily or permanently defer the donor from the blood donation system.[18]

Following the start of the COVID-19 outbreak in the United States, additional screening questions and requirements were implemented. Although not standardized across all blood collection organizations, the American Red Cross implemented new deferral policies in February 2020 before regional and national shutdown. All donors with a recent travel history to China, Hong Kong, Macau, Iran, Italy, and South Korea were deferred for 28 days. Donors diagnosed or suspected to have COVID-19 or had contact with a COVID-19–positive patient were also deferred for 28 days despite the absence of any data or evidence as of yet that SARS-CoV-2 can be transmitted through blood products.[19]

Several measures were adopted by all blood donation centers and blood drives to prevent transmission of SARS-CoV-2. Measures included temperature screening for all donors and staff before entry into the donation centers, social distancing (>6 feet) when possible, disinfecting machines and surfaces between donations, having donors and staff wear face masks, use of hand sanitizer before and during the donation process, and increased spacing between beds. These preventative practices echoed the Centers of Disease Control (CDC) guidelines and were similarly implemented in other blood donation centers.[20–23]

As these policies were put into place, blood donations began to decrease as the COVID-19 pandemic grew and blood drive cancellation increased. Regionally, one of the hospitals affected was University of Washington Medical Center, which reported a blood supply shortfall as early as February 29, 2020.[24] Nationally blood collections dropped and in a press release by the American Red Cross on March 17, 2020, approximately 2700 Red Cross blood drives were canceled across the country, resulting in 86,000 fewer donations. Evidently, more than 80% of their usual blood supply comes from these blood drives.[25] Of note, as per the American Association of Blood Banks (AABB), 33,000 units of blood are needed daily to meet patient need before the pandemic.[26]

As a result, hospitals needed to develop strategies to adapt to these blood supply shortages. Mitigation strategies that were proposed included additional criteria for transfusion orders review with more stringent guidelines. Splitting platelet units into 2 doses each were also considered to minimize platelet shortage. Hospitals increasingly adopted these measures over the course of a few weeks starting in March 2020.[27]

On April 2, 2020, the FDA issued new blood donation guidance to address the need for blood and blood components. They no longer required collections to be discarded due to errors in vital signs or donation intervals and added a 72-hour window to allow a donor to respond to questions about eligibility and component suitability.[28] The FDA changed deferral guidelines and a previous guidance that deferred many donors for up to 12 months due to various reasons was revised to a deferral of 3 months (**Table 1**).[29] In addition, donors who were previously permanently deferred between 1980 to 1986 due to spending more than 3 months in specified European countries were allowed to be reconsidered for donation. Exceptions and alternatives were also issued under 21 CFR 640.120(b) to address blood and blood component shortages.[30]

Concurrently, the CDC and Centers for Medicare and Medicaid Services recommended rescheduling elective surgeries as needed and shifting elective urgent inpatient surgical procedures to outpatient settings when feasible. The American College of Surgeons similarly recommended the same guidelines.[31] They stated surgeries should be reviewed with "a plan to minimize, postpone, or cancel electively scheduled operations, endoscopies, or other invasive procedures."[32] These policies were initiated by hospitals such as University of Washington Medical Center where elective surgeries and procedures were postponed starting March 7, 2020. During that time, blood usage and blood demand reached parity at Washington Medical Center.[24] This decrease in elective surgery was echoed in many hospitals, with one report citing a 71.7% decrease in surgical volume.[33]

Nationally, elective surgery cancellation and blood mitigation strategies became ubiquitous as seen by the AABB survey. The week of March 23, 2020, most of the hospitals reported they were no longer performing elective surgeries, with only 10.6% of

Table 1	
Updated blood collection policies and Federal Drug Administration regulatory changes	
New Screening Measures and Changes	**Deferral**
Persons who traveled in COVID-19 endemic areas [a] Persons diagnosed with COVID-19, contact with people with the virus, and those suspected of having it [a]	14–28 d[a]
For male donors who would have been deferred for having sex with another man For female donors who would have been deferred for having sex with a man who had sex with another man For those with recent tattoos and piercings For those who have traveled to malaria-endemic areas (and are residents of malaria nonendemic countries): the agency is changing the recommended deferral period from 12 to 3 mo. In addition, the guidance provides notice of an alternate procedure that permits the collection of blood and blood components from such donors without a deferral period, provided the blood components are pathogen-reduced using an FDA-approved pathogen reduction device.	From 12 mo to 3 mo
For those who spent time in certain European countries or on military bases in Europe who were previously considered to have been exposed to a potential risk of transmission of Creutzfeldt-Jakob disease or variant Creutzfeldt-Jakob disease, the agency is eliminating the recommended deferrals and is recommending allowing reentry of these donors.	From indefinite deferral to no deferral

[a] Policy of various blood centers.[20–23]
Data from Refs.[19–23,29]

hospitals still conducting elective surgeries.[34] Blood usage mitigation techniques as mentioned earlier became more prevalent.[27] In fact, blood wastage increased the following week, March 30th, with 25% of hospitals reporting increased blood wastage due to cancellation of elective surgeries and nonurgent medical procedures.[35] Wastage peaked the week of May 4 at 54% and the subsequent week, May 11, decreased to 52% as many hospitals started to resume elective procedures (**Fig. 1**).[36,37]

PATIENT BLOOD MANAGEMENT DURING COVID-19 PANDEMIC
General Principles

Blood transfusion is considered one of the most common hospital procedures performed in the United States. The safety of blood products and the appropriateness of transfusion are significant and timely issues. Over the last 3 decades, studies have shown that transfusion of one red blood cell (RBC) unit increases wound complications by 4%, hospital length of stay (LOS) by 1.5 days, and mortality by 0.9%.[38–40] In nonbleeding patients, restricting blood transfusions by using a hemoglobin trigger of less than 7 g/dL significantly reduces cardiac events, rebleeding, bacterial infections, and total mortality.[41] Other blood components carry similar risks. Plasma is frequently misused, and its benefits are overestimated particularly in nonbleeding patients. In a retrospective cohort study, Warner and colleagues[42] found that prophylactic administration of plasma in the critically ill was not associated with improved clinical outcomes. Similar studies on prophylactic preprocedure platelet transfusion showed an increase in risk of thrombosis and mortality.[43]

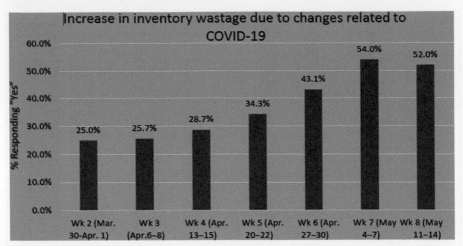

Fig. 1. As elective surgical cases were canceled and blood utilization decreased in much of the United States, a trend of increased wastages was seen. (*From* AABB. COVID-19 weekly hospital transfusion services survey: week 8 snapshot. Available at: http://www.aabb.org/research/hemovigilance/bloodsurvey/Docs/AABB-COVID-19-Impact-Survey-Snapshot-Week-8.pdf.)

Patient blood management (PBM) is a multidisciplinary, evidence-based strategy in which the need for blood products is managed in order to provide better patient outcomes and appropriate stewardship of a limited resource while reducing health care costs (**Table 2**). The primary goal of PBM program is to ensure optimal decision support using evidence-based guidelines and transfusing the most appropriate blood products with a minimum dose required for the clinical situation.[44] In addition, pharmaceutical products such as desmopressin and antifibrinolytics (such as Amicar or Tranexamic acid) have been shown to reduce bleeding.[45–48] Prothrombin complex concentrates and vitamin K may also be effective in warfarin reversal and correcting international normalized ratio.[49–51] Iron supplements, oral or intravenous preparations, and erythropoiesis-stimulating agents are proved to be useful in repleting iron stores and thus increasing hemoglobin levels.[52] PBM and bloodless medicine programs is now a priority throughout national and international health systems (**Fig. 2**).[53] Hospitals and academic medical centers across the nation are beginning to develop bloodless medicine and PBM programs in response to the favorable evidence.

PATIENT BLOOD MANAGEMENT STRATEGIES USED IN COVID-19 PANDEMIC

During the 2020 COVID-19 pandemic, blood supply shortages were observed worldwide, including the United States. The major blood suppliers and hospitals across the country issued emergency pleas for donations and reports significant numbers of blood drives were canceled due to school and workplace closures, which resulted in thousands of fewer blood donations typically collected.[19] In Beijing, China during the 2003 SARS epidemic, blood products shortages necessitated importation of blood products from other Chinese provinces to supply needs for clinical use in patients.[54,55] Similarly, the COVID-19 pandemic has had a major ripple effect on the number of eligible blood donors, blood supply, and on blood safety.

Therefore, PBM strategies are imperative in order to manage shortages during natural disaster or disease pandemics as well as long-term socioeconomic effects

Table 2 University of Rochester Medical Center evidence-based transfusion guideline		
Product	Clinical Indication	Transfusion Trigger
Red blood cells	Anemia Anemia with acute coronary syndromes	Hct <21%; Hgb <7 g/dL Hct <24%; Hgb <8 g/dL
Platelets	High risk of bleeding Fever or sepsis Acute bleeding Intracranial hemorrhage Documented platelet dysfunction	Platelet count <10,000 Platelet count<20,000 Platelet count<50,000 Platelet count<100,000 Per platelet function test
Plasma	Urgent need for warfarin reversal Clinical coagulopathy Acute bleeding Plasma exchange for TTP Factor V or XI deficiency	INR >1.7 Based on relevant laboratory and TEG values To maintain the RBC to plasma ratio of our MTP
Cryoprecipitate	Low fibrinogen level Documented dysfibrinogenemia Uremic coagulopathy unresponsive to DDAVP Factor VIII deficiency	<150 and bleeding Clinically significant bleeding without obvious causation

Abbreviations: DDAVP, desmopressin; Hct, hematocrit; Hgb, hemoglobin; INR, international normalized ratio; MTP, massive transfusion policy; TEG, thromboelastography; TTP, thrombotic thrombocytopenic purpura.

following these crises. Implementation of the most recent evidence-supported transfusion guidelines and eliminating unnecessary transfusions are considered the main goals of PBM programs during major disasters. Some effective strategies are as follows:

- Evaluation of appropriateness of transfusion orders and further discussion with clinical team if needed.
- Use of other pharmaceutical products such as desmopressin, antifibrinolytics, vitamin K, prothrombin complex concentrates, or intravenous iron if appropriate.

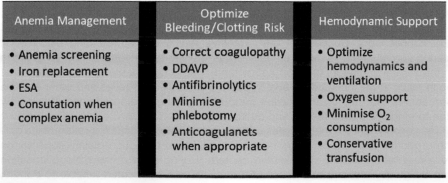

Anemia Management	Optimize Bleeding/Clotting Risk	Hemodynamic Support
• Anemia screening • Iron replacement • ESA • Consutation when complex anemia	• Correct coagulopathy • DDAVP • Antifibrinolytics • Minimise phlebotomy • Anticoagulanets when appropriate	• Optimize hemodynamics and ventilation • Oxygen support • Minimise O$_2$ consumption • Conservative transfusion

Fig. 2. Patient blood management strategies.

- Blood-sparing strategies during surgery such as implementation of normovolemic or hemodilution measures or usage of cell salvage.
- Staff education and open communication is imperative.

CHALLENGES OF MANAGING RESUMPTION OF NORMAL HOSPITAL SURGICAL OCCUPANCY

Although the demand for blood products during the COVID-19 pandemic has decreased due to postponement of elective surgeries, hospitals must have an emergency blood management plan. This plan should be in place and ready to be implemented during and following any natural crisis in order to maintain sustainability of a safe blood supply. As hospitals resume elective surgery and see increases in non-COVID-19 admissions, long-term shortages beyond the pandemic peak persist. At this time, blood collection centers and donors are still required to avoid large gatherings and follow all safety measures. Thus, a significant blood supply shortage may be present beyond the pandemic peak. In addition, due to the prolonged incubation period (up to 14 days) of SARS-CoV-2 and the potential of asymptomatic carriers, recruitment of blood donors as well as maintaining safety in the blood collection process remains a major concern.

EFFECT OF COVID-19 PANDEMIC ON TRANSFUSION SERVICE AND BLOOD BANK OPERATIONS

Being prepared to face a pandemic ensures that blood products are available to those patients requiring transfusion support, and a robust plan helps to protect the safety and health of the transfusion service professionals needed to perform testing and prepare blood products.[56] The effects of any pandemic on transfusion service and blood bank operations are 2-fold the work force and the blood supply.

Although many employees were encouraged or required to work remotely during the COVID-19 pandemic, this is not an option for laboratory professionals working in an academic medical center transfusion service and blood bank. To provide necessary transfusion support and to prepare and modify blood products, blood bank employees must be physically present in the laboratory at all times. Thus, for employees' safety and to prevent the spread of infection, repeated cleaning and disinfection of the work environment should be undertaken in conjunction with universal masking of employees and meticulous handwashing. To promote social distancing, separating staff by off-setting shift hours across the operation will more evenly distribute the staff across a 24-hour period. Depending on the physical layout of the work area it may be possible to set up workstations in different areas of the laboratory so that the staff is physically separated from each other as much as possible. That being said, plans must be in place to continue operations if multiple staff members become infected and cannot work. Because of the extensive regulations surrounding blood bank testing and competency requirements, cross-training technologists from other areas in the clinical laboratory on short notice tends not to be a viable option. A plan must be in place at the institutional level to postpone elective surgeries and other elective procedures that rely on transfusion support if staffing levels become critically low due to employee absenteeism and quarantine.

The second concern that transfusion services and blood banks may experience during a pandemic is the blood products supply. Blood collection mainly depends on volunteer blood donors at collection centers. During such a crisis blood donation can be greatly reduced as a result of donors becoming infected, unable to donate, or avoiding public gatherings.[57] Several conservation options should be considered by the transfusion service in order to conserve a rapidly dwindling blood supply along with additional measures promoted by a PBM program, when available.

- The blood type of trauma patients should be determined as rapidly as possible so that transfusion can be performed using type-specific RBC, thereby conserving the supply of group "O" RBC, a universal donor type. Group "O−" RBC should be reserved for women of childbearing age (<50 years) and female children. All other group "O" individuals should receive group "O+" RBC.
- If platelet availability is constrained, units can be split into 2 doses. At the authors' facility they found that one-half unit of platelets is sufficient to provide clinical benefit to most patients. However, based on the patient's clinical condition, a full dose can be transfused if required.
- Because of decreased blood utilization as a result of elective procedures withholding, reducing standing orders and managing blood product standing orders with the blood supplier is essential to minimize waste, particularly in multisite hospital systems with transfusion services located at each hospital. Transferring RBC to the highest transfusion volume facility in the health care system could be an option as well to reduce wastage.
- Inventory levels of reagents and supplies must be closely monitored. The transfusion service must work closely with the supply chain to ensure that critical reagents and supplies are available throughout the pandemic to perform critical testing. This may involve placing orders to bring levels to a level sufficient to perform testing for 3 months or more if availability or delivery could potentially be a problem.
- To assist the blood supplier, facilities could host additional blood drives either at the facility itself (if there is sufficient room to ensure adequate social distancing) or supporting drives in a larger venue (such as a mall closed due to the pandemic or a government building not currently or minimally occupied).
- If the hospital blood bank is FDA registered or licensed, the collection of convalescent plasma could be undertaken to provide a possible course of treatment either alone or in combination with other treatments to infected patients.[58]

Although blood conservation measures may be necessary, there likely will be a decrease in demand for RBC resulting from canceling elective surgical procedures. In the COVID-19 pandemic a reduction in blood orders from our blood supplier reduced spending at our facility by approximately 50%. Blood bank serologic testing was reduced by approximately 30% during the same time period but without the associated decrease in budget due to the advanced purchase of reagents and supplies. Close monitoring of testing volumes, blood product purchases, and waste is important to determine how the pandemic will affect cost projections.

CONVALESCENT PLASMA
Blood-Based Therapeutics for COVID-19

Unlike other subspecialties in pathology and laboratory medicine, transfusion medicine/blood banking is almost exclusively focused on therapeutics, including hands on treatment of patients. Thus it is understandable that physicians, nurses, and medical technologists in this area of medicine have been focused on possible treatment approaches for COVID-19. In the absence of effective and safe antiviral treatments, the strategy of transfusing convalescent plasma has long attracted interest and has been used in treatment of infectious disease, most recently in viral diseases.[59] The interest is due to the abundant evidence that humoral immunity plays a role in resolution of viral infection and prevention of reinfection after primary infection or vaccination. Convalescent plasma has a long history but almost no quality evidence for its efficacy and safety, as its use has often been reserved for last ditch efforts in desperately ill patients. In addition, much of the history of its use antedates the recognition that randomized trials are needed for ultimate proof of efficacy and safety due to the highly variable course of many illnesses, including COVID-19.[60]

In the current pandemic, early case reports of convalescent plasma usage reported that some patients who were seriously ill, requiring ICU care and mechanical ventilation,[61] cleared virus more rapidly than expected and made sufficient recovery and shorter LOS. Thousands of units of plasma, almost all untested for antiviral neutralizing titers, have been transfused in the United States using FDA-approved emergency investigational new drug and expanded access protocols.[62] Many small randomized trials and a few larger multicenter trials are underway a few months into the epidemic in the United States. These include some trials in patients with critical illness, using primary endpoints for efficacy such as ability to be weaned from mechanical ventilation, discharge from hospital, and survival. Other trials target prevention of infection in exposed individuals or prevention of hospitalization in newly SARS-CoV-2 RNA–positive individuals with mild or moderate symptoms. In most cases, given the uncertainty of whether antibody is protective, no specific titer or neutralizing titer of antibody in the plasma is specified. In other trials, high titers of antibody are required (eg, reactive at >1:320). Donors must meet standard FDA and state safety requirements for blood donation and be either RNA negative or greater than 28 days past clinical recovery in order to donate.[63] Donation can be by manual plasmapheresis or machine apheresis, with the former considerably less efficient but less costly.

There are many unresolved issues concerning convalescent plasma efficacy and safety, for example,[59] does antibody clearance of virus lead to clinical improvement in moderately to severely ill patients?,[60] does antibody prevent clinical deterioration in recently infected, asymptomatic or mildly symptomatic patients?, and[61] are there mid- to longer-term consequences of transfusing allogeneic plasma? Many statements have been made that allogeneic plasma transfusion is a common therapy with only rare acute complications (acute lung injury, volume overload, hemolysis, anaphylaxis, etc.). However, recent observational literature in critically ill patients demonstrate that allogeneic plasma transfusion is associated with nosocomial bacterial infection,[64] organ failure, and thrombosis.[65] The role of transfusing ABO "compatible plasma," an accepted practice, in worsening the risk of bleeding,[66] infection/sepsis,[67] organ failure,[67] and mortality[66] is not proved, but transfusion of ABO compatible, but not identical, plasma is likely not immunologically neutral. Immune complexes between antibody and soluble antigen form after transfusion and, at least in model systems, can activate monocytes, interfere with platelet and coagulation factor function, and may injure endothelial cells.[68]

A likely more efficacious and safer product than convalescent plasma being considered for use in COVID-19 disease and its prevention is hyperimmune immunoglobulin G (IgG). Intravenous IgG (IVIgG) made from multiple donors with detectable titers of anti-SARS-CoV-2 antibody would be expected to be more potent and carry fewer risks than convalescent allogeneic plasma that has not been processed.[69] However, it will be many months before such products are routinely available and much less proven effective and safe in patients. One clear cut benefit of IVIgG is a reduced risk of some adverse immune effects (acute lung injury, hemolysis, organ failure) because no single donor is heavily represented. Infectious disease transmission, although uncommon, after plasma that has been tested for HIV, hepatitis C, etc. is in general not a risk with use of IVIgG preparations. Both convalescent plasma and hyperimmune IgG may carry risks of antibody enhancement of viral infection.[70]

Finally, although not a blood product, humanized monoclonals to proteins and glycoproteins that are necessary for viral entry and replication hold some promise as preventive and therapeutic strategies in COVID-19.

BLOOD SAFETY DURING COVID-19
Steps Taken to Protect Blood Supply

In general, blood donors must be healthy on the day of donation and meet existing FDA donor screening measures. Typically, these measures should prevent individuals with any respiratory symptoms or infection from donation. Donors are also instructed to contact the blood collection center if any signs or symptoms developed within the next few days of donation. The collected blood or blood components will then be discarded and any distributed products will be recalled. Nevertheless, to date no transfusion-transmitted COVID-19 cases have been reported.

RISK OF BLOOD PRODUCTS CONTAMINATION WITH COVID-19

Overall, respiratory viruses are not known to be transmitted via blood transfusions. Thus far, there are no reported cases of transfusion-transmitted COVID-19 nor any type of the other coronaviruses. As a precaution measure to the blood safety, particularly after the rapid increase in COVID-19 infection rates in China, Chang and colleagues[71] screened all donations collected at the Wuhan Blood Center over 2 months (January through March 2020). RT-PCR testing for SARS-CoV-2 RNA was performed on pools of 6 to 8 plasma samples. Out of the screened 2430 donations, one donor tested positive for SARS-CoV-2. This donor was positive for COVID-19 previously and was quarantined appropriately in a cabin hospital in Wuhan until 2 consecutive negative throat swab results 3 days apart were obtained. At the time of donation, the donor displayed no symptoms. However, his plasma SARS-CoV-2 was still detectable. Later on, in a retrospective testing of 4995 donations collected between December 2019 and January 2020, plasma samples of 3 more healthy donors from Wuhan were also found to be positive for SARS-CoV-2. However, specific IgG and IgM against SARS-CoV-2 by enzyme-linked immunosorbent assay were negative, indicating the possibility of infection in the early stage. The investigator concluded that because of the asymptomatic COVID-19 cases, screening donors for SARS-CoV-2 will be critical to ensure blood safety.

Hence, to date there are no FDA requirements in place to screen blood donors or test blood components for COVID-19. Individuals with COVID-19 infection do not meet the blood donation guidelines.

DISCLOSURE

Dr. Majed A. Refaai has received consulting fees and/or research funding from CSL Behring, Octapharma, Bayer, Instrumentation Laboratory, and iLine microsystems and has received speaking fees from CSL Behring. The other Authors have nothing to disclose.

REFERENCES

1. Wu F, Zhao S, Yu B, et al. A new coronavirus associated with human respiratory disease in China. Nature 2020;579(7798):265–9.

2. Paules CI, Marston HD, Fauci AS. Coronavirus infections—more than just the common cold. JAMA 2020;323(8):707–8.
3. Sultan S, Altayar O, Siddique SM, et al. AGA Institute rapid review of the gastro-intestinal and liver manifestations of COVID-19, meta-analysis of international data, and recommendations for the consultative management of patients with COVID-19. Gastroenterology 2020;159(1):320–34.e27.
4. Huang C, Wang Y, Li X, et al. Clinical features of patients infected with 2019 novel coronavirus in Wuhan, China. Lancet 2020;395(10223):497–506.
5. Chan JF, Yuan S, Kok KH, et al. A familial cluster of pneumonia associated with the 2019 novel coronavirus indicating person-to-person transmission: a study of a family cluster. Lancet 2020;395(10223):514–23.
6. Coronavirus (COVID-19). 2020. Available at: https://www.cdc.gov/coronavirus/2019-ncov/index.html. Accessed May 28, 2020.
7. Oran DP, Topol EJ. Prevalence of Asymptomatic SARS-CoV-2 Infection: A Narrative Review [published online ahead of print, 2020 Jun 3]. Ann Intern Med 2020. M20-3012. https://doi.org/10.7326/M20-3012.
8. Guan WJ, Ni ZY, Hu Y, et al. Clinical characteristics of coronavirus disease 2019 in China. N Engl J Med 2020;382(18):1708–20.
9. Nomoto H, Ishikane M, Katagiri D, et al. Cautious handling of urine from moderate to severe COVID-19 patients. Am J Infect Control 2020;48(8):969–71.
10. Killerby ME, Biggs HM, Haynes A, et al. Human coronavirus circulation in the United States 2014-2017. J Clin Virol 2018;101:52–6.
11. Wang W, Xu Y, Gao R, et al. Detection of SARS-CoV-2 in different types of clinical specimens. JAMA 2020;323(18):1843–4.
12. Chen W, Lan Y, Yuan X, et al. Detectable 2019-nCoV viral RNA in blood is a strong indicator for the further clinical severity. Emerg Microbes Infect 2020;9(1):469–73.
13. Pascarella G, Strumia A, Piliego C, et al. COVID-19 diagnosis and management: a comprehensive review. J Intern Med 2020;288(2):192–206.
14. Liu T, Zhang J, Yang Y, et al. The role of interleukin-6 in monitoring severe case of coronavirus disease 2019. EMBO Mol Med 2020;12(7):e12421.
15. Tan L, Wang Q, Zhang D, et al. Lymphopenia predicts disease severity of COVID-19: a descriptive and predictive study. Signal Transduct Target Ther 2020;5(1):33.
16. Zhang L, Yan X, Fan Q, et al. D-dimer levels on admission to predict in-hospital mortality in patients with Covid-19. J Thromb Haemost 2020;18(6):1324–9.
17. Jean SS, Lee PI, Hsueh PR. Treatment options for COVID-19: the reality and challenges. J Microbiol Immunol Infect 2020;53(3):436–43.
18. CFR - code of federal regulations title 21. 2019. Available at: https://www.accessdata.fda.gov/scripts/cdrh/cfdocs/cfcfr/cfrsearch.cfm?fr=630.10. Accessed May 15, 2020.
19. What to know about the coronavirus and blood donation. 2020. Available at: https://www.redcrossblood.org/donate-blood/dlp/coronavirus–covid-19–and-blood-donation.html. Accessed May 15, 2020.
20. Coronavirus and blood donation. 2020. Available at: https://www.mbc.org/coronavirus-blood-donation/. Accessed May 15, 2020.
21. COVID-19 and the blood supply. 2020. Available at: https://www.carterbloodcare.org/covid-19-and-the-blood-supply/. Accessed May 15, 2020.
22. COVID Info. 2020. Available at: https://www.vitalant.org/COVID-Info. Accessed May 15, 2020.
23. COVID-19 response. 2020. Available at: https://www.bloodcenter.org/donate/donor/covid19-response/. Accessed May 15, 2020.

24. Pagano MB, Hess JR, Tsang HC, et al. Prepare to adapt: blood supply and transfusion support during the first 2 weeks of the 2019 novel coronavirus (COVID-19) pandemic affecting Washington State. Transfusion 2020;60(5):908–11.
25. American red cross faces severe blood shortage as coronavirus outbreak threatens availability of nation's supply. 2020. Available at: https://www.redcross.org/about-us/news-and-events/press-release/2020/american-red-cross-faces-severe-blood-shortage-as-coronavirus-outbreak-threatens-availability-of-nations-supply.html. Accessed May 15, 2020.
26. Message to blood donors during the COVID-19 pandemic. AABB: Bethesda, MD; 2020. p. 2.
27. COVID-19 impact on hospital practices: week 1-4 survey snapshot. AABB: Bethesda, MD; 2020. Available at: http://www.aabb.org/research/hemovigilance/bloodsurvey/Docs/AABB-COVID-19-Impact-Survey-Snapshot-Week-1-4.pdf. Accessed May 15, 2020.
28. Alternative Procedures for Blood and Blood Components during the COVID-19 Public Health Emergency. U.S. Department of Health and Human Services Food and Drug Administration Center for Biologics Evaluation and Research. p. 8. Available at: https://www.fda.gov/regulatory-information/search-fda-guidance-documents/alternative-procedures-blood-and-blood-components-during-covid-19-public-health-emergency. Accessed May 15, 2020.
29. Coronavirus (COVID-19) update: FDA provides updated guidance to address the urgent need for blood during the pandemic. 2020. Available at: https://www.fda.gov/news-events/press-announcements/coronavirus-covid-19-update-fda-provides-updated-guidance-address-urgent-need-blood-during-pandemic. Accessed May 15, 2020.
30. Alternative procedures for blood and blood components during the COVID-19 public health emergency. 2020. Available at: https://www.fda.gov/regulatory-information/search-fda-guidance-documents/alternative-procedures-blood-and-blood-components-during-covid-19-public-health-emergency. Accessed May 15, 2020.
31. Healthcare facilities: preparing for community transmission. 2020. Available at: https://www.cdc.gov/coronavirus/2019-ncov/hcp/guidance-hcf.html. Accessed May 15, 2020.
32. COVID-19: recommendations for management of elective surgical procedures. 2020. Available at: https://www.facs.org/covid-19/clinical-guidance/elective-surgery. Accessed May 15, 2020.
33. Hemingway JF, Singh N, Starnes BW. Emerging practice patterns in vascular surgery during the COVID-19 pandemic. J Vasc Surg 2020;72(2):396–402.
34. AABB survey COVID-19 impact on care of patients requiring transfusion: week 1 snapshot. 2020. 1. Available at: http://www.aabb.org/research/hemovigilance/bloodsurvey/Docs/AABB-COVID-19-Impact-Survey-Snapshot-Week-1.pdf. Accessed May 16, 2020.
35. AABB survey COVID-19 impact on care of patients requiring transfusion: week 2 snapshot. 2020. 1. Available at: http://www.aabb.org/research/hemovigilance/bloodsurvey/Docs/AABB-COVID-19-Impact-Survey-Snapshot-Week-2.pdf. Accessed May 16, 2020.
36. AABB COVID-19 weekly hospital transfusion services survey: week 7 snapshot. 2020. 1. Available at: http://www.aabb.org/research/hemovigilance/bloodsurvey/Docs/AABB-COVID-19-Impact-Survey-Snapshot-Week-7.pdf. Accessed May 16, 2020.

37. AABB COVID-19 weekly hospital transfusion services survey: week 8 snapshot. 2020. 1. Available at: http://www.aabb.org/research/hemovigilance/bloodsurvey/Docs/AABB-COVID-19-Impact-Survey-Snapshot-Week-8.pdf. Accessed May 16, 2020.

38. Ferraris VA, Davenport DL, Saha SP, et al. Surgical outcomes and transfusion of minimal amounts of blood in the operating room. Arch Surg 2012;147(1):49–55.

39. Bernard AC, Davenport DL, Chang PK, et al. Intraoperative transfusion of 1 U to 2 U packed red blood cells is associated with increased 30-day mortality, surgical-site infection, pneumonia, and sepsis in general surgery patients. J Am Coll Surg 2009;208(5):931–7, 937.e1-2; [discussion: 938–9].

40. Ferraris VA, Ferraris VA, Brown JR, et al. 2011 update to the Society of Thoracic Surgeons and the Society of Cardiovascular Anesthesiologists blood conservation clinical practice guidelines. Ann Thorac Surg 2011;91(3):944–82.

41. Hajjar LA, Vincent JL, Galas FR, et al. Transfusion requirements after cardiac surgery: the TRACS randomized controlled trial. JAMA 2010;304(14):1559–67.

42. Warner MA, Chandran A, Jenkins G, et al. Prophylactic plasma transfusion is not associated with decreased red blood cell requirements in critically ill patients. Anesth Analg 2017;124(5):1636–43.

43. Schmidt AE, Henrichs KF, Kirkley SA, et al. Prophylactic preprocedure platelet transfusion is associated with increased risk of thrombosis and mortality. Am J Clin Pathol 2017;149(1):87–94.

44. Mehra T, Seifert B, Bravo-Reiter S, et al. Implementation of a patient blood management monitoring and feedback program significantly reduces transfusions and costs. Transfusion 2015;55(12):2807–15.

45. Twum-Barimah E, Abdelgadir I, Gordon M, et al. Systematic review with meta-analysis: the efficacy of tranexamic acid in upper gastrointestinal bleeding. Aliment Pharmacol Ther 2020;51(11):1004–13.

46. Myles PS, Smith JA, Forbes A, et al. Tranexamic acid in patients undergoing coronary-artery surgery. N Engl J Med 2017;376(2):136–48.

47. Dunn CJ, Goa KL. Tranexamic acid: a review of its use in surgery and other indications. Drugs 1999;57(6):1005–32.

48. Lim CC, Tan HZ, Tan CS, et al. Desmopressin acetate (DDAVP) to prevent bleeding in percutaneous kidney biopsy: a systematic review. Intern Med J 2020. https://doi.org/10.1111/imj.14774.

49. Refaai MA, Kothari TH, Straub S, et al. Four-factor Prothrombin complex concentrate reduces time to procedure in vitamin K antagonist-treated patients experiencing gastrointestinal bleeding: a post hoc analysis of two randomized controlled trials. Emerg Med Int 2017;2017:8024356.

50. Polito NB, Kanouse E, Jones CMC, et al. Effect of vitamin K administration on rate of warfarin reversal. Transfusion 2019;59(4):1202–8.

51. Mazur H, Young S, McGraw M, et al. 471: efficacy and safety of 4F-PCC VS. FFP for warfarin reversal in emergent surgery/invasive procedure. Crit Care Med 2019;47(1):216.

52. Cho BC, Serini J, Zorrilla-Vaca A, et al. Impact of preoperative erythropoietin on allogeneic blood transfusions in surgical patients: results from a systematic review and meta-analysis. Anesth Analg 2019;128(5):981–92.

53. Tokin C, Almeda J, Jain S, et al. Blood-management programs: a clinical and administrative model with program implementation strategies. Perm J 2009; 13(1):18–28.

54. Cai X, Ren M, Chen F, et al. Blood transfusion during the COVID-19 outbreak. Blood Transfus 2020;18(2):79–82.

55. Raturi M, Kusum A. The active role of a blood center in outpacing the transfusion transmission of COVID-19. Transfus Clin Biol 2020;27(2):96–7.
56. AABB Interorganizational Task Force on Pandemic Influenza and the Blood Supply, in Pandemic influenza issues outline. AABB. p. 16. Bethesda, MD;2020.
57. Maintaining a Safe and Adequate Blood Supply during Pandemic Influenza, in Guidelines for Blood Transfusion Services. World Health Organization (WHO). Geneva, Switzerland;2011.
58. Roback JD, Guarner J. Convalescent Plasma to Treat COVID-19: Possibilities and Challenges [published online ahead of print, 2020 Mar 27]. JAMA 2020. https://doi.org/10.1001/jama.2020.4940.
59. Bloch EM, Shoham S, Casadevall A, et al. Deployment of convalescent plasma for the prevention and treatment of COVID-19. J Clin Invest 2020;130(6):2757–65.
60. Dzik S. COVID-19 Convalescent Plasma: Now Is the Time for Better Science [published online ahead of print, 2020 Apr 23]. Transfus Med Rev. 2020;S0887-7963(20)30026-2. http://doi.org/10.1016/j.tmrv.2020.04.002.
61. Zeng F, Chen X, Deng G. Convalescent plasma for patients with COVID-19. Proc Natl Acad Sci U S A 2020;117(23):12528.
62. Joyner M. 2020. Available at: https://www.uscovidplasma.org/#workflow. Accessed May 22, 2020.
63. Available at: https://www.fda.gov/emergency-preparedness-and-response/coronavirus-disease-2019-covid-19/donate-covid-19-plasma.
64. Subramanian A, Berbari EF, Brown MJ, et al. Plasma transfusion is associated with postoperative infectious complications following esophageal resection surgery: a retrospective cohort study. J Cardiothorac Vasc Anesth 2012;26(4): 569–74.
65. Bence CM, Traynor MD Jr, Polites SF, et al. The incidence of venous thromboembolism in children following colorectal resection for inflammatory bowel disease: A multi-center study [published online ahead of print, 2020 Feb 20]. J Pediatr Surg. 2020;S0022-3468(20)30121-4. http://doi.org/10.1016/j.jpedsurg.2020.02.020.
66. Refaai MA, Fialkow LB, Heal JM, et al. An association of ABO non-identical platelet and cryoprecipitate transfusions with altered red cell transfusion needs in surgical patients. Vox Sang 2011;101(1):55–60.
67. Inaba K, Branco BC, Rhee P, et al. Impact of ABO-identical vs ABO-compatible nonidentical plasma transfusion in trauma patients. Arch Surg 2010;145(9): 899–906.
68. Refaai MA, Cahill C, Masel D, et al. Is it time to reconsider the concepts of "universal donor" and "ABO compatible" transfusions? Anesth Analg 2018;126(6): 2135–8.
69. Nguyen AA, Habiballah SB, Platt CD, et al. Immunoglobulins in the treatment of COVID-19 infection: proceed with caution! Clin Immunol 2020;216:108459.
70. Liu L, Wei Q, Lin Q, et al. Anti-spike IgG causes severe acute lung injury by skewing macrophage responses during acute SARS-CoV infection. JCI Insight 2019; 4(4):e123158.
71. Chang L, Zhao L, Gong H, et al. Severe acute respiratory syndrome coronavirus 2 RNA detected in blood donations. Emerg Infect Dis 2020;26(7):1631–3.

Clinical Features and Management of COVID-19–Associated Hypercoagulability

Gianluca Massaro, MD[a], Dalgisio Lecis, MD[a],
Eugenio Martuscelli, MD[a,b], Gaetano Chiricolo, MD[a,b,*],
Giuseppe Massimo Sangiorgi, MD[a,b]

KEYWORDS

- COVID-19 coagulopathy • Hypercoagulability • Venous thromboembolism
- Arterial thrombosis • Antithrombotic therapy

KEY POINTS

- COVID-19 is associated with blood coagulation changes leading to a prothrombotic state.
- Thrombotic complications affect more the venous than the arterial district.
- The incidence of thrombosis increases in more severe forms of the disease and is associated with high mortality.
- Management of hypercoagulability in COVID-19 is based on preventive measures in patients at risk or the treatment of manifest thrombotic complications.
- Anticoagulation is the most widely used therapy for the prevention and treatment of thrombosis associated with SARS-CoV-2 infection. Numerous trials are ongoing to define the best therapeutic strategy in the different clinical presentations of the disease.

INTRODUCTION

Coronavirus disease 2019 (COVID-19) is a viral illness caused by the severe acute respiratory syndrome coronavirus 2 (SARS-CoV-2). COVID-19 carries several important cardiovascular implications.[1,2] Since this pandemic disease broke out, it has been observed an increasing occurrence of thromboembolic events in patients without a history of cardiovascular disease.[3] The progressive acquisition of knowledge on the

This article previously appeared in *Cardiac Electrophysiology Clinics*, Volume 14, Issue 1, March 2022.

G. Massaro and D. Lecis contributed equally to the article conception and writing.

[a] Division of Cardiology, "Tor Vergata" University Hospital, v.le Oxford 81, Rome 00133, Italy;
[b] Department of Biomedicine and Prevention, "Tor Vergata" University of Rome, Rome 00133, Italy
* Corresponding author. Division of Cardiology, "Tor Vergata" University Hospital, v.le Oxford 81, Rome 00133, Italy.
E-mail address: nucciochiricolo@gmail.com

Clinics Collections 12 (2022) 159–175
https://doi.org/10.1016/j.ccol.2021.12.012
2352-7986/22/© 2021 Elsevier Inc. All rights reserved.

pathogenetic effects of SARS-CoV-2 infection has found a prominent role of the venous and arterial vascular system in the disease. Accumulated evidence has shown that coagulopathy is frequently observed in COVID-19 patients, especially in those with critical illness.[4] Han and colleagues[5] reported increased D-dimer values and fibrin/fibrinogen degradation products and reduced prothrombin time (PT)-activity in patients with COVID-19. The increase in D-dimer is particularly marked in severe patients and can be used in patient triaging and disease monitoring. SARS-CoV-2 infection in severe forms triggers a vicious cycle that includes hypercoagulability, endothelial cell activation, and massive release of inflammatory mediators[6] (Fig. 1). All this leads to an increased incidence of pulmonary and systemic thrombotic phenomena. A large series of autopsies documented an incidence of venous thromboembolism (VTE) of 42.5% and pulmonary embolism (PE) of 21%.[7] Among the most feared systemic complications of SARS-CoV-2 infection is disseminated intravascular coagulation (DIC), primarily characterized by thrombotic phenomena, with a lower incidence of bleeding and thrombocytopenia than other viral infections. Autopsies also revealed thrombotic microangiopathy observed in the lungs, termed "pulmonary intravascular coagulopathy".[7] In severe COVID-19, the "cytokine storm" is associated with abnormal coagulation parameters. It has been noticed that, in COVID-19 patients, higher interleukin (IL)-6 blood levels are directly related to fibrinogen levels predisposing to a hypercoagulable state and thromboembolic events.[8] COVID-19–associated

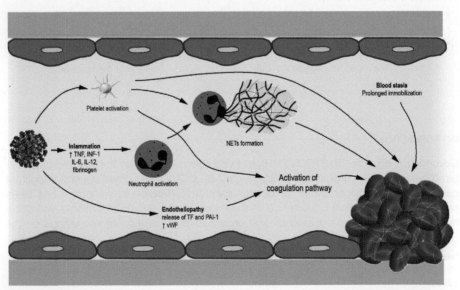

Fig. 1. Major mechanisms associated with the procoagulative state of COVID-19. SARS-CoV-2 exerts multiple effects systemically. Activation of the inflammatory response results in the recruitment of immune cells, including neutrophils. The virus can lead to a pathologic hyperactivation of platelets and endothelial damage that triggers the coagulation pathway.[17] Some evidence points to a role of activated platelets in stimulating NETosis. NETs contribute to the onset of thrombotic phenomena. All this is favored by blood stasis, due to prolonged immobilization typical of the most severe forms of the disease.[87] IL-6, interleukin-6; IL-12, interleukin-12; INF-1, interferon-1; NET, neutrophil extracellular trap; PAI-1, plasminogen activator inhibitor-1; TNF, tumor necrosis factor; TF, tissue factor; vWF, Von-Willebrand factor.

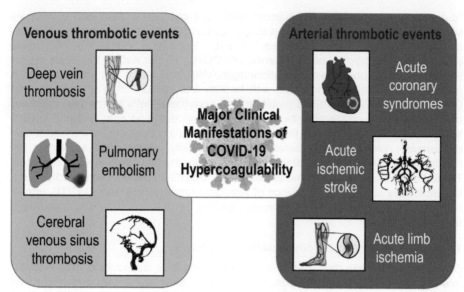

Fig. 2. Major thrombotic complications associated with COVID-19. Thromboses affect both arterial and venous districts. The latter are more frequent.

hypercoagulability can essentially be grouped into two main clinical manifestations: venous thrombotic events and arterial thrombotic events (ATEs) **(Fig. 2)**.

PATHOPHYSIOLOGY OF HYPERCOAGULABILITY

A major cause of morbidity and mortality in COVID-19 patients is thromboinflammation (the coordinated activation of thrombosis and inflammation). Laboratory tests revealed, in a great percentage of patients hospitalized with COVID-19, the evidence of a coagulopathy resembling DIC with marked elevated levels of D-dimers in the plasma, a mild prolongation of the PT, and borderline thrombocytopenia.[9] The postmortem examinations of COVID-19 patients showed extensive endothelial injury and diffuse microthrombosis.[10–12] However, the etiology of COVID-19–associated coagulopathy is still controversial and is likely to be heterogeneous, involving many different cell types. Indeed, observational studies and case series showed that not all the COVID-19 patients admitted to the ICU fulfilled the ISTH criteria for DIC (elevation of D-dimer levels, moderate-to-severe thrombocytopenia, prolongation of PT time, and decreased fibrinogen levels). Goshua and colleagues observed that, in a cohort of critically ill patients with COVID-19, the platelet counts were typically normal or mildly elevated and fibrinogen levels were markedly increased: findings that are inconsistent with coagulopathy of consumption such as DIC.[13] The global interpretation from these diverse reports is that although COVID-19–associated coagulopathy has some shared pathophysiological features with DIC, the coagulopathy observed in patients with COVID-19 can be considered as a distinct entity. In COVID-19, the variable state of hypercoagulability depends both on the type of cell involvement (eg, endothelial cells, platelets, leukocytes) and the time of sample collection during the disease process. In patients with severe COVID-19, elevated levels of inflammatory markers (such as C-reactive protein, ferritin, erythrocyte sedimentation rate, and cytokines, including IL-1β, IL-6, and TNF) lead to a hyperinflammatory response known as "cytokine storm," which is associated with poor outcomes. Jose and colleagues showed the correlation between elevated circulating levels of inflammatory cytokines and abnormal coagulation parameters.[14] The IL-6 levels have been shown to correlate directly with fibrinogen levels in patients with COVID-19,[8] as well as the levels of pro-thrombotic acute phase reactants (fibrinogen, vWF, and factor VIII) are increased in patients with COVID-19 compared with healthy individuals.[15,16] In a recent review, Gu and colleagues[17] identified platelets and endothelial cells as the two main cell types whose dysfunction contributes to the inflammation and coagulopathy associated with COVID-19, leading to thrombosis and eventually death. In the context of cardiovascular risk factors (diabetes mellitus, obesity, aging, and smoking), the mechanism of thrombocytopathy and endotheliopathy has been well represented. These findings are in line with the evidence that COVID-19 patients with cardiovascular risk factors have a high incidence of vascular complications (such as VTE, arterial thrombosis, and thrombotic microangiopathy), which contribute to the high mortality.[18–20]

Thrombocytopathy and Endotheliopathy in COVID-19

Contrary to what was thought in the past regarding their limited functions, platelets interact with many other cell types, including circulating blood cells and endothelial cells, either directly or through the release of signaling molecules, thus functioning as a blood component that bridges the immune system (through interactions with various leukocytes) and thrombosis (via platelet activation and release of hemostatic and inflammatory mediators).[21] Manne and colleagues demonstrated that platelets are hyperactivated in patients with COVID-19.[22] Activated platelets express on their surface some molecules involved in the stimulation of the immune system (such as P-selectin and CD40 L). Moreover, activated platelets can release α-granules, complement C3, and various cytokines (CCL2, IL-1β, IL-7, and IL-8), thus triggering the immune system activation camp.[23,24] Another cause of platelets hyperactivation is hypoxia,[25] a condition widely documented in COVID-19 patients who develop mild to severe hypoxia with peripheral blood oxygen desaturation. In addition, platelets dysfunction could be associated with a direct viral infection. ACE2, the cell-entry receptor for SARS-CoV-2, is expressed in the respiratory epithelium and endothelial cells,[26] but SARS-CoV-2 RNA traces were detected in platelet.[22] Other potential methods of SARS-CoV-2 entry into platelets independent of ACE2 are emerging.[27] At last, a potential mechanism for platelet hyperactivation and thrombocytopenia consists in the formation of immune complexes similar to that seen in heparin-induced thrombocytopenia (HIT) with the consequence of an increased platelet clearance.[28]

Endotheliopathy is a critical feature of severe COVID-19 across multiple studies. The endothelial damage and microvascular thrombosis are the results of both the direct viral infection of endothelial cells by SARS-CoV-2 and the endothelial cell response to the inflammatory process associated with COVID-19. In critically ill patients with COVID-19, it is possible to reveal increased circulating levels of markers of endothelial cell damage, including thrombomodulin, angiopoietin 2, and vWF.[29] Della Rocca and colleagues showed an increased number of schistocytes in the peripheral blood smear of patients hospitalized with COVID-19 at different stages of disease severity, thus identifying a new biomarker to reveal a high-risk subpopulation with latent systemic microvascular damage irrespective of respiratory symptoms.[30] It has been well documented that age is the major risk factor for COVID-19–related death. Aging is strictly associated with endothelial dysfunction because of oxidative and nitrosative stress. In aged endothelial cells, the accumulation of reactive oxygen species can decrease the availability of nitric oxide (NO), a potent vasodilator with antiplatelet properties and cardioprotective effects.[31] One of the most important functions of the vascular endothelium is to maintain a balance between proinflammatory and anti-inflammatory factors. In the elderly, the simultaneous invasion of the endothelium by SARS-CoV-2 via the angiotensin-converting enzyme 2 (ACE2) receptor can exacerbate endothelial dysfunction and damage, further promoting vascular inflammation and thrombosis.

VENOUS THROMBOTIC EVENTS IN COVID-19

A high incidence of thrombotic events, particularly deep vein thrombosis (DVT) and PE, has been documented in COVID-19 patients. As described in many studies, elevated D-dimer level is a common finding in COVID-19 patients. Anyway, high D-dimer levels meet low specificity in the absence of overt VTE clinical manifestations. Then, it is essential to recognize some "red flags" that can increase VTE suspicion in COVID-19 patients. The occurrence of typical DVT symptoms (asymmetric limb pain or edema), the increasing supplemental oxygen requirement, and hemodynamic instability in the setting of imaging findings inconsistent with worsening COVID-19 pneumonia or the onset of acute unexplained right ventricular dysfunction can be considered clinical manifestations of VTE.[32] Several scoring risk systems have been developed to help the clinician in the identification of VTE (**Table 1**). The most used are the Padua prediction score (including factors such as previous VTE, active cancer, reduced mobility, known thrombophilic condition, recent trauma or surgery, age $\geq$ 70 years, respiratory/cardiac failure, acute myocardial infarction/stroke, acute infection, obesity, and ongoing hormonal treatment; <4: low risk of VTE; $\geq$4: high risk of VTE), the International Medical Prevention Registry on Venous Thromboembolism (IMPROVE) score (7 risk factors: active cancer, previous VTE, thrombophilia, lower limb paralysis, immobilization < 7 days, intensive care unit/coronary care unit stay, age > 60 years; more than one positive factor increases the risk of symptomatic VTE to 7.2%), and the Wells' score (clinical signs/symptoms of DVT, PE most likely diagnosis, tachycardia [>100 bpm], immobilization/surgery in previous 4 weeks, prior DVT/PE, hemoptysis, active malignancy).[33] These tools are helpful to identify patients estimated at a higher risk for VTE and start prevention with a standard dose of subcutaneous unfractionated heparin (UFH) or low-molecular-weight heparin (LMWH) according to the published guidelines.

Laboratory Parameters in VTE

The most consistent hemostatic abnormalities with COVID-19 include, as mentioned earlier, increased D-dimer levels.[34] A prospective study comparing coagulation parameter disorders among patients with COVID-19 and healthy controls suggested that the D-dimer levels (10.36 vs 0.26 ng/L; $P < .001$), fibrin/fibrinogen degradation products (33.83 vs 1.55 mg/L; $P < .001$), and fibrinogen (5.02 vs 2.90 g/L; $P < .001$), in all SARS-CoV-2 cases, were substantially higher than those in healthy controls. Moreover, these biomarkers, especially D-dimer and fibrinogen degradation products, were higher in patients with severe SARS-CoV-2 infection than those with mild disease.[5] Another common finding is mild thrombocytopenia. A meta-analysis showed that patients with severe disease were found to have a significantly lower platelet count (mean difference: -31×10^9/L; 95% confidence interval [CI], -35 to -29×10^9/L), and thrombocytopenia was associated with a 5-fold higher odds of having the severe disease (odds ratio: 5.13; 95% CI, 1.81–14.58).[35] Other hemostatic abnormalities variably associated with COVID-19 severity are the prolongation of the PT, international normalized ratio (INR),[13,14] and thrombin time.[36] A trend toward shortened activated partial thromboplastin time (aPTT) is variably associated with

Table 1
Scoring systems commonly used for the assessment of the risk of venous thromboembolism and pulmonary embolism.

Items	Score
Padua Risk Score	
Active cancer (metastases and/or chemoradiotherapy in the previous 6 mo)	3
Previous VTE (with the exclusion of superficial vein thrombosis)	3
Bedrest for $\geq$ 3 d	3
Thrombophilia	3
Recent ($\leq$1 mo) trauma and/or surgery	2
Elderly age ($\geq$70 y)	1
Heart and/or respiratory failure	1
Acute myocardial infarction or ischemic stroke	1
Acute infection and/or rheumatologic disorder	1
Obesity (BMI $\geq$ 30 kg/m^2)	1
Ongoing hormonal treatment	1
High risk of VTE: $\geq$ 4 points	
IMPROVE score	
Previous VTE	3
Known thrombophilia	2
Current lower limb paralysis or paresis	2
History of cancer	2
ICU/CCU stay	1
Complete immobilization $\geq$ 1 d	1
Age $\geq$ 60 y	1
High-risk indication for prophylaxis if score $\geq$ 3	
Well's score	
Clinical signs/symptoms of DVT	3
PE is most likely diagnosis	3
Tachycardia (>100 bpm)	1.5
Immobilization/surgery in previous 4 wk	1.5
Prior DVT/PE	1.5
Hemoptysis	1
Active malignancy (trt w/in 6 mo)	1
Total score > 4: PE likely Total score < 4: PE unlikely	

Abbreviations: BMI, body mass index; CCU, cardiac care unit; DVT, deep venous thrombosis; ICU, intensive care unit; PE, pulmonary embolism; VTE, venous thromboembolism.

the disease severity.[37,38] Tang and colleagues[39] assessed 183 patients with COVID-19, 21 (11.5%) of whom died. The patients who died showed increased levels of D-dimer and fibrin degradation products (w3.5- and w1.9-fold, respectively) and PT prolongation (by 14%) (P < .001) when compared with survivors. Among the patients who died, 71% fulfilled the International Society on Thrombosis and Haemostasis (ISTH) criteria[40] for DIC, compared with only 0.6% among survivors. Taken all together, these hemostatic abnormalities indicate some forms of coagulopathy that may predispose to thrombotic events. However, the underlying mechanism leading to the clinical manifestations of VTE is still unknown.

Nevertheless, it is uncertain whether these hemostatic changes are a specific effect of SARS-CoV-2 infection or are a consequence of the cytokine storm that precipitates the onset of systemic inflammatory response syndrome (SIRS) as documented in other severe viral diseases.[41,42] A recent study reported 3 cases with severe COVID-19 and cerebral infarction, with one associated with bilateral limb ischemia, in the setting of elevated antiphospholipid antibodies.[43] The presence of antiphospholipid antibodies (eg, anticardiolipin IgA, anti–β2-glycoprotein I IgA, and IgG) has been described in the serum of COVID-19 patients. This finding may contribute to an increased risk of both venous and arterial thrombosis.[44,45] However, some studies have highlighted that in setting a high degree of inflammation, like in SIRS, and an increased level of inflammatory markers, those antibodies can be falsely positive.[46] Whether antiphospholipid antibodies play a significant role in the pathophysiology of thrombosis associated with COVID-19 requires further investigation.

Imaging for VTE

To yield a definitive diagnosis of VTE, imaging studies can be helpful. The American Heart Association guidelines on managing massive and submassive PE recommend performing computed tomography pulmonary angiography (CTPA) in all patients with intermediate or high pretest probability or a positive D-dimer.[47] Referring to COVID-19, some studies have shown the usefulness of compression ultrasonography and CTPA in this setting of patients.[48,49] An Italian study showed that 16 (36%) of 44 consecutive symptomatic patients had VTE on imaging, and 10 (33%) of 30 patients had a PE at CTPA. Half of the thromboembolic events were diagnosed within 24 h of hospital admission, highlighting the significance of early diagnosis and treatment in patients with COVID-19.[50] The decision to perform an imaging study for diagnosing DVT should be based on clinical judgment. The feasibility of these imaging modalities (mainly ultrasound imaging) in COVID-19 is a matter of concern because of the prolonged health care assistants' exposition time. Therefore, the role of bedside point-of-care ultrasound is essential in aiding diagnosis, reducing the exposition time. In a recent multicenter study, a 100% sensitivity and a 95.8% specificity have been showing resorting to point-of-care ultrasound for the diagnosis of DVT.[51] At last, in patients with high clinical suspicion of PE, a bedside cardiac ultrasound also assists with the diagnosis by rapid assessment of right ventricular size and function.

ATEs IN COVID-19

The relationship between viral respiratory infections and arterial thrombosis, especially acute coronary syndrome (ACS), is clearly described[52] Cases of ACS have been previously described with influenza or other viral illness. They have been attributed to a combination of SIRS as well as localized vascular or plaque inflammation.[53] During the COVID-19 pandemics, small series of patients with coronary, cerebrovascular, and peripheral ATEs have also been reported, but their true incidence and consequences are not well described. In a series of 18 patients with COVID-19 and ST-segment elevation, in more than 50% of them, the origin was considered to be noncoronary.[54] Acute limb ischemia has been reported in 2 young COVID-19 patients with occlusion of major arteries of the upper and lower limbs.[55] In the systematic review and meta-summary of Tan and colleagues, it has been reported that the incidence of acute ischemic stroke in COVID-19 patients ranges from 0.9% to 2.7%. From this meta-summary, it has been observed that acute ischemic stroke severity in COVID-19 patients is typically at least moderate (NIHSS score 19 ± 8), with a high prevalence (40.9%) of large vessel occlusion. Notably, a significant number of cases tested positive for antiphospholipid antibodies. Although it is reported that antiphospholipid antibodies are commonly found in COVID-19 infections, the true prevalence of antiphospholipid-antibody positivity in the general population is not known. It has also been detected in healthy individuals. Hence, the significance of antiphospholipid antibodies in the pathogenesis of acute ischemic stroke in COVID-19 patients remains uncertain. It may be worthwhile for future studies to repeat and trend these serologic markers after the acute thrombotic setting.

At last, the mortality rate of COVID-19 patients experiencing acute ischemic stroke has been reported high (38.0%).[56] Recently, Cantador and colleagues[57] observed the 1% incidence of systemic ATEs in a large cohort of 1419 COVID-19 patients, with a death rate of 28.6%. In this study, the incidence of thrombotic events, at least for cerebrovascular, seems to be higher than expected with very serious consequences. A meta-analysis conducted by Lippi and colleagues showed that cTnI concentration is only marginally increased in all patients with SARS-CoV-2 infection, whereby values exceeding the 99th percentile in the upper reference limit can only be observed in 8% to 12% of positive cases. Furthermore, higher troponin levels are associated with severe COVID-19.[58] Hence, it is reasonable to hypothesize that initial measurement of cardiac damage biomarkers immediately after hospitalization for SARS-CoV-2 infection, and longitudinal monitoring during the hospital stay may help identify a subset of patients with possible cardiac injury and thereby predict the progression of COVID-19 toward a worse clinical picture.[59] However, not all such events are due to thrombotic ACS. These data, taken all together, suggest that, although COVID-19 may favor the occurrence of thrombotic events, the destabilization and thrombosis of atherosclerotic plaques do not seem to be a frequent mechanism that warrants the need for specific systematic preventive measures. Nevertheless, a high level of suspicion and clinical surveillance should undoubtedly be maintained.

MANAGEMENT OF COVID-19–ASSOCIATED HYPERCOAGULABILITY

Coagulopathy associated with SARS-CoV-2 infection has peculiar characteristics compared with that associated with conventional sepsis, as evidenced by the difference in coagulation parameters described earlier. This is confirmed by the evidence of reduced mortality in patients with COVID-19 and elevated D-dimer undergoing anticoagulation than non–COVID-19 patients.[60]

COVID-19 disease is associated with a higher incidence of thrombotic than hemorrhagic complications, which is the rationale for pharmacologic schemes targeting the coagulation pathway.

In the early stages of the pandemic, the absence of randomized clinical trials (RCTs) forced physicians to take an empirical approach to the use of anticoagulant regimens. Early evidence of different clinical pictures and numerous variables characterizing COVID-19 disease led to the realization that the "one-size-fits-all" strategy was not feasible.

To date, more than 75 RCT testing anticoagulant regimens in different clinical settings have been designed.[61] The choice of drug and dosage in RCTs depends on the expected rate of thrombotic events in the study population: the use of prophylactic or intermediate doses has been preferred in trials of patients with mild COVID-19, whereas patients with critical illness or requiring intensive care have been treated with higher-dose regimens.

Given the higher incidence of thrombosis in venous versus arterial districts,[48,62] clinical trials have tested more pharmacologic regimens to prevent and treat VTE. The use of such strategies in different types of patients will be discussed in the following section.

Pharmacologic Approaches

The main approaches used in RCTs for the prevention and treatment of thrombotic complications of COVID-19 include UFH, LMWH, fondaparinux, direct oral anticoagulants (DOACs), antiplatelet drugs, direct parenteral thrombin inhibitors, fibrinolytic agents, and drugs less commonly used in clinical practice such as dociparstat, dipyridamole, and nafamostat. The most significant evidence is with heparins and antiplatelet drugs.

Data on head-to-head comparisons between different drugs are lacking, so the choice is often driven by practical considerations.

Their wide use, mainly in the hospital setting, has made heparins the most studied anticoagulant drugs to treat COVID-19 coagulopathy. In addition to its anticoagulant effect, heparin also has anti-inflammatory properties and protective effects on the endothelium.[63]

In prophylactic anticoagulation, once-daily LMWH is preferred over twice-daily subcutaneous UFH administration to reduce health care worker exposure. Therapeutic anticoagulation with UHF has the advantage that it can be temporarily discontinued and shows utility, especially in patients who are candidates for invasive procedures. However, frequent blood draws to check that aPTT is in the therapeutic range favor LMWH for the reasons already stated.

The antiviral and anti-inflammatory effects of heparin provide the rationale for the use of nebulized forms of UFH. Three trials are ongoing to test the efficacy and safety of this formulation compared to standard-of-care (INHALE-HEP and PACTR2020076032743) or prophylactic LMWH (NEBU-HEPA)

Direct anticoagulants represent an unquestionable advantage, especially in outpatients, to reduce the continuous recourse to INR assessment. However, their intrahospital use is limited by numerous interactions with other medications that are used to treat COVID-19 disease and the inability to use them in patients under orotracheal intubation or with dysphagia.

The use of antiplatelet drugs in the prophylaxis of thrombotic complications in patients with COVID-19 disease has been evaluated in both mild and severe forms of the disease. However, unlike heparins, antiplatelet drugs have not demonstrated effects on "endotheliopathy."[17]

Prevention of VTE in Patients with Mild COVID-19

Patients with mild COVID-19 generally do not require hospitalization and should maintain home isolation. There are several ongoing clinical trials on the use of LMWH,[61] DOAC, or aspirin in these patients. The only clinical trial published to date tested the use of sulodexide in the early stages of the disease in 243 patients in preventing hospitalizations and the use of oxygen therapy. The treatment arm showed a reduction in hospitalizations (relative risk: 0.60; 95% CI, 0.37–0.96; P = .03) and in the need for oxygen support (relative risk: 0.71; 95% CI, 0.50–1.00; P = .05) compared with placebo, with no significant difference in mortality.

Current recommendations do not indicate antithrombotic prophylaxis in all patients. However, in subjects at high risk of VTE (immobility, procoagulative status, previous VTE), antithrombotic prophylaxis should be considered, also taking into account the risk of bleeding.

Prevention and Treatment of VTE in Hospitalized Patients

When the pandemic began its spread in Europe, in China, Tang and colleagues[64] demonstrated that, in patients hospitalized for COVID-19 and with high D-dimer or high sepsis-induced coagulopathy (SIC) score, 28-day mortality was lower among those receiving anticoagulation than among those not receiving it. Most of the treated patients had received LMWH at prophylactic doses. Therefore, the international societies agreed that prophylactic dose LMWH should be considered in all patients (including noncritically ill) who require hospital admission for COVID-19 infection in the absence of any contraindications.[65]

Anticoagulant dosing for the prevention of VTE is not well defined. Some clinicians use a therapeutic-dose anticoagulant regimen in the prevention of thrombotic complications in all hospitalized patients, whereas others reserve it for patients at high thrombotic risk, based on D-dimer or SIC score values. As already discussed, some evidence shows that SARS-CoV-2 disease has distinctive features compared with other forms of sepsis. Hadid and colleagues[66] have proposed a specific score for COVID-19 called CIC (COVID-19–induced coagulopathy) score, which adds the D-dimer value to the previous SIC score. Although not yet validated, this score can be helpful to estimate the risk of thrombotic complications and start more intensive anticoagulation in patients with severe disease.

An observational study in the United States showed a better outcome in hospitalized patients treated with treatment-dose of anticoagulants than in those treated with prophylactic-dose.[67] HESACOVID, a randomized phase 2 clinical trial, showed improved gas exchange and reduced need for mechanical ventilation in patients with severe COVID-19 receiving therapeutic enoxaparin compared with the group receiving prophylactic anticoagulation.[68]

Numerous clinical trials are ongoing to evaluate the use of different anticoagulant regimens in patients with severe disease. The design of the trials involves the use of more intense anticoagulation. In some studies, the administration of fibrinolytic agents is tested in patients with very severe forms, despite the rather limited sample size.

A complication observed in patients with severe forms of COVID-19 is DIC. Traditionally, DIC is characterized by thrombotic and hemorrhagic complications, whereas in the specific setting of SARS-CoV-2 disease, the former is more frequent than the latter. In patients with COVID-19 and DIC, prophylactic anticoagulation should be administered in the absence of overt bleeding. There is a tendency to recommend a less intense anticoagulation regimen in these patients; however, the individual risk of VTE and significant bleeding must be weighed.

Prevention of VTE in Postdischarge Patients

Some trials in acutely ill medical patients have shown that the extension of anticoagulation therapy after discharge is associated with reducing thromboembolic events at the cost of increased bleeding.[69] Given the particular tendency to hypercoagulability of patients with COVID-19, some trials evaluate the use of different pharmacologic regimens, including DOACs.[70,71]

Treatment of Arterial Thromboembolic Complications

Arterial complications of SARS-CoV-2 infection have received less attention because of their lower incidence compared with their venous counterparts.[48,62] A report from the New York City area shows that 57% of arterial thromboses, in patients with COVID-19 (upper- and lower limb ischemia, bowel ischemia, and cerebral ischemia), were treated with systemic anticoagulant therapy alone, 6% with administration of systemic tissue-plasminogen activator, 27% with revascularization, and 10% with amputation.[72]

Patients with acute coronary thrombosis and concomitant SARS-CoV-2 infection have a higher thrombotic burden and a worse prognosis.[73] Hospital admissions for

ST-segment elevation myocardial infarction (STEMI) were reduced during the pandemic, with a more extended treatment delay and hospitalization.[74] The treatment of patients with STEMI and established or suspected COVID-19 raised essential questions. The proposal to increase thrombolysis to protect health care workers[75] was not adopted by the European Association of Percutaneous Cardiovascular Interventions (EAPCI). Primary percutaneous coronary intervention (PCI) was confirmed as the gold-standard therapy for STEMI, whereas thrombolysis can be helpful when the catheterization laboratory is not available or timely primary PCI cannot be achieved.[76]

For patients with COVID-19 and ischemic stroke, the use of thrombolysis and thrombectomy should be continued. There are some difficulties in managing neurologic rehabilitation, mostly related to organizational issues and risk of infection.[77]

Acute limb thrombosis associated with COVID-19 is characterized by greater clot burden and increased rate of amputation and death.[78] As for myocardial infarction and ischemic stroke, treatment involves prompt intervention, characterized first by therapeutic anticoagulation, preferably with UFH, and then by an assessment based on the stability and viability of the limb on the most appropriate approach.

COAGULOPATHY AND VACCINES

A turning point in the fight against COVID-19 has been the development of vaccines, whose efficacy, especially against severe forms of the disease, and safety profile has led to a rapid "conditional marketing authorization" by the main regulatory agencies.[79]

Abnormal activation of the coagulation system has been implicated in the pathogenesis of some severe adverse reactions related to the administration of anti–COVID-19 vaccines. After the marketing authorization, there have been increasing reports, albeit rare, of thrombotic complications at unusual sites, associated with thrombocytopenia, arising mainly after the administration of viral vector vaccines (Vaxzevria by AstraZeneca AB and COVID-19 Vaccine Janssen by Janssen-Cilag International NV). The incidence of this complication, named Vaccine-associated Immune Thrombosis and Thrombocytopenia (VITT) syndrome, remains largely unknown and appears to be between 1 in 125,000 and 1 in 1,000,000.[80]

In April 2021, the New England Journal of Medicine reports a total of 39 cases of thrombosis, observed after administration of the Vaxzevria vaccine, in different descriptive studies.[81–83] Clinical manifestations appear between 5 and 24 days after the first administration of the AstraZeneca serum. The affected population is predominantly female with an age of less than 50 years. In some cases (25.9%), affected women were using oral contraceptives. In most cases, thrombosis involved cerebral veins, although cases of involvement of the splanchnic venous district and PE have been described. Of note, severe thrombocytopenia (platelet count <25,000/mm^3) was present in 52.6% of the cases evaluated. The concomitance of thrombocytopenia and thrombosis suggested an autoimmune mechanism in the pathogenesis of the syndrome. A German group led by Andreas Greinacher shed light on the pathogenesis of VITT, highlighting its similarities to the condition known as HIT.[84] HIT is due to the formation of autoantibodies directed against a complex epitope formed by platelet-derived factor 4 (PF4) and heparin or another polyanionic molecule. These autoantibodies can bind the Fcγlla receptor (FcRγlla) present at the platelet surface causing intense intravascular platelet activation and aggregation.[85] They have also been found in VITT, even in the absence of previous heparin exposure.[81] The cause of the formation of these antibodies in patients with VITT is unclear.

Cases of platelet count reduction associated with bleeding in the absence of thrombotic phenomena have been described in persons vaccinated with mRNA vector vaccines (Comirnaty by BioNTech Manufacturing GmbH and COVID-19 Vaccine Moderna by Moderna Biotech Spain, SL). Although it is not yet clear whether there is a causal link between this condition and the vaccine, an autoimmune-type mechanism has been hypothesized here too.[86]

SUMMARY

Coagulopathy is common in acute sepsis. However, hypercoagulability associated with SARS-CoV-2 infection has peculiar features.

COVID-19 is associated with a high rate of thrombotic complications, mainly in the venous district. The "thromboinflammation" that characterizes the disease is evident in the alterations of laboratory parameters and some clinical manifestations characterized by a high mortality rate. Numerous clinical trials are ongoing to define the best preventive and therapeutic strategy in the management of thrombosis from COVID-19.

CLINICS CARE POINTS

- In the management of patients with COVID-19, attention must be paid to the occurrence of arterial and venous thromboembolic complications, which appear to be frequently associated with the disease

- COVID-19 is associated with changes in coagulation parameters, which are more evident in severe forms of the disease (increased D-dimer, lengthening of PT and INR, thrombocytopenia, and shortening or sometimes lengthening of aPTT).

- The diagnosis of thrombotic complications such as DVT or PE cannot be derived solely from laboratory parameters but needs to be correlated with symptoms and must be supported by imaging methods such as CT angiography or ultrasound. Some scoring systems can be useful (see **Table 1**)

- Current recommendations do not indicate antithrombotic prophylaxis in all COVID-19 patients. However, in subjects at high risk of VTE (immobility, procoagulative status, and previous VTE), antithrombotic prophylaxis should be considered.

- Low-molecular-weight heparin at prophylactic dosage should be considered in all patients (including noncritically ill) who require hospital admission for COVID-19 infection in the absence of any contraindications.

- The rare cases of thrombotic complications related to the administration of anti–COVID-19 vaccines, especially those using a viral vector, should not cast doubt on the advantages of vaccination. Epidemiologic data on adverse reactions and an understanding of the pathogenetic mechanisms may be helpful in limiting the incidence of such complications.

DISCLOSURE

The authors have nothing to disclose.

REFERENCES

1. Clerkin KJ, Fried JA, Raikhelkar J, et al. COVID-19 and cardiovascular disease. Circulation 2020;141(20):1648–55.
2. Madjid M, Safavi-Naeini P, Solomon SD, et al. Potential effects of coronaviruses on the cardiovascular system: a review. 2020. JAMA Cardiol 2020;5(7):831–40.
3. Driggin E, Madhavan MV, Bikdeli B, et al. Cardiovascular considerations for patients, health care workers, and health systems during the COVID-19 pandemic 2020;75:21.

4. Iba T, Levy JH, Levi M, et al. Coagulopathy in COVID-19. J Thromb Haemost 2020;18:2103–9.
5. Han H, Yang L, Liu R, et al. Prominent changes in blood coagulation of patients with SARS-CoV-2 infection. Clin Chem Lab Med CCLM 2020;58:1116–20.
6. Gerotziafas GT, Catalano M, Colgan M-P, et al, Scientific Reviewer Committee. Guidance for the management of patients with vascular disease or cardiovascular risk factors and COVID-19: position paper from VAS-European independent Foundation in Angiology/vascular medicine. Thromb Haemost 2020;120:1597–628.
7. Edler C, Schröder AS, Aepfelbacher M, et al. Dying with SARS-CoV-2 infection— an autopsy study of the first consecutive 80 cases in Hamburg, Germany. Int J Legal Med 2020;134:1275–84.
8. Ranucci M, Ballotta A, Di Dedda U, et al. The procoagulant pattern of patients with COVID-19 acute respiratory distress syndrome. J Thromb Haemost 2020;18:1747–51.
9. Guan W, Ni Z, Hu Y, et al. Clinical characteristics of coronavirus disease 2019 in China. N Engl J Med 2020;382:1708–20.
10. Dolhnikoff M, Duarte-Neto AN, Almeida Monteiro RA, et al. Pathological evidence of pulmonary thrombotic phenomena in severe COVID-19. J Thromb Haemost 2020;18:1517–9.
11. Carsana L, Sonzogni A, Nasr A, et al. Pulmonary post-mortem findings in a series of COVID-19 cases from northern Italy: a two-centre descriptive study. Lancet Infect Dis 2020;20:1135–40.
12. Menter T, Haslbauer JD, Nienhold R, et al. Postmortem examination of COVID-19 patients reveals diffuse alveolar damage with severe capillary congestion and variegated findings in lungs and other organs suggesting vascular dysfunction. Histopathology 2020;77:198–209.
13. Goshua G, Pine AB, Meizlish ML, et al. Endotheliopathy in COVID-19-associated coagulopathy: evidence from a single-centre, cross-sectional study. Lancet Haematol 2020;7:e575–82.
14. Jose RJ, Manuel A. COVID-19 cytokine storm: the interplay between inflammation and coagulation. Lancet Respir Med 2020;8:e46–7.
15. Panigada M, Bottino N, Tagliabue P, et al. Hypercoagulability of COVID-19 patients in intensive care unit: a report of thromboelastography findings and other parameters of hemostasis. J Thromb Haemost 2020;18:1738–42.
16. Escher R, Breakey N, Lämmle B. Severe COVID-19 infection associated with endothelial activation. Thromb Res 2020;190:62.
17. Gu SX, Tyagi T, Jain K, et al. Thrombocytopathy and endotheliopathy: crucial contributors to COVID-19 thromboinflammation. Nat Rev Cardiol 2021;18:194–209.
18. Cui S, Chen S, Li X, et al. Prevalence of venous thromboembolism in patients with severe novel coronavirus pneumonia. J Thromb Haemost 2020;18:1421–4.
19. Zhang L, Feng X, Zhang D, et al. Deep vein thrombosis in hospitalized patients with COVID-19 in Wuhan, China: prevalence, risk factors, and outcome. Circulation 2020;142:114–28.
20. Nahum J, Morichau-Beauchant T, Daviaud F, et al. Venous thrombosis among critically ill patients with coronavirus disease 2019 (COVID-19). JAMA Netw Open 2020;3:e2010478.
21. Koupenova M, Freedman JE. Platelets and immunity: going viral. Arterioscler Thromb Vasc Biol 2020;40:1605–7.
22. Manne BK, Denorme F, Middleton EA, et al. Platelet gene expression and function in patients with COVID-19. Blood 2020;136:1317–29.

23. Fitch-Tewfik JL, Flaumenhaft R. Platelet granule exocytosis: a comparison with chromaffin cells. Front Endocrinol, 2013;4(77).
24. Sut C, Tariket S, Aubron C, et al. The non-hemostatic aspects of transfused platelets. Front Med 2018;5:42.
25. Tyagi T, Ahmad S, Gupta N, et al. Altered expression of platelet proteins and calpain activity mediate hypoxia-induced prothrombotic phenotype. Blood 2014;123:1250–60.
26. Ackermann M, Verleden SE, Kuehnel M, et al. Pulmonary vascular endothelialitis, thrombosis, and angiogenesis in covid-19. N Engl J Med 2020;383:120–8.
27. Hoffmann M, Kleine-Weber H, Schroeder S, et al. SARS-CoV-2 cell entry depends on ACE2 and TMPRSS2 and is blocked by a clinically proven Protease inhibitor. Cell 2020;181:271–80.e8.
28. Perdomo J, Leung HHL, Ahmadi Z, et al. Neutrophil activation and NETosis are the major drivers of thrombosis in heparin-induced thrombocytopenia. Nat Commun 2019;10:1322.
29. Pine AB, Meizlish ML, Goshua G, et al. Circulating markers of angiogenesis and endotheliopathy in COVID-19. Pulm Circ 2020;10. 204589402096654.
30. Della Rocca DG, Magnocavallo M, Lavalle C, et al. Evidence of systemic endothelial injury and microthrombosis in hospitalized COVID-19 patients at different stages of the disease. J Thromb Thrombolysis 2021;51:571–6.
31. Lakatta EG, Levy D. Arterial and cardiac aging: major Shareholders in cardiovascular disease enterprises: Part II: the aging Heart in health: links to Heart disease. Circulation 2003;107:346–54.
32. Bikdeli B, Madhavan MV, Jimenez D, et al. COVID-19 and thrombotic or thromboembolic disease: implications for prevention, antithrombotic therapy, and follow-up. J Am Coll Cardiol 2020;75:2950–73.
33. Obi AT, Barnes GD, Wakefield TW, et al. Practical diagnosis and treatment of suspected venous thromboembolism during COVID-19 pandemic. J Vasc Surg Venous Lymphat Disord 2020;8:526–34.
34. Lippi G, Favaloro EJ. D-Dimer is associated with severity of coronavirus disease 2019: a pooled analysis. Thromb Haemost 2020;120:876–8.
35. Lippi G, Plebani M, Henry BM. Thrombocytopenia is associated with severe coronavirus disease 2019 (COVID-19) infections: a meta-analysis. Clin Chim Acta 2020;506:145–8.
36. Gao Y, Li T, Han M, et al. Diagnostic utility of clinical laboratory data determinations for patients with the severe COVID-19. J Med Virol 2020;92:791–6.
37. Huang C, Wang Y, Li X, et al. Clinical features of patients infected with 2019 novel coronavirus in Wuhan, China. The Lancet 2020;395:497–506.
38. Lippi G, Salvagno GL, Ippolito L, et al. Shortened activated partial thromboplastin time: causes and management. Blood Coagul Fibrinolysis 2010;21:459–63.
39. Tang N, Li D, Wang X, et al. Abnormal coagulation parameters are associated with poor prognosis in patients with novel coronavirus pneumonia. J Thromb Haemost 2020;18:844–7.
40. Levi M, Toh CH, Thachil J, et al. Guidelines for the diagnosis and management of disseminated intravascular coagulation. Br J Haematol 2009;145:24–33.
41. Ramacciotti E, Agati LB, Aguiar VCR, et al. Zika and Chikungunya virus and risk for venous thromboembolism. Clin Appl Thromb 2019;25. 107602961882118.
42. Smither S, O'Brien L, Eastaugh L, et al. Haemostatic changes in five patients infected with Ebola virus. Viruses 2019;11:647.
43. Zhang Y, Xiao M, Zhang S, et al. Coagulopathy and antiphospholipid antibodies in patients with Covid-19. N Engl J Med 2020;382:e38.

44. Mendoza-Pinto C, García-Carrasco M, Cervera R. Role of infectious diseases in the antiphospholipid syndrome (including its Catastrophic variant). Curr Rheumatol Rep 2018;20:62.

45. Abdel-Wahab N, Talathi S, Lopez-Olivo MA, et al. Risk of developing antiphospholipid antibodies following viral infection: a systematic review and meta-analysis. Lupus 2018;27:572–83.

46. Salluh JIF, Soares M, Meis ED. Antiphospholipid antibodies and multiple organ failure in critically ill cancer patients. Clinics 2009;64:79–82.

47. Jaff MR, McMurtry MS, Archer SL, et al. Management of massive and submassive pulmonary embolism, iliofemoral deep vein thrombosis, and chronic thromboembolic pulmonary hypertension: a scientific statement from the American Heart association. Circulation 2011;123:1788–830.

48. Klok FA, Kruip MJHA, van der Meer NJM, et al. Confirmation of the high cumulative incidence of thrombotic complications in critically ill ICU patients with COVID-19: an updated analysis. Thromb Res 2020;191:148–50.

49. Grillet F, Behr J, Calame P, et al. Acute pulmonary embolism associated with COVID-19 pneumonia detected with pulmonary CT angiography. Radiology 2020;296:E186–8.

50. Lodigiani C, Iapichino G, Carenzo L, et al. Venous and arterial thromboembolic complications in COVID-19 patients admitted to an academic hospital in Milan, Italy. Thromb Res 2020;191:9–14.

51. Fischer EA, Kinnear B, Sall D, et al. Hospitalist-operated compression ultrasonography: a point-of-care ultrasound study (HOCUS-POCUS). J Gen Intern Med 2019;34:2062–7.

52. Kwong JC, Schwartz KL, Campitelli MA, et al. Acute myocardial infarction after laboratory-confirmed influenza infection. N Engl J Med 2018;378:345–53.

53. Corrales-Medina VF, Madjid M, Musher DM. Role of acute infection in triggering acute coronary syndromes. Lancet Infect Dis 2010;10:83–92.

54. Bangalore S, Sharma A, Slotwiner A, et al. ST-segment elevation in patients with covid-19 — a case series. N Engl J Med 2020;382:2478–80.

55. Perini P, Nabulsi B, Massoni CB, et al. Acute limb ischaemia in two young, non-atherosclerotic patients with COVID-19. The Lancet 2020;395:1546.

56. Tan Y-K, Goh C, Leow AST, et al. COVID-19 and ischemic stroke: a systematic review and meta-summary of the literature. J Thromb Thrombolysis 2020;50:587–95.

57. Cantador E, Núñez A, Sobrino P, et al. Incidence and consequences of systemic arterial thrombotic events in COVID-19 patients. J Thromb Thrombolysis 2020;50:543–7.

58. Yang X, Yu Y, Xu J, et al. Clinical course and outcomes of critically ill patients with SARS-CoV-2 pneumonia in Wuhan, China: a single-centered, retrospective, observational study. Lancet Respir Med 2020;8:475–81.

59. Lippi G, Lavie CJ, Sanchis-Gomar F. Cardiac troponin I in patients with coronavirus disease 2019 (COVID-19): evidence from a meta-analysis. Prog Cardiovasc Dis 2020;63:390–1.

60. Yin S, Huang M, Li D, et al. Difference of coagulation features between severe pneumonia induced by SARS-CoV2 and non-SARS-CoV2. J Thromb Thrombolysis 2021;51:1107–10.

61. Talasaz AH, Sadeghipour P, Kakavand H, et al. Recent randomized trials of antithrombotic therapy for patients with COVID-19: JACC state-of-the-art review. J Am Coll Cardiol 2021;77:1903–21.

62. Fournier M, Faille D, Dossier A, et al. Arterial thrombotic events in Adult Inpatients with COVID-19. Mayo Clin Proc 2021;96:295–303.
63. Poterucha TJ, Libby P, Goldhaber SZ. More than an anticoagulant: do heparins have direct anti-inflammatory effects? Thromb Haemost 2017;117:437–44.
64. Tang N, Bai H, Chen X, et al. Anticoagulant treatment is associated with decreased mortality in severe coronavirus disease 2019 patients with coagulopathy. J Thromb Haemost 2020;18:1094–9.
65. Thachil J, Tang N, Gando S, et al. ISTH interim guidance on recognition and management of coagulopathy in COVID-19. J Thromb Haemost 2020;18:1023–6.
66. Hadid T, Kafri Z, Al-Katib A. Coagulation and anticoagulation in COVID-19. Blood Rev 2021;47:100761.
67. Paranjpe I, Fuster V, Lala A, et al. Association of treatment dose anticoagulation with in-hospital Survival among hospitalized patients with COVID-19. J Am Coll Cardiol 2020;76:122–4.
68. Lemos ACB, do Espírito Santo DA, Salvetti MC, et al. Therapeutic versus prophylactic anticoagulation for severe COVID-19: a randomized phase II clinical trial (HESACOVID). Thromb Res 2020;196:359–66.
69. Schindewolf M, Weitz JI. Broadening the categories of patients eligible for extended venous thromboembolism treatment. Thromb Haemost 2020;120:014–26.
70. Available at: https://clinicaltrials.gov/ct2/show/NCT04662684. Accessed September 25, 2021.
71. Available at: https://clinicaltrials.gov/ct2/show/NCT04650087. Accessed September 25, 2021.
72. Etkin Y, Conway AM, Silpe J, et al. Acute arterial thromboembolism in patients with COVID-19 in the New York city area. Ann Vasc Surg 2021;70:290–4.
73. Choudry FA, Hamshere SM, Rathod KS, et al. High thrombus burden in patients with COVID-19 presenting with ST-segment elevation myocardial infarction. J Am Coll Cardiol 2020;76:1168–76.
74. De Luca G, Verdoia M, Cercek M, et al. Impact of COVID-19 pandemic on mechanical reperfusion for patients with STEMI. J Am Coll Cardiol 2020;76:2321–30.
75. Zeng J, Huang J, Pan L. How to balance acute myocardial infarction and COVID-19: the protocols from Sichuan Provincial People's Hospital. Intensive Care Med 2020;46:1111–3.
76. Chieffo A, Stefanini GG, Price S, et al. EAPCI position statement on invasive management of acute coronary syndromes during the COVID-19 pandemic. Eur Heart J 2020;41:1839–51.
77. Venketasubramanian N, Anderson C, Ay H, et al. Stroke care during the COVID-19 pandemic: international expert panel review. Cerebrovasc Dis Basel Switz 2021;50:245–61.
78. Goldman IA, Ye K, Scheinfeld MH. Lower-extremity arterial thrombosis associated with COVID-19 is characterized by greater Thrombus burden and increased rate of amputation and death. Radiology 2020;297:E263–9.
79. Available at: https://www.ema.europa.eu/en/human-regulatory/overview/public-health-threats/coronavirus-disease-covid-19/treatments-vaccines-covid-19. Accessed September 28 2021.
80. Franchini M, Liumbruno GM, Pezzo M. COVID-19 vaccine-associated immune thrombosis and thrombocytopenia (VITT): Diagnostic and therapeutic recommendations for a new syndrome. Eur J Haematol 2021;107:173–80.
81. Greinacher A, Thiele T, Warkentin TE, et al. Thrombotic thrombocytopenia after ChAdOx1 nCov-19 vaccination. N Engl J Med 2021;384:2092–101.

82. Schultz NH, Sørvoll IH, Michelsen AE, et al. Thrombosis and thrombocytopenia after ChAdOx1 nCoV-19 vaccination. N Engl J Med 2021;384:2124–30.
83. Scully M, Singh D, Lown R, et al. Pathologic antibodies to platelet factor 4 after ChAdOx1 nCoV-19 vaccination. N Engl J Med 2021;384:2202–11.
84. Oldenburg J, Klamroth R, Langer F, et al. Diagnosis and management of vaccine-related thrombosis following AstraZeneca COVID-19 vaccination: guidance statement from the GTH. Hämostaseologie. 2021;41:184–9.
85. Linkins L-A. Heparin induced thrombocytopenia. BMJ 2015;350:g7566.
86. Lee E, Cines DB, Gernsheimer T, et al. Thrombocytopenia following Pfizer and Moderna SARS-CoV-2 vaccination. Am J Hematol 2021;96:534–7.
87. Ortega-Paz L, Capodanno D, Montalescot G, et al. Coronavirus Disease 2019–Associated Thrombosis and Coagulopathy: Review of the Pathophysiological Characteristics and Implications for Antithrombotic Management [cited 2021 Jul 15];10. J Am Heart Assoc 2021. Available at: https://www.ahajournals.org/doi/10.1161/JAHA.120.019650.

COVID-19–Associated Endothelial Dysfunction and Microvascular Injury

From Pathophysiology to Clinical Manifestations

Maria Paola Canale, MD[a,b], Rossella Menghini, PhD[a],
Eugenio Martelli, MD[c,d], Massimo Federici, MD[a,b],*

KEYWORDS

- Covid-19 clinical manifestations • Endothelial dysfunction • Systemic inflammation
- ACE2 • ADAM17

KEY POINTS

- The broad spectrum of clinical manifestations, affecting almost all organs and systems, is a consequence of the endothelial dysfunction and systemic inflammatory response.
- Endothelial cells activated by a hyperinflammatory state induced by viral infection may promote localized inflammation, increase reactive oxidative species production, and alter dynamic interplay between the procoagulant and fibrinolytic factors in the vascular system, leading to thrombotic disease not only in the pulmonary circulation but also in peripheral veins and arteries.
- Several data support the involvement of an increased activity of ADAM17 in both COVID-19's comorbidities and SARS-CoV-2 infection. In fact, the ADAM17 upregulation leads to the angiotensin-converting enzyme 2 (ACE2) ectodomain proteolytic cleavage, facilitating viral entry, and to the cleavage of tumor necrosis factor alpha and interleukin-6 receptor and other proinflammatory molecules, contributing to the "cytokine storm" and reinforcing the inflammatory process during SARS-CoV-2 infection.
- The molecular interaction of SARS-CoV-2 with the ACE2 receptor located in the endothelial cell surface, either at the pulmonary and systemic level, leads to early impairment of endothelial function, which, in turn, is followed by vascular inflammation and thrombosis of peripheral blood vessels.

This article previously appeared in *Cardiac Electrophysiology Clinics*, Volume 14, Issue 1, March 2022.

[a] Department of Systems Medicine, University of Rome Tor Vergata, Rome, Italy; [b] Center for Atherosclerosis, Policlinico Tor Vergata, Rome, Italy; [c] Department of General and Specialist Surgery "P. Stefanini", Sapienza University of Rome, Italy; [d] Division of Vascular Surgery, S. Anna and S. Sebastiano Hospital, Caserta, Italy
* Corresponding author. Department of Systems Medicine, Via Montpellier 1, Roma 00133, Italy.
E-mail address: federicm@uniroma2.it

2352-7986/22/© 2021 Elsevier Inc. All rights reserved.

INTRODUCTION

Coronavirus-19 disease (COVID-19) affects more people than previous coronavirus infections, namely severe acute respiratory syndrome (SARS) and middle east respiratory syndrome (MERS) and has a higher mortality. Higher incidence and mortality can probably be explained by COVID-19 causative agent's greater affinity (about 10–20 times) for angiotensin-converting enzyme 2 (ACE2) receptor compared with other coronaviruses.[1,2] According to the World Health Organization's (WHO) recent data "there have been 199.466.211 confirmed cases of COVID-19, including 4.244.541 deaths" (source: WHO data, August 4, 2021). In the same way as SARS and MERS, it affects the respiratory system. Nevertheless, because of the viral rapid diffusion and the increased numbers of infected people, many extra respiratory system manifestations have been documented.[3–5] Severe symptoms result from hyperinflammatory response, which in turn causes systemic cytokine release and endothelial damage, and several clinical and laboratory findings support the role of endothelial dysfunction in the pathophysiology of disease, suggesting that the endothelium may represent an attractive target for new treatments.[6]

In this review, the authors first summarize clinical manifestations, then present symptoms of COVID-19 and the pathophysiological mechanisms underlying specific organ/system disease. After, they review current understanding of key pathophysiological mechanisms with particular regard to the role of endothelial dysfunction, microvascular injury, and systemic inflammatory response in disease progression and severity. Finally, they illustrate possible novel mechanisms and treatments aimed at protecting the endothelium.

COVID-19 CLINICAL MANIFESTATIONS

COVID-19 transmission mainly occurs directly via respiratory and saliva droplets from person to person. Indirect transmission, through fomites, may also occur. Airborne transmission only occurs when procedures generate aerosol. Incubation period is usually less than 1 week (about 5–6 days) but may last longer up to 2 weeks. Initial symptoms are nonspecific and similarly to other virosis such as influenza: fatigue, myalgias, dry cough, and low-grade fever.[7] Symptoms improve in most of the cases or progress to dyspnea in fewer ones.[3] Zeng and colleagues reviewed the symptomatology of COVID-19: the commonest signs/symptoms were fever (90%) and cough (68%) followed by dyspnea (22%), headache (12%), and sore throat (14%). Diarrhea was present in only about 4% of patients. Mean duration of fever in survivors is about 12 days, whereas mean duration of cough is slightly longer (19 days).[8] Although fever is a very common finding, its absence does not rule out the diagnosis.[9] Longer duration of fever is proportionate to disease's severity (31 days for patients admitted to the intensive care unit vs 9 days for those hospitalized in a different setting)[10]. As mentioned earlier, in about one-fifth of patients disease progresses to dyspnea.[3,7] Rapid progression to respiratory failure requiring noninvasive and invasive ventilation may occur. Viral respiratory invasion alone is insufficient to explain these findings. Endothelial dysfunction, subsequent inflammation, and lung injury with diffuse alveolar damage leading in some cases to acute distress respiratory syndrome is the underlying pathophysiological mechanism responsible for respiratory failure.[7] Patients may experience other clinical features that strongly suggest endothelial dysfunction and microvascular thrombosis. Pain, warmth, and localized limb swelling are consistent with deep venous thrombosis, and acute onset tachycardia, dyspnea, and chest pain strongly suggest pulmonary embolism.[5]

The alterations of the coagulation mechanisms observed in COVID-19 can lead to acute thrombotic phenomena of the arteries of the lower limbs, curiously even in patients with healthy arteries (ie, in the absence of underlying peripheral arterial disease) or without atrial fibrillation or preexisting coagulation disorders. The most severe acute ischemia occurs in patients admitted to intensive care units for severe forms of COVID-19 pneumonia: they rarely represent the only clinical manifestation of the infection. The conservative approach with medical therapy alone may be the most appropriate, considering the poor results of surgical revascularization. This latter, on the contrary, has always been characterized by excellent results in non-COVID patients operated on within a few hours of the onset of acute symptoms. The rate of limb loss/amputation is dramatically high in patients with COVID affected by acute limb ischemia.[11]

Concomitant oliguria and general symptoms (ie, nausea and vomiting) deserve urgent renal function testing and raise the possibility of uremia in the setting of acute kidney injury. In addition, new-onset generalized edema reflects heart failure and/or heavy proteinuria. Moreover, the presence/absence of associated signs/symptoms may further contribute to orient the diagnosis during patient's physical examination. For instance, the coexistence of dyspnea, new-onset generalized edema with symmetric periorbital involvement, and negative hepatojugular reflux indicates concomitant respiratory and renal rather than cardiac involvement. Laboratory tests would eventually show abnormal renal function, hypoalbuminemia, and heavy proteinuria, and transthoracic echocardiography confirms normal systolic function and absence of valves abnormalities. Severe headache may reflect central venous thrombosis or intracerebral hemorrhage. Finally, systemic inflammatory response may indirectly cause neurologic signs/symptoms such as headache, encephalopathy, or seizures.[5]

COVID-19 is characterized by a wide spectrum of clinical severity. Asymptomatic persons experience no symptoms and have normal chest radiographs but play an important role in disease transmission to others. Mild illness is characterized by general symptoms common to other virosis; gastrointestinal symptoms may be present too (abdominal pain, nausea, vomiting, and diarrhea). In moderate illness, symptoms of pneumonia are present with still normal blood gases, and interstitial ground-glass opacities appear on high-resolution computed tomography scan. Severe illness is characterized by pneumonia with hypoxemia (peripheral oxygen saturation is <92% in ambient air). Finally, critical state is characterized by the presence of acute distress respiratory syndrome, coagulation disorders, cardiac failure, acute renal injury, and shock.[7,9,12–17] Patients with comorbidities have a worse disease course and prognosis compared with healthy ones, as observed in previous coronavirus infections.[1] Advanced age, male sex, diabetes, hypertension, ischemic heart disease, cancer, chronic obstructive pulmonary disease, and chronic renal insufficiency are risk factors for developing a severe form of COVID-19.[18–20] These conditions affect negatively patient's immune system.[1,21]

A full description of the COVID-19 treatment by organ/system involvement is beyond the scope of this review. Most suitable treatment should be prescribed depending on disease's severity and organ involvement. At the present time, treatment encompasses oxygen (when required); symptomatic, antiinflammatory, antiviral, and anticoagulant drugs (prophylactic or therapeutic, with low-molecular-weight heparin); and monoclonal antibodies. Moreover, in selected patients resistant to treatment, plasma exchange therapy and immunomodulatory medications may be required.[7] Updated COVID-19 treatment guidelines by disease's severity are provided by national and international institutions at their Web sites. Finally, major concern has been raised about the use of renin-angiotensin blocking agents in patients with

COVID-19. Routine discontinuation is not recommended by the guidelines of international cardiology societies.[22,23]

A Molecular Perspective to Explain Endothelial Cell Activation in COVID 19

The COVID-19 clinical manifestations by organ/system and the underlying pathophysiological mechanisms of disease are summarized in **Tables 1–3**. Mechanisms that specifically contribute to determine a clinical manifestation are also reported. Endothelium represents an interface between blood and body's tissues.[24] The broad spectrum of clinical manifestations, affecting almost all organs and systems, is a consequence of the endothelial dysfunction and systemic inflammatory response. As shown in **Tables 1–3**, endothelial dysfunction's different components and systemic inflammatory response, namely "cytokine storm," play a pivotal role in determining most of the clinical manifestations of COVID-19 (left column) and always underlie severe manifestations.[4,5]

Recent findings suggest that endothelial dysfunction represents a crucial pathologic characteristic in COVID19, being implicated in microvascular and macrovascular complications associated with the infection, including myocardial infarction and stroke.[25] Biomarkers of endothelial dysfunction are increased in patients with COVID-19 and are associated with more severe forms of the disease and high mortality.[26] Endothelial dysfunction may result from a combination of direct viral effects, as

Table 1
COVID-19 clinical manifestations by system and pathophysiological mechanism

Clinical Manifestations (Refs.[1–5])	Pathophysiological Mechanisms (Refs.[1–5])

Respiratory
  Pneumonia
  Acute respiratory distress syndrome
  Microvascular lung thrombosis
  Respiratory failure
	Multifactorial
	Direct viral injury and inflammation
	Endothelial dysfunction
	• proinflammatory
	• procoagulant
	• proaggregating
	• capillary leakage
	• increased vascular permeability
	Systemic inflammatory response
	("cytokine storm")

Cardiac
  Myocarditis/pericarditis
  Arrhythmias
  Right or/and left heart failure
  Acute coronary syndrome
  Cardiogenic shock
	Multifactorial
	Direct viral injury and inflammation
	Endothelial dysfunction
	• proinflammatory
	• procoagulant
	High ACE2 levels
	Systemic inflammatory response
	("cytokine storm")
	Hypoxemia
	Oxygen supply mismatch

Arterial
  Large vessel occlusion: clinical presentation depending on the affected artery (cerebral, cardiac, mesenteric, renal, limb)
  Central nervous system vasculitis
	Multifactorial
	Direct viral injury
	Endothelial dysfunction
	• proinflammatory
	• procoagulant
	• proaggregating
	Hypoxia

Table 2
COVID-19 clinical manifestations by system and pathophysiological mechanism

Clinical Manifestations (Refs.[1–5])	Pathophysiological Mechanisms (Refs.[1–5])

Venous thromboembolism
  Deep vein thrombosis
  Pulmonary embolism
  Intravenous/intraarterial catheters and
    extracorporeal circuit thrombosis
  Central venous thrombosis
	Multifactorial
	Endothelial dysfunction
	• proinflammatory
	• prooxidant
	• procoagulant
	• proaggregating
	Hypoxia

Renal
  Hematuria/proteinuria
  Electrolyte abnormalities
  Acute tubular necrosis
  Acute kidney injury
	Multifactorial
	Direct viral injury
	Endothelial dysfunction leading to
	• vasoconstriction
	• microvascular dysfunction
	Systemic inflammatory response ("cytokine storm")
	Immune complexes
	Hypovolemia

Hepatic/Gastrointestinal
  Liver function tests abnormalities
  Gastrointestinal symptoms (diarrhea,
    abdominal pain, nausea, vomiting)
	Multifactorial
	Direct viral injury
	Endothelial dysfunction
	• proinflammatory
	• procoagulant
	• proaggregating
	Microvascular small bowel injury
	Systemic inflammatory response ("cytokine storm")
	Hypoxia-associated metabolic abnormalities

Neurologic/ocular
  Ageusia, anosmia
  Dizziness, headache, seizures
  Guillain-Barré syndrome
  Encephalitis/meningoencephalitis
  Encephalomyelitis
  Acute hemorrhagic necrotizing
    encephalopathy
  Conjunctivitis and retinal changes
	Multifactorial
	Direct nervous system invasion for ageusia, anosmia, encephalitis, meningoencephalitis
	Direct viral injury
	Endothelial dysfunction
	• proinflammatory
	• procoagulant
	Systemic inflammatory response ("cytokine storm")
	Postinfectious/immune-mediated for Guillain-Barré syndrome, encephalomyelitis, acute hemorrhagic-necrotizing encephalopathy
	Direct viral injury and inflammation for conjunctivitis

suggested by the presence of viral elements within the endothelium in autopsies from patients who died of COVID19, and a consequence of virus-dependent activation of inflammatory response.[27] Moreover, endothelial changes are multiorgan, indicating that endothelial dysfunction may be involved in numerous symptoms of SARS-CoV-2-positive patients.[28] Injury of endothelial cells is involved in several pathophysiological mechanisms that may promote the occurrence of micro- and macrovascular involvement in COVID19 infection. Endothelial cells activated by a hyperinflammatory state induced by viral infection may promote localized inflammation, increase reactive

Table 3
COVID-19 clinical manifestations by system and pathophysiological mechanism

Clinical Manifestations (Refs.[1-5])	Pathophysiological Mechanisms (Refs.[1-5])

Dermatologic
  Acrocutaneous lesions
  Erythematous and maculopapular rash
  Vesicles
  Livedoid, necrotic lesions, petechiae
	Multifactorial
	  Endothelial dysfunction with deposition of microthrombi
	  Systemic inflammatory response ("cytokine storm")
	  Immune response sensitivity
	  Vasculitis

Hematologic
  Blood cell count abnormalities (lymphopenia, leukocytosis neutrophilia, thrombocytopenia)
  Increased inflammatory markers
  Increased coagulation markers
	Multifactorial
	  Direct viral injury and inflammation and endothelial dysfunction proinflammatory for lymphopenia
	  Systemic inflammatory response and/or bacterial infection for leukocytosis
	  Systemic inflammatory response (early phase) for increased inflammatory markers and increased coagulation makers

Miscellaneous
  Fever
  Fatigue
  Myalgias
  Endocrine (new-onset diabetes, severe illness in diabetic/obese patients, ketoacidosis)
  High-grade fever
  Hypotension
  Multiorgan dysfunction
  Disseminated intravascular coagulation
  Long-term COVID-19 syndrome
	Cytokine release common to other virus for fever, fatigue, and myalgias
	Direct viral injury, lactate level increase, low oxygen, and low pH for myalgias
	Multifactorial for endocrine
	Endothelial dysfunction leading to systemic inflammatory response ("cytokine storm")
	ACE2 viral binding on beta cells
	Impaired counter-regulation (not specific to COVID-19)
	Altered immune response (not specific to COVID-19)
	Systemic inflammatory response for high-grade fever, hypotension, and multiorgan dysfunction
	Endothelial dysfunction leading to coagulation/fibrinolytic abnormalities, macro- and microthrombosis, bleeding for disseminated intravascular coagulation
	Multifactorial for long-term COVID
	Virus-specific pathophysiologic changes
	Inflammatory damage and immunologic aberrations
	Sequelae of postcritical illness

oxidative species production, and alter dynamic interplay between the procoagulant and fibrinolytic factors in the vascular system, leading to thrombotic disease not only in the pulmonary circulation but also in peripheral veins and arteries.[29] It was proposed that mitochondrial dysfunction and oxidative stress, induced by viral infection, can initiate a feedback loop, promoting a chronic state of inflammatory cytokine production and endothelial alteration even after the viral particles have been eliminated from the body.[30] Agents that limit endothelial dysfunction may mitigate the proinflammatory and prothrombotic state induced by COVID-19 infection; therefore, targeted inhibition of cytokines, major effectors of endothelial activation, represents a more focused approach than generalized antiinflammatory agents. Some clinical trials that use strategies aimed to have inhibit the inflammasome–interleukin-1β (IL-1β)–IL-6 pathway already yielded preliminary results; some, but not all, indicate signals of efficacy being a critical aspect in the maintaining of the balance between the potential benefits versus the potential of lowering immunologic defences.[24]

ADAM17 Abridges COVID19 and Endothelial Dysfunction

ADAM17 (a disintegrin and a metalloproteinase 17) is a type I transmembrane protein that belongs to a superfamily of Zn-dependent metalloproteases. ADAM17 plays a key role in the regulation of the proteolytic release from cellular membranes of some cytokines, chemokines, growth factors, and their receptors, affecting downstream signaling and cellular responses. Increased ADAM17-mediated shedding has been described in a variety of diseases such as ischemia, heart failure, arthritis, atherosclerosis, diabetes, cancer, neurologic, and immune diseases. Tissue inhibitor of metalloproteinase 3 (TIMP3), a key endogenous inhibitor involved in regulation of the activity of matrix metalloproteinases and ADAMs, is the only known physiologic inhibitor of ADAM17. Previous reports have implicated the ADAM17/TIMP3 dyad as a mediator between metabolic stimuli, inflammation, and innate immunity.[31] The increased activity of ADAM17 has been correlated with increased insulin resistance and hyperglycemia. Furthermore, the upregulation of ADAM17 activity increased insulin receptor resistance in patients with type 2 diabetes.[32] Several data support the involvement of an increased activity of ADAM17 in both COVID-19's comorbidities and SARS-CoV-2 infection. In fact, the ADAM17 upregulation leads to the ACE2 ectodomain proteolytic cleavage, facilitating viral entry, and to the cleavage of tumor necrosis factor alpha and IL-6R and other proinflammatory molecules, contributing to the "cytokine storm" and reinforcing the inflammatory process during SARS-CoV-2 infection. This hyperinflammatory state has deleterious effects on the vascular system with resulting endothelial cell dysfunction and not only affects local endothelial function but can also provoke a prothrombotic and antifibrinolytic imbalance in blood that favors thrombus accumulation.[33] Coagulation abnormalities and disruption of factors released by endothelial cells represent also the common pathophysiological link between SARS-CoV-2 infection and the cardiovascular events, including acute cardiac injury, stroke, heart failure, arrhythmias, and cardiomyopathies. In particular, the molecular interaction of SARS-CoV-2 with the ACE2 receptor located in the endothelial cell surface, either at the pulmonary and systemic level, leads to early impairment of endothelial function, which, in turn, is followed by vascular inflammation and thrombosis of peripheral blood vessels.[34]

In this context, the worse clinical outcome observed in patients with COVID-19 with diabetes may be in part related to the increased ADAM17 activity and its unbalanced interplay with ACE2. Therefore, strategies aimed to inhibit ADAM17 activity may be explored to develop new effective therapeutic approaches.

SUMMARY

In the last 2 years a great progress had been made to provide mechanisms explaining how Sars-COV-2 affects human health. Data point to endothelium as a major site of action of the virus. The overactivation of the physiologic functions of endothelium such as control of vasomotion, vascular permeability, fibrinolysis and hemostasis, inflammation, and oxidative stress may contribute to the COVID19 disease and provide a framework to develop new therapeutics against Sars-COV-2 in the future.

CLINICS CARE POINTS

- Endothelial dysfunction represents a crucial pathologic characteristic in COVID19, being implicated in microvascular and macrovascular complications associated with the infection, including myocardial infarction and stroke.

- Endothelial dysfunction may result from a combination of direct viral effects, as suggested by the presence of viral elements within the endothelium in autopsies from patients who died of COVID19, and a consequence of virus-dependent activation of inflammatory response.

- Treatment encompasses oxygen (when required); symptomatic, antiinflammatory, antiviral, and anticoagulant drugs (prophylactic or therapeutic, with low-molecular-weight heparin), and monoclonal antibodies.

CONFLICTS OF INTEREST/DISCLOSURES

This work was in part supported by PRIN 2017FM74HK (to M.F.).

REFERENCES

1. Johnson KD, Harris C, Cain JK, et al. Pulmonary and extra-pulmonary clinical manifestations of COVID-19. Front Med (Lausanne) 2020;7:526.
2. Wrapp D, Wang N, Corbett KS, et al. Cryo-EM structure of the 2019-nCoV spike in the prefusion conformation. Science 2020;367:1260–3.
3. Canatan D, Vives Corrons JL, De Sanctis V. The multifacets of COVID-19 in adult patients: a concise clinical review on pulmonary and extrapulmonary manifestations for healthcare physicians. Acta Biomed 2020;91:e2020173.
4. Gupta A, Madhavan MV, Sehgal K, et al. Extrapulmonary manifestations of COVID-19. Nat Med 2020;26:1017–32.
5. Gavriilaki E, Anyfanti P, Gavriilaki M, et al. Endothelial dysfunction in COVID-19: lessons learned from coronaviruses. Curr Hypertens Rep 2020;22:63.
6. Castro P, Palomo M, Moreno-Castaño AB, et al. Is the endothelium the missing link in the pathophysiology and treatment of COVID-19 complications? Cardiovasc Drugs Ther 2021;1–14.
7. Parasher A. COVID-19: current understanding of its pathophysiology, clinical presentation and treatment. Postgrad Med J 2021;97:312–20.
8. Zheng J. SARS-CoV-2: an emerging coronavirus that causes a global threat. Int J Biol Sci 2020;16:1678–85.
9. Guan WJ, Ni ZY, Hu Y, et al. China medical treatment expert group for Covid-19. Clinical characteristics of coronavirus disease 2019 in China. N Engl J Med 2020; 382:1708–20.
10. Chen J, Qi T, Liu L, et al. Clinical progression of patients with COVID-19 in Shanghai, China. J Infect 2020;80:e1–6.
11. Etkin Y, Conway AM, Silpe J, et al. Acute arterial thromboembolism in patients with COVID-19 in the New York City Area. Ann Vasc Surg 2021;70:290–4.
12. Li Q, Guan X, Wu P, et al. Early transmission dynamics in Wuhan, China, of novel coronavirus-infected pneumonia. N Engl J Med 2020;382:1199–207.
13. Yuki K, Fujiogi M, Koutsogiannaki S. COVID-19 pathophysiology: a review. Clin Immunol 2020;215:108427.
14. Donnelly CA, Ghani AC, Leung GM, et al. Epidemiological determinants of spread of causal agent of severe acute respiratory syndrome in Hong Kong. Lancet 2003;361:1761–6.

15. Goyal P, Choi JJ, Pinheiro LC, et al. Clinical characteristics of covid-19 in New York City. N Engl J Med 2020;382:2372–4.
16. Young BE, Ong SWX, Kalimuddin S, et al. Singapore 2019 Novel coronavirus outbreak research team. epidemiologic features and clinical course of patients infected with SARS-CoV-2 in Singapore. JAMA 2020;323:1488–94.
17. Cheung KS, Hung IFN, Chan PPY, et al. Gastrointestinal manifestations of SARS-CoV-2 infection and virus load in fecal samples from a Hong Kong Cohort: systematic review and meta-analysis. Gastroenterology 2020;159:81–95.
18. Liu X, Zhou H, Zhou Y, et al. Risk factors associated with disease severity and length of hospital stay in COVID-19 patients. J Infect 2020;81:e95–7.
19. Wynants L, Van Calster B, Collins GS, et al. Prediction models for diagnosis and prognosis of covid-19: systematic review and critical appraisal. BMJ 2020;369: m1328.
20. Pijls BG, Jolani S, Atherley A, et al. Demographic risk factors for COVID-19 infection, severity, ICU admission and death: a meta-analysis of 59 studies. BMJ Open 2021;11:e044640.
21. Park J, Lee DS, Christakis NA, et al. The impact of cellular networks on disease comorbidity. Mol Syst Biol 2009;5:262.
22. European Society of Cardiology Position statement of the ESC Council on hypertension on ACE-Inhibitors and angiotensin receptor blockers. Eur Heart J 2021 Nov 16;ehab696. https://doi.org/10.1093/eurheartj/ehab696.
23. Bozkurt B, Kovacs R, Harrington B. Joint HFSA/ACC/AHA statement Addresses concerns Re: Using RAAS Antagonists in COVID-19. J Card Fail 2020;26:370.
24. Libby P, Lüscher T. COVID-19 is, in the end, an endothelial disease. Eur Heart J 2020;41:3038–44.
25. Gu SX, Tyagi T, Jain K, et al. Thrombocytopathy and endotheliopathy: crucial contributors to COVID-19 thromboinflammation. Nat Rev Cardiol 2021;18:194–209.
26. Pine AB, Meizlish ML, Goshua G, et al. Circulating markers of angiogenesis and endotheliopathy in COVID-19. Pulm Circ 2020;10. 204589402096654.
27. Varga Z, Flammer AJ, Steiger P, et al. Endothelial cell infection and endotheliitis in COVID-19. Lancet 2020;395:1417–8.
28. Fodor A, Tiperciuc B, Login C, et al. Endothelial dysfunction, inflammation, and oxidative stress in COVID-19-mechanisms and therapeutic targets. Oxid Med Cell Longev 2021;2021:8671713.
29. Siddiqi HK, Libby P, Ridker PM. COVID-19 - a vascular disease. Trends Cardiovasc Med 2021;31:1–5.
30. Chang R R, Mamun A A, Dominic A A, et al. SARSCoV-2 mediated endothelial dysfunction: the potential role of chronic oxidative stress. Front Physiol 2021; 11:605908.
31. Menghini R, Fiorentino L, Casagrande V, et al. The role of ADAM17 in metabolic inflammation. Atherosclerosis 2013;228:12–7.
32. Cardellini M, Menghini R, Luzi A, et al. Decreased IRS2 and TIMP3 expression in monocytes from offspring of type 2 diabetic patients is correlated with insulin resistance and increased intima-media thickness. Diabetes 2011;60:3265–70.
33. Zipeto D, Palmeira JDF, Argañaraz GA, et al. ACE2/ADAM17/TMPRSS2 interplay may be the main risk factor for COVID-19. Front Immunol 2020;11:576745.
34. Maiuolo J, Mollace R, Gliozzi M, et al. The contribution of endothelial dysfunction in systemic injury subsequent to SARS-Cov-2 infection. Int J Mol Sci 2020;21: 9309.

COVID-19, Acute Myocardial Injury, and Infarction

Armando Del Prete, MD[a,b,*], Francesca Conway, MD[c],
Domenico G. Della Rocca, MD, PhD[d],
Giuseppe Biondi-Zoccai, MD, MStat[a,e,f], Francesco De Felice, MD[g],
Carmine Musto, MD, PhD[g], Marco Picichè, MD[h],
Eugenio Martuscelli, MD, PhD[i], Andrea Natale, MD[d,j,k],
Francesco Versaci, MD[a]

KEYWORDS

• COVID-19 • Myocardial injury • Myocardial infarction • SARS-CoV-2

Continued

INTRODUCTION

The new coronavirus-associated disease 2019 (COVID-19), due to severe acute respiratory syndrome coronavirus-2 (SARS-CoV-2), represents an unprecedented public health emergency that has been accompanied by a global health crisis. Although SARS-CoV-2 primarily infects the respiratory system, causing a variety of clinical presentations, from asymptomatic infection to interstitial pneumonia and severe acute respiratory distress syndrome (ARDS), the cardiovascular implications are also significant, especially in their contribution to disease morbidity and mortality.

When the cardiovascular system is affected, complications can include myocardial injury, acute myocardial infarction (MI), heart failure, myocarditis, dysrhythmias, and

This article previously appeared in *Cardiac Electrophysiology Clinics*, Volume 14, Issue 1, March 2022.

[a] Division of Cardiology, Santa Maria Goretti Hospital, Via Guido Reni 1, 04100 Latina, Italy; [b] Department of Systems Medicine, University of Rome "Tor Vergata", Via Montpellier 1, 00133 Rome, Italy; [c] London School of Hygiene and Tropical Medicine, Keppel St, London WC1E 7HT, United Kingdom; [d] Texas Cardiac Arrhythmia Institute, St. David's Medical Center, 000 N Interstate Hwy 35 Suite 720, Austin, TX 78705, USA; [e] Department of Medical-Surgical Sciences and Biotechnologies, Sapienza University, Corso della Repubblica 79, 04100 Latina, Italy; [f] Mediterranea Cardiocentro, Via Ponte di Tappia 82, 80133 Naples, Italy; [g] Division of Cardiology, San Camillo Hospital, Circonvallazione Gianicolense 87, 00152 Rome, Italy; [h] Department of Cardiac Surgery, San Bortolo Hospital, Viale Ferdinando Rodolfi 37, 36100 Vicenza, Italy; [i] Department of Biomedicine and Prevention, University of Rome "Tor Vergata", Via Montpellier 1, 00133 Rome, Italy; [j] Interventional Electrophysiology, Scripps Clinic, 9898 Genesee Ave Fl 3, La Jolla, CA 92037, USA; [k] Metro Health Medical Center, Case Western Reserve University School of Medicine, 9501 Euclid Ave, Cleveland, OH 44106, USA

* Corresponding author. Division of Cardiology, Santa Maria Goretti Hospital, Via Guido Reni 1, Latina, Italy.
E-mail address: armando.delprete85@gmail.com

Clinics Collections 12 (2022) 187–201
https://doi.org/10.1016/j.ccol.2021.12.014
2352-7986/22/© 2021 Elsevier Inc. All rights reserved.

Continued

KEY POINTS

- Severe acute respiratory syndrome coronavirus-2 (SARS-CoV-2) primarily infects the respiratory tract but can broadly affect the cardiovascular system too.
- SARS-CoV-2 can damage the myocardium by direct viral invasion or indirectly through inflammation, endothelial activation, and microvascular thrombosis.
- Myocardial injury affects about one-quarter of patients with COVID-19, even those without prior cardiovascular disease.
- Patients with COVID-19 who experience myocardial injury have higher hospital mortality rates and can present long-term complications.
- The diagnosis of myocardial injury can be particularly challenging in the context of COVID-19, particularly in patients with advanced disease.

venous thromboembolic events.[1] Although various studies have demonstrated an association between preexisting cardiovascular disease and severe COVID-19 manifestations, it is possible that the viral infection itself may lead to cardiac complications or exacerbate preexisting cardiovascular conditions.[2,3]

Acute myocardial injury is not uncommon in patients with COVID-19 and correlates with disease severity.[4] In addition, patients with long-term coronary artery disease or risk factors for atherosclerotic disease are at heightened risk of acute coronary syndromes (ACS) if infected with SARS-CoV-2. Acute coronary events in patients with COVID-19 may be the result of the systemic inflammatory hyperactivity, triggered by the viral infection and mediated by circulating cytokines that interact with preexisting atherosclerotic plaques, potentially causing plaque instability and rupture, ultimately leading to a type 1 MI.[5] In patients who eventually overcome myocardial injury and SARS-CoV-2 infection, there is evidence of long-term cardiovascular complications, although the magnitude of these sequelae is still unclear.

PHYSIOPATHOLOGICAL INVOLVEMENT OF THE CARDIOVASCULAR SYSTEM

SARS-CoV-2 primarily infects cells in the respiratory tract, causing a wide spectrum of respiratory manifestations, from asymptomatic or mild infection to bilateral interstitial pneumonia and severe ARDS.[1] There is also evidence supporting the affinity of the virus for multiple tissues, suggesting that SARS-CoV-2 has an organotropism that extends beyond the respiratory system, involving the brain, the liver, the kidney, and the cardiovascular district.[6] When the cardiovascular system is affected a vast range of complications can occur, from myocardial injury and acute MI to heart failure, myocarditis, dysrhythmias, and venous thromboembolic events.[1]

Previously published reports have described increased incidence of myocardial injury among patients with COVID-19.[7] During SARS-COV-2 infection the myocardium may be damaged by the viral invasion of cardiac muscle cells, inflammation and production of free radicals and reactive oxygen species, microvascular thrombosis, and a disproportion between oxygen supply and demand.[8] As a result, myocardial dysfunction, heart failure, myocardial injury, and both type 1 and type 2 MI may manifest, mediated by these one or more of these underlying mechanisms. Cardiac tissue tropism of SARS-CoV-2 is supported by the findings of an autopsy series of 20 patients: detectable viral SARS-CoV genome was found in 7 of the 20 heart samples, along with increased myocardial fibrosis and inflammation.[9]

Direct viral invasion is not the only mechanism through which SARS-CoV-2 can damage the heart. A particularly interesting interaction has been described between SARS-CoV-2 and the renin angiotensin system (RAS).[10] The main hypothesis is that the RAS may be involved in the pathophysiology of COVID-19 via activation of the classic pathway. The angiotensin-converting enzyme 2 (ACE2) serves as a master regulator of the RAS. By metabolizing the vasoconstricting and proinflammatory angiotensin II (Ang II), ACE2 generates Ang 1 to 7, which counteracts the proinflammatory and prooxidant effects of Ang II.[11] Molecular studies have demonstrated that ACE2 is the SARS-CoV-2 cell entry receptor, through the activation of the viral outer membrane spike protein S by transmembrane protease serine 2 (TMPRSS2).[12] SARS-CoV-2 uses ACE2 as the port of entry by binding the extracellular domain of the host receptor through the S1/s2 subunits of the transmembrane spike glycoprotein.[13,14] Once a cell becomes infected with SARS-CoV-2, ACE2 is internalized, the virus can enter the cell and release its RNA to initiate replication and transcription of the viral genome. After synthesis and assembly of structural proteins, new virus is released from the cell by exocytosis, whereas host cells may be disabled or destroyed in the process.[15] Beyond causing direct cell damage through viral infiltration, SARS-CoV-2 downregulates ACE 2 expression and Ang 1 to 7 production, leading to the loss of the RAS counterregulatory protective arm.[16] By hampering the expression of ACE2, the beneficial degradation of Ang II to the counterregulatory Ang^{1-7} decreases, leading to unopposed Ang II effects, mediated by the receptor AT1. The AngII/AT1 activation yields several unfavorable effects, which include vasoconstrictive effects, but also host potentially detrimental effects on the endothelium, inflammation, and coagulation, ultimately increasing vascular permeability and promoting organ damage (**Fig. 1**).[17,18] These findings are supported by the fact that COVID-19 patients often present with increased AngII levels.[19,20] ACE2 is widely expressed in the lung but can also be found in high concentrations in the circulatory system at the level of arterial and venous endothelium as well as largely expressed by myocardial pericytes.[21,22]

Cardiovascular damage mediated by SARS-CoV-2 may therefore be the result of 3 different pathways:

- Direct myocardial damage due to viral entry through ACE2, resulting in myocardial cell destruction and inflammation;
- Indirect injury due to ACE2 downregulation following viral replication, with subsequent hyperactivation of the Ang II/AT1 system, responsible of vasoconstrictive, proinflammatory, and prooxidant effects
- Indirect injury through the activation of B and T immune cells, leading to a systemic inflammatory response and increased cardiac stress due to hypoxemia.[23,24]

The immune-mediated pathway can generate a cytokine storm with high circulating levels of interleukin-2 (IL-2), IL-7, IL-10, and tumor necrosis factor, as a result of alternate immune response. This mechanism has been observed in severe forms of COVID-19 and can mediate myocardial injury as well as lung injury (particularly diffuse alveolar damage), finally leading to multiorgan failure. Components of the systemic inflammatory response can exert a negative inotropic effect, promote cardiomyocyte apoptosis and fibrosis, and induce the release of procoagulant factors.[25] The high plasma levels of activated macrophages that usually accompany conditions of hypercytokinemia can lead to further release of cytokines, including IL-1β and IL-6, which promote the expression of adhesion molecules, inflammatory cell infiltration, and vascular inflammation, contributing to formation and propagation of microcirculatory lesions and endothelial dysfunction.[26] Macrophages can also release procoagulant

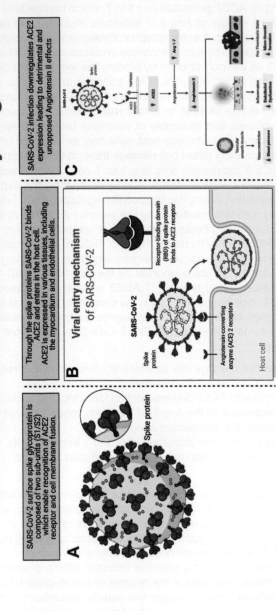

Fig. 1. SARS-CoV-2 entry in host cells (*A*, *B*) and downregulation of ACE2 expression (*C*).

factors, further accelerating inflammation and augmenting a prothrombotic condition and thrombotic microangiopathy.[27] High circulating levels of macrophages might also interact with preexisting atherosclerotic plaques, leading to rupture of the fibrous cap and possibly causing type 1 MI.[28] These pathways are not unique to SARS-CoV-2, as viral infections are known to determine adverse cardiovascular events by precipitating plaque rupture in the setting of inflammation and a prothrombotic state.[29] It is also possible that hyperinflammation may generate a supply-demand mismatch at the level of the myocardium. SARS-CoV-2 infection can therefore precipitate myocardial injury by determining an oxygen supply–demand imbalance, either with or without acute coronary plaque pathology (type 1 and 2 MI).

SARS-CoV-2 can attack the cardiovascular system through different strategies: through direct damage of myocytes mediated by the virus as well as indirect mechanisms due to RAS pathway dysregulation, hyperinflammation leading to endothelial disfunction in different districts, and activation of procoagulant factors with microvascular thrombosis and oxygen supply–demand imbalance (**Fig. 2**). These mechanisms can take place in the presence of preexisting cardiovascular conditions or in patients without a clinical history of cardiovascular disease (CVD). Nonetheless, individuals with cardiovascular comorbidities or diabetes are at greater risk of experiencing a more aggressive SARS-CoV2 infection and the related cardiovascular complications.[30]

PREVALENCE AND CLINICAL OUTCOME OF MYOCARDIAL INJURY IN COVID-19

The detection of least one elevated cardiac troponin value greater than the 99th percentile upper reference limit defines myocardial injury. Although MI represents a manifestation of myocardial injury, it requires clinical evidence of acute myocardial ischemia in order to perform the diagnosis. There are various subtypes of MI, the most common being type 1 infarction (characterized by plaque rupture, ulceration, erosion, or dissection resulting in coronary thrombosis) and type 2 infarction (secondary to myocardial oxygen supply–demand mismatch in the absence of coronary thrombosis).[31] Individuals infected with SARS-CoV-2 seem to be in a condition of increased susceptibility to various forms of myocardial injury.[32]

A study conducted in Wuhan showed evidence of cardiac damage with high levels of circulating troponin in up to 28% of patients with SARS-CoV-2. Furthermore, patients with evidence of cardiac injury had higher mortality rates compared with those without (51.2% vs 4.55%, $P < 0.001$). Complications such as acute respiratory syndrome distress, electrolyte alteration, and acute kidney injury were prevalent in patients with cardiac injury, suggesting how the cardiac involvement plays a detrimental effect in the prognosis of these patients[33]

A recently published review, composed of 26 studies including a total of 11,685 patients, estimated a lower prevalence of acute myocardial injury among SARS-CoV-2–infected patients, with around 20% showing evidence of myocardial injury (detected through the sample of troponin and/or creatine-kinase MB). In discussing the physiopathological mechanisms, the investigators also suggest a possible clinical role of cardiac biomarkers in the risk stratification of COVID-19.[34,35]

A systematic review published in 2021 estimated the rate of new cardiac injury between 7.2% and 77%, respectively, in live and dead SARS-CoV-2–infected cases, reiterating the concept that cardiac injury is associated to worse outcomes and higher rates of mortality, predominantly driven by development of shock and malignant arrythmias. In fact, about 46.3% of patients with cardiac injury required mechanical ventilation, 58.5% experienced acute respiratory distress syndrome, and 15.9%

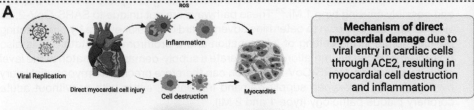

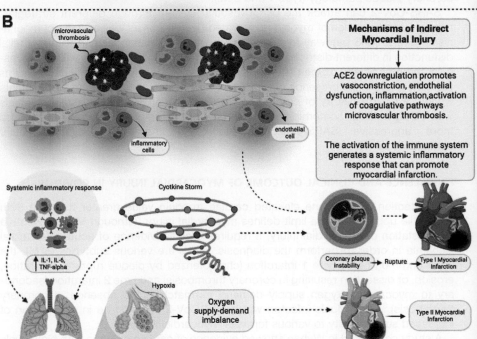

Fig. 2. Direct (*A*) and indirect (*B*) mechanisms of acute myocardial injury during SARS-CoV-2 infection and clinical outcomes.

suffered from electrolyte disturbance. In addition, the levels of troponin I seemed to be inversely correlated with the days of survival.[36]

In a multicenter retrospective cohort study including 2736 patients, 36% were found to have elevated troponin concentration. Even small increases in troponin I levels (ranging from 0.03 to 0.09 ng/mL), found in the 16% of the entire cohort of patients, were significantly associated with the death of the patients (adjusted hazard ratio: 1.75; 95% confidence interval [CI]: 1.37–2.24; *P* < .001). Patients with evidence of more robust damage to the myocardium may experience more than a 3-fold increase in the risk of mortality. Patients with preexisting CVD are more likely to experience myocardial injury compared with those without.[37]

PRINCIPAL IMAGING FINDINGS IN PATIENTS WITH COVID-19 WITH MYOCARDIAL INJURY

The clinical presentation of myocardial injury in patients with COVID-19 is usually atypical and therefore hard to diagnose. The cause of the increase in troponin levels in patients with COVID-19 has not been clearly defined. Cardiac damage can arise in patients with no previous history of CVD and in the absence of chest pain. Diagnosing pathologies such as myocarditis in patients with COVID-19 and increased levels of troponin is quite challenging, given the scarcity of studies that correlate the evidence from imaging techniques such as cardiac MRI or invasive methods such as endomyocardial biopsy to the clinical and echocardiographic findings in these patients. In addition, the latency between the onset of symptoms and the evidence of myocardial injury (about 14 days) raises doubts as to whether myocyte damage can be considered only as a marker of advanced disease severity or if it directly implies a greater risk of COVID-19 mortality.[8,38–40] A recent study evaluating a total of 201 patients with COVID-19 with critical and noncritical clinical conditions and with myocardial injury, detected through an elevation of CK-MB and troponin I levels, reported 18.7% of cases showing evidence of echocardiographic abnormalities. The main abnormalities were right ventricular dilatation and dysfunction (prevalent in critical patients). The investigators were able to highlight the direct contribution of COVID-19 to the myocardial injury of these patients. In addition, 43.7% of patients had new changes at electrocardiography and 36.3% had signs of ST depression.[41]

Cardiac MRI (CMR) represents the hallmark of the morphologic definition and classification of myocardial tissue pathology, especially in patients with myocardial edema. In a systematic review by Ojha and colleagues including 199 patients from 34 studies, myocarditis was the most common diagnosis at cardiac MRI in patients with evidence of myocardial injury (40.2% of cases). Mapping abnormalities, edema, and late gadolinium enhancement (LGE) represented the most frequently detected myocardial findings.[42] In a prospective observational trial by Puntmann and colleagues including 100 recently recovered COVID-19 cases, abnormal findings at CMR were found in 78% of patients, of which 60% showed ongoing myocardial inflammation with an increased native T2 (in a minority of cases regional scar and pericardial enhancement were detected), regardless of preexisting conditions and COVID-19 severity, raising concerns on the long-term consequences of SARS-CoV-2.[43] Most of the patients experienced only mild forms of illness.[43]

The prevalence of cardiac damage at CMR was quite lower in another recent multicenter trial involving 148 cases of severe COVID-19 recruited from 6 different facilities and with laboratory evidence of troponin elevation. The trial evaluated patients after discharge through CMR. The CMR protocol included adenosine stress perfusion (where clinically appropriate) and was performed at a median of 68 days postdischarge. Twenty-six percent of CMRs showed evidence of a myocarditis-like scar, 22% of infarction or ischemia, and 6% characterized by combination of both. Most of the myocarditis-like lesions involved 3 or less segments and was not accompanied by left ventricular dysfunction, although 30% of these patients had active myocarditis. Stress perfusion revealed inducible ischemia in 26% of cases and myocardial infarction findings in 19%. These findings suggest how even after discharge the rate of cardiac injury remains high. About a quarter of all patients included in the trial experienced ischemic heart disease (in the absence of previous CVD history in two-thirds of cases).[44] The discrepancy in prevalence of cardiac abnormalities at CMR that emerges from the 2 previously cited studies can be explained by differences in the selection of study participants and in the definition of myocardial injury and inflammation using isolated or combined CMR parameters and, in addition, by the different latency periods between the acute phase of COVID-19 and the timing of CMR. Moreover, abnormal T1 sequences and LGE may overdiagnose myocardial inflammation if used alone. The studies did not investigate the possibility of underlying and silent pathologic cardiac conditions not directly related to COVID-19. Several limitations affected these studies, including the absence of a description of patients' symptoms and their correlation to imaging findings.[45] A recent literature review examining 277 patients with COVID-19 undergoing autopsy showed that the true prevalence of myocarditis was lower than 2%. Cardiovascular histopathologic findings potentially related to COVID-19 infections were found in the 47.8% of cases. The findings included myocardial microvascular thrombi, inflammation, or intraluminal megakaryocytes The investigators specified that the wide differences in histology reports found in the studies may be a marker of observer bias.[46] There are several ongoing studies with larger sample sizes, an accurate standard protocol of imaging assessment, and longer follow-up periods that aim to explore the mid- and long-term cardiac sequelae following COVID-19 and identify factors that could significantly affect the outcomes of these patients.

MYOCARDIAL INFARCTION TYPE 1, 2, AND 3

This paragraph explores the challenges in the management of the different types of MI and the possible overlap of acute pathologies (whether myocardial, pulmonary, or systemic) that further nuance the diagnosis.[47,48]

The largest study investigating COVID-19 and acute cardiovascular events is a Swedish study involving 86,742 patients diagnosed with COVID-19 and a matched population of controls (348,481 patients). The investigators calculated the incidence rate ratio (IRR) of acute MI following COVID-19. The IRR was calculated in 2 separate analyses: including the day of exposure to SARS-CoV-2 (day 0) and excluding day 0. Excluding day 0 from the analysis led to the estimation of the IRR of acute MI of 2.89 (95% CI 1.51–5.55) in the first week of infection and 2.53 (95% CI 1.29–4.94), and 1.60 (95% CI 0.84–3.04), respectively, in the second week and in the third and fourth weeks. The inclusion of day 0 in the analysis resulted in a significant increase in the IRR during the first week (IRR 8.44; 95% CI 5.45–13.08) followed by comparable rate ratios in the remaining weeks. The analysis that excludes the day of viral exposure ensures potential elimination of testing bias because there is a possibility of a higher likelihood of detecting even asymptomatic forms of SARS-COV-2 in patients who are admitted to the hospital for MI or ischemic stroke. On the other hand, the exclusion of the day of viral exposure may lead to an underestimation of the true risk of cardiovascular events.[49] These results seem to clash with the significant reduction in hospital admission rates for acute ischemic cardiovascular events (both acute coronary syndromes and ischemic strokes) that has been described during the initial phases of the pandemic.[50,51] A possible explanation of this discrepancy is that particularly during the first wave of the pandemic several patients experiencing ACS and acute ischemic stroke did not seek timely medical attention for fear of exposure to SARS-CoV-2 at the hospital or to respect measures of physical distancing. Another possible explanation is related to the clinical instability of patients with COVID-19 and the rapid deterioration of the conditions of patients with severe forms, preventing a complete diagnostic evaluation.[49,52]

There are also certain characteristics of patients hospitalized for STEMI and affected by COVID-19 that have been recently described in the literature and that raise concern among providers. Specifically, a study including a nationwide registry of 1010 consecutive patients treated within 42 specific STEMI care networks investigated the clinical, procedural, and in-hospital prognostic features of COVID-19 patients affected by STEMI. This population showed a significant increase in stent thrombosis (3.3% vs 0.8%, P = .020), cardiogenic shock (9.9% vs 3.8%, P = .007), and in-hospital mortality compared with non-COVID-19 STEMI patients (23.1% vs 5.7%, P < .0001).[53]

A single-center observational study of 115 consecutive patients with STEMI managed by primary percutaneous coronary intervention (PCI) showed a higher thrombus burden and higher rates of multivessel thrombosis (17.9% vs 0%, P = .003) and stent thrombosis (10.3% vs 1.2%, P = .04) in patients with COVID-19 compared with non-COVID patients. Although the thrombolysis in MI flow and thrombus grade were similar in the 2 groups, the modified thrombus grade after first device resulted higher in patients with COVID-STEMI (75% vs 31%; P = 1⁄4 0.0006). Of these cases of COVID-STEMI a high percentage (about 60% vs 9.2% P = .002) received a Gp IIb/IIIa and underwent thrombectomy (17.9% vs 1.3%) when compared with non-COVID patients. The patients in the COVID-19 group had higher proportions of hypertension, diabetes, dyslipidemia, and previous PCI. The myocardial blush grade (MBG) resulted significantly lower in the COVID-STEMI (MBG of 2–3 in 54% vs 93%, P < .0001); the postprocedural median left ventricular ejection fraction resulted lower in COVID-STEMI patients (42.5% vs 45.0%; P = .019) as well as higher peak plasma troponin levels. The higher thrombus burden found in the COVID-STEMI group may represent a requirement for a more aggressive antithrombotic therapy in selected cases, although the actual evidence supporting this conduct is still poor.[54]

Data investigating ACS and COVID-19 remain conflictual, and the association is still uncertain. A systematic review and meta-analysis including 50,123 patients from 10 studies revealed a nonstatistically significant difference in admission rates of patients with STEMI during the pandemic compared with the previous year (IRR = 0.789, 95% CI 0.730–0.852 P = .01) and no increases in mortality for STEMI patients treated during the pandemic (odds ratio [OR] = 1.178, 95% CI 0.926–1.498, P = .01). What emerged from this review is that door-to-balloon time was significantly prolonged in STEMIs treated during the pandemic. Although these results harbor uncertainty regarding the impact of the pandemic on STEMI admission rates or mortality, they shed light on the organizational strain that facilities faced in the midst of the pandemic response.[55]

Diagnosis and management in patients with type 2 MI and COVID-19 are challenging, with repercussions on time to coronary angiographic evaluation. Inaccurate diagnosis of type 1 MI instead of type 2 and difficulties with differential diagnosis between MI and myocarditis might lead to an overestimation of acute MI. In a study by Stefanini and colleagues conducted on 28 patients with a diagnosis of STEMI that were promptly referred to the catheterization laboratory for urgent coronary angiography, 60.7% had a culprit lesion requiring urgent percutaneous treatment, whereas 39.3% did not show any signs of coronary obstructive lesion at angiography.[56]

Unfortunately the investigators did not investigate if the clinical presentation was attributable to a type 2 MI or to myocarditis or to SARS-CoV-2–related endothelial dysfunction. It is reasonable to hypothesize that a type 2 MI due to demand ischemia might be much more common in patients experiencing COVID-19. The condition of systemic inflammation triggered by viral infections, such as coronavirus and influenza virus,[57] may lead to oxygen supply–demand mismatch in the myocardium. It is also critical to highlight that it is clinically challenging to perform a correct differential diagnosis between non-STEMI ACS from other conditions that imply a form of myocardial injury such as hypoxemia, arrhythmias, sepsis, or myocarditis. To further complicate the matter, it is possible that these conditions may overlap, particularly in complex patients experiencing severe COVID-19. Sudden cardiac deaths or unexplained deaths have been reported in patients with SARS-CoV-2 infection and a previously diagnosed coronary artery disease. In this subset of patients it is possible to speculate a type 3 MI as the cause of the demise.[58–60]

The Takotsubo syndrome (TTS) is another cardiomyopathy that may determine myocardial injury in patients with COVID-19. TTS consists in a transient acute myocardial dysfunction, often characterized by circumferential myocardial regional akinesia/hypokinesia, leading to clinical acute heart failure, and in some cases mimicking an acute MI. Although the definite physiopathology of TTS has not yet been totally clarified, it is known that the sympathetic stimulation (ie, catecholamine-induced microvascular impairment) driven by sudden stress represents a trigger, and other evidences suggest how ongoing inflammation, infections, and other clinical conditions such as respiratory failure may be involved in the etiology.[61]

A case series of 118 consecutive patients with COVID-19 undergoing transthoracic evaluation found ultrasound features of TTS in 4.2%. These patients also had higher level of plasmatic troponin compared with patients without TTS myocardial injury and high rates of in-hospital complications and mortality.[62] These findings are in line with the findings of other investigators who reported high rates of severe respiratory and cardiac insufficiency eventually leading to greater oxygen requirements, use of vasopressors, and cardiac ventricular support devices in patients with TTS myocardial injury associated with COVID-19.[63–65]

The available evidence on COVID-19 and myocardial injury highlights the necessity to perform an accurate evaluation of the troponin elevation (ie, of the myocardial injury), the patients' clinical features, and an appropriate risk stratification. Direct invasive testing should be reserved for patients with a high pretest probability of coronary artery disease (CAD), whereas computed tomography scan or CMR is the appropriate test for patients with an intermediate probability of CAD, in order to evaluate either epicardial arteries or coronary arteries and rule out myocarditis. Patients with a low risk of CAD should be referred to strict follow-up.

Patients with COVID-19 that in addition experience an STEMI or very high-risk NSTEMI should be referred to the catheterization laboratory within the timeframe suggested by the current guidelines. Fibrinolysis should be considered only in case of difficulties in patients' transfer to a hub center in order to perform timely PCIs.[66,67]

MULTISYSTEM INFLAMMATORY SYNDROME IN CHILDREN

Although COVID-19 usually represents a mild entity among children, with approximately 2% to 6% requiring intensive care, the infection should not be underestimated in the pediatric population.[68] A multisystem inflammatory syndrome (MIS-C) caused by SARS-CoV-2 has been reported among the pediatric population from several countries. MIS-C can lead to a large spectrum of symptoms that mimic a Kawasaki-like disease. Clinical manifestations range from persistent pyrexia to polymorphic rash, conjunctivitis, mucosal abnormalities, and myocardial involvement (including acute myocardial dysfunction, arrythmias, and acute pericarditis).[68]

Once again the cytokine storm plays a role in the pathogenesis of MIS-C. The condition of hyperinflammation can generate multiple consequences within the cardiac district. In severe cases there have been reports of coronary artery dilatation and aneurysm (8%–24% of patients), which may be due to the state of hyperinflammation with disruption of the arterial wall, as seen in Kawasaki disease (KD).[69]

Other clinical features described in children affected by MIS-C are acute myocardial dysfunction, hypotension requiring fluid resuscitation, and, in some cases, cardiogenic shock requiring cardiac inotropic support, mechanical ventilation, and extracorporeal membrane oxygenation.[69]

A key clinical difference between MIS-C and KD is represented by the fact that ventricular dysfunction and eventually shock are common presentations in MIS-C (50% of cases) and occur less frequently in children with KD (5%–10%).[69]

Recent evidence suggests that the administration of immunomodulatory drugs during the acute phase of the illness, such as intravenous immunoglobulins and steroids, may reverse the dysregulated inflammatory response yielding to recovery within days or a few weeks. Anticoagulation therapy is also suggested in the pediatric patients presenting with severe ventricular dysfunction and in case of evidence of giant coronary aneurysm.[69]

Although MIS-C is associated to low mortality, nothing is known of its mid- and long-term sequelae.

SUMMARY

Based on the current literature on myocardial injury during COVID-19, it is possible to conclude that this association is not uncommon. Myocardial injury can be considered as a concerning complication of SARS-CoV-2 infection, which can eventually lead to a large spectrum of myocardial pathologies (ie, myocarditis, myocardial infarction, Takotsubo syndrome) through the interaction between the virus and myocardial and endothelial cells, mediated by direct viral invasion or indirect mechanisms such as the downregulation of ACE2 receptor expression. Immune-mediated overresponse, cytokine storm, and activation of prothrombotic pathways are further mechanisms of myocardial damage that contribute to the various forms of myocardial injury that have been described.[22,23,70]

Although a trend of reduction in the number of hospital admissions for MI has been described, particularly during the first wave of pandemic, it is necessary to interpret these findings with caution and to consider the weight of other factors such as patient's reluctance to seek medical attention due to fear of in-hospital SARS-CoV-2 exposure or the strain on the organizational capacity of facilities in building the response to the pandemic.[49,52,71]

The direct impact of acute myocardial injury on the mortality of patients with COVID-19 has been described, whereas there is also evidence of long-term sequelae of myocardial injury (both inflammatory and ischemic) that are particularly concerning in older patients and in patients with cardiovascular comorbidities.[72]

There is therefore a pressing need to continue investigating these new and complex clinical entities in order to understand how to treat and manage these patients. It is possible to hypothesize the need for dedicated protocols that involve a strict cardiovascular follow-up through both clinical and sequential imaging evaluation, based on the patients' comorbidities and overall risk stratification.

CLINICS CARE POINTS

- Myocardial injury during COVID-19 can manifest through a large spectrum of pathologies (myocarditis, myocardial infarction, Takostubo Syndrome and MIS-C).

- Cardiac damage during SARS-CoV-2 infection can arise in patients with no previous hystory of heart disease or in the absence of symptoms and is therefore challenging to diagnose.
- There is evidence of long-term effects in patients affected by myocardial injury during SARS-CoV-2 infection, although the impact and reversibility of these sequelae is still not fully understood.
- Patients that experience myocardial injury during COVID-19 should undergo regular follow-up through clinical and imaging evaluation and dedicated protocols should be designed, based on their individual risk.

CONFLICT OF INTEREST

All the authors report no conflict of interest.

REFERENCES

1. Long B, Brady WJ, Koyfman A, et al. Cardiovascular complications in COVID-19. Am J Emerg Med 2020 Jul;38(7):1504–7.
2. Huang C, Wang Y, Li X, et al. Clinical features of patients infected with 2019 novel coronavirus in Wuhan, China. Lancet 2020;395:497–506.
3. Guan WJ, Ni ZY, Hu Y, et al. China medical treatment expert group for covid-19. Clinical characteristics of coronavirus disease 2019 in China. N Engl J Med 2020; 382(18):1708–20.
4. Efros O, Barda N, Meisel E, et al. Myocardial injury in hospitalized patients with COVID-19 infection-Risk factors and outcomes. PLoS One 2021;16(2):e0247800.
5. Sheth AR, Grewal US, Patel HP, et al. Possible mechanisms responsible for acute coronary events in COVID-19. Med Hypotheses 2020;143:110125.
6. Puelles VG, Lütgehetmann M, Lindenmeyer MT, et al. Multiorgan and renal tropism of SARS-CoV-2. N Engl J Med 2020;383(6):590–2.
7. Gu ZC, Zhang C, Kong LC, et al. Incidence of myocardial injury in coronavirus disease 2019 (COVID-19): a pooled analysis of 7,679 patients from 53 studies. Cardiovasc Diagn Ther 2020;10(4):667–77.
8. Giustino G, Croft LB, Stefanini GG, et al. Characterization of myocardial injury in patients with COVID-19. J Am Coll Cardiol 2020;76(18):2043–55.
9. Oudit GY, Kassiri Z, Jiang C, et al. SARS-coronavirus modulation of myocardial ACE2 expression and inflammation in patients with SARS. Eur J Clin Invest 2009;39:618–25.
10. Babapoor-Farrokhran S, Gill D, Walker J, et al. Myocardial injury and COVID-19: possible mechanisms. Life Sci 2020;253:117723.
11. Laghlam D, Jozwiak M, Nguyen LS. Renin-angiotensin-aldosterone system and immunomodulation: a state-of-the-art review. Cells 2021;10(7):1767.
12. Hoffmann M, Kleine-Weber H, Schroeder S, et al. SARS-CoV-2 cell entry depends on ACE2 and TMPRSS2 and is blocked by a clinically proven protease inhibitor. Cell 2020;181(2):271–80, e8.
13. Li W, Moore MJ, Vasllieva N, et al. Angiotensin-converting enzyme 2 is a functional receptor for the SARS coronavirus. Nature 2003;426(6965):450–4.
14. Huang Y, Yang C, Xu XF, et al. Structural and functional properties of SARS-CoV-2 spike protein: potential antivirus drug development for COVID-19. Acta Pharmacol Sin 2020;41(9):1141–9.
15. Liu PP, Blet A, Smyth D, et al. The science underlying COVID-19: implications for the cardio- vascular system. Circulation 2020;142:68–78.

16. Sankrityayan H, Kale A, Sharma N, et al. Evidence for use or disuse of renin-angiotensin system modulators in patients having COVID-19 with an underlying cardiorenal disorder. J Cardiovasc Pharmacol Ther 2020;25(4):299–306.

17. Walls AC, Park YJ, Tortorici MA, et al. Structure, function, and antigenicity of the SARS-CoV-2 spike glycoprotein. Cell 2020;181(2):281–92.e6.

18. Kuba K, Imai Y, Penninger JM. Angiotensin-converting enzyme 2 in lung diseases. Curr Opin Pharmacol 2006;6(3):271–6.

19. Arentz M, Yim E, Klaff L, et al. Characteristics and outcomes of 21 critically ill patients with COVID-19 in Washington State. JAMA 2020;323:1612–4.

20. Liu Y, Yang Y, Zhang C, et al. Clinical and biochemical indexes from 2019-nCoV infected patients linked to viral loads and lung injury. Sci China Life Sci 2020;63: 364–74.

21. Zhou F, Yu T, Du R, et al. Clinical course and risk factors for mortality of adult inpatients with COVID-19 in Wuhan, China: a retrospective cohort study. The Lancet 2020;395:1054–62.

22. Chen L, Li X, Chen M, et al. The ACE2 expression in human heart indicates new potential mechanism of heart injury among patients infected with SARS-CoV-2. Cardiovasc Res 2020;116(6):1097–100.

23. Mehta P, McAuley DF, Brown M, et al. HLH across Speciality Collaboration, UK. COVID-19: consider cytokine storm syndromes and immunosuppression. Lancet 2020;395(10229):1033–4.

24. Clerkin KJ, Fried JA, Raikhelkar J, et al. COVID-19 and cardiovascular disease. Circulation 2020;141(20):1648–55.

25. Moccia F, Gerbino A, Lionetti V, et al. COVID-19-associated cardiovascular morbidity in older adults: a position paper from the Italian Society of Cardiovascular Researches. Geroscience 2020;42(4):1021–49.

26. Tay MZ, Poh CM, Rénia L, et al. The trinity of COVID-19: immunity, inflammation and interven- tion. Nat Rev Immunol 2020;20:363–74.

27. Ramadan MS, Bertolino L, Marrazzo T, et al. The Monaldi Hospital Cardiovascular Infection Study Group. Cardiac complications during the active phase of COVID-19: review of the current evidence. Intern Emerg Med 2021;1–11.

28. Nencioni A, Trzeciak S, Shapiro NI. The microcirculation as a diagnostic and therapeutic target in sepsis. Intern Emerg Med 2009;4(5):413–8.

29. Xiong TY, Redwood S, Prendergast B, et al. Coronaviruses and the cardiovascular system: acute and long-term implications. Eur Heart J 2020;41(19):1798–800.

30. Perrotta F, Corbi G, Mazzeo G, et al. COVID-19 and the elderly: insights into pathogenesis and clinical decision-making. Aging Clin Exp Res 2020;32(8): 1599–608.

31. Thygesen K, Alpert JS, Jaffe AS, et al. Executive group on behalf of the Joint European Society of Cardiology (ESC)/American College of Cardiology (ACC)/ American heart association (AHA)/World heart Federation (WHF) Task Force for the Universal definition of myocardial infarction. Fourth universal definition of myocardial infarction (2018). J Am Coll Cardiol 2018;72(18):2231–64.

32. Bonow RO, Fonarow GC, O'Gara PT, et al. Association of coronavirus disease 2019 (COVID-19) with myocardial injury and mortality. JAMA Cardiol 2020;5(7): 751–3.

33. Shi S, Qin M, Shen B, et al. Association of cardiac injury with mortality in hospitalized patients with COVID-19 in Wuhan, China [published online March 25, 2020]. JAMA Cardiol 2020;5(7):802–10.

34. Bavishi C, Bonow RO, Trivedi V, et al. Special article—acute myocardial injury in patients hospitalized with COVID-19 infection: a review. Prog Cardio-vasc Dis 2020;63:682–9.

35. Nishiga M, Wang DW, Han Y, et al. COVID- 19 and cardiovascular disease: from basic mechanisms to clinical perspectives. Nat Rev Cardiol 2020;17:543–58.

36. Moayed MS, Rahimi-Bashar F, Vahedian-Azimi A, et al. Cardiac injury in COVID-19: a systematic review. Adv Exp Med Biol 2021;1321:325–33.

37. Lala A, Johnson KW, Januzzi JL, et al. Preva- lence and impact of myocardial injury in patients hospitalized with COVID-19 infection. J Am Coll Cardiol 2020; 76:533–46.

38. Guo T, Fan Y, Chen M, et al. Cardiovascular implications of fatal outcomes of patients with coronavirus disease 2019 (COVID-19). JAMA Cardiol 2020;27:1–8.

39. Shi S, Qin M, Shen B, et al. Association of cardiac injury with mortality in hospitalized patients with COVID-19 in Wuhan, China. JAMA Cardiol 2020;25:802–10.

40. Romero J, Alviz I, Parides M, et al. T-wave inversion as a manifestation of COVID-19 infection: a case series. J Interv Card Electrophysiol 2020;59(3):485–93.

41. Liaqat A, Ali-Khan RS, Asad M, et al. Evaluation of myocardial injury patterns and ST changes among critical and non-critical patients with coronavirus-19 disease. Sci Rep 2021;4828.

42. Ojha V, Verma M, Pandey NN, et al. Cardiac magnetic resonance imaging in coronavirus disease 2019 (COVID-19): a systematic review of cardiac magnetic resonance imaging findings in 199 patients. J Thorac Imaging 2021;36:73–83.

43. Puntmann VO, Carerj ML, Wieters I, et al. Outcomes of cardiovascular magnetic resonance imaging in patients recently recov- ered from coronavirus disease 2019 (COVID-19). JAMA Cardiol 2020;5:1265–73.

44. Kotecha T, Knight DS, Razvi Y, et al. Patterns of myocardial injury in recovered troponin-positive COVID-19 patients assessed by cardiovascular magnetic resonance European Heart. Journal 2021;42(Issue 19):1866–78.

45. Friedrich MG, Cooper LT. What we (don't) know about myocardial injury after COVID-19. Eur Heart J 2021;42(Issue 19):1879–82.

46. Halushka MK, Vander Heide RS. Myocarditis is rare in COVID-19 autopsies: cardiovascular findings across 277 postmortem examinations. Cardiovasc Pathol 2021;50:107300.

47. Solomon MD, McNulty EJ, Rana JS, et al. The COVID-19 pandemic and the incidence of acute myocardial infarction. N Engl J Med 2020;383:691–9.

48. Tejada Meza H, Lambea Gil Á, Saldaña AS, et al. Impact of COVID-19 outbreak on ischemic stroke admissions and in-hospital mortality in North-West Spain. Int J Stroke 2020;15:755–62.

49. Katsoularis I, Fonseca-Rodriguez O, et al. Risk of acute myocardial infarction and ischaemic stroke following COVID-19 in Sweden: a self-controlled case series and matched cohort study Lancet 2021;398(10300):599–607.

50. Mafham MM, Spata E, Goldacre R, et al. COVID-19 pandemic and admission rates for and management of acute coronary syndromes in England. Lancet 2020;396:381–9.

51. D'Anna L, Brown M, Oishi S, et al. Impact of national lockdown on the hyperacute stroke care and rapid transient ischaemic attack outpatient service in a comprehensive tertiary stroke centre during the COVID-19 pandemic. Front Neurol 2021; 12:627493.

52. Rudilosso S, Laredo C, Vera V, et al. Acute stroke care is at risk in the era of COVID-19: experience at a comprehensive stroke center in Barcelona. Stroke 2020;51:1991–5.

53. Rodriguez-Leor O, Cid Alvarez AB, Pérez de Prado A. In-hospital outcomes of COVID-19 ST-elevation myocardial infarction patients. EuroIntervention 2021;16: 1426–33.
54. Choudry FA, Hamshere SM, Rathod KS, et al. High thrombus burden in patients with COVID-19 presenting with ST-Segment elevation myocardial infarction. J Am Coll Cardiol 2020;76(10):1168–76.
55. Rattka M, Dreyhaupt J, Winsauer C, et al. Effect of the COVID- 19 pandemic on mortality of patients with STEMI: a systematic review and meta-analysis. Heart 2020;107:482–7.
56. Stefanini GG, Montorfano M, Trabattoni D, et al. ST-elevation myocardial infarction in patients with COVID-19: clinical and angiographic outcomes. Circulation 2020; 141:2113–6.
57. Smeeth L, Thomas SL, Hall AJ, et al. Risk of myocardial infarction and stroke after acute infection or vaccination. N Engl J Med 2004;351:2611–8.
58. Ebinger JE, Shah PK. Declining admissions for acute cardiovascular illness: the Covid-19 paradox. J Am Coll Cardiol 2020;76:289–91.
59. Metzler B, Siostrzonek P, Binder RK, et al. Decline of acute coronary syn- drome admissions in Austria since the outbreak of COVID-19: the pandemic response causes cardiac collateral damage. Eur Heart J 2020;41:1852–3.
60. De Rosa S, Spaccarotella C, Basso C, et al. Reduction of hospitalizations for myocardial infarction in Italy in the COVID-19 era. Eur Heart J 2020;41:2083–8.
61. Medina de Chazal H, Del Buono MG, Keyser-Marcus L, et al. Stress cardiomyopathy diagnosis and treatment: JACC state-of-the-art review. J Am Coll Cardiol 2018;72:1955–71.
62. Giustino G, Croft LB, Oates CP, et al. Takotsubo cardiomyopathy in males with Covid-19. J Am Coll Cardiol 2020;76:628–9.
63. Roca E, Lombardi C, Campana M, et al. Takotsubo syndrome associated with COVID-19. Eur J Case Rep Intern Med 2020;7:001665.
64. Park JH, Moon JY, Sohn KM, et al. Two fatal cases of stress-induced cardiomyopathy in COVID-19 patients. J Cardio- Vasc Imaging 2020;28:300–3.
65. Nguyen D, Nguyen T, De Bels D, et al. A case of Takotsubo cardiomyopathy with COVID 19. Eur Heart J Cardiovasc Imaging 2020;21:1052.
66. Cameli M, Pastore MC. Giulia Elena Mandoli et al COVID-19 and Acute Coronary Syndromes: current Data and Future Implications. Front Cardiovasc Med 2021;7: 593496.
67. Impact of COVID-19 pandemic on mechanical reperfusion for patients with STEMI. De Luca G, Verdoia M, Cerchek M et al. Am Coll Cardiol 2020;76(20): 2321–30.
68. Sperotto F, Friedman K, Son MB, et al. Cardiac manifestations in SARS-CoV-2-associated multisystem inflammatory syndrome in children: a comprehensive review and proposed clinical approach. Eur J Pediatr 2021;180(2):307–22.
69. Alsaied T, Tremoulet AH, Burns JC, et al. Review of cardiac involvement in multisystem inflammatory syndrome in children. Circulation 2021;143(1):78–88.
70. Della Rocca DG, Magnocavallo M, Lavalle C, et al. Evidence of systemic endothelial injury and microthrombosis in hospitalized COVID-19 patients at different stages of the disease. J Thromb Thrombolysis 2021;51(3):571–6.
71. Versaci F, Scappaticci M, Calcagno S, et al. ST-elevation myocardial infarction in the COVID-19 era. Minerva Cardiol Angiol 2021;69(1):6–8.
72. De Luca G, Cercek M, Jensen LO, et al. Impact of COVID-19 pandemic and diabetes on mechanical reperfusion in patients with STEMI: insights from the ISACS STEMI COVID 19 Registry. Cardiovasc Diabetol 2020;19(1):215.

Innovation in Ambulatory Care of Heart Failure in the Era of Coronavirus Disease 2019

Orly Leiva, MD[a,1], Ankeet S. Bhatt, MD, MBA[b,1],
Muthiah Vaduganathan, MD, MPH[b,*]

KEYWORDS

- Ambulatory • Care optimization • COVID-19 • Guideline-directed medical therapy
- Heart failure

KEY POINTS

- Major gaps exist in the implementation of guideline-directed medical therapy for heart failure (HF). Ambulatory care optimization should focus on rapid and successful implementation of effective therapies.
- HF is associated with high comorbid disease burden. Ambulatory management of comorbidities should be incorporated into HF disease management programs.
- Optimizing ambulatory HF care will require a multidisciplinary team to address therapeutic optimization, active comorbid disease management, and nutrition and structured exercise-based interventions.

INTRODUCTION

Heart failure (HF) is a chronic disease state that affects up to 6 million Americans; the prevalence is poised to rise in upcoming years given population aging and adverse trends in cardiometabolic comorbidities.[1] HF is a major contributor of morbidity and mortality in the United States, with 1 in 9 death certificates mentioning HF and more than 58,000 deaths attributed to HF annually.[1] The natural history of HF with reduced ejection fraction (HFrEF) has been significantly disrupted with the sequential development and demonstration of benefit of 6 distinct classes of disease-modifying therapies: angiotensin-converting enzyme inhibitors (ACEi), angiotensin II receptor blockers (ARB), angiotensin receptor-neprilysin inhibitors (ARNI), β-blockers,

This article previously appeared in *Heart Failure Clinics*, Volume 16, Issue 4, October 2020.
[a] Department of Medicine, Brigham and Women's Hospital, Boston, MA, USA; [b] Division of Cardiovascular Medicine, Brigham and Women's Hospital, Boston, MA, USA
[1] Co-first authors.
* Corresponding author. 75 Francis Street, Boston, MA 02215.
E-mail address: mvaduganathan@bwh.harvard.edu
Twitter: @LeivaOrly (O.L.); @ankeetbhatt (A.S.B.); @mvaduganathan (M.V.)

2352-7986/22/© 2021 Elsevier Inc. All rights reserved.

mineralocorticoid receptor antagonists (MRA), and most recently, the sodium glucose cotransporter-2 inhibitors (SGLT2i). However, despite these recent advances, fewer than 1% of patients with HF are simultaneously treated with target doses of multiple evidence-based classes (ACEi/ARB/ARNI, β-blockers, and MRA).[2–4] In addition, as there are currently no approved therapies for patients with HF with preserved ejection fraction, its management has relied on the rigorous targeting of key comorbidities and effective hemodynamic and volume-control strategies.

Although focus on optimization around the time of hospitalization represents an important target of care efforts, a large segment of the HF population lives in community settings, at times with limited care access. Most patient-physician interactions occur in ambulatory clinics, including those that span primary care, cardiology, and advanced HF. As such, optimizing care pathways in the ambulatory setting is a particularly promising area of care innovation. In addition, the emergence of the Coronavirus Disease 2019 (COVID-19) pandemic has threatened traditional care approaches, limiting health care access and interactions. The introduction of new technologies and expansion in insurance coverage of telehealth options, combined with team-based multidisciplinary efforts, have the potential to provide a lasting impact on care delivery in ambulatory practice.

GAPS IN PROVISION OF EVIDENCE-BASED THERAPIES

Data from the Changing the Management of Patients with Heart Failure (CHAMP-HF), Contemporary Drug Treatment of Chronic HF (CHECK-HF), and Quality of Adherence to guideline recommendations for life-saving treatment in HF survey (QUALIFY) registries suggest there are important gaps in the use and dosing of key elements of guideline-directed medical therapy (GDMT) in clinical practice.[5–9] Despite a robust evidence base and guideline documents supporting full implementation of GDMT at target doses, the administration and uptitration of these therapies in patients with HFrEF are suboptimal[10] (Table 1).

IMPLEMENTING GUIDELINE-DIRECTED MEDICAL THERAPY

Given the multifaceted interactions between patients with HF and the health care system, team-based care approaches to GDMT optimization may be particularly

Table 1
Incomplete use and target dose achievement of guideline-directed medical therapy for heart failure with reduced ejection fraction in usual care settings globally

Registry	On/Adherent to Therapy, %			≥50% Target Dose,[a] %			≥100% Target Dose,[a] %		
	ACEi/ARB/ARNI	Beta Blocker	MRA	ACEi/ARB/ARNI	Beta Blocker	MRA	ACEi/ARB/ARNI	Beta Blocker	MRA
CHAMP-HF	73.4	67	33.4	83.1	72.5	98.2	16.8	27.5	76.6
CHECK-HF	84	86	56	76	55	97.9	43.6	18.9	52
QUALIFY	62	79	86	74	60	76	22.7	14.8	70.8

Abbreviations: ACEi, angiotensin-converting enzyme inhibitor; ARB, angiotensin receptor blocker; ARNI, angiotensin receptor-neprilysin inhibitor; CHAMP-HF, changing the management of patients with heart failure; CHECK-HF, Contemporary Drug Treatment of Chronic HF; MRA, mineralocorticoid receptor antagonist; QUALIFY, quality of adherence to guideline recommendations for life-saving treatment in HF survey.
[a] Percentages reported as a proportion of patients on therapy.

valuable.[11] One strategy to improve delivery of GDMT is using non-physician medical staff under the guidance of HF specialists to engage in more active and frequent therapeutic changes. For instance, clinical pharmacists are experienced members of inpatient and outpatient interdisciplinary care teams and may serve as an important resource to aid in earlier initiation and uptitration. A model of pharmacist involvement in HF consult services in the inpatient setting has led to increased use of GDMT.[12] In the outpatient setting, one small pilot study used pharmacists to help manage dose titrations of GDMT. Despite small sample size, this intervention led to target dose β-blocker titration in 78% of patients and a significant reduction in all-cause hospital admissions.[13] Other studies have also shown reduction in hospital readmissions for HF when pharmacists are used to assist GDMT implementation in the outpatient setting.[14] Similarly, nursing-directed clinics have also been shown to increase adherence and optimize titration of GDMT.[15,16] Organizing these non-physician providers in GDMT-specific clinics (**Fig. 1**) represents a strategy to de-link usual care (which may focus on acute care needs and decongestion) and therapeutic optimization.[17,18] Randomized clinical trials examining an early intensive GDMT uptitration strategy as compared with usual care are under way (NCT03412201).

High-Quality Transitions in Care

Quality improvement programs have been previously implemented to attempt to improve GDMT uptake in patients admitted with HF. The American Heart Association's Get with the Guidelines Heart Failure (GWTG-HF) program is one such example.[19] Hospitals participating in the GWTG-HF program had higher use of GDMT (notably ACEi) and slightly improved readmission rates.[20,21] The GWTG-HF program expands on the progress of preceding initiatives including the Organized Program to Initiate Lifesaving Treatment in Hospitalized Patients with Heart Failure (OPTIMIZE-HF) program, which focused on implementing high-quality care at hospital discharge.[22] Process improvement initiatives embedded within OPTIMIZE-HF were shown to be associated with reduced HF and cardiovascular readmission rates.[23] In parallel with these "real-world" clinical programs, traditional randomized trials have demonstrated that in-hospital initiation of evidence-based therapies is not only safe, but may lead to improved postdischarge use and therapeutic persistence.[24–26] However, patient-centered transitional care alone, such as evaluated in the Patient-Centered Care Transitions in HF (PACT-HF) service model, has not been associated with improved postdischarge outcomes.[27] In the PACT-HF trial the intervention group incorporated a hospital nurse navigator to facilitate a needs-based assessment and intervention reflecting self-reported quality of life, education, patient-centered discharge summary, multidisciplinary referrals, and family physician follow-up at the time of discharge. These findings highlight the importance of linked programs specifically designed to improve GDMT uptake during HF hospitalization, which seamlessly continue acceleration of therapy in the post-hospitalization period.

Telemedicine and Remote Health Management

Telemedicine represents an emerging strategy for optimizing GDMT and HF care at a more rapid pace, especially for patients who live in rural settings or those with limited access or high barriers to traditional clinical visits. These approaches may be particularly relevant in an era of COVID-19 and associated need for social distancing, further limiting contact with traditional ambulatory clinic settings. Indeed, the Centers for Medicare and Medicaid Services has expanded coverage to Medicare telehealth services in March 2020 in response to the escalating COVID-19 pandemic.

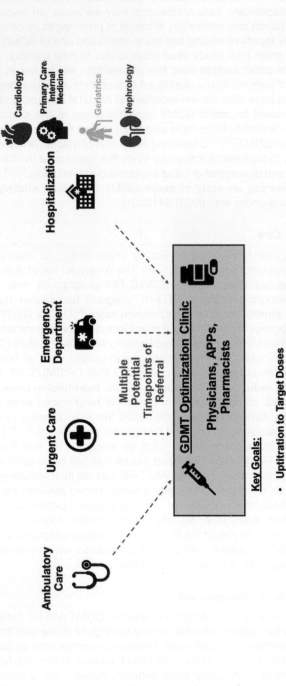

Fig. 1. Innovative care delivery pathway to optimize GDMT in HF. APP, advanced practice provider. (*From* Myhre PL, Januzzi JL Jr, Butler J, et al. De novo heart failure: where the journey begins. Eur J Heart Fail 2019, 21(10):1245–7; with permission.)

Although the results have been mixed in other clinical settings, studies suggest that telemedicine may facilitate improved patient interaction that may in turn promote GDMT initiation and uptitration at a scale difficult to obtain with traditional in-person visits.[28–30] A meta-analysis of 8323 patients across 25 randomized controlled trials suggested a reduction in all-cause mortality with telemonitoring (monitoring blood pressure, weight, electrocardiographic strips) compared with usual care among patients with HF.[31] In the Telemedical Interventional Management in Heart Failure II (TIM-HF2) trial conducted in Germany, patients with HF were randomized to telemonitoring strategy or usual care.[29] The telemonitoring group was given an electrocardiogram device, blood pressure measuring device, electronic scale, oximeter, and a mobile phone to communicate remotely with the clinic. The telemedical data were transmitted daily and the patient was managed according to a set algorithm. Telemonitoring reduced cardiovascular mortality and hospitalization for HF after 12 months of follow-up.[29] Given improvement in technology and continuous assessment, using wearable technology offers a new and convenient method for managing HF in the outpatient setting and particularly alerting providers when hemodynamics may allow for more aggressive GDMT. For example, one study provided participants a smartphone and a smartwatch along with an application that tracked participant activity data and required them to input daily self-measured blood pressure and body weight. Although this study was limited in size, a significant increase in quality of life and performance status was reported.[32] In patients with advanced HF, monitoring of pulmonary artery (PA) and intracardiac pressures via implantable devices has already been shown to reduce HF hospitalizations.[33,34] For example, the CardioMEMS Heart Sensor Allows Monitoring of Pressure to Improve Outcomes in NYHA Class III Heart Failure Patients (CHAMPION) trial showed improved clinical outcomes with longitudinal assessment and access to real-time PA pressure measurements that may be due to improved GDMT in the monitored group.[33] Given interconnectivity and telecommunication advances in the modern era, telemedicine is poised to become increasingly important in the management of chronic diseases such as HF. For example, the upcoming HF Study to Evaluate Vital Signs and Overcome Low Use of GDMT by Remote Monitoring (HF-eVOLUTION) trial will be evaluating the effectiveness of vital signs monitoring via wrist watch on GDMT use and may shed light on this novel strategy (NCT04292275). Similar telehealth solutions should be developed and empirically evaluated to determine if implementation may help improve GDMT use.

COMORBIDITY MANAGEMENT IN HEART FAILURE

Patients with HF often have comorbid noncardiac conditions that contribute to morbidity, mortality, and impaired health-related quality of life. In one study, more than 80% of patients with HF had at least 1 noncardiovascular comorbid condition and 25% had more than 3.[35] Patients with HF and comorbid conditions have worse outcomes, including increased mortality and HF admissions.[35] Chronic obstructive lung disease (COPD) and anemia have independently been associated with increased HF admissions and poorer outcomes.[36] Patients with comorbid conditions also had more severe HF symptoms, including fatigue, dyspnea, pain, and anxiety, which may collectively contribute to worse quality of life.[37] Therefore, comprehensive ambulatory management of patients with HF should include active surveillance and management of comorbid conditions. In addition, added comorbidity burden increased polypharmacy and may adversely affect adherence. Evaluation and early treatment or prevention of comorbid conditions are crucial to prevent potential exacerbation of HF and provide comprehensive cardiopulmonary and systemic care.

The most commonly identified comorbidities in patients with HF are diabetes mellitus, COPD, chronic kidney disease, and anemia.[35,37–39] In patients with diabetes mellitus (both with and without HF), new therapeutic options have emerged, including SGLT2i. SGLT2i has been found to decrease HF events in patients with type 2 diabetes mellitus.[40–44] The landmark Dapagliflozin in Patients with Heart Failure and Reduced Ejection Fraction (DAPA-HF) trial additionally demonstrated that dapagliflozin may be helpful in the treatment of patients with established HFrEF.[45] Cardiologists will need to take a more active role in prescribing these therapies, which have traditionally been considered only for their glucose-lowering potential. COPD is comorbid with HF and has been associated with increased mortality and hospitalization.[46,47] In the context of multiple intersecting comorbidities, programs designed to aid patients in medication adherence (and avoidance of potentially harmful or unnecessary therapies) will become increasingly important, particularly as medication burden increases.[48]

Last, depression is an often-overlooked comorbidity in patients with HF. Depression is comorbid in approximately 22% of patients with HF and has been associated with poor health-related quality of life and is an independent risk factor for subsequent cardiovascular events.[49,50] Importantly, depression may adversely impact therapeutic and lifestyle adherence.[51] Therefore, early screening and mental health support may be an additional avenue to improve adherence in patients with HF with concomitant depression.

VACCINATION

Vaccination is an important part of global prevention, even more so in patients with chronic diseases such as HF. In particular, vaccination against pulmonary pathogens (influenza and pneumococcus) in HF has some promise in improving outcomes, although no large clinical trials have been reported yet.[52] There are many plausible mechanisms by which influenza infection may promote worsening HF, including proinflammatory acceleration of atherogenesis in addition to direct myocardial depressant effects of inflammatory cytokines. Routine early influenza vaccination has been shown to be effective in patients with atherosclerotic vascular disease and recent acute coronary syndrome.[53] In addition, recent data suggest that early, well-matched consistent influenza vaccination in patients with HF may improve clinical outcomes and reduce rehospitalization rates.[54] Data from a large randomized clinical trial also showed an association between influenza vaccination and improved cardiovascular events.[55] Despite this, usual care evidence suggests major gaps in influenza vaccination rates in the United States, with increasing refusal rates.[56] In addition, centers performing well with respect to influenza vaccination in patients with HF also performed well with respect to other HF quality measures, suggesting that particular centers may have integrated structured approaches to influenza vaccination administration into traditional HF disease management programs. Despite common sense indication for influenza vaccination and clear biological plausibility for benefit in patients with established cardiopulmonary disease, a focal antivaccination contingent and strong personal feelings and fears with regard to influenza vaccination may, in part, explain disappointing vaccination rates among patients with cardiovascular disease. New implementation avenues, particular those that may involve direct, patient-facing behavioral economic nudges, are needed to better understand barriers for nonvaccination and strategies for improvement. These learnings from vaccination efforts for seasonal influenza may be effectively translated to overcome upcoming challenges in disseminating effective vaccines against COVID-19 (once developed and available).

LIFESTYLE INTERVENTIONS IN AMBULATORY PRACTICE

As with many chronic cardiometabolic diseases, lifestyle modification is critical as a central tenet of disease management. HF is no exception, and thus lifestyle modification interventions should be part of every outpatient HF program and clinic. Structured exercise programs are one such intervention that has been proposed in HF, particularly given the overlap among HF, metabolic syndrome, and obesity, all of which are potentially mitigated by exercise and accelerated basal metabolic rates.[57] The Heart Failure: A Controlled Trial Investigating Outcomes of Exercise Training (HF-ACTION) trial investigated the health effects of an exercise training program in patients with HFrEF.[58] This trial showed that an exercise training program in patients with HF is safe and may have modest reductions in all-cause and cardiovascular mortality and hospitalization.[58] Patients in the exercise group also had improved 6-minute walk distance and cardiopulmonary exercise duration. Furthermore, this improvement in 6-minute walk distance and cardiopulmonary exercise duration was similar across baseline physical activity levels.[59] One small study showed that a multidisciplinary clinic with cardiac rehabilitation, dieticians, psychologists, and nurse educators reduced HF hospitalization.[60] In addition to exercise, diet is important for HF and health overall.[61] HF is a catabolic state and malnutrition and cachexia are poor prognostic factors in HF.[62] One small upcoming study will investigate the role of diet optimization via nutrition education on nutritional and quality-of-life outcomes in patients with HF (NCT03845309), although larger trials are needed to investigate disruptive nutritional programs that may benefit patients with HF.

SUMMARY

Advancement in therapeutic options in recent decades have afforded us several avenues and tools for care optimization, including pharmacologic therapies, novel technology-based monitoring, and nonpharmacological interventions, such as vaccination, nutrition, and structured exercise-based approaches. Delivering high-quality HF care in a fragmented health system is increasingly challenging and likely ineffective; integrated ambulatory clinics designed around multidisciplinary teams including physicians, advanced practice providers, clinical pharmacists, nurses, nutritionists, exercise physiologists, and social workers, among others, are needed to provide care that is effective and optimal. These approaches, coupled with telehealth solutions, may minimize multiple health care interactions and travel for patients at risk for COVID-19. Furthermore, greater study is needed with regard to how these teams may effectively partner and engage patients to be champions of their own health, empowering them to seek new interventions, technologies, and lifestyle changes. Overall, the ambulatory setting (extending well beyond the walls of a single clinic) offers a comprehensive environment for care optimization. Ambulatory innovations in HF care must focus not only on disease-modifying interventions, but also on comprehensive HF and comorbid care designed to relieve symptoms, improve functional status, and optimize nutrition and weight management.

DISCLOSURE

O. Leiva and A.S. Bhatt have no relevant disclosures. M. Vaduganathan is supported by the KL2/Catalyst Medical Research Investigator Training award from Harvard Catalyst (NIH/NCATS Award UL 1TR002541); serves on advisory boards for Amgen, AstraZeneca, Baxter Healthcare, Bayer AG, Boehringer Ingelheim, Cytokinetics, and

Relypsa; and participates on clinical endpoint committees for studies sponsored by Novartis and the National Institutes of Health.

REFERENCES

1. Mozaffarian D, Benjamin EJ, Go AS, et al. Heart disease and stroke statistics–2015 update: a report from the American Heart Association. Circulation 2015; 131(4):e29–322.
2. Greene SJ, Fonarow GC, DeVore AD, et al. Titration of medical therapy for heart failure with reduced ejection fraction. J Am Coll Cardiol 2019;73(19):2365–83.
3. Peri-Okonny PA, Mi X, Khariton Y, et al. Target doses of heart failure medical therapy and blood pressure: insights from the CHAMP-HF registry. JACC Heart Fail 2019;7(4):350–8.
4. Bress AP, King JB. Optimizing medical therapy in chronic worsening HFrEF: a long way to go. J Am Coll Cardiol 2019;73(8):945–7.
5. DeVore AD, Thomas L, Albert NM, et al. Change the management of patients with heart failure: rationale and design of the CHAMP-HF registry. Am Heart J 2017; 189:177–83.
6. Greene SJ, Butler J, Albert NM, et al. Medical therapy for heart failure with reduced ejection fraction: the CHAMP-HF registry. J Am Coll Cardiol 2018; 72(4):351–66.
7. Brunner-La Rocca HP, Linssen GC, Smeele FJ, et al. Contemporary drug treatment of chronic heart failure with reduced ejection fraction: the CHECK-HF registry. JACC Heart Fail 2019;7(1):13–21.
8. Komajda M, Cowie MR, Tavazzi L, et al. Physicians' guideline adherence is associated with better prognosis in outpatients with heart failure with reduced ejection fraction: the QUALIFY international registry. Eur J Heart Fail 2017;19(11): 1414–23.
9. Komajda M, Anker SD, Cowie MR, et al. Physicians' adherence to guideline-recommended medications in heart failure with reduced ejection fraction: data from the QUALIFY global survey. Eur J Heart Fail 2016;18(5):514–22.
10. Yancy CW, Januzzi JL Jr, Allen LA, et al. 2017 ACC expert consensus decision pathway for optimization of heart failure treatment: answers to 10 pivotal issues about heart failure with reduced ejection fraction: a report of the American College of Cardiology Task Force on Expert Consensus Decision Pathways. J Am Coll Cardiol 2018;71(2):201–30.
11. Wagner EH. The role of patient care teams in chronic disease management. BMJ 2000;320(7234):569–72.
12. Blizzard S, Verbosky N, Stein B, et al. Evaluation of pharmacist impact within an interdisciplinary inpatient heart failure consult service. Ann Pharmacother 2019; 53(9):905–15.
13. Ingram A, Valente M, Dzurec MA. Evaluating pharmacist impact on guideline-directed medical therapy in patients with reduced ejection fraction heart failure. J Pharm Pract 2019. 897190019866930.
14. McKinley D, Moye-Dickerson P, Davis S, et al. Impact of a pharmacist-led intervention on 30-day readmission and assessment of factors predictive of readmission in African American men with heart failure. Am J Mens Health 2019;13(1). 1557988318814295.
15. Andersson B, Kjork E, Brunlof G. Temporal improvement in heart failure survival related to the use of a nurse-directed clinic and recommended pharmacological treatment. Int J Cardiol 2005;104(3):257–63.

16. Balakumaran K, Patil A, Marsh S, et al. Evaluation of a guideline directed medical therapy titration program in patients with heart failure with reduced ejection fraction. Int J Cardiol Heart Vasc 2019;22:1–5.

17. O'Connor CM. Guideline-directed medical therapy clinics: a call to action for the heart failure team. JACC Heart Fail 2019;7(5):442–3.

18. Myhre PL, Januzzi JL Jr, Butler J, et al. De novo heart failure: where the journey begins. Eur J Heart Fail 2019;21(10):1245–7.

19. Hong Y, LaBresh KA. Overview of the American Heart Association "Get with the Guidelines" programs: coronary heart disease, stroke, and heart failure. Crit Pathw Cardiol 2006;5(4):179–86.

20. Heidenreich PA, Hernandez AF, Yancy CW, et al. Get with the guidelines program participation, process of care, and outcome for Medicare patients hospitalized with heart failure. Circ Cardiovasc Qual Outcomes 2012;5(1):37–43.

21. Bergethon KE, Ju C, DeVore AD, et al. Trends in 30-day readmission rates for patients hospitalized with heart failure: findings from the get with the guidelines-heart failure registry. Circ Heart Fail 2016;9(6).

22. Fonarow GC, Abraham WT, Albert NM, et al. Organized program to initiate life-saving treatment in hospitalized patients with heart failure (OPTIMIZE-HF): rationale and design. Am Heart J 2004;148(1):43–51.

23. Curtis LH, Greiner MA, Hammill BG, et al. Representativeness of a national heart failure quality-of-care registry: comparison of OPTIMIZE-HF and non-OPTIMIZE-HF Medicare patients. Circ Cardiovasc Qual Outcomes 2009;2(4):377–84.

24. Mentz RJ, DeVore A, Tasissa G, et al. Predischarge initiation of ivabradine in the management of heart failure: results of the PRIME-HF trial. Circ Cardiovasc Qual Outcomes 2019;12:A252.

25. Gattis WA, O'Connor CM, Gallup DS, et al. Predischarge initiation of carvedilol in patients hospitalized for decompensated heart failure: results of the initiation management predischarge: process for Assessment of Carvedilol Therapy in Heart Failure (IMPACT-HF) trial. J Am Coll Cardiol 2004;43(9):1534–41.

26. Velazquez EJ, Morrow DA, DeVore AD, et al. Angiotensin-neprilysin inhibition in acute decompensated heart failure. N Engl J Med 2019;380(6):539–48.

27. Van Spall HGC, Lee SF, Xie F, et al. Effect of patient-centered transitional care services on clinical outcomes in patients hospitalized for heart failure: the PACT-HF randomized clinical trial. JAMA 2019;321(8):753–61.

28. Chaudhry SI, Mattera JA, Curtis JP, et al. Telemonitoring in patients with heart failure. N Engl J Med 2010;363(24):2301–9.

29. Koehler F, Koehler K, Deckwart O, et al. Efficacy of telemedical interventional management in patients with heart failure (TIM-HF2): a randomised, controlled, parallel-group, unmasked trial. Lancet 2018;392(10152):1047–57.

30. Eurlings C, Boyne JJ, de Boer RA, et al. Telemedicine in heart failure-more than nice to have? Neth Heart J 2019;27(1):5–15.

31. Inglis SC, Clark RA, McAlister FA, et al. Structured telephone support or telemonitoring programmes for patients with chronic heart failure. Cochrane Database Syst Rev 2010;(8):CD007228.

32. Werhahn SM, Dathe H, Rottmann T, et al. Designing meaningful outcome parameters using mobile technology: a new mobile application for telemonitoring of patients with heart failure. ESC Heart Fail 2019;6(3):516–25.

33. Givertz MM, Stevenson LW, Costanzo MR, et al. Pulmonary artery pressure-guided management of patients with heart failure and reduced ejection fraction. J Am Coll Cardiol 2017;70(15):1875–86.

34. Abraham WT, Adamson PB, Bourge RC, et al. Wireless pulmonary artery haemo-dynamic monitoring in chronic heart failure: a randomised controlled trial. Lancet 2011;377(9766):658–66.

35. Sharma A, Zhao X, Hammill BG, et al. Trends in noncardiovascular comorbidities among patients hospitalized for heart failure: insights from the get with the guidelines-heart failure registry. Circ Heart Fail 2018;11(6):e004646.

36. Guder G, Brenner S, Stork S, et al. Chronic obstructive pulmonary disease in heart failure: accurate diagnosis and treatment. Eur J Heart Fail 2014;16(12): 1273–82.

37. Lawson CA, Solis-Trapala I, Dahlstrom U, et al. Comorbidity health pathways in heart failure patients: a sequences-of-regressions analysis using cross-sectional data from 10,575 patients in the Swedish Heart Failure Registry. PLoS Med 2018;15(3):e1002540.

38. Adams KF Jr, Fonarow GC, Emerman CL, et al. Characteristics and outcomes of patients hospitalized for heart failure in the United States: rationale, design, and preliminary observations from the first 100,000 cases in the Acute Decompen-sated Heart Failure National Registry (ADHERE). Am Heart J 2005;149(2): 209–16.

39. O'Connor CM, Abraham WT, Albert NM, et al. Predictors of mortality after discharge in patients hospitalized with heart failure: an analysis from the Orga-nized Program to Initiate Lifesaving Treatment in Hospitalized Patients with Heart Failure (OPTIMIZE-HF). Am Heart J 2008;156(4):662–73.

40. Zinman B, Wanner C, Lachin JM, et al. Empagliflozin, cardiovascular outcomes, and mortality in type 2 diabetes. N Engl J Med 2015;373(22):2117–28.

41. Neal B, Perkovic V, Mahaffey KW, et al. Canagliflozin and cardiovascular and renal events in type 2 diabetes. N Engl J Med 2017;377(7):644–57.

42. Wiviott SD, Raz I, Bonaca MP, et al. Dapagliflozin and cardiovascular outcomes in type 2 diabetes. N Engl J Med 2019;380(4):347–57.

43. Zelniker TA, Braunwald E. Cardiac and renal effects of sodium-glucose co-trans-porter 2 inhibitors in diabetes: JACC state-of-the-art review. J Am Coll Cardiol 2018;72(15):1845–55.

44. Pasternak B, Ueda P, Eliasson B, et al. Use of sodium glucose cotransporter 2 inhibitors and risk of major cardiovascular events and heart failure: Scandinavian register based cohort study. BMJ 2019;366:l4772.

45. McMurray JJV, Solomon SD, Inzucchi SE, et al. Dapagliflozin in patients with heart failure and reduced ejection fraction. N Engl J Med 2019;381:1995–2008.

46. Canepa M, Temporelli PL, Rossi A, et al. Prevalence and prognostic impact of chronic obstructive pulmonary disease in patients with chronic heart failure: data from the GISSI-HF trial. Cardiology 2017;136(2):128–37.

47. Hawkins NM, Virani S, Ceconi C. Heart failure and chronic obstructive pulmonary disease: the challenges facing physicians and health services. Eur Heart J 2013; 34(36):2795–803.

48. Allen LA, Fonarow GC, Liang L, et al. Medication initiation burden required to comply with heart failure guideline recommendations and hospital quality mea-sures. Circulation 2015;132(14):1347–53.

49. Newhouse A, Jiang W. Heart failure and depression. Heart Fail Clin 2014;10(2): 295–304.

50. Rutledge T, Reis VA, Linke SE, et al. Depression in heart failure a meta-analytic review of prevalence, intervention effects, and associations with clinical out-comes. J Am Coll Cardiol 2006;48(8):1527–37.

51. Jeyanantham K, Kotecha D, Thanki D, et al. Effects of cognitive behavioural therapy for depression in heart failure patients: a systematic review and meta-analysis. Heart Fail Rev 2017;22(6):731–41.
52. Bhatt AS, DeVore AD, Hernandez AF, et al. Can vaccinations improve heart failure outcomes?: contemporary data and future directions. JACC Heart Fail 2017;5(3): 194–203.
53. Udell JA, Zawi R, Bhatt DL, et al. Association between influenza vaccination and cardiovascular outcomes in high-risk patients: a meta-analysis. JAMA 2013; 310(16):1711–20.
54. Modin D, Jorgensen ME, Gislason G, et al. Influenza vaccine in heart failure. Circulation 2019;139(5):575–86.
55. Vardeny O, Claggett B, Udell JA, et al. Influenza vaccination in patients with chronic heart failure: the PARADIGM-HF trial. JACC Heart Fail 2016;4(2):152–8.
56. Bhatt AS, Liang L, DeVore AD, et al. Vaccination trends in patients with heart failure: insights from get with the guidelines-heart failure. JACC Heart Fail 2018; 6(10):844–55.
57. McKelvie RS. Exercise training in patients with heart failure: clinical outcomes, safety, and indications. Heart Fail Rev 2008;13(1):3–11.
58. O'Connor CM, Whellan DJ, Lee KL, et al. Efficacy and safety of exercise training in patients with chronic heart failure: HF-ACTION randomized controlled trial. JAMA 2009;301(14):1439–50.
59. Mediano MFF, Leifer ES, Cooper LS, et al. Influence of baseline physical activity level on exercise training response and clinical outcomes in heart failure: the HF-ACTION trial. JACC Heart Fail 2018;6(12):1011–9.
60. Chen SM, Fang YN, Wang LY, et al. Impact of multi-disciplinary treatment strategy on systolic heart failure outcome. BMC Cardiovasc Disord 2019;19(1):220.
61. Butler T. Dietary management of heart failure: room for improvement? Br J Nutr 2016;115(7):1202–17.
62. Rahman A, Jafry S, Jeejeebhoy K, et al. Malnutrition and cachexia in heart failure. JPEN J Parenter Enteral Nutr 2016;40(4):475–86.

Neurologic Emergencies during the Coronavirus Disease 2019 Pandemic

Julie G. Shulman, MD[a],*, Thomas Ford, MD[a],
Anna M. Cervantes-Arslanian, MD[a,b,c]

KEYWORDS

- COVID-19 • Neurologic emergencies • Cerebrovascular disease • Thrombolysis
- Seizure

KEY POINTS

- Institutions should create protocols for managing neurologic emergencies during the pandemic that allow for rapid and thorough evaluation of patients while also minimizing viral exposure to other patients and staff.
- Less than 5% of patients with coronavirus disease 2019 will have cerebrovascular complications and these typically occur in patients who are critically ill.
- Persons with epilepsy may face significant challenges with regards to care and prevention of seizures, although there does not seem to be an increase in emergency department presentations with seizure.
- Seizure is a rare complication of coronavirus disease 2019 with antiepileptic drug selection impacted by concurrent organ failure, drug–drug interactions with coronavirus disease 2019 therapies, and ongoing drug shortages.

As the coronavirus disease 2019 (COVID-19) pandemic continues, the scientific community is working diligently to rapidly expand knowledge of the disease and disseminate this knowledge worldwide. As of January 2021, there have been more than 90,000 scientific publications relating to COVID-19.[1] The rapid expansion of data on this topic has led to novel means of interpretation and dissemination, including expedited reviews for publication in peer-reviewed journals, open source platforms for review of article preprints, widespread use of social media, and protocol sharing among academic institutions.[2] The literature regarding neurologic features of COVID-19 specifically has been primarily in the form of case reports and a few case series, limiting

This article previously appeared in *Neurologic Clinics*, Volume 39, Issue 2, May 2021.

[a] Department of Neurology, Boston University School of Medicine, 72 East Concord Street, Suite C3, Boston, MA 02118, USA; [b] Department of Neurosurgery, Boston University School of Medicine, 725 Albany St, Suite 7C, Boston, MA 02118, USA; [c] Department of Medicine (Infectious Diseases), Boston University School of Medicine, 801 Massachusetts Avenue, Crosstown, 2nd floor, Boston MA 02118, USA
* Corresponding author.
E-mail address: Julie.Shulman@bmc.org

the generalizability of this information owing to the inherent heterogeneity of these studies and patients.[3] Here, we review what has thus far been published about the intersection of COVID-19 and neurology with particular attention to cerebrovascular disease and seizure. Considerations in managing the acute presentations of these conditions in the context of the pandemic can serve as a model for management of other neurologic emergencies.

CONSIDERATIONS FOR MANAGING ACUTE STROKE DURING THE PANDEMIC
Initial Evaluation

Given the rapid sequence of events that unfold upon the activation of a stroke alert, it is critical that hospitals have standardized measures in place to protect staff from potential exposure when patients are known or suspected to be infected with severe acute respiratory syndrome novel coronavirus 2(SARS-CoV-2). Many groups have proposed adjustments to institutional stroke protocols to continue to offer timely stroke care while preserving personal protective equipment (PPE) and limiting provider exposure.[4–6] For regions with high community prevalence of COVID-19, it is reasonable to consider all patients undergoing stroke alerts to be persons under investigation. A surgical mask should be placed on the patient and 1 member of the stroke team should be designated to don PPE and enter the patient's room for the evaluation. This provider, who is charged with interviewing the patient and performing the initial examination, is then able to communicate with other members of the team (either by phone or tablet computer already placed within the room) to facilitate joint decision-making on eligibility for acute intervention. Although it is common practice at many institutions for the stroke team to accompany patients to neuroimaging studies, it is recommended that, in the case of patients with suspected or confirmed COVID-19, the initial evaluator remain in the patient's room with PPE donned to limit PPE use and accidental exposure while doffing. Upon the patient's return to their room, further examination by the designated team member can be used to guide decision-making on thrombolysis and mechanical thrombectomy.

Mechanical Thrombectomy

Unfortunately, a number of centers have seen significant delays in the delivery of mechanical thrombectomy during the pandemic, particularly for those patients arriving from another facility.[7,8] As a result, measures that simultaneously conserve PPE and maintain provider safety while still providing timely interventional therapy during the ongoing pandemic are necessary. In a recent consensus statement, the Society of Vascular and Interventional Neurology outlined several recommendations on the periprocedural management of patients who are deemed candidates for mechanical thrombectomy.[9] Before mechanical thrombectomy, it is recommended that all patients undergo screening (and testing if feasible) for COVID-19 and be placed in negative-pressure isolation if warranted. The Society of Vascular and Interventional Neurology also recommends that the number of involved personnel be limited and endotracheal intubation be avoided if possible to conserve ventilator capacity and decrease the risk of ventilator-associated injury in patients who may be managed with conscious sedation. For those requiring intubation, centers have adapted techniques (such as the use of negative-pressure rooms and barrier enclosure) to minimize the circulation of respiratory droplets.[10,11] After completion of the procedure, the Society of Vascular and Interventional Neurology recommends that initial neurologic and puncture site evaluations take place in the interventional suite while the patient awaits bed placement elsewhere in the hospital to limit donning and doffing of PPE.

Postacute Stroke Care

For acute ischemic stroke patients not meeting criteria for intervention with intravenous (IV) tissue plasminogen activator (tPA) or mechanical thrombectomy, priorities generally shift to postevent monitoring for clinical progression, as well as workup of potential etiologies and initiation of secondary prevention measures. Some institutions have moved toward the use of video evaluation by nursing staff and/or the stroke team to decrease PPE use and limit provider exposure, as well as deferring diagnostic testing that is not thought to impact inpatient management.[4] An example of a modified approach to monitoring poststroke patients who do not undergo thrombolysis or mechanical thrombectomy is shown in **Fig. 1**.

For patients undergoing acute intervention with IV tPA and/or mechanical thrombectomy, postintervention monitoring before the pandemic was largely centered around frequent examination by both bedside nursing and members of the stroke team.[12] A recent study (albeit one conducted before the pandemic) evaluated the safety of a low-intensity monitoring protocol for patients meeting a predefined threshold for low risk for neurologic decompensation and found that selected patients who underwent less frequent neurologic and vital sign checks in the 24 hours after the administration of IV tPA did not see an increased incidence of clinical worsening requiring transfer to an intensive care unit.[13] Similarly, investigations questioning the usefulness of routine surveillance neuroimaging in otherwise stable postintervention patients have called into question their necessity.[14,15] These findings have been extrapolated to inform policy about post-thrombolysis and post-thrombectomy care in the COVID-19 pandemic, when intensive care unit beds have been in short supply and frequent evaluations by providers increase the risk of exposure.[4,16,17] Examples of this process of risk stratification and disposition decision-making are shown in **Figs. 2** and **3**.

Impact on Stroke-Related Outcomes

Hospitals across the world have reported significant reductions in admissions for all types of stroke patients during the pandemic, with the most impact usually occurring during times of local government restrictions on activities and in patients with a transient ischemic attack or minor stroke. Specifically, this phenomenon has been reported in the United States,[18–22] Canada,[23] China,[24] Spain,[25] Amsterdam,[26] Brazil,[27] Bangladesh,[28]

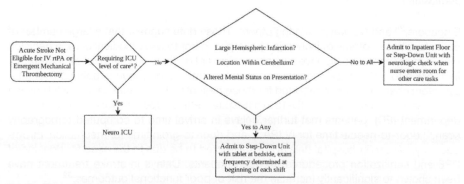

Fig. 1. Neurologic monitoring frequency in patients not receiving IV tPA or emergent mechanical thrombectomy. [a]Indications including (but not limited to) vasoactive medications, insulin drip for hyperglycemia, need for mechanical ventilation. ICU, intensive care unit. (*Adapted from* Optimization of Resources and Modifications in Acute Ischemic Stroke Care in Response to the Global COVID-19 Pandemic. J Stroke Cerebrovas Dis 2020 Aug;29(8):104980, with permission.)

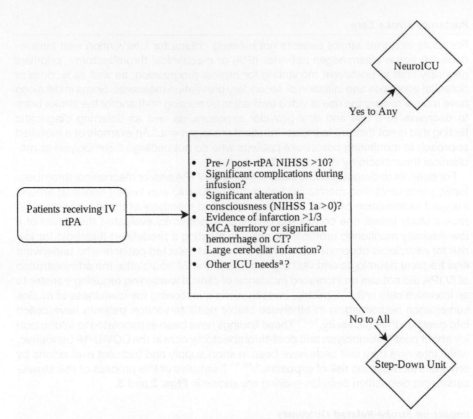

Fig. 2. Disposition determination algorithm after the administration of IV tPA. [a]Indications including (but not limited to) vasoactive medications, insulin drip for hyperglycemia, need for mechanical ventilation. CT, computed tomography; ICU, intensive care unit; MCA, middle cerebral artery; NIHSS, National Institutes of Health Stroke Scale. (*Adapted from* Optimization of Resources and Modifications in Acute Ischemic Stroke Care in Response to the Global COVID-19 Pandemic. J Stroke Cerebrovas Dis 2020 Aug;29(8):104980, with permission.)

Singapore,[29] and Norway,[30] among others. These data suggest that a large number of patients with symptoms of ischemic stroke chose not to seek medical care, a decision that, in many cases, could have a significant impact on their long-term functional status. In addition to a decrease in acute stroke presentations, delays in hospital arrival after symptom onset have been reported for those patients who do seek care,[21] likely owing to the fear of exposure to COVID-19 in a hospital setting. Upon arrival to the emergency department (ED), patients met further delays in arrival time to computed tomography scan,[21] door-to-needle time for IV tPA,[31] and door-to-groin time for mechanical thrombectomy.[8] These in-hospital delays are suspected to be due to the need for donning of PPE and sanitization procedures between patients. Delays in stroke treatment have been shown to significantly increase the risk of poor functional outcomes.[32]

CORONAVIRUS DISEASE 19–ASSOCIATED CEREBROVASCULAR DISEASE
Epidemiology

Infection with SARS-CoV-2 has been associated with a myriad of neurologic complications (**Table 1**) and the presence of neurologic symptoms seem to be quite

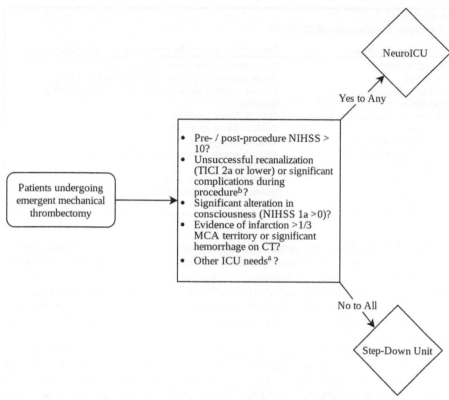

Fig. 3. Disposition determination algorithm after emergent mechanical thrombectomy. [a] Indications including (but not limited to) vasoactive medications, insulin drip for hyperglycemia, need for mechanical ventilation. [b] including (but not limited to) dissection, hemodynamic instability, and respiratory decompensation requiring intubation. CT, computed tomography; ICU, intensive care unit; MCA, middle cerebral artery; NIHSS, National Institutes of Health Stroke Scale; TICI, thrombolysis in cerebral infarction. (*Adapted from* Optimization of Resources and Modifications in Acute Ischemic Stroke Care in Response to the Global COVID-19 Pandemic. J Stroke Cerebrovas Dis 2020 Aug;29(8):104980, with permission.)

common, occurring in up to 84% of those with critical illness.[33] The majority of acute cerebrovascular disease associated with COVID-19 infection is acute ischemic stroke, but there have been reports of intracerebral hemorrhage,[34] venous sinus thrombosis,[35] posterior reversible encephalopathy syndrome (PRES),[36] reversible cerebral vasoconstriction syndrome,[37] and endotheliitis without parenchymal infarction.[38]

Ischemic stroke has been reported in 1% to 5% of patients hospitalized with COVID-19, with the higher end of that range coming from very early reports out of Wuhan, China, in predominantly critically ill patients.[39–45] Although nonspecific neurologic symptoms (such as headache, dizziness, and fatigue) are frequently reported early in the course of infection,[3] there is a suggestion that cerebrovascular disease tends to occur an average of 10 days (range, 0–33 days) after the onset of respiratory illness.[39] Most studies report that COVID-19–associated cerebrovascular disease occurs in predominantly male patients who are more than 60 years of age and have known vascular risk factors.[40,41,43–45] However, several studies reported out of New

Table 1
Neurologic complications of COVID-19

Acute Complications	Parainfectious and Postinfectious Complications
Encephalopathy	Acute disseminated encephalomyelitis
Myalgias	Acute necrotizing hemorrhagic encephalopathy
Anosmia/dysgeusia	Steroid responsive (autoimmune) encephalopathy
Headache	Myositis
Cerebrovascular complications	Critical illness neuromyopathy
Seizures	Guillain-Barre syndrome
Meningoencephalitis	Transverse myelitis
Cranial and peripheral neuropathies	Myalgic encephalomyelitis, with or without dysautonomia
Myoclonus	Sudden sensorineural hearing loss
Movement disorders	Unknown late neurologic complications
Psychosis	

York City[42,46] found strokes, particularly large vessel occlusion (LVO) strokes, occurring in younger patients. The majority of strokes reported are attributed to cardioembolism, many considered cryptogenic.[43–47] In the United States, cerebrovascular disease seems to be a complication of COVID-19 seen more commonly in racial minorities (Blacks and Hispanics),[42–44] but this may be due to more data coming from larger urban hospitals and the disproportionate effect COVID-19 has had on minority communities overall.

The mortality of ischemic stroke in COVID-19 is high (25%–44%),[40–45] leading to some speculation that stroke is predominantly associated with preexisting critical illness. Patients admitted with COVID-19 and neurologic disease have been found to have a higher in-hospital mortality (37.5% vs 4.3%) and greater disability at discharge (modified Rankin Scale of 5 vs 2) compared with patients admitted with the same neurologic diagnoses without COVID-19.[48] Similarly, when patients with COVID-19–associated ischemic stroke were compared with propensity score matched patients with stroke alone, they were found to have greater stroke severity (National Institutes of Health Stroke Scale 10 vs 6), higher risk for severe disability (modified Rankin Scale 4 vs 2; $P<.001$), and higher mortality (odds ratio, 4.3).[49] These findings suggest that COVID-19–associated cerebrovascular disease is more severe with worse functional outcomes and higher mortality than non-COVID-19–associated cerebrovascular disease.

Intracerebral hemorrhage occurs less commonly in patients with COVID-19 than acute ischemic stroke. Several reports in the spring in the United States noted that hemorrhage occurred predominantly in hospitalized patients on anticoagulation, often prescribed for elevated D-dimer levels.[34,44,50,51] Other risk factors associated with intracerebral hemorrhage include a prolonged international normalized ratio and partial thromboplastin time independent of anticoagulation use, thrombocytopenia, older age, non-White race, and mechanical ventilation.[34,50,51] Patients with COVID-19 and intracerebral hemorrhage experienced very high in-hospital mortality, up to 84.6% in 1 center.[51]

Cerebral venous sinus thromboses have been infrequently reported despite an abundance of evidence reporting deep vein thromboses elsewhere. Unlike other cerebrovascular complications, cerebral venous sinus thromboses seems to occur more often in females, with a wide age range reported. This finding is similar to patterns seen in non–COVID-associated cerebral venous sinus thromboses. It seems that cerebral venous sinus thromboses associated with COVID-19 may occur at the same time as typical respiratory or gastrointestinal symptoms, but may also occur in a delayed fashion, up to weeks after initial infection.[35]

Thirteen cases of PRES in the setting of COVID-19 have been reported as of June 30, 2020.[36] Unlike the majority of patients with PRES outside of COVID-19, these patients had only modest fluctuations in blood pressure. Risk factors for COVID-19–associated PRES include an underlying infection or immunomodulatory agents with endothelial effects. In general, as with other associated etiologies, the neurologic prognosis for COVID-19–associated PRES is favorable.[36]

Pathophysiology

Several mechanisms may lead to ischemic stroke in patients with COVID-19 (**Box 1**). One of the more widely accepted hypotheses is that SARS-CoV-2 causes damage to endothelial cells, which leads to activation of inflammatory and thrombotic pathways, microvascular and macrovascular injury, and ultimately coagulopathy similar to that seen in sepsis, characterized by elevated fibrinogen, partial thromboplastin time, D-dimer, and sometimes thrombocytopenia.[3,39] Some studies have also noted a high prevalence of antiphospholipid antibodies[52,53] in critically ill patients with COVID-19. SARS-CoV-2 can also trigger a hyperinflammatory state and cytokine storm similar to that which occurs in hemophagocytic lymphohistiocytosis.[54,55] Cellular entry of SARS-CoV-2 via the angiotensin-converting enzyme 2 receptor leads to the downregulation of receptors with consequent overactivation of the classic renin–angiotensin system axis causing vasoconstriction and a prothrombotic state.[56] Other investigators have suggested a possible direct endothelial invasion and replication within the arterial wall,[57] a process previously described in varicella zoster virus.[58] Finally, the inherent increased risk of stroke in all critically ill patients can also apply to patients with COVID-19, with potential mechanisms including destabilization of atherosclerotic plaque, triggering of atrial fibrillation, or increasing thrombus formation in conditions of hypoxia.[3]

Acute Stroke Treatment for Coronavirus Disease 19–Associated Stroke

In light of the finding that patients with COVID-19 are at risk of mixed hematologic complications,[59–61] the efficacy and safety of administration of IV tPA in this subset of acute ischemic stroke patients has been a topic of debate. Although the efficacy of thrombolysis outside of the context of the COVID-19 pandemic in decreasing

---

Box 1
Mechanisms of stroke in COVID-19

- Exacerbation of underlying risk factors
- Viral mediated hematologic derangement/hypercoagulable state
- Effects on the renin–angiotensin system
- Hyperinflammatory condition (cytokine storm)
- Complication of COVID treatments
- General critical illness, hypoxia, hypotension
- Myocarditis, stress cardiomyopathy
- Atrial fibrillation
- Endotheliitis/vasculitis

long-term disability from acute ischemic stroke has been demonstrated clearly,[62,63] there are limited data that address whether this specific patient population is at an increased risk of clinically significant hemorrhagic transformation compared with the general population, thereby altering the risk:benefit relationship. Data on this topic are limited in quality and provide mixed results. One review found that 10.3% of patients with COVID-19 (3/29) receiving IV tPA had clinically significant hemorrhagic transformation,[64] although another did not report any instances (0/13).[65] In the absence of a true consensus regarding the risk of symptomatic hemorrhage in patients with COVID-19 with suspected acute ischemic stroke, the decision to administer tPA is provider-dependent and should be made with consideration of non–COVID-specific contraindications to thrombolysis and other patient-specific factors.

In addition to increased severity of stroke, presentation with LVO stroke has been observed in patients infected with COVID-19.[42,64,66,67] Although emergent mechanical thrombectomy in a patient with confirmed COVID-19 is feasible[11] with appropriate modifications as described elsewhere in this article,[9] the limited data available thus far have unfortunately shown poor outcomes with increased mortality in patients with LVO stroke and COVID-19 compared with LVO stroke alone.[68,69] Specifically, there have been reports of increased procedural complications including clot fragmentation, downstream emboli, and distal emboli to a new vascular territory.[70] An increase in postprocedural complications, including early cerebral reocclusion[69] and deep venous thrombosis and/or pulmonary emboli,[68] has also been reported. Despite these risks, mechanical thrombectomy is recommended in patients with COVID-19 and LVO stroke, with appropriate precautions.

CONSIDERATIONS FOR MANAGING EPILEPSY DURING THE PANDEMIC

Like many chronic illnesses, medical care for persons with epilepsy (PWE) has been impacted by the pandemic. With the shutdowns seen in many countries, there has been a dramatic reduction in the availability of outpatient care such as visits with a neurologist/epileptologist and electroencephalograms (EEGs). Even when in-person visits have been available, many patients chose to defer medical care owing to the fear of viral exposure in the clinic. The advent of widely available telehealth has improved access to care but cannot entirely replicate an in-person evaluation or EEG monitoring. With overcrowding and concerns about infection control, many hospitals have canceled elective admissions and surgeries, delaying care for those awaiting characterization of epileptic spells in epilepsy monitoring units or epilepsy surgery.

The American Epilepsy Society has reported survey data of their membership indicating that 10% of PWE have noted worsening in seizure frequency unrelated to COVID-19 infection during the pandemic, with increased stress, sleep deprivation, and decreased access to medical care and pharmacies cited as potential contributors.[71] This phenomenon has been seen in previous coronavirus outbreaks as well. During the 2003 SARS epidemic in Taiwan, 1 epilepsy center noted that 22% of PWE experienced inability to access antiepileptic drugs (AEDs) owing to lack of access to health care providers and/or pharmacies, leading to increased seizure frequency in 12% (including 2 patients with status epilepticus [SE] who required intensive care unit admission).[72]

However, not all reports about epilepsy care during the pandemic have been negative. Some epileptologists have noted improvement in seizure control in PWE during the pandemic owing to better medication adherence and increased sleep.[71] Despite concerns that ED visits for seizures would increase if patients were not accessing outpatient care, 1 health system in Italy actually observed a decrease in visits for seizures during the height of the pandemic in their country.[73] Limited evidence has also suggested that PWE without other comorbidities are not at higher risk for acquiring COVID-19 or suffering from more severe complications,[74] unlike patients with a history of cerebrovascular disease.[75,76]

Approach to Managing Seizures and Status Epilepticus During the Pandemic

For the most part, the evaluation and treatment of patients with seizures and/or SE during the pandemic should be unchanged with regard to general management principles, such as those outlined in the Neurocritical Care Society Guidelines.[77] However, there are some key, novel considerations regarding infection control, medications, and resource use.

Convulsive SE should be considered aerosol generating and appropriate PPE should be used for all treating staff. This point is most critical for physicians performing endotracheal intubation. Although debate exists about whether early versus delayed intubation is superior for patient outcomes in severe COVID-19 infection,[78,79] infection control may be considered in some centers. Some centers advocate for earlier intubation in respiratory failure given the potential for increased aerosolization associated with the use of noninvasive ventilation (bilevel or continuous positive airway pressure) and to a lesser extent high-flow nasal cannula, especially in the context of lack of negative pressure rooms and sufficient PPE.[80,81] These factors may influence decision-making for patients with mild respiratory distress after a seizure.

During the pandemic, there have been several shortages of medications frequently used for continuous sedation (IV midazolam, propofol) and AEDs (valproic acid, levetiracetam) that have impacted the care of hospitalized epilepsy patients and in the emergent management of seizures and SE. The main driver for these drug shortages has been the massive increase in simultaneous worldwide need; up to one-third of hospitalized patients with COVID-19 have severe respiratory distress requiring prolonged intubation and sedation.[82] In addition, manufacturing shutdowns in China and closure of exportation from India interrupted the usual supply chain to the United States.[83] Thus, it is important for health care systems to develop alternative sedation and SE treatment protocols to account for potential shortages. In particular, ketamine has experienced a recent resurgence for use in sedation as well as seizures and SE. There may be a particular role in SARS-CoV-2 infection, because ketamine has an anti-inflammatory effect, in particular lowering levels of IL-6, which are often increased in COVID-19 infection.[84,85]

Some patients may present to the ED with seizure or SE as the presenting feature of COVID-19.[86,87] Therefore, it may be reasonable to consider all patients with seizure or SE presenting to the ED as persons under investigation. Irrespective of COVID-19 status, a typical diagnostic work-up for new seizure involves obtaining MRI and EEG. Many investigators suggest the postponement of these studies during the pandemic unless they might provide urgent information that would change management.[74] Because seizure in COVID-19 may occur secondary to conditions like stroke, cerebral venous sinus thromboses, or meningoencephalitis, in our center we advocate for obtaining these studies during admission for a new seizure diagnosis, especially if there are no other provoking factors present.

Electroencephalography

Many health care systems decreased the use of EEG during the initial surge for all patients or modified indications and restricted access. Some eliminated the use of EEG for inpatients suspected to have COVID-19 altogether or created treatment algorithms which modified the standard of care for typical evaluations such as myoclonus, encephalopathy, and nonconvulsive SE.[88]

Pursuing EEG for patients with COVID-19 requires consideration of the risk:benefit ratio, given the risk of potential viral transmission to the technologist. If the study is unlikely to change management decisions for the patient, strong consideration should be given to foregoing the study. Most studies require prolonged set-up times and close proximity to patients' faces, which increase the risk of viral transmission (which may be lessened by proper use of PPE). Although an EEG in itself is not an aerosolizing procedure, the patient population requiring EEG may have behavioral unpredictability with the potential for yelling or coughing. For this reason, we recommend the use of N95 respirators, face shields, gowns, and gloves for all technologists during EEG lead placement and adjustment of all patients. Other infection control measures may include having a dedicated machine exclusively for patients with COVID-19 or using only disposable electrodes and cables.[89]

We recommend obtaining an EEG in cases of known SE who remain encephalopathic or comatose after the initial treatment of the seizure, for myoclonus and encephalopathy that has not responded to an empiric trial of an AED,[88] and for encephalopathy or coma evaluation when other explanations have been excluded. If EEG is pursued, a standard 10 to 20 EEG complement of electrodes with electrocardiogram should be used. Expedited studies with simplified montages to screen for SE (generalized and most regional or focal types), encephalopathy, and reactivity may be helpful in the intensive care unit setting if there are concerns about resource use.[90] The interpretation of specific patterns on the intensive care unit EEG suggestive of encephalopathy, nonconvulsive SE, focal slowing (suggestive of a lesion, such as a stroke), and postanoxic changes are beyond the scope of this article, but we recommend EEG scoring as per the American Clinical Neurophysiology Society guidance.[91] We suggest continuous video EEG monitoring to limit technologist active hands-on time in the room as well as to allow the electroencephalographer to make clinical correlations with the EEG findings. With reduced montages, however, there may be difficulty in identifying artifacts and a failure to identify lateralized periodic discharges. Most societies have recommended against the use of hyperventilation during EEG to decrease the risk of viral transmission.[89,90]

Because patients with COVID-19 are often intubated (sometimes with less common ventilation strategies), the electroencephalographer may be aided in interpretation of the study if the mode and rate of ventilation is recorded. There is no reason why EEG cannot be used for patients requiring the prone position, but experience with interpretation is very limited. When prone, the typical artifacts that are usually seen in the occipital leads (representing contact with bedding for supine patients) would instead be in the frontopolar leads.[90] Furthermore, positioning affects the cerebrospinal fluid (CSF) layer surrounding the brain parenchyma and shifts from supine to prone will redistribute CSF by up to 30% owing to gravity. As CSF is more conductive than brain parenchyma, and this factor will change the scalp potentials with thicker CSF layers associated with a decreased EEG signal.[92]

CORONAVIRUS DISEASE 19–ASSOCIATED SEIZURES AND STATUS EPILEPTICUS

Seizures seem to be an infrequent complication in patients with COVID-19, with a reported incidence of less than 1.6% in single health system studies[40,93–95] There are many mechanisms by which seizures may occur in COVID-19 (**Box 2**). PWE may be at greater risk of seizure during COVID-19 (similar to other common

---

Box 2
Mechanisms of seizure in COVID-19

- Exacerbation of underlying epilepsy
- Metabolic derangements
- Hypoxia
- Hyperinflammatory condition (cytokine storm)
- Complication of COVID treatments
- General critical illness
- Meningoencephalitis, infectious, or parainfectious
- Secondary consequence of cerebrovascular disease

---

infections), although the American Epilepsy Society reported survey data indicating that most PWE (>80%) did not experience worsening of seizure frequency, although they had symptoms of COVID-19 infection.[71] Metabolic derangements, organ failure, hypoglycemia, hypoxia, and some medications used during critical illness may all lower the seizure threshold. Moreover, subclinical seizures or nonconvulsive SE are common in patients with other forms of critical illness and depressed mental status.[96] There have been reports of new-onset epilepsy in COVID-19, most of which have been described in patients with a preexisting risk factor that lowered their seizure threshold. However, not all patients have a history of epilepsy, identified preexisting risk factor, or current metabolic derangement to explain new-onset seizures.[86,97] Some of these patients have been determined to have meningoencephalitis either from SARS-CoV-2 infection or as a parainfectious process.[88,97–99] Finally, COVID-related cerebrovascular complications may also lead to seizures.

The management of seizures and SE in COVID-19 may have some notable differences with regard to AED selection. In general, we advocate for the use of an IV AED formulation to avoid concerns of malabsorption. Critically ill patients with COVID-19 are at risk for multiple organ system failures. Cardiac complications in COVID-19 may be exacerbated by the combined effects of both COVID treatments and AEDs that lead to PR and/or QT prolongation (such as hydroxychloroquine and phenytoin). Hepatic injury and potential anticoagulation use may limit the use of phenytoin, valproate, and carbamazepine. Acute kidney injury leading to the need for renal replacement therapy or placement of patients on extracorporeal membrane oxygenation may require dose adjustments to maintain therapeutic concentrations of AEDs in serum.[100] Finally, as noted elsewhere in this article, key drug shortages may influence management decisions.

SUMMARY

Significant attention must be paid to the logistical challenges of managing neurologic emergencies in the setting of the COVID-19 pandemic. Thoughtful modifications of protocols allow for efficient delivery of high-quality care for all patients while protecting health care providers from viral exposure during the pandemic. Although the percentage of SARS-CoV-2 infections associated with neurologic emergencies is small, the large and still growing number of total infected individuals will likely result in a high burden of COVID-19 associated neurologic disease.[39] COVID-19–associated cerebrovascular disease and seizure are areas of active research that require further investigation to clarify their pathophysiology and determine optimal treatment measures.

CLINICS CARE POINTS

- Institutions should create protocols for managing neurologic emergencies during the pandemic that allow for rapid and thorough evaluation of patients while also minimizing viral exposure to other patients and staff.

- Less than 5% of patients with COVID-19 will have cerebrovascular complications and these typically occur in patients who are critically ill.

- PWE may face significant challenges with regards to care and prevention of seizures, but thus far there does not seem to be an increase in ED presentations with seizure

- Seizure is a rare complication of COVID-19 with AED selection impacted by concurrent organ failure, drug–drug interactions with COVID therapies, and ongoing drug shortages.

DISCLOSURE

The authors have nothing to disclose.

REFERENCES

1. LitCovid. Available at: https://www.ncbi.nlm.nih.gov/research/coronavirus/. Accessed November 10, 2020.
2. Cervantes-Arslanian A, Lau KHV, Anand P, et al. Rapid dissemination of protocols for managing neurology inpatients with COVID-19. Ann Neurol 2020; 88(2):211–4.
3. Pezzini A, Padovani A. Lifting the mask on neurological manifestations of COVID-19. Nat Rev Neurol 2020. https://doi.org/10.1038/s41582-020-0398-3.
4. Ford T, Curiale G, Nguyen TN, et al. Optimization of resources and modifications in acute ischemic stroke care in response to the global COVID-19 pandemic. J Stroke Cerebrovasc Dis 2020. https://doi.org/10.1016/j.jstrokecerebrovasdis. 2020.104980.
5. Khosravani H, Rajendram P, Notario L, et al. Protected code stroke: hyperacute stroke management during the coronavirus disease 2019 (COVID-19) pandemic. Stroke 2020. https://doi.org/10.1161/STROKEAHA.120.029838.
6. On Behalf of the AHA/ASA Stroke Council Leadership. Temporary emergency guidance to US stroke centers during the coronavirus disease 2019 (COVID-19) pandemic: on behalf of the American Heart Association/American Stroke Association Stroke Council Leadership. Stroke 2020;51(6):1910–2.
7. Yang B, Wang T, Chen J, et al. Impact of the COVID-19 pandemic on the process and outcome of thrombectomy for acute ischemic stroke. J Neurointerv Surg 2020. https://doi.org/10.1136/neurintsurg-2020-016177.
8. Kerleroux B, Fabacher T, Bricout N, et al. Mechanical thrombectomy for acute ischemic stroke amid the COVID-19 outbreak: decreased activity, and increased care delays. Stroke 2020. https://doi.org/10.1161/STROKEAHA.120. 030373.
9. Nguyen T, Abdalkader M, Jovin T. Mechanical thrombectomy in the era of COVID-19. Emergency preparedness for the neuroscience teams. Stroke 2020;51(6):1896–901.

10. Canelli R, Connor CW, Gonzalez M, et al. Barrier enclosure during endotracheal intubation. N Engl J Med 2020;382(20):1957–8.

11. Mansour OY, Malik AM, Linfante I. Mechanical Thrombectomy of COVID-19 positive acute ischemic stroke patient: a case report and call for preparedness. BMC Neurol 2020. https://doi.org/10.1186/s12883-020-01930-x.

12. Powers WJ, Rabinstein AA, Ackerson T, et al. Guidelines for the Early Management of Patients With Acute Ischemic Stroke: 2019 Update to the 2018 Guidelines for the Early Management of Acute Ischemic Stroke: a guideline for healthcare professionals from the American Heart Association/American Stroke Association. Stroke 2019;50(12). https://doi.org/10.1161/STR.0000000000000211.

13. Faigle R, Butler J, Carhuapoma JR, et al. Safety trial of low-intensity monitoring after thrombolysis: optimal post tpa-iv monitoring in ischemic STroke (OPTIMIST). Neurohospitalist 2020;10(1):11–5.

14. George AJ, Boehme AK, Dunn CR, et al. Trimming the fat in acute ischemic stroke: an assessment of 24-h CT Scans in tPA Patients. Int J Stroke 2015; 10(1):37–41.

15. Guhwe M, Utley-Smith Q, Blessing R, et al. Routine 24-hour computed tomography brain scan is not useful in stable patients post intravenous tissue plasminogen activator. J Stroke Cerebrovasc Dis 2016;25(3):540–2.

16. Dafer RM, Osteraas ND, Biller J. Acute stroke care in the coronavirus disease 2019 pandemic. J Stroke Cerebrovasc Dis 2020. https://doi.org/10.1016/j.jstrokecerebrovasdis.2020.104881.

17. Gioia LC, Poppe AY, Laroche R, et al. Streamlined Poststroke Treatment Order Sets During the SARS-CoV-2 pandemic: simplifying while not compromising care. Stroke 2020. https://doi.org/10.1161/STROKEAHA.120.031008.

18. Esenwa C, Parides MK, Labovitz DL. The effect of COVID-19 on stroke hospitalizations in New York City. J Stroke Cerebrovasc Dis 2020. https://doi.org/10.1016/j.jstrokecerebrovasdis.2020.105114.

19. Cummings C, Almallouhi E, Al Kasab S, et al. Blacks are less likely to present with strokes during the COVID-19 pandemic: observations from the buckle of the stroke belt. Stroke 2020. https://doi.org/10.1161/STROKEAHA.120.031121.

20. de Havenon A, Ney J, Callaghan B, et al. A Rapid Decrease in Stroke, Acute Coronary Syndrome, and Corresponding Interventions at 65 United States Hospitals Following Emergence of COVID-19. medRxiv 2020. https://doi.org/10.1101/2020.05.07.20083386.

21. Ghanchi H, Takayanagi A, Savla P, et al. Effects of the COVID-19 pandemic on stroke patients. Cureus 2020. https://doi.org/10.7759/cureus.9995.

22. Sharma M, Lioutas V-A, Madsen T, et al. Decline in stroke alerts and hospitalisations during the COVID-19 pandemic. Stroke Vasc Neurol 2020. https://doi.org/10.1136/svn-2020-000441.

23. Bres Bullrich M, Fridman S, Mandzia JL, et al. COVID-19: stroke admissions, emergency department visits, and prevention clinic referrals. Can J Neurol Sci 2020. https://doi.org/10.1017/cjn.2020.101.

24. Wang J, Chaudhry SA, Tahsili-Fahadan P, et al. The impact of COVID-19 on acute ischemic stroke admissions: analysis from a community-based tertiary care center. J Stroke Cerebrovasc Dis 2020. https://doi.org/10.1016/j.jstrokecerebrovasdis.2020.105344.

25. Meza HT, Lambea GÁ, Saldaña AS, et al. Impact of COVID-19 outbreak on ischemic stroke admissions and in-hospital mortality in North-West Spain. Int J Stroke 2020;15(7):755–62.

26. Rinkel LA, Prick JCM, Slot RER, et al. Impact of the COVID-19 outbreak on acute stroke care. J Neurol 2020. https://doi.org/10.1007/s00415-020-10069-1.
27. Diegoli H, Magalhães PSC, Martins SCO, et al. Decrease in hospital admissions for transient ischemic attack, mild, and moderate stroke during the COVID-19 era. Stroke 2020. https://doi.org/10.1161/STROKEAHA.120.030481.
28. Hasan ATMH, Das SC, Islam MS, et al. Impact of COVID-19 on hospital admission of acute stroke patients in Bangladesh. PLoS One 2020. https://doi.org/10.1101/2020.09.28.316448.
29. Paliwal PR, Tan BYQ, Leow AST, et al. Impact of the COVID-19 pandemic on hyperacute stroke treatment: experience from a comprehensive stroke centre in Singapore. J Thromb Thrombolysis 2020. https://doi.org/10.1007/s11239-020-02225-1.
30. Saxhaug Kristoffersen E, Holt Jahr S, Thommessen B, et al. Effect of COVID-19 pandemic on stroke admission rates in a Norwegian population. Acta Neurol Scand 2020. https://doi.org/10.1111/ane.13307.
31. Neves Briard J, Ducroux C, Jacquin G, et al. Early impact of the COVID-19 pandemic on acute stroke treatment delays. Can J Neurol Sci 2020. https://doi.org/10.1017/cjn.2020.160.
32. Darehed D, Blom M, Glader E-L, et al. In-hospital delays in stroke thrombolysis: every minute counts. Stroke 2020;51(8):2536–9.
33. Helms J, Kremer S, Merdji H, et al. Neurologic Features in Severe SARS-CoV-2 Infection. N Engl J Med 2020;382(23):2268–70.
34. Melmed KR, Cao M, Dogra S, et al. Risk factors for intracerebral hemorrhage in patients with COVID-19. J Thromb Thrombolysis 2020. https://doi.org/10.1007/s11239-020-02288-0.
35. Nwajei F, Anand P, Abdalkader M, et al. Cerebral Venous Sinus Thromboses in Patients with SARS-CoV-2 infection: three cases and a review of the literature. J Stroke Cerebrovasc Dis 2020. https://doi.org/10.1016/j.jstrokecerebrovasdis.2020.105412.
36. Anand P, Lau KHV, Chung DY, et al. Posterior reversible encephalopathy syndrome in patients with coronavirus disease 2019: two cases and a review of the literature. J Stroke Cerebrovasc Dis 2020;29(11):105212.
37. Dakay K, Kaur G, Gulko E, et al. Reversible cerebral vasoconstriction syndrome and dissection in the setting of COVID-19 infection. J Stroke Cerebrovasc Dis 2020;29(9):105011.
38. Pugin D, Vargas M-I, Thieffry C, et al. COVID-19–related encephalopathy responsive to high-dose glucocorticoids. Neurology 2020;95(12):543–6.
39. Ellul MA, Benjamin L, Singh B, et al. Neurological associations of COVID-19. Lancet Neurol 2020;19(9):767–83.
40. Mao L, Jin H, Wang M, et al. Neurologic manifestations of hospitalized patients with coronavirus disease 2019 in Wuhan, China. JAMA Neurol 2020. https://doi.org/10.1001/jamaneurol.2020.1127.
41. Li Y, Li M, Wang M, et al. Acute cerebrovascular disease following COVID-19: a single center, retrospective, observational study. Stroke Vasc Neurol 2020;5(3):279–84.
42. Majidi S, Fifi JT, Ladner TR, et al. Emergent large vessel occlusion stroke during New York City's COVID-19 outbreak: clinical characteristics and paraclinical findings. Stroke 2020. https://doi.org/10.1161/STROKEAHA.120.030397.
43. Kihira S, Schefflein J, Mahmoudi K, et al. Association of Coronavirus Disease (COVID-19) with large vessel occlusion strokes: a case-control study. AJR Am J Roentgenol 2020;29:1–6.

44. Rothstein A, Oldridge O, Schwennesen H, et al. Acute cerebrovascular events in hospitalized COVID-19 patients. Stroke 2020. https://doi.org/10.1161/STROKEAHA.120.030995.

45. Jillella DV, Janocko NJ, Nahab F, et al. Ischemic stroke in COVID-19: an urgent need for early identification and management. PLoS One 2020. https://doi.org/10.1371/journal.pone.0239443.

46. Yaghi S, Ishida K, Torres J, et al. SARS-CoV-2 and Stroke in a New York Healthcare System. Stroke 2020;51(7):2002–11.

47. Siegler JE, Cardona P, Arenillas JF, et al. Cerebrovascular events and outcomes in hospitalized patients with COVID-19: the SVIN COVID-19 Multinational Registry. Int J Stroke 2020. https://doi.org/10.1177/1747493020959216. 174749302095921.

48. Benussi A, Pilotto A, Premi E, et al. Clinical characteristics and outcomes of inpatients with neurologic disease and COVID-19 in Brescia, Lombardy, Italy. Neurology 2020;95(7):e910–20.

49. Ntaios G, Michel P, Georgiopoulos G, et al. Characteristics and outcomes in patients with COVID-19 and acute ischemic stroke: the Global COVID-19 Stroke Registry. Stroke 2020. https://doi.org/10.1161/STROKEAHA.120.031208.

50. Dogra S, Jain R, Cao M, et al. Hemorrhagic stroke and anticoagulation in COVID-19. J Stroke Cerebrovasc Dis 2020;29(8):104984.

51. Kvernland A, Kumar A, Yaghi S, et al. Anticoagulation use and Hemorrhagic Stroke in SARS-CoV-2 Patients Treated at a New York Healthcare System. Neurocrit Care 2020. https://doi.org/10.1007/s12028-020-01077-0.

52. Beyrouti R, Adams ME, Benjamin L, et al. Characteristics of ischaemic stroke associated with COVID-19. J Neurol Neurosurg Psychiatry 2020;91(8):889–91.

53. Zhang Y, Xiao M, Zhang S, et al. Coagulopathy and antiphospholipid antibodies in patients with Covid-19. N Engl J Med 2020;382(17):e38.

54. Bhaskar S, Sinha A, Banach M, et al. Cytokine storm in COVID-19-immunopathological mechanisms, clinical considerations, and therapeutic approaches: the REPROGRAM Consortium position paper. Front Immunol 2020;11:1648.

55. Divani AA, Andalib S, Di Napoli M, et al. Coronavirus disease 2019 and stroke: clinical manifestations and pathophysiological insights. J Stroke Cerebrovasc Dis 2020;29(8):104941.

56. South AM, Tomlinson L, Edmonston D, et al. Controversies of renin-angiotensin system inhibition during the COVID-19 pandemic. Nat Rev Nephrol 2020;16(6):305–7.

57. Gulko E, Overby P, Ali S, et al. Vessel Wall Enhancement and Focal Cerebral Arteriopathy in a Pediatric Patient with Acute Infarct and COVID-19 Infection. AJNR Am J Neuroradiol 2020;41(12):2348–50.

58. Shulman JG, Cervantes-Arslanian AM. Infectious Etiologies of Stroke. Semin Neurol 2019;39(4):482–94.

59. Bhattacharjee S, Banerjee M. Immune thrombocytopenia secondary to COVID-19: a systematic review. SN Compr Clin Med 2020;1–11. https://doi.org/10.1007/s42399-020-00521-8.

60. Tang N, Li D, Wang X, et al. Abnormal coagulation parameters are associated with poor prognosis in patients with novel coronavirus pneumonia. J Thromb Haemost 2020;18(4):844–7.

61. Thachil J, Tang N, Gando S, et al. ISTH interim guidance on recognition and management of coagulopathy in COVID-19. J Thromb Haemost 2020;18(5):1023–6.

62. National Institute of Neurological Disorders and Stroke rt-PA Stroke Study Group. Tissue plasminogen activator for acute ischemic stroke. N Engl J Med 1995;333(24):1581–7.
63. Hacke W, Kaste M, Bluhmki E, et al. Thrombolysis with alteplase 3 to 4.5 hours after acute ischemic stroke. N Engl J Med 2008;359(13):1317–29.
64. Tan Y-K, Goh C, Leow AST, et al. COVID-19 and ischemic stroke: a systematic review and meta-summary of the literature. J Thromb Thrombolysis 2020. https://doi.org/10.1007/s11239-020-02228-y.
65. Carneiro T, Dashkoff J, Leung LY, et al. Intravenous tPA for Acute Ischemic Stroke in Patients with COVID-19. J Stroke Cerebrovasc Dis 2020. https://doi.org/10.1016/j.jstrokecerebrovasdis.2020.105201.
66. Oxley TJ, Mocco J, Majidi S, et al. Large-vessel stroke as a presenting feature of Covid-19 in the young. N Engl J Med 2020;382(20):e60.
67. Baracchini C, Pieroni A, Viaro F, et al. Acute Stroke Management Pathway During Coronavirus-19 Pandemic. Neurol Sci 2020;41:1003–5.
68. Pop R, Hasiu A, Bolognini F, et al. Stroke thrombectomy in patients with COVID-19: initial experience in 13 cases. AJNR Am J Neuroradiol 2020. https://doi.org/10.3174/ajnr.A6750. ajnr;ajnr.A6750v1.
69. Escalard S, Maïer B, Redjem H, et al. Treatment of acute ischemic stroke due to large vessel occlusion with COVID-19: experience from Paris. Stroke 2020;51(8):2540–3.
70. Wang A, Mandigo GK, Yim PD, et al. Stroke and mechanical thrombectomy in patients with COVID-19: technical observations and patient characteristics. J Neurointerv Surg 2020;12(7):648–53.
71. Albert DVF, Das RR, Acharya JN, et al. The Impact of COVID-19 on epilepsy care: a survey of the American Epilepsy Society membership. Epilepsy Curr 2020;20(5):316–24.
72. Lai S-L, Hsu M-T, Chen S-S. The impact of SARS on epilepsy: the experience of drug withdrawal in epileptic patients. Seizure 2005;14(8):557–61.
73. Cheli M, Dinoto A, Olivo S, et al. SARS-CoV-2 pandemic and epilepsy: the impact on emergency department attendances for seizures. Seizure 2020;82:23–6.
74. French JA, Brodie MJ, Caraballo R, et al. Keeping people with epilepsy safe during the COVID-19 pandemic. Neurology 2020;94(23):1032–7.
75. Florez-Perdomo WA, Serrato-Vargas SA, Bosque-Varela P, et al. Relationship between the history of cerebrovascular disease and mortality in COVID-19 patients: a systematic review and meta-analysis. Clin Neurol Neurosurg 2020;197:106183.
76. Pranata R, Huang I, Lim MA, et al. Impact of cerebrovascular and cardiovascular diseases on mortality and severity of COVID-19-systematic review, meta-analysis, and meta-regression. J Stroke Cerebrovasc Dis 2020;29(8):104949.
77. Brophy GM, Bell R, Claassen J, et al. Guidelines for the evaluation and management of status epilepticus. Neurocrit Care 2012;17(1):3–23.
78. Rola P, Farkas J, Spiegel R, et al. Rethinking the early intubation paradigm of COVID-19: time to change gears? Clin Exp Emerg Med 2020;7(2):78–80.
79. Matta A, Chaudhary S, Bryan Lo K, et al. Timing of Intubation and Its Implications on Outcomes in Critically Ill Patients With Coronavirus Disease 2019 Infection. Crit Care Explorations 2020;2(10):e0262.
80. Tran K, Cimon K, Severn M, et al. Aerosol generating procedures and risk of transmission of acute respiratory infections to healthcare workers: a systematic review. PLoS One 2012;7(4):e35797.

81. Schünemann HJ, Khabsa J, Solo K, et al. Ventilation techniques and risk for transmission of coronavirus disease, including COVID-19: a living systematic review of multiple streams of evidence. Ann Intern Med 2020;173(3):204–16.
82. Wunsch H. Mechanical ventilation in COVID-19: interpreting the current epidemiology. Am J Respir Crit Care Med 2020;202(1):1–4.
83. Choo EK, Rajkumar SV. Medication shortages during the COVID-19 crisis: what we must do. Mayo Clin Proc 2020;95(6):1112–5.
84. Ortoleva J. Consider Adjunctive Ketamine in Mechanically Ventilated Coronavirus Disease-2019 Patients. J Cardiothorac Vasc Anesth 2020;34(10):2580.
85. Dale O, Somogyi AA, Li Y, et al. Does intraoperative ketamine attenuate inflammatory reactivity following surgery? A systematic review and meta-analysis. Anesth Analg 2012;115(4):934–43.
86. Anand P, Al-Faraj A, Sader E, et al. Seizure as the presenting symptom of COVID-19: a retrospective case series. Epilepsy Behav 2020;112:107335.
87. Vollono C, Rollo E, Romozzi M, et al. Focal status epilepticus as unique clinical feature of COVID-19: a case report. Seizure 2020;78:109–12.
88. Anand P, Zakaria A, Benameur K, et al. Myoclonus in patients with coronavirus disease 2019: a multicenter case series. Crit Care Med 2020. https://doi.org/10.1097/CCM.0000000000004570.
89. Alotaibi F, Althani Z, Aljaafari D, et al. Saudi Epilepsy Society consensus on epilepsy management during the COVID-19 Pandemic. Neurosciences (Riyadh) 2020;25(3):222–5.
90. Gélisse P, Rossetti AO, Genton P, et al. How to carry out and interpret EEG recordings in COVID-19 patients in ICU? Clin Neurophysiol 2020;131(8):2023–31.
91. Hirsch LJ, LaRoche SM, Gaspard N, et al. American Clinical Neurophysiology Society's Standardized Critical Care EEG Terminology: 2012 version. J Clin Neurophysiol 2013;30(1):1–27.
92. Rice JK, Rorden C, Little JS, et al. Subject position affects EEG magnitudes. Neuroimage 2013;64:476–84.
93. Lu L, Xiong W, Liu D, et al. New onset acute symptomatic seizure and risk factors in coronavirus disease 2019: a retrospective multicenter study. Epilepsia 2020;(6):61. https://doi.org/10.1111/epi.16524.
94. Narula N, Joseph R, Katyal N, et al. Seizure and COVID-19: association and review of potential mechanism. Neurol Psychiatry Brain Res 2020;38:49–53.
95. Anand P, Zhou L, Bhadelia N, et al. Neurologic findings among inpatients with COVID-19 at a safety-net US hospital. Neurol Clin Pract 2020. https://doi.org/10.1212/CPJ.0000000000001031.
96. Claassen J, Mayer SA, Kowalski RG, et al. Detection of electrographic seizures with continuous EEG monitoring in critically ill patients. Neurology 2004;62(10):1743–8.
97. Sohal S, Mansur M. COVID-19 presenting with seizures. IDCases 2020;20:e00782.
98. Moriguchi T, Harii N, Goto J, et al. A first case of meningitis/encephalitis associated with SARS-Coronavirus-2. Int J Infect Dis 2020;94:55–8.
99. Karimi N, Sharifi Razavi A, Rouhani N. Frequent convulsive seizures in an adult patient with COVID-19: a case report. Iranian Red Crescent Med J 2020;22(3). https://doi.org/10.5812/ircmj.102828.
100. Asadi-Pooya AA, Attar A, Moghadami M, et al. Management of COVID-19 in people with epilepsy: drug considerations. Neurol Sci 2020;41(8):2005–11.

Changes in Clinical Care of the Newborn During COVID-19 Pandemic
From the Womb to First Newborn Visit

Pezad N. Doctor, MBBS[a],*, Deepak Kamat, MD, PhD[b],
Beena G. Sood, MD, MS[c]

KEYWORDS

• SARS-CoV-2 • Newborn • Perinatal transmission • Pandemic

KEY POINTS

- Perinatal transmission of SARS-CoV-2 is mainly horizontal, necessitating strict control measures for preventing spread of infection to newborns.
- Universal screening for SARS-CoV-2 for all pregnant women is necessary to guide delivery room preparation and postdelivery care of newborns and mothers.
- Newborns infected with SARS-CoV-2 are usually asymptomatic or have mild clinical disease; therefore, other causes need to be investigated in case of severe illness.
- Breast feeding and bonding between newborn and SARS-CoV-2 infected mother can be encouraged with proper education and infection control measures.
- All newborns should have routine newborn care irrespective of their SARS-CoV-2 status as early discharge has not shown to reduce the spread of infection.

INTRODUCTION

Coronavirus disease 2019 (COVID-19), caused by severe acute respiratory syndrome coronavirus 2 (SARS-CoV-2), which was first reported in the Wuhan region of China in December in 2019 has struck the world, affecting humans across all age groups.[1] Initially, it was thought to affect mainly the respiratory system causing a "pneumonia of unknown etiology,"[2] but it was soon discovered that it affects multiple organ systems with significant morbidity and mortality. SARS-CoV-2 has been demonstrated to be transmitted by respiratory droplets, contact, and fomites.[3–5] SARS-CoV-2 has

This article previously appeared in *Pediatric Clinics*, Volume 68, Issue 5, October 2021.
[a] Department of Pediatrics, Children's Hospital of Michigan, 3901, Beaubien Boulevard, Detroit, MI 48201, USA; [b] Department of Pediatrics, UT Health Science Center, UT Health San Antonio, San Antonio, TX 78229, USA; [c] Department of Pediatrics, Wayne State University School of Medicine, 540E Canfield Street, Detroit, Michigan 48201, USA
* Corresponding author. Office of Pediatric education, 3901 Beaubien, Detroit, MI 48201.
E-mail address: pezaddoctor@gmail.com

Clinics Collections 12 (2022) 233–248
https://doi.org/10.1016/j.ccol.2021.12.017
2352-7986/22/© 2021 Elsevier Inc. All rights reserved.

proven to be highly contagious with a reproduction number of 2.2 to 5.7, which means that 1 person with SARS-CoV-2 infection can infect on an average 2 to 5 people around him or her if no precautions are followed.[6] SARS-CoV-2 gains entry into the lungs and gut by binding to the angiotensin-converting enzyme receptor 2 present abundantly on the type 2 pneumocytes and gastrointestinal epithelium. There is controversy regarding in utero transmission of SARS-CoV-2. However, there is increasing evidence of horizontal transmission from mother to neonate. There is a scarcity of data regarding pregnant women affected with COVID-19, and its implications during pregnancy: prenatal visits, antenatal scans, testing, and management of symptomatic women, and delivery, as well as delivery room preparedness, logistics, and postnatal care of newborns.[7–10] In this review, we highlight major changes in clinical practice implemented during delivery and postnatal care of newborns born to mothers with confirmed or suspected SARS-CoV-2 infection during the pandemic, based on various expert opinions and evolving evidence.

SARS-CoV-2 INFECTION IN PREGNANCY

Early speculations regarding SARS-CoV-2 infection in pregnancy were concerning owing to changes in cellular immunity during pregnancy along with an array of physiologic changes in the cardiovascular, respiratory, and coagulation systems. Few studies have investigated whether SARS-CoV-2 infection poses additional risk during pregnancy.[11] Studies so far have shown similar COVID-19 symptoms in pregnant and nonpregnant women.[12,13] Surveillance data from the Centers for Disease Control and Prevention (CDC) including 91,412 women of reproductive age group (15–45 years of age) with laboratory-confirmed SARS-CoV-2 infection showed no difference between pregnant (8207) and nonpregnant women (83,205) in terms of cough and shortness of breath.[14] Headache, fever, chills, diarrhea, and muscle aches were in fact less frequently noted in pregnant women compared with nonpregnant women. Initial studies from New York showed a significant asymptomatic carrier rate ($\leq$33%) in pregnant women.[15,16] Therefore, universal screening for SARS-CoV-2 infection in all pregnant women during hospitalization or at the time of delivery was proposed and soon became the standard of care. In a series of 54 pregnant women with confirmed (n = 38) and suspected (n = 16) SARS-CoV-2 infections reported by Sentilhes and colleagues,[17] oxygen supplementation was required in 24.1%, intensive care unit admission in 9.3%, and severe illness was observed in those over the age of 35 years or those with comorbidities, such as asthma and obesity. A recent report by the CDC's Coronavirus Disease 19-Associated Hospitalization Surveillance Network surveillance team found that, of the 598 pregnant women hospitalized in 13 states across the country with COVID-19 between March 1 and August 22, 2020, the majority of them (55%) were asymptomatic.[18] However, severe illness was observed In symptomatic women that included intensive care admission in 16%, mechanical ventilation in 8%, and mortality in 1%.[18] In an analysis of approximately 400,000 women aged 15 to 44 years with symptomatic COVID-19 by the CDC's Surveillance for Emerging Threats to Mothers and Babies Network (SET-NET), intensive care unit admission, invasive ventilation, extracorporeal membrane oxygenation, and death were more likely in pregnant women than in nonpregnant women.[19] In a 35-year-old woman infected with COVID-19, placental pathology showed inflammation and the presence of SARS-CoV-2 by immunohistochemistry at 22 weeks gestation, possibly contributing to the development of early-onset preeclampsia, hypertension, and disseminated coagulopathy.[20] Hence, a multidisciplinary team of maternal and fetal medicine specialists and neonatologists is essential in the care of pregnant women with SARS-CoV-2 infection and their infants.

IMPACT ON ROUTINE ANTENATAL VISIT AND SCANS

Since the declaration of SARS-CoV-2 as a pandemic by World health Organization (WHO), the American College of Obstetrics and Gynecology (ACOG) has proposed various modifications in the existing guidelines of antenatal visits and ultrasounds. These modifications were primarily made to decrease the amount contact between the pregnant women and health care facilities as well as to decrease the transmission of SARS-CoV-2 throughout the general population.[21] Minimal data are available on the impact on maternal and fetal health after these guideline changes. In a 28-year-old pregnant woman with gestational diabetes mellitus and chronic hypertension who was found to be COVID-19 positive at 34 weeks gestation, her routine nonstress testing and amniotic fluid index testing were delayed owing to her COVID-19–positive status. Ultimately, her nonstress testing revealed category 2 tracing persistently, requiring urgent cesarean section.[22] This case highlights that the frequency of antenatal visits and testing should be decided on an individualized basis, especially for high-risk pregnancies.

TRANSMISSION FROM MOTHER TO NEWBORN

The first case of SARS-CoV-2 infection in a neonate was reported in February 2020. The infant presented at 17 days of age with a fever, cough, runny nose, and vomiting.[23] This presentation led to suspicion of vertical transmission in utero because the mother of the newborn had tested positive for SARS-CoV-2. Early studies conducted in China were unable to isolate SARS-CoV-2 from amniotic fluid, vaginal mucus, cord blood, placenta, urine, feces, or breast milk. Similarly, Silva and colleagues did not find SARS-CoV-2 by reverse transcriptase polymerase chain reaction (RT-PCR) in 18 samples of amniotic fluid, umbilical cord, and placenta obtained from COVID-19–positive mothers.[24] Therefore, the risk of vertical transmission was considered highly unlikely.[25–29] However, in a retrospective cohort study of 3497 respiratory, urine, stool, and serum samples from adults analyzed for SARS-CoV-2 viral load, the median duration of the virus in stools (22 days; interquartile range [IQR], 17–31 days) was significantly longer than in respiratory (18 days; IQR, 13–29 days; $P = .02$) and serum samples (16 days; IQR, 11–21 days; $P < .001$).[30] In a study by Zeng and colleagues,[9] 3 of the 33 neonates born to COVID-19–positive mothers tested positive by RT-PCR from nasopharyngeal and anal swabs by 2 days of age despite strict isolation of the newborn soon after delivery. Two of the 3 neonates were born at full term with mild symptoms such as fever, vomiting, and lethargy; the third neonate was born at 31 weeks of gestation and developed respiratory distress syndrome and pneumonia, along with leukocytosis and thrombocytopenia requiring noninvasive positive pressure ventilation and antibiotics because his blood culture was positive for *Enterobacter* spp. Hence, the contribution of SARS-CoV-2 in causing symptoms in the third neonate was dubious. However, in a case reported by Dong and colleagues[31] of a neonate born to a SARS-CoV-2–positive mother was found to have high levels of SARS-CoV-2–specific IgM antibodies at 2 hours of age despite negative pressure room delivery and strict adherence to precautions. Her PCR results were negative on 5 consecutive samples during the first 16 days of life. Her IgM and IgG levels were still elevated at 16 days of life, but were trending down. Because IgM antibodies are elevated only after 3 to 7 days after the infection, high IgM levels in the infant only at the 2 hours of age strongly suggested an intrauterine infection. In a review of 217 neonates born to SARS-CoV-2–infected mothers, only 7 (3%) tested positive.[32] Of the 7, 3 had positive serum IgM and IgG levels with negative PCR and the remaining 4 had a positive PCR from nasopharyngeal or anal swabs. In the national registry of perinatal

COVID-19 infection established by the American Academy of Pediatrics Section on Neonatal Perinatal Medicine (AAP SONPM NPC-19 registry), which includes 295 centers, 139 of 6229 infants (2.2%) born to COVID-19–positive mothers tested positive as of February 20, 2021.[33] More than one-third (2888) of these newborns had contact, droplet, and air-borne isolation, 2303 (28%) had contact and droplet isolation, 1677 (20%) had contact, droplet, air-borne, and negative pressure isolation, 466(6%) had unspecified form of isolation, and 873 (11%) had no isolation.[33] Because the evidence for vertical transmission is weak, newborns are most likely infected via horizontal transmission after delivery from mother or other caregivers. Therefore, implementing strict infection control measures during and after delivery, quarantine of infected mothers, and close monitoring of neonates in the perinatal period was essential in decreasing horizontal transmission. The CDC's SET-NET had information of 2869 newborns delivered from 13 jurisdictions between March 29 and October 14, 2020. They reported 610 infants (21.3%) who were tested and 16 (2.6%) of them were positive for SARS-CoV-2. They were primarily those born to women with infection at delivery.[34] This result led to the development and implementation of essential delivery preparedness strategies across various birthing centers to curb the spread of SARS-CoV-2.

COVID-19 VACCINATION DURING PREGNANCY

The US Food and Drug Administration recently approved 2 vaccines against SARS-CoV-2 (Pfizer-BioNtech mRNA vaccine and Moderna mRNA-1273 vaccine) under the context of an Emergency Use Authorization in high-risk priority groups. The CDC's Advisory Committee on Immunization Practices and the ACOG have recommended their use in pregnant and lactating women.[35,36] However, the data are lacking regarding the benefits (to the mother and transplacental passage of passive immunity to the fetus) and side effects of these vaccines in this subset of patients because pregnant women were not involved in the studies during vaccine development.[37] In a study by Flannery and colleagues[38] involving 1714 mothers who delivered from April to August 2020 in the northeastern United States, 83 (6%) had detectable IgG and/or IgM antibodies at delivery. However, the majority of infants born to these seropositive mothers (72/83) had detectable IgG levels at birth, suggesting transplacental transfer during pregnancy. For Moderna mRNA-1273 vaccine, the WHO revised the recommendation on January 29, 2021, stating that "pregnant women at high risk of exposure to SARS CoV-2 (e.g. health workers) or who have comorbidities which add to their risk of severe disease, may be vaccinated in consultation with their health care provider."[39] Although immunization may be the best available options for pregnant and lactating mothers to protect themselves and their infants, longitudinal clinical studies are necessary to implement safe vaccination guidelines.

DELIVERY ROOM AND NEWBORN RESUSCITATION PRACTICES

Much of delivery room preparedness recommendations depended on the COVID-19 status of the mother. Therefore, a short turnaround time of the test was crucial for optimal preparedness during delivery. If resources were available, all mothers were tested for SARS-CoV-2 at delivery, regardless of their clinical profile, to prevent nosocomial spread to other patients and health care workers.[40] All mothers whose COVID-19 status was unknown either owing to a lack of resources, testing refusal, or in whom the test results were not back by the time they delivered were considered positive owing to the high asymptomatic carrier state.[15] Important aspects of delivery room preparedness included the availability of KN95 masks, appropriate personal protective equipment, medical professionals experienced in neonatal resuscitation to minimize aerosolization during newborn resuscitation, and separation of the mother from the newborn.[15,40] Discussion and planning between the obstetric and neonatal teams guided maternal and newborn care, such as the use of maternal steroids (dexamethasone for COVID-19–related lung injury in mother vs betamethasone for fetal lung maturity), magnesium sulfate for preterm delivery, unfractionated heparin for thromboembolism prophylaxis, and the use of remdesivir.[41] Positive pressure ventilation using bag and mask, endotracheal intubations, and high-flow nasal cannula have the potential to aerosolize the respiratory droplets, allowing SARS-CoV-2 to remain in air for more than 3 hours and propagate for more than 2 months.[42] Pregnant women who are COVID-19 positive or unknown should deliver preferably in a negative pressure room, if available, with an adjoining room for neonatal resuscitation.[40,43,44] If not available, a single room with minimal entry and exit of essential caregivers from the room is paramount.[43,44] Earlier, delayed cord clamping was deferred owing to the unknown risk of vertical transmission.[8] However, according to recent recommendations from the ACOG and the AAP SONPM, delayed cord clamping can be practiced in suspected or confirmed COVID-19–positive mothers because there is no strong evidence to suggest transplacental viral transmission at this time.[43,45]

Mode of Delivery

Varied speculations have been made on the mode of delivery in pregnant women with SARS-CoV-2.[46–49] Cesarean section was performed for routine obstetric indications or worsening respiratory distress and exhaustion owing to COVID-19.[40] Some centers also preferred cesarean section for decreasing the total hospital stay of the mother and to minimize cross-infection.[40,47] However, in a case reported by Iqbal and colleagues,[48] a full-term female infant who was born by vaginal delivery to a SARS-CoV-2–infected mother was asymptomatic and discharged home on the 6th day of life. A retrospective cohort study among adults found that SARS-CoV-2 was present in stool samples for a longer duration compared with serum and respiratory mucosa.[30] Therefore, caution should be taken in mothers with diarrhea during vaginal delivery. In a systematic review by Khan and colleagues49 that which included 8 studies, comprising a total of 100 women with COVID-19, cesarean section was noted in 85%, premature deliveries in 29%, and low birthweight infants in 16%. However, there is a shift in this trend; recent data from the AAP SONPM NPC-19 registry showed that of 7486 suspected or confirmed COVID-19–positive pregnant women, 4872 (65%) delivered vaginally and the remaining 2614 (35%) underwent cesarean section as of February 20, 2021.[33]

BREAST MILK AND BREASTFEEDING

The AAP, along with other academic organizations such as the Academy of Breast Feeding, the CDC, and the WHO recommend breastfeeding in mothers with confirmed or suspected COVID-19 while taking the necessary precautions.[45,50–53] Mothers can either pump breast milk or directly nurse the baby while wearing a face mask and performing breast and hand hygiene.[52] The mother can either wash her hands with soap and water or use sanitizer with at least 60% alcohol before touching the baby. Preferably, expressed breast milk should be fed by an uninfected healthy caregiver not at risk of developing severe illness from SARS-CoV-2.[54] Earlier studies were unable to detect SARS-CoV-2 in breast milk.[13,25,27,55,56] However, in few studies SARS-CoV-2 was detected in breast milk.[57,58] A case was reported of a 32-week gestational age preterm baby who was breastfed SARS-CoV-2–positive breast milk but did not become infected. The baby was inadvertently fed expressed breast milk from the mother who later tested positive for SARS-CoV-2. Her expressed milk also tested positive by RT-PCR despite using a face mask and standard personal protective equipment while expressing the milk. However, the newborn tested negative for SARS-CoV-2 nasopharyngeal swab as well as for antibodies at 30 days after the exposure.[59] Similarly, in a series of 14 infants breast fed by SARS-CoV-2–positive mothers, breast milk tested positive in only 1 case. Four of the 14 infants (including the one fed the infected breast milk) tested positive for SARS-CoV-2, but the clinical course of all the infants was uneventful. The repeat testing of these 4 infants was negative for SARS-CoV-2 at 6 weeks.[60] Although there is no clear evidence that infants fed breast milk from COVID-19–positive mothers are protected from SARS-CoV-2 infection, breast milk may contain antibodies against SARS-CoV-2 providing passive immunity and protecting the baby. The Human Milk Banking Association of North America milk banks provide heat-treated pasteurized donor breast milk that has been shown to inactivate viruses similar to SARS-CoV-2.[61] Hence, human donor milk could be used in preterm and term neonates admitted to the nursery and neonatal intensive care unit (NICU) for longer durations.

MOTHER AND NEWBORN SEPARATION

Owing to the unknown infective properties of the virus, the Chinese Neonatal 2019-nCoV expert working Group published its first consensus statement in February 2020 soon after the first case of SARS-CoV-2 was reported in a neonate.[8] They recommended separation of mother and child based on a systematic review of the adult literature on SARS-CoV-2 as well as previous reports of Middle East respiratory syndrome-related coronavirus and severe acute SARS-CoV infections.[8] As more cases were reported from China and around the world affecting newborns as early as few hours, separation of the mother with suspected or confirmed SARS-CoV-2 from newborn was strongly recommended by other health organizations such as the AAP, ACOG, and CDC.[43,45,62] However, separation may not be always feasible owing to the lack of infrastructure and resources available in other parts of the world. Recent amendments to the CDCs guidelines allow a case-by-case approach and takes into account decision made between the health care provider and mother, the clinical condition of the mother and infant, availability of testing, staffing, space, personal protective equipment, and test results of the newborn.[62] As of August 3, 2020, the CDC recommends mothers to remain separated for at least 10 days after the occurrence of first symptoms (20 days if critically ill or the mother is immunocompromised), and at least 24 hours after the last fever without use of antipyretics and improvement in other symptoms.[62] If the newborn is tested COVID-19 positive, there is no need for separation. If the mother refuses separation, the newborn and mother should be placed in a negative pressure room with 6 feet or more distance between the two. In addition, the newborn should be placed in a temperature-regulated isolette to minimize droplet spread from mother. The Italian Society of Neonatology guidelines endorsed by the Union of European Neonatal and Perinatal Societies suggest that rooming-in of mother and newborn is workable if a mother is SARS-CoV-2 positive, or is a person under investigation, or is asymptomatic, or has minimal symptoms at delivery, but with strict infection control measures.[63] Ample research-based evidence has concluded that early maternal–newborn bonding positively impacts the growth and development in term and preterm neonates.[64,65] Early separation may negatively affect the bonding, breast milk production, and mental health of the mother during the hospital stay and after discharge with uncertain short- and long-term implications. In a recent study of 45 newborns born to SARS-CoV-2–positive mothers, 33 (73%) roomed-in with the mother. Thirty-one of the 33 newborns were breastfed within the 1 hour of birth. All 33 newborns tested negative for SARS-CoV-2, did not require NICU admission, and remained asymptomatic at their 2-week telemedicine follow-up visit.[66]

CLINICAL FEATURES OF SARS-CoV-2 INFECTION IN NEONATES

Various clinical studies have concluded that newborns and infants are less susceptible to SARS-CoV-2 infection and have a fairly mild clinical course with lower mortality compared with adults. A few theories have been proposed explaining this difference in clinical susceptibility. These include immature angiotensin-converting enzyme receptor 2 in neonates, which may prevent or decrease binding of the virus to the epithelial cells and naïve immune system of newborn mounting a poor inflammatory response.[67,68] However, the exact pathogenesis of COVID-19 is still being investigated. Neonates and children are usually asymptomatic or develop mild symptoms such as respiratory distress and feeding difficulties. A clinical finding of COVID-19 specific to newborns has not been recognized. The first few case series from China reported that the majority of newborns born to SARS-CoV-2–confirmed positive mothers were unaffected.[25,26] Later, a few publications reported varied presentations such as respiratory distress, shock, tachycardia, sepsis, thrombocytopenia, and occasionally death in neonates.[8,9,32,69] Other presenting symptoms include temperature instability, poor feeding, diarrhea, vomiting, and abdominal distension. Associated risk factors such as prematurity, prolonged rupture of membranes, and sepsis were also present in these neonates. In another case series of 4 neonates ranging between 30 hours and 17 days of age with a confirmed SARS-CoV-2 positive result by nucleic acid testing, 2 had fever, 1 developed respiratory distress, 1 had cough, and 1 had no symptoms.[69] Recently, another case of a SARS-CoV-2–positive neonate was reported who developed cyanosis and hypoxemia with respiratory distress at 48 hours of life. His chest radiograph showed ground glass opacity and he improved on high-flow nasal cannula with a 30% Fio_2.[70] Aghdam and colleagues[71] reported a 15-day-old neonate who presented with fever, tachycardia, and respiratory distress who improved quickly and was discharged 6 days later. In China, a greater proportion of infants less than 1 year of age had severe or critical disease compared with older children (10.6% vs 4.8%).[72] Owing to the high incidence of asymptomatic cases, other causes should be investigated in newborns with confirmed SARS-CoV-2 infection who demonstrate clinical deterioration. However, in a recent review of 18 PubMed articles that included 25 SARS-CoV-2–positive confirmed newborns less than 28 days of age, with a mean age of 8.2 ± 8.5 days, a gestational age of 37.4 ± 4.0 weeks, and a birth weight of 3041.6 ± 866.0 grams, the clinical features included fever in 28%, vomiting in 16%, cough or shortness of breath in 12%, diarrhea, lethargy or respiratory difficulty in 8% or cyanosis, feeding intolerance, hyperpnea, mild intercostal retractions, mottling, sneezing, nasal stuffiness, and paroxysmal episodes in 4%; only 16% of these newborns were completely asymptomatic.[73] Deaths were not reported in any of the newborns and 8 of 25 (32%) required intensive care. The mean length of hospital stays of 15.8 ± 10.8 days.[73] In another review of 26 articles published from December 1, 2019, to May 12, 2020, that included 38 SARS-CoV-2–positive confirmed neonates, 26 (68%) were symptomatic at a median age of 10 days (IQR, 2–19 days).[74] Clinical findings included fever in 50%, gastrointestinal symptoms in 26%, hypoxia in 20%, and cough in 20%. All newborns were discharged home after a median length of stay of 10 days (IQR, 6–14 days).[74] In a study by the national surveillance registry of

UK that included 66 newborns who tested positive, 16 (24%) were born preterm. The incidence of SARS-CoV-2 was estimated to be 5.6 per 10,000 live births. The most common symptoms were hyperthermia (35%), poor feeding/vomiting (33%), and coryza (26%). In terms of respiratory support, 33% required supplemental oxygen, 15% required noninvasive ventilation, and 5% required intubation.[75] In a large single-center study in New York including 101 newborns born to SARS-CoV-2–positive mothers, maternal severe or critical COVID-19 disease was associated with birth approximately 1 week before the due date (median gestational age, 37.9 weeks [IQR, 37.1–38.4 weeks] vs median, 39.1 weeks [IQR, 38.3–40.2 weeks]; $P = .02$) and an increased risk of requiring phototherapy (3 of 10 [30.0%] vs 6 of 91 [7.0%]; $P = .04$) compared with newborns of mothers with asymptomatic or mild COVID-19.[76] Interestingly, a preterm newborn delivered at 34 weeks of gestation developed late-onset fever, thrombocytopenia, and elevated inflammatory markers concerning for fetal inflammatory response syndrome, which was attributed to maternal SARS-CoV-2 infection. The neonate tested negative for SARS-CoV-2 by RT-PCR twice 24 hours apart. He subsequently developed pulmonary hypertension requiring inhaled nitric oxide with significant improvement and discharge home at 22 days of age.[77]

DEFINITION OF COVID-19 IN NEONATES

In February 2020, the Chinese Perinatal-neonatal 2019-nCoV Committee proposed the definition of suspected and confirmed neonatal cases after a systematic review of current and previous literature in their consensus statement.

Suspected COVID-19

All newborns born to SARS-CoV-2–positive confirmed mothers within 14 days before birth and 28 days after birth or newborns exposed directly to SARS-CoV-2–infected individuals (including family members, caregivers, medical staff, and visitors) are considered to be suspected cases.[8]

Confirmed COVID-19

Newborn in whom respiratory tract or blood specimens tested by RT-PCR are positive for SARS-CoV-2;
OR
Virus gene sequencing of the respiratory tract or blood specimens is highly homologous to that of the known SARS-CoV-2 specimens.[8]

Management

The majority of newborns with suspected and confirmed SARS-CoV-2 who require medical attention do so because of associated comorbidities of the perinatal period. All newborns with suspected or confirmed SARS-CoV-2 should be quarantined with droplet and contact precautions for at least 14 days. The management of these newborns is mainly supportive. Owing to a lack of evidence of the efficacy and safety profile of pharmaceutical agents such as hydroxychloroquine, azithromycin, and remdesivir in newborns, their use is not recommended.[5,8] Similarly, there is no evidence for the effectiveness of gamma globulin, hormonal therapy or interferon therapy.[8] However, owing to the widespread use of the COVID-19 vaccine, we expect to see an increase in the titers of anti-COVID-19 antibodies in intravenous immunoglobulin pooled from plasma donors that could be used for treating SARS-CoV-2 in the near future. Modifications in clinical practice made while caring for newborns with SARS-CoV-2 in terms of respiratory support, isolation, appropriate use of personal protective equipment, and KN95 masks by health care providers, laboratory and radiology staff and for discharge planning is summarized elsewhere in this article.

Respiratory support, personal protective equipment, and isolation

There are few neonates reported with suspected or confirmed SARS-CoV-2 requiring respiratory support so far.[9,78] Aerosolization of SARS-CoV-2 can be decreased by limiting and/or cautiously performing procedures such as ventilation (bag and mask, invasive and noninvasive), endotracheal intubation, and insertion of orogastric or nasogastric tubes.[5,15,40,79] For bag and mask ventilation, high-efficiency particulate air filters should be used between the mask and CO_2 detector to minimize aerosolization.[80,81] Dual limb conventional ventilators are a closed circuit containing in-built high-efficiency particulate air filters near the endotracheal tube and, therefore, are safer than bag and mask ventilation.[80,81] Suctioning should be performed using an in-line suction catheter.[80] The use of personal protective equipment, including a face mask, face shield, and gloves, while performing these aerosolization procedures and even otherwise is essential for health care workers to protect themselves and minimize spread while taking care of these newborns as recommended by the CDC.[82] Depending on the availability of infrastructure and resources, isolation or cohorting of confirmed newborns in a designated enclosed space in NICU is recommended.[8,40] Reusable monitoring tools such as stethoscope and thermometers should not be shared among patients.

Laboratory evaluation

Both the AAP and the CDC recommend testing for SARS-CoV-2 for all newborns delivered by suspected or confirmed SARS-CoV-2–positive mothers because it guides ongoing infection prevention and control, clinical observation of newborn, the need for isolation, discharge planning, and newborn outpatient follow-up visits.[45,82] The timing of first testing is usually between 24 and 48 hours after delivery, depending on the discharge plan for the newborn. If the results of the first test at 24 hours are negative, the AAP recommends repeat testing at 24 hours or later after the first test result because some tests in newborns become positive at a later time. If the first test performed at 24 hours is positive, then repeat testing at least 24 hours apart should be performed until 2 test results are negative.[45,82] This process will suggest clearance of the virus from the mucosal sites. RT-PCR from nasopharyngeal and throat swabs are recommended. Presently, the diagnostic role of antibody testing has not been well-established owing to inconclusive data.

Radiologic studies

A chest radiograph should be performed if clinically indicated. Radiologic findings in newborns are not specific and may include ground glass opacities, unilateral and bilateral subsegmental opacities and pneumothorax.[8,9,26] In a national surveillance registry from the UK, of the 26 newborns who were SARS-CoV-2 positive and had chest radiographs, 14 (56%) had abnormal findings, with ground-glass changes reported in 7 (28%); in addition. 4 of these 7 babies were born preterm.[75]

ROUTINE NEWBORN SURVEILLANCE AND NEWBORN/NEONATAL INTENSIVE CARE UNIT VISITATION BY FAMILY MEMBERS

In April 2020, the Vermont Oxford Network, in partnership with the AAP SONPM, conducted an audit to assess the impact of SARS-CoV-2 on neonates and their families.[83] Of the 332 hospitals, 54% reported shortages of equipment, testing, or personnel, 73% reported minor disruptions to care for infants and families, and 3% reported an inability to provide care to some, most, or all infants.[84] Owing to the ever-evolving evidence of SARS-CoV-2 transmission between asymptomatic carriers, varying policy changes have been made by many NICUs and newborn nurseries across the world to limit the entry of healthy family members. Owing to vulnerability of the infant's health in the NICU, the AAP recommends restricting parents and family members with COVID-19 for 14 to 20 days from the onset of disease symptoms or the first positive test.[45] Some NICUs made strict visitation policies with exceptions on a case-by-case basis. This difference led to disparities in the NICU visitation by family members and lack of parental participation in family-centered rounds.[83] The AAP strongly advocated that "any policy restricting visitors for pediatric patients should be applied equally regardless of children's race, ethnicity, socioeconomic status, culture, and religion" to minimize health disparities.[85] Nonetheless, various social, emotional, and psychological challenges were faced by family members during the separation of neonates staying for an extended duration in the NICU.[83] Parental stress arising from NICU admission has been associated with poor neurodevelopmental outcomes in preterm babies.[86] Especially in the pandemic, parental stress can worsen owing to restricted visitation. Owing to growing evidence of low transmission risk in the NICU, these restrictions have been alleviated to some extent in most NICUs and newborn nurseries across the country.[87] In a center where universal screening of neonates, parents, and staff was practiced, no SARS-CoV-2 infection among the neonates admitted to the NICU was noted in an area with a high incidence of SARS-CoV-2.[88] If parental visitation is restricted, the NICU should provide numerous ways to best support infants and their families to cope within this stressful environment.[89] As the literature on SARS-CoV-2 in neonates accumulates, evidence-based policies should be formulated to prevent horizontal spread of SARS-CoV-2 in the NICU that can be applicable universally.[90]

DISCHARGE PLANNING AND FOLLOW-UP

Routine newborn care including physical examination, vitamin K injection, administration of erythromycin eye ointment, performing hearing and critical congenital heart disease screens, and administering hepatitis B vaccine per the institutional policies should be completed before discharge, regardless of SARS-CoV-2 testing. If the newborn tests positive, remains positive on repeat testing, and is asymptomatic, then the newborn can be discharged with home quarantine for 10 days from the first positive test.[45] Care should be taken to prevent spread from the newborn to other members at home. Newborn visits can be arranged by telemedicine or phone. In-office visits should be avoided as far as possible to prevent spread. Some hospital centers, through charitable organizations, have been arranging and distributing electronic scales at discharge for assessing weight gain at home.[40] This practice may decrease the need for newborn in-office visits. If an in-office visit is necessary, parents should inform the clinic about the COVID-19 status of the newborn and the accompanying parent before arrival so that necessary precautions can be in place at the pediatrician's office. If the newborn is tested negative at discharge, then thorough parental counseling and additional infection prevention education should be provided to all the possible caregivers and household members after discharge. Other household members who may have been exposed to COVID-19 should maintain 6 or more feet of distance with the use of facemasks and adequate hand hygiene.[45] In a cohort analysis of 101 neonates born to mothers with perinatal SARS-CoV-2 infections at a single institution in New York, 55 who were seen at the newborn COVID-19 follow-up clinic remained healthy at 2 weeks of life. The appropriate duration of infection control practiced by the breastfeeding mother is unknown because a varying duration of viral shedding has been shown from different sites.[30] However, the AAP recommends that infection control be practiced for at least 10 days from the onset of symptoms and at least 24 hours from being afebrile without antipyretics.[7] Other precautionary measures as mentioned elsewhere in this article should be followed by mothers while breast-feeding. Parents should be educated regarding normal newborn care and common red flags concerning illness in newborns.[45]

CLINICS CARE POINTS

- While extensive research suggest horizontal transmission of COVID-19 from caregivers to neonates, there are few case reports demonstrating the rare possibility of vertical transmission.

- Although most of the neonates with SARS-CoV2 are asymptomatic or have a mild clinical course, there are rare case reports of severe disease manifestation in this age group.

- Most governing agencies have recommended mothers with COVID-19 to continue breast feeding, considering its long-term benefits.

DISCLOSURE

The authors have nothing to disclose.

REFERENCES

1. Lu R, Zhao X, Li J, et al. Genomic characterisation and epidemiology of 2019 novel coronavirus: implications for virus origins and receptor binding. Lancet 2020;395(10224):565–74.
2. Hui DS, E IA, Madani TA, et al. The continuing 2019-nCoV epidemic threat of novel coronaviruses to global health - The latest 2019 novel coronavirus outbreak in Wuhan, China. Int J Infect Dis 2020;91:264–6.
3. Li Q, Guan X, Wu P, et al. Early Transmission Dynamics in Wuhan, China, of Novel Coronavirus–Infected Pneumonia. N Engl J Med 2020;382(13):1199–207.
4. Shen K, Yang Y, Wang T, et al. Diagnosis, treatment, and prevention of 2019 novel coronavirus infection in children: experts' consensus statement. World J Pediatr 2020;16(3):223–31.
5. World Health Organization. Clinical management of COVID-19 2020. https://www.who.int/publications-detail/clinical-management-of-severe-acute-respiratory-infection-when-novel-coronavirus-(ncov)-infection-is-suspected.
6. Uddin M, Mustafa F, Rizvi TA, et al. SARS-CoV-2/COVID-19: viral genomics, epidemiology, vaccines, and therapeutic interventions. Viruses 2020;12(5).
7. Puopolo KM, Hudak ML, Kimberlin DW, et al. American Academy of pediatrics committee on fetus and newborn, section of neonatal-perinatal medicine & committee on infectious disease 2020. Initial guidance: management of infants born to mothers with COVID-19. Available at: https://downloads.aap.org/AAP/PDF/COVID%2019%20Initial%20Newborn%20Guidance.pdf. Accessed October 2, 2020.
8. Wang L, Shi Y, Xiao T, et al. Chinese expert consensus on the perinatal and neonatal management for the prevention and control of the 2019 novel coronavirus infection (First edition). Ann Transl Med 2020;8(3):47.

9. Zeng L, Xia S, Yuan W, et al. Neonatal Early-Onset Infection With SARS-CoV-2 in 33 Neonates Born to Mothers With COVID-19 in Wuhan, China. JAMA Pediatr 2020;174(7):722–5.

10. Shalish W, Lakshminrusimha S, Manzoni P, et al. COVID-19 and neonatal respiratory care: current evidence and practical approach. Am J Perinatol 2020;37(8): 780–91.

11. Juan J, Gil MM, Rong Z, et al. Effect of coronavirus disease 2019 (COVID-19) on maternal, perinatal and neonatal outcome: systematic review. Ultrasound Obstet Gynecol 2020;56(1):15–27.

12. Lim WS, Macfarlane JT, Colthorpe CL. Pneumonia and pregnancy. Thorax 2001; 56(5):398–405.

13. Schwartz DA. An analysis of 38 pregnant women with COVID-19, their newborn infants, and maternal-fetal transmission of SARS-CoV-2: maternal coronavirus infections and pregnancy outcomes. Arch Pathol Lab 2020;144(7):799–805.

14. Ellington S, Strid P, Tong VT, et al. Characteristics of Women of Reproductive Age with Laboratory-Confirmed SARS-CoV-2 Infection by Pregnancy Status - United States, January 22-June 7, 2020. MMWR Morb Mortal Wkly Rep 2020;69(25): 769–75.

15. Perlman J, Oxford C, Chang C, et al. Delivery Room Preparedness and Early Neonatal Outcomes During COVID-19 Pandemic in New York City. Pediatrics 2020;146(2).

16. Breslin N, Baptiste C, Gyamfi-Bannerman C, et al. Coronavirus disease 2019 infection among asymptomatic and symptomatic pregnant women: two weeks of confirmed presentations to an affiliated pair of New York City hospitals. Am J Obstet Gynecol MFM 2020;2(2):100118.

17. Sentilhes L, De Marcillac F, Jouffrieau C, et al. Coronavirus disease 2019 in pregnancy was associated with maternal morbidity and preterm birth. Am J Obstet Gynecol 2020;223(6):914 e911–5.

18. Delahoy MJ, Whitaker M, O'Halloran A, et al. Characteristics and Maternal and Birth Outcomes of Hospitalized Pregnant Women with Laboratory-Confirmed COVID-19 - COVID-NET, 13 States, March 1-August 22, 2020. MMWR Morb Mortal Wkly Rep 2020;69(38):1347–54.

19. Zambrano LD, Ellington S, Strid P, et al. Update: characteristics of symptomatic women of reproductive age with laboratory-confirmed SARS-CoV-2 infection by pregnancy status - United States, January 22-October 3, 2020. MMWR Morb Mortal Wkly Rep 2020;69(44):1641–7.

20. Hosier H, Farhadian SF, Morotti RA, et al. SARS-CoV-2 infection of the placenta. J Clin Invest 2020;130(9):4947–53.

21. Boelig RC, Saccone G, Bellussi F, et al. MFM guidance for COVID-19. Am J Obstet Gynecol MFM 2020;2(2):100106.

22. Suresh SC, MacGregor CA, Ouyang DW. Urgent Cesarean Delivery Following Nonstress Test in a Patient with COVID-19 and Pregestational Diabetes. Neoreviews 2020;21(9):e625–30.

23. Zeng LK, Tao XW, Yuan WH, et al. [First case of neonate with COVID-19 in China]. Zhonghua er ke Za Zhi Chin J Pediatr 2020;58(4):279–80.

24. Simões E, Silva AC, Leal CRV. Is SARS-CoV-2 vertically transmitted? Front Pediatr 2020;8:276.

25. Chen H, Guo J, Wang C, et al. Clinical characteristics and intrauterine vertical transmission potential of COVID-19 infection in nine pregnant women: a retrospective review of medical records. Lancet 2020;395(10226):809–15.

26. Zhu H, Wang L, Fang C, et al. Clinical analysis of 10 neonates born to mothers with 2019-nCoV pneumonia. Transl Pediatr 2020;9(1):51–60.
27. Fan C, Lei D, Fang C, et al. Perinatal transmission of 2019 coronavirus disease–associated severe acute respiratory syndrome coronavirus 2: should we worry? Clin Infect Dis 2021;72(5):862–4.
28. Chen R, Zhang Y, Huang L, et al. Safety and efficacy of different anesthetic regimens for parturients with COVID-19 undergoing Cesarean delivery: a case series of 17 patients. Can J Anaesth 2020;67(6):655–63.
29. Mullins E, Evans D, Viner RM, et al. Coronavirus in pregnancy and delivery: rapid review. Ultrasound Obstet Gynecol 2020;55(5):586 92.
30. Zheng S, Fan J, Yu F, et al. Viral load dynamics and disease severity in patients infected with SARS-CoV-2 in Zhejiang province, China, January-March 2020: retrospective cohort study. BMJ 2020;369:m1443.
31. Dong L, Tian J, He S, et al. Possible Vertical Transmission of SARS-CoV-2 From an Infected Mother to Her Newborn. JAMA 2020;323(18):1846–8.
32. Wang S, Guo L, Chen L, et al. A Case Report of Neonatal 2019 Coronavirus Disease in China. Clin Infect Dis 2020;71(15):853–7.
33. NPC-19 Registry update: AAP SONPM National Registry of Perinatal COVID 19 infection. 2020. Available at: https://my.visme.co/view/ojq9qq8e-npc-19-registry. Accessed February 20, 2021.
34. Woodworth KR, Olsen EO, Neelam V, et al. Birth and Infant Outcomes Following Laboratory-Confirmed SARS-CoV-2 Infection in Pregnancy - SET-NET, 16 Jurisdictions, March 29-October 14, 2020. MMWR Morb Mortal Wkly Rep 2020; 69(44):1635–40.
35. Centers for Disease Control and Prevention. COVID-19 ACIP vaccine recommendations. 2020. Available at: https://www.cdc.gov/vaccines/hcp/acip-recs/vacc-specific/covid-19.html. Accessed February 20, 2021.
36. American College of Obstetricians and Gynecologists' Immunization, Infectious Disease, and Public Health Preparedness Expert Work Group. Practice Advisory. Vaccinating pregnant and lactating patients against COVID-19 2021. Available at: https://www.acog.org/clinical/clinical-guidance/practice-advisory/articles/2020/12/vaccinating-pregnant-and-lactating-patients-against-covid-19. Accessed February 21, 2021.
37. Adhikari EH, Spong CY. COVID-19 Vaccination in Pregnant and Lactating Women. JAMA 2021;325(11):1039–40.
38. Flannery DD, Gouma S, Dhudasia MB, et al. Assessment of Maternal and Neonatal Cord Blood SARS-CoV-2 Antibodies and Placental Transfer Ratios. JAMA Pediatr 2021;175(6):594–600.
39. World Health Organization. The Moderna COVID-19 (mRNA-1273) vaccine: what you need to know 2021. Available at: https://www.who.int/news-room/feature-stories/detail/the-moderna-covid-19-mrna-1273-vaccine-what-you-need-to-know. Accessed February 2, 2021.
40. Amatya S, Corr TE, Gandhi CK, et al. Management of newborns exposed to mothers with confirmed or suspected COVID-19. J Perinatol 2020;40(7):987–96.
41. Altendahl M, Afshar Y, De St, et al. Perinatal maternal-fetal/neonatal transmission of COVID-19: a guide to safe maternal and neonatal care in the era of COVID-19 and physical distancing. NeoReviews 2020;21(12):e783–94.
42. van Doremalen N, Bushmaker T, Morris DH, et al. Aerosol and surface stability of HCoV-19 (SARS-CoV-2) compared to SARS-CoV-1 2020. 2020.2003.2009.20033217.

43. American College of Obstetricians and Gynecologists. COVID-19 FAQs for Obstetrician-Gynecologists, Obstetrics 2020. Available at: https://www.acog.org/clinical-information/physician-faqs/covid-19-faqs-for-ob-gyns-obstetrics. Accessed July 3, 2020.

44. Ovalı F. SARS-CoV-2 infection and the newborn. Front Pediatr 2020;8(294).

45. American Academy of Pediatrics Section on Neonatal-Perinatal Medicine. COVID-19 clinical guidance FAQs 2020. Available at: https://services.aap.org/en/pages/2019-novel-coronavirus-covid-19-infections/clinical-guidance/faqs-management-of-infants-born-to-covid-19-mothers/.

46. Zhang L, Jiang Y, Wei M, et al. Analysis of the pregnancy outcomes in pregnant women with COVID-19 in Hubei Province. Zhonghua fu chan ke za zhi 2020; 55(3):166–71.

47. Qi H, Luo X, Zheng Y, et al. Safe delivery for pregnancies affected by COVID-19. BJOG 2020;127(8):927–9.

48. Iqbal SN, Overcash R, Mokhtari N, et al. An Uncomplicated Delivery in a Patient with Covid-19 in the United States. N Engl J Med 2020;382(16):e34.

49. Ali Khan MM, Khan MN, Mustagir MG, et al. COVID-19 infection during pregnancy: a systematic review to summarize possible symptoms, treatments, and pregnancy outcomes 2020. 2020.2003.2031.20049304.

50. Academy of breastfeeding medicine statement on coronavirus 2019 (COVID-19). Available at: https://www.bfmed.org/abm-statement-coronavirus. Accessed February 20, 2021.

51. Pregnancy, Breastfeeding, and Caring for Newborns. 2020. Available at: https://www.cdc.gov/coronavirus/2019-ncov/need-extra-precautions/pregnancy-breastfeeding.html. Accessed January 2, 2021.

52. World Health Organization. Breastfeeding advice during the COVID-19 outbreak 2020. Available at: http://www.emro.who.int/nutrition/nutrition-infocus/breastfeeding-advice-during-covid-19-outbreak.html.

53. Davanzo R, Moro G, Sandri F, et al. Breastfeeding and coronavirus disease-2019: ad interim indications of the Italian Society of Neonatology endorsed by the Union of European Neonatal & Perinatal Societies. Matern Child Nutr 2020;16(3): e13010.

54. Sullivan SE, Thompson LA. Best Practices for COVID-19–Positive or Exposed Mothers—Breastfeeding and Pumping Milk. JAMA Pediatr 2020;174(12):1228.

55. Liu W, Wang J, Li W, et al. Clinical characteristics of 19 neonates born to mothers with COVID-19. Front Med 2020;14(2):193–8.

56. Li Y, Zhao R, Zheng S, et al. Lack of Vertical Transmission of Severe Acute Respiratory Syndrome Coronavirus 2, China. Emerg Infect Dis 2020;26(6):1335–6.

57. Wu Y, Liu C, Dong L, et al. Coronavirus disease 2019 among pregnant Chinese women: case series data on the safety of vaginal birth and breastfeeding. BJOG 2020;127(9):1109–15.

58. Groß R, Conzelmann C, Müller JA, et al. Detection of SARS-CoV-2 in human breastmilk. Lancet 2020;395(10239):1757–8.

59. Lugli L, Bedetti L, Lucaccioni L, et al. An Uninfected Preterm Newborn Inadvertently Fed SARS-CoV-2–Positive Breast Milk. Pediatrics 2020. e2020004960.

60. Bertino E, Moro GE, De Renzi G, et al. Detection of SARS-CoV-2 in Milk From COVID-19 Positive Mothers and Follow-Up of Their Infants. Front Pediatr 2020;8.

61. Darnell MER, Taylor DR. Evaluation of inactivation methods for severe acute respiratory syndrome coronavirus in noncellular blood products. Transfusion 2006; 46(10):1770–7.

62. Centers for Disease Control. Interim considerations for infection prevention and control of coronavirus disease 2019 (COVID-19) in inpatient obstetric healthcare settings 2020. Available at: https://www.cdc.gov/coronavirus/2019-ncov/hcp/inpatient-obstetric-healthcare-guidance.html.

63. Union of European Neonatal and Perinatal Societies. Breastfeeding and SARS-CoV infection 2020. Available at: https://www.uenps.eu/2020/03/16/sars-cov-2-infection-sin-recommendations-endorsed-by-uenps/. Accessed January 25, 2021.

64. Gonya J, Ray WC, Rumpf RW, et al. Investigating skin-to-skin care patterns with extremely preterm infants in the NICU and their effect on early cognitive and communication performance: a retrospective cohort study. BMJ Open 2017; 7(3):e012985.

65. Weber A, Harrison TM, Sinnott L, et al. Associations Between Nurse-Guided Variables and Plasma Oxytocin Trajectories in Premature Infants During Initial Hospitalization. Adv Neonatal Care 2018;18(1):E12–23.

66. Patil UP, Maru S, Krishnan P, et al. Newborns of COVID-19 mothers: short-term outcomes of colocating and breastfeeding from the pandemic's epicenter. J Perinatol 2020;40(10):1455–8.

67. Hoffmann M, Kleine-Weber H, Schroeder S, et al. SARS-CoV-2 Cell Entry Depends on ACE2 and TMPRSS2 and Is Blocked by a Clinically Proven Protease Inhibitor. Cell 2020;181(2):271–80.e278.

68. Diaz JH. Hypothesis: angiotensin-converting enzyme inhibitors and angiotensin receptor blockers may increase the risk of severe COVID-19. J Travel Med 2020;27(3).

69. Zhang ZJ, Yu XJ, Fu T, et al. Novel coronavirus infection in newborn babies aged <28 days in China. Eur Respir J 2020;55(6).

70. Rappaport L. Neonatal SARS-CoV-2 May Present With Hypoxemia Without Respiratory Distress. Medscape 2020.

71. Kamali Aghdam M, Jafari N, Eftekhari K. Novel coronavirus in a 15-day-old neonate with clinical signs of sepsis, a case report. Infect Dis (Lond) 2020; 52(6):427–9.

72. Dong Y, Mo X, Hu Y, et al. COVID-19 among child China. Epidemiol 2020;145(6): e20200702.

73. De Bernardo G, Giordano M, Zollo G, et al. The clinical course of SARS-CoV-2 positive neonates. J Perinatol 2020;40(10):1462–9.

74. Trevisanuto D, Cavallin F, Cavicchiolo ME, et al. Coronavirus infection in neonates: a systematic review. Arch Dis Child Fetal Neonatal Ed 2021;106(3):330–5.

75. Gale C, Quigley MA, Placzek A, et al. Characteristics and outcomes of neonatal SARS-CoV-2 infection in the UK: a prospective national cohort study using active surveillance. Lancet Child Adolesc Health 2021;5(2):113–21.

76. Dumitriu D, Emeruwa UN, Hanft E, et al. Outcomes of Neonates Born to Mothers With Severe Acute Respiratory Syndrome Coronavirus 2 Infection at a Large Medical Center in New York City. JAMA Pediatr 2021;175(2):157–67.

77. McCarty KL, Tucker M, Lee G, et al. Fetal Inflammatory Response Syndrome Associated with Maternal SARS-CoV-2 Infection. Pediatrics 2020. e2020010132.

78. Yu N, Li W, Kang Q, et al. Clinical features and obstetric and neonatal outcomes of pregnant patients with COVID-19 in Wuhan, China: a retrospective, single-centre, descriptive study. Lancet Infect Dis 2020;20(5):559–64.

79. Gupta M, Zupancic JAF, Pursley DM. Caring for newborns born to mothers with COVID-19: more questions than answers. Pediatrics 2020;146(2). e2020001842.

80. Cook TM, El-Boghdadly K, McGuire B, et al. Consensus guidelines for managing the airway in patients with COVID-19: guidelines from the Difficult Airway Society, the Association of Anaesthetists the Intensive Care Society, the Faculty of Intensive Care Medicine and the Royal College of Anaesthetists. Anaesthesia 2020; 75(6):785–99.

81. Edelson DP, Sasson C, Chan PS, et al. Interim guidance for basic and advanced life support in adults, children, and neonates with suspected or confirmed COVID-19: from the Emergency Cardiovascular Care Committee and Get With The Guidelines-Resuscitation Adult and Pediatric Task Forces of the American Heart Association. Circulation 2020;141(25):e933–43.

82. Centers for Disease Control. Evaluation and management considerations for neonates at risk for COVID-19 2020. Available at: https://www.cdc.gov/coronavirus/2019-ncov/hcp/caring-for-newborns.html. Accessed February 20, 2021.

83. Pang EM, Sey R, De Beritto T, et al. Advancing Health Equity by Translating Lessons Learned from NICU Family Visitations During the COVID-19 Pandemic. Neoreviews 2021;22(1):e1–6.

84. Horbar JD, Edwards EM, Soll RF, et al. COVID-19 and newborn care: April 2020. Pediatrics 2020. e2020002824.

85. Virani AK, Puls HT, Mitsos R, et al. Benefits and risks of visitor restrictions for hospitalized children during the COVID pandemic. Pediatrics 2020;146(2).

86. Turpin H, Urben S, Ansermet F, et al. The interplay between prematurity, maternal stress and children's intelligence quotient at age 11: a longitudinal study. Sci Rep 2019;9(1):450.

87. Salvatore CM, Han JY, Acker KP, et al. Neonatal management and outcomes during the COVID-19 pandemic: an observation cohort study. Lancet Child Adolesc Health 2020;4(10):721–7.

88. Cavicchiolo ME, Trevisanuto D, Lolli E, et al. Universal screening of high-risk neonates, parents, and staff at a neonatal intensive care unit during the SARS-CoV-2 pandemic. Eur J Pediatr 2020;179(12):1949–55.

89. Murray PD, Swanson JR. Visitation restrictions: is it right and how do we support families in the NICU during COVID-19? J Perinatol 2020;40:1576–81.

90. de Winter JP, De Luca D, Tingay DG. COVID-19 surveillance for all newborns at the NICU; conditio sine qua non? Eur J Pediatr 2020;179(12):1945–7.

The Impact of Coronavirus Disease 2019 on Pediatric Asthma in the United States

Aishwarya Navalpakam, MD[a], Elizabeth Secord, MD[b],
Milind Pansare, MD[c],*

KEYWORDS

• COVID-19 • Pediatric asthma • United States

KEY POINTS

• The COVID-19 pandemic caused morbidities and mortalities of historic proportion and disrupted health-care delivery in the United States.
• The elderly and patients with chronic illnesses including asthma are at increased risks of poor outcomes.
• Limited data in the United States indicate children with asthma have done well despite multiple challenges to health-care delivery.
• It is important to adhere to asthma treatment guidelines to maintain asthma control in children during the pandemic.

INTRODUCTION

Coronaviruses are a common cause of upper respiratory infections in children.[1] A novel human coronavirus, severe acute respiratory syndrome coronavirus 2 (SARS-CoV-2), mutated in bats in Wuhan, China, and has been attributed to be the cause of a global pandemic leading to illness and death in 2020.[2] Initially, asthma was thought to be a risk factor for poor clinical outcomes in adult patients with coronavirus disease 2019 (COVID-19). However, limited data currently available have not shown significant COVID-19 illness or increase in asthma exacerbations in children during the pandemic. In this article, we aim to outline impact of COVID-19 on pediatric asthma in the United States and current recommendations for asthma care.

This article previously appeared in *Pediatric Clinics*, Volume 68, Issue 5, October 2021.
[a] Division of Allergy and Immunology, Department of Pediatrics, Pediatric Specialty Center, Children's Hospital of Michigan, 4th Floor, 3950 Beaubien Boulevard, Detroit, MI 48236, USA;
[b] Department of Pediatrics, Wayne State University, Detroit, MI, USA; [c] Department of Pediatrics, Division of Allergy and Immunology, Pediatric Specialty Center, Children's Hospital of Michigan, Central Michigan University, Suite # 4018, 4th Floor, 3950 Beaubien Boulevard, Detroit, MI 48236, USA
* Corresponding author.
E-mail address: mpansare@dmc.org

Clinics Collections 12 (2022) 249–261
https://doi.org/10.1016/j.ccol.2021.12.018
2352-7986/22/© 2021 Elsevier Inc. All rights reserved.

IMPACT OF COVID-19 IN THE UNITED STATES

The United States has become an epicenter during the pandemic, reporting the highest number of cases and deaths due to COVID-19. In the United States alone by December 31, 2020, a total aggregate count of COVID-19 cases of 19,663,976 and total deaths of 341,199 were reported by states and territorial jurisdictions to the Centers for Disease Control and Prevention (CDC). These numbers continue to increase. In the age-group of 0 to 17 years, the total number of reported COVID-19 cases was 1,500,972 (10.5% estimated from the age reported in 14,226,540 cases) and the death count was 211 (<0.2% estimated from the age reported in 237,889 deaths) during the same period.[3] The CDC had listed asthma as a risk factor for COVID-19 outcomes, particularly morbidity and mortality.[4] Asthma is the most common chronic respiratory disease in children, affecting about 6 million children in the United States in ages 0 to 17 years. Every year, one in 6 children with asthma visits the ED and about 1 in 20 children with asthma is hospitalized for the same condition (https://cdc.gov.asthma). Practitioners and parents alike anticipated and rapidly prepared for the significant impact of SARS-CoV-2 infections in children with asthma. The reality was not what was anticipated.

RESPIRATORY VIRUSES AND ASTHMA

Asthma in children is often triggered by respiratory viruses. It is theorized that the type I interferon production, which is important for defense against viruses, is decreased in asthmatic individuals and is inhibited by Th2 inflammation seen in allergic asthma.[5] Studies also suggest that in atopic individuals, certain respiratory viruses such as respiratory syncytial virus (RSV) or human rhinovirus (RV), owing to the formation of specific IgE, may cause exacerbations.[5] RSV and RV have actually been implicated in the development of asthma. Other viruses such as influenza, coronavirus, adenovirus, parainfluenza virus, and metapneumovirus are considered risk factors for asthma exacerbations. At the advent of the COVID-19 pandemic, there was a concern that SARS-CoV-2 infection may also result in increased asthma exacerbations in children, which surprisingly did not occur.

PATHOPHYSIOLOGY OF SEVERE ACUTE RESPIRATORY SYNDROME CORONAVIRUS-2

COVID-19 is caused by the novel coronavirus SARS-CoV-2. It is a single-stranded RNA virus (ssRNA) that contains a spike protein (S protein) that binds to angiotensin-converting enzyme 2 (ACE2) receptors found on human cells. The ssRNA is inserted into the airway epithelial cells, where it replicates causing local inflammation, tissue damage, and cytokine release. The majority of these ACE2 receptors are located on type II alveolar epithelial cells. There are other associated receptors such as type II cellular transmembrane serine protease (TMPRSS2) that activate S protein and allow for the fusion of the viral membrane into the host cell.[6]

POTENTIAL ASTHMA-PROTECTIVE FACTORS AGAINST COVID-19

The pathophysiologic hallmark of asthma is chronic airway inflammation. Generally, two types of inflammatory asthma are described: type 2-high (T2) asthma and type 2-low (T1) asthma, based on the expression of T helper cell type 2 (TH2) cytokines. Type 2-high asthma is characterized by eosinophilic airway inflammation, elevated levels of cytokines such as interleukin (IL) 4, IL-5, and IL-13, and elevated levels of IgE. This is also known as allergic asthma that appears earlier in life, is responsive to corticosteroids, and is a common phenotype in children. The type 2 low asthma phenotype is more common in adults, has later disease onset, has less allergic comorbidities, and is less responsive to corticosteroids.

ACE2 receptor expression appears to vary with asthma phenotype. A study of two large adult asthma cohorts identified increased expression of the ACE2 gene in the bronchial epithelium of patients with type 2-low or T1-high asthma.[7] Interestingly, these patients also tended to have higher known risk factors for COVID-19 including hypertension, lymphopenia, and male gender.[7,8] This suggests that the T2-low phenotype is likely associated with higher risk of COVID-19. Another study of cohort of children with asthma, the Urban Environment and Childhood Asthma (URECA) cohort, revealed that allergic sensitization in children (positive IgE tests for allergens, either skin or serum testing) with asthma was associated with decreased ACE2 expression in children.[9] The type 2-high asthma phenotype characterized by the elevated serum IgE level, fractional exhaled nitric oxide (FeNO), and IL-13 expression was associated with decreased ACE2 receptor expression in this URECA cohort.[9] It suggests that T2 high-asthma and allergic sensitization is associated with decreased ACE2 receptor expression and may be a cause of decreased SARS-CoV-2 infection in these patients. This may be important to pediatric patients with asthma who tend to have the T2-high asthma phenotype. Children, when compared to adults, have lower ACE2 receptors in their nasal epithelium. This may account for the decreased incidence of COVID-19 in children.[10]

The use of inhaled corticosteroids (ICSs) may also provide a protective role for asthma from COVID-19. Cultures of human nasal and tracheal epithelial cells reveal that the combination of glycopyrronium, a long-acting muscarinic antagonist, formoterol, a long-acting beta-2 agonist, and budesonide, an ICS, inhibits replication of HCoV-229E, a virus that causes common cold by preventing receptor expression and decreases virus-induced airway inflammation.[11] When gene expression of ACE2 and TMPRSS2 was analyzed in sputum cells from patients with severe asthma, it was found that the use of ICSs was associated with lower expression of these receptors.[12] These studies suggests patients with asthma who are adherent to their ICSs thus may have decreased risk of COVID-19.

COVID-19 AND ASTHMA PREVALENCE

The number of adult patients with asthma hospitalized owing to COVID-19 across the world is low, with incidence reported from 1% to 2.7%.[13] An online questionnaire sent to 91 pediatric practitioners in 27 countries attempted to estimate the incidence of clinically relevant COVID-19 in pediatric patients with asthma. They noted that incidence is 12.8 times less frequent in children than in adults.[14] A retrospective study of a large cohort in Israel also showed that patients with asthma have a lower susceptibility for COVID-19 in pediatric and adult patients. The study did not find any difference in the rate of hospitalization in patients with COVID-19 with or without asthma.[15] A nationwide study in Japan examining asthma during the COVID-19 outbreak found decreased asthma admissions in 2020 compared with previous years for children and adults.[16] A study of 212 children with allergic asthma in Spain found no significant difference in asthma control or severity between patients with and without COVID-19.[17]

In the United States, adult data suggest that there is no significant increased risk of mortality associated with a history of asthma. A matched cohort study of adult patients with asthma admitted to Massachusetts General Hospital with COVID-19 found that patients with asthma were less likely to require intensive care and mechanical ventilation and did not have increased risk of mortality.[18] A large COVID-19 registry with 11,405 patients from the Mount Sinai Health System in NYC revealed that of the

54.8% of patients who were COVID-19 positive, only 4.4% had asthma, suggesting there was no significant association between asthma history and disease.[19]

The early data from Wuhan regarding hospitalized pediatric patients and those with severe COVID-19 do not list asthma as a risk factor.[20,21] As per the CDC, in the United States, as of January 2021, 10.8% of 16,212,877 COVID-19 cases are found in children. However, these data are changing and not necessarily accurate of the true incidence in children owing to lack of prioritization of testing in this population. Hospitalization is reported to be low among children when compared with adults (CDC). Owing to a paucity of data, there has been an urgent call for further studies in childhood asthma in the current pandemic.[22]

Asthma exacerbations have a seasonal pattern, generally have increased prevalence in the late fall and spring, and are seen across North America and known as the September peak or asthma epidemic.[23,24] This is attributed to viral upper respiratory infections (URI), air pollutants, weather changes, and increase in aeroallergens.[25] Viral infections particularly account for asthma exacerbations in children during the start of school in early fall. Although respiratory viruses are a risk factor for asthma exacerbations, this did not seem to pertain to the current SARS-CoV-2 infection outbreak. Previously, SARS-CoV infection, which caused the first SARS outbreak in 2002, did not appear to be associated with an increase in asthma exacerbations in children.[26] However, there are very few studies published evaluating incidence, trends, hospitalization, and mortality related to pediatric asthma with COVID-19 in the United States. Some of the published studies in the US population are summarized in **Table 1**.[27–31]

IMPACT ON PEDIATRIC ASTHMA: MORBIDITY AND MORTALITY

Various studies from around the world, including China, Brazil, Italy, Switzerland, and the United States, reveal that asthma is not associated with increased risk of mortality in adult patients with COVID-19.[13] The Morbidity and Mortality Weekly Report from October 2020 that evaluated COVID-19 trends among school-age children (N = 277, 285) noted that 1.2% were hospitalized, 0.1% had intensive care unit (ICU) admissions, and less than 0.1% died. Of those patients (hospitalized, ICU admissions, died owing to COVID-19), each had at least one underlying medical condition, and 55% of the underlying conditions were accounted for by chronic lung disease including asthma, emphysema, and chronic obstructive pulmonary disease (COPD).[32] The final determination of COVID-19 impact toward pediatric asthma morbidity and mortality remains to be seen owing to lack of sufficiently powered studies providing significant data.

IMPACT ON PEDIATRIC ASTHMA: CLINICAL CARE

As the pandemic surged worldwide, international and governmental agencies of countries across all the continents responded by implementing control measures to contain the spread of virus. In the United States, federal, state, and local governments passed many unprecedented regulations including stay-at-home orders; the closing of local businesses, universities, and schools; social distancing; and face mask mandates. In the initial surge of disease, health resources were targeted toward the care of seriously ill patients with COVID-19, and nonurgent care was deferred to the alternate delivery model. The federal government declared a public health emergency and also allocated resources to provide medical care. The Health Insurance Portability and Accountability Act was relaxed, which allowed physicians to use their personal electronic devices to communicate with their patients during the pandemic.[33] The Centers

Table 1
Summary of pediatric asthma and COVID-19 studies

Study	Timeline	Asthma Findings
Kenyon et al,[27] 2020 Initial ED impact of COVID-19 in pediatric asthma • Retrospective chart review • Compared daily ED visits for asthma for the January–April period in 2020 to years 2016–2019	January to April from years 2016 to 2020	• ED utilization for asthma decreased by 3 standard deviations below the mean in year 2020 as compared with years 2016–2019. • Decreased ED visits by 76% in March–April 2020 (COVID) as compared with January–March 2020 (pre–COVID-19)
Taquechel et al,[28] 2020 Asthma health-care utilization during COVID-19 • Retrospective chart review • Compared outpatient, inpatient, and ED visits for asthma for the January to May period from years 2015–2020	January to May from years 2015 to 2020	Until March 17, 2020, similar visits (when compared with 2015–2019) After March 17, 2020: • Outpatient in-person asthma encounters decreased by 87%. • Hospital encounters decreased by 84%. • Telephone encounters increased by 19%. • TM visits increased by 61%. Other findings: • Decreased asthma-related steroid prescriptions. • Decreased frequency of rhinovirus infections.

Bandi et al,[29] 2020
Risks of COVID-19 in asthma in children aged <18 y evaluated by the TM clinic
• Tested for SARS-CoV-2 (PCR)
• Documented asthma status
	March 12, 2020, to April 20, 2020	474 patients tested → 5.2% tested positive for SARS-CoV-2
		• Rate of asthma in SARS-CoV-2-positive cases: 12%
		• Rate of asthma in SARS-CoV-2-negative cases:10%
		  ○ No significant difference
		  ○ Asthma not a risk factor for infection

Bailey et al,[30] 2020 SARS-CoV-2 testing in US children • Retrospective cohort study	January 1, 2020, to September 8, 2020	135794 patients tested for SARS-COV-2 → 4% positive • 7% had severe illness (ICU care, increased length of stay, ventilation). • 0.2% died. • Asthma had a negative association with SARS-CoV-2 positive test results (SR, 0.86 [95% CI, 0.80–0.91]).

(continued on next page)

Table 1
(continued)

Study	Timeline	Asthma Findings
Secord et al,[31] 2021 ED visits for pediatric asthma • Retrospective chart review	March 15 to May 31 in 2019 and in 2020	Asthma ED visits significantly decreased during school closure from March 15 to May 31, 2020, when compared with the same period in 2019. • Average daily ED visits for asthma of 17 in 2019 vs 3.5 in 2020 • Total ED visits for asthma of 1304 in 2019 vs 260 in 2020 ($P = .001$)

Abbreviations: ED, emergency department; PCR, polymerase chain reaction; SR, standardized ratio.

for Medicare & Medicaid Services also promoted telemedicine (TM) by waiving previous restrictions of patient qualification for TM visits, by permitting office-based and home-based video encounters on personal devices with patients, and by improving reimbursements.[34]

In the United States, practitioners actively responded by establishing virtual clinics and using telehealth tools in all medical specialties to curb the pandemic.[35] An ad hoc expert panel of allergy/immunology specialists from the United States and Canada developed a consensus document to guide specialists in lieu of reduced services due to the pandemic.[36] The guidelines on COVID-19 and allergy contingency planning noted "If the allergy/immunology office does not have personal protective equipment available, it would be recommended that no patients with co-potential for asthma exacerbation and COVID-19 be seen at the office; the patient should instead be seen at a facility capable of isolation and equipped for asthma care." These recommendations are expected to be adjusted based on disease prevalence. Most ambulatory allergy services in the country restricted new patient appointments and procedures. The established patients were evaluated in virtual platforms. Sick patients were referred to facilities equipped with personnel protection, laboratory testing for SARS-CoV-2, and high acuity care treatments. Diagnostic testing and therapeutic interventions for allergic disease and asthma were restricted owing to concerns of the spread of the virus. This included testing for allergic sensitization, lung functions, FeNO, and nebulized treatments and allergy injections.[36,37] Clinicians considered health-care delivery during the pandemic to be suboptimal and are eager to resume face-to-face encounters as soon as possible. Parents were also unwilling to bring their children to hospitals and clinics for fear of contracting the virus during the pandemic. Many raised concerns about inhaled or oral steroids and risks of COVID-19 infections. Despite the multiple challenges of wildly spreading disease and misinformation, the patient outcomes with asthma were not worse and have been better than expected, generally. This is likely due to initial fear of susceptibility to severe COVID-19 with asthma, which prompted families to adopt health safety measures and improve adherence to asthma medications. A study at a health system in Wisconsin using electronic medication monitors noted a 14.5% relative increase in asthma controller adherence across all age-groups from January to March 2020.[38] The increased adherence is due to parental concern about asthma control during the outbreak.[39] School closures in particular also reduced exposures to allergens and viruses among children, which are important triggers of asthma, thus enabling improved asthma control.

COVID-19 AND ASTHMA TREATMENT GUIDELINES

There were some initial concerns about continuing ICSs and oral corticosteroids for asthma owing to fear of contracting the virus because steroids can impair immune responses. A meta-analysis of 39 trials revealed that ICS use was not associated with higher risk of pneumonia or respiratory infection due to COVID-19.[40] A study of RNA expression in bronchial brushes of a cohort of adult patients with asthma in the United Kindgom found that there was no significant difference in expression of ACE2 receptor and TMPRSS between healthy controls and patients with moderate and severe asthma undergoing varying corticosteroid treatment.[41] There was no greater risk for asthmatics than the general population for risk of COVID-19, regardless of the severity of asthma and various corticosteroid treatment intensities. This supports the use of inhaled steroids in the management of asthma.

In response to the pandemic, the Global Initiative for Asthma (GINA) updated guidelines on asthma care during the pandemic.[42] The guideline emphasized the importance of optimal asthma management and medication adherence in reducing the risk of asthma exacerbations. The guidelines also recommend continuing prescribed medications including daily ICSs and biologic therapy.[42] The American Academy of Allergy, Asthma, and Immunology also reiterated that patients with asthma should continue to use their medications and aim for good control.[43] Both recommended the controller medication dose not be reduced or discontinued during the pandemic unless there is clear-cut benefit after careful consideration of risk/benefit for the child.[36,42,43] Systemic or oral steroids are recommended for use in moderate to severe asthma exacerbations that are unimproved with bronchodilators.[42,43] There is no evidence to suggest impairment of immune response to COVID-19 in patients treated with biologics for asthma. It is reasonable to continue administration of these agents during the pandemic.[42–44] Allergen immunotherapy used as an adjunct is also recommended to be continued with adjustment in doses and duration.[43]

COVID-19: USE OF NEBULIZERS AND SPIROMETRY

Many national and international societies including the GINA, National Asthma Council Australia, and American College of Allergy, Asthma and Immunology recommend against using nebulizers to reduce the risk of spreading the virus, with a preference for pressurized metered dose inhalers (MDIs).[42,43] SARS-CoV-2 is transmitted via droplets and aerosols. Owing to aerosol treatments, SARS-CoV-2 may persist in the air for up to 2 hours and may be recirculated and remain on dependent surfaces, promoting virus spread.[45] There is also concern that the particles that are generated with nebulization may stimulate cough in patients, which can spread the pathogen.[46] Use of the albuterol MDI (90 mcg/puff), 4 to 8 puffs every 20 minutes for 3 doses and then inhalation using the valved holding chamber every 1 to 4 hours, has shown to be as effective as nebulized therapy for mild to moderate asthma exacerbation in children.[47] MDIs with spacers have comparable efficacy with nebulizers, take shorter time for delivery, are more portable, and are less likely to spread the virus during the pandemic. Nebulizer treatments may still be necessary in very young or sick children and are

---

Box 1
Guidelines for minimizing risk of SARS-CoV-2 transmission[42]

Follow CDC guidelines[a]

Follow state and local directives on public health measures to control disease.

CDC guidelines for schools and childcare program.

Social and physical distancing measures
- Avoid close contact from other people—remain six feet away from others at all times.
- Practice self-isolation if you are in a high-risk group or if you are sick.
- Stay home and avoid large crowds and indoor spaces.

Face mask and personal protection measures:
- Wash hands using a sanitizing handwash containing at least 60% alcohol.
- Refrain from touching your face.
- Cover your mouth/nose when coughing with your elbow or a tissue.
  - Dispose of your tissue immediately afterward.
- Wear a face mask or face covering in public settings (now recommended by the CDC).
- Clean and disinfect surfaces regularly.

[a]https://www.cdc.gov/coronavirus/2019-ncov/prevent-getting-sick/prevention.html.

preferred in settings equipped with infection control measures. Most hospitals and clinics have rapidly adapted to the change of using MDIs to help control the pandemic without compromising asthma outcomes.

Spirometry is an important tool of asthma management but poses a considerable risk for the spread of infection to individuals and the surrounding surfaces within and around the test areas. The American Thoracic Society recommends prioritizing patients' clinical status by screening for urgent cases, ensuring protection of the health-care worker, and using in-line filters for spirometry.[48] The full operation of lung function services can resume when virus prevalence is low.[48] General guidelines for infection control and daily asthma management adapted from GINA guidelines are highlighted in **Box 1** and **Table 2**. The Food and Drug Administration under the Emergency Use Authorization approved two mRNA vaccines for ages more than 18 years in December 2020 for control of the pandemic.[47] Many other vaccines are in the research pipeline and under investigation for use in children.

Table 2 General guidance for care of patients with asthma during the COVID-19 pandemic[36]	
Asthma Medications	• Continue daily controller (inhaled corticosteroids) as prescribed • Step down in treatment only in cases risk/benefit is carefully evaluated • For severe asthma: continue biologic therapy or oral corticosteroids if prescribed. • Close monitoring—use control tests such as the ACT, peak flow meter, and periodic virtual or clinic visits • Provide all patients with a written asthma action plan ○ Recommend that patients do not share inhalers and spacer devices

Acute Exacerbations	• Use a short course of OCS when appropriate for severe asthma exacerbations
	• Avoid nebulizers where possible to reduce the risk of spreading virus.
	  ○ Nebulizers may be required for:
	    ■ Severe or life-threatening exacerbation
	    ■ Young children (<4 y)
	    ■ Patients who are unable to use MDIs even with a valved holding chamber.
	  ○ Strict infection control procedures if aerosol-generating procedures are needed
	• A pressurized metered dose inhaler (MDI) via a spacer is preferred for mild to moderate asthma exacerbation.

Spirometry	• Avoid in patients with confirmed or suspected COVID-19 or if COVID-19 cases are high in community ○ Practice appropriate aerosol, droplet, and contact precautions if spirometry is needed. • Consider home peak flow monitoring • Follow local public health measures to control spread of infection—including personal hygiene and use of PPE.
Vaccination	• Recommend the annual influenza vaccine. • Follow CDC guidelines for COVID-19 vaccination. • After obtaining COVID-19 vaccines, continue to wear a mask and avoid close contact with others.

Abbreviations: ACT, asthma control test; OCS, oral corticosteroid; PPE, personal protection equipment.

SUMMARY

The COVID-19 pandemic has had a severe economic and health impact all over the world, including the United States, in particular. The available data, albeit limited, suggest that the initial concerns of the serious impact of COVID-19 illness in children with asthma are not evident to date. The reduction in asthma morbidities is likely due to a combination of improved adherence and decreased exposure to both allergens and viral infections in children. International guidelines are updated to guide physicians in the midst of the pandemic. In the face of unprecedented time, it is important to be vigilant, adhere to treatment guidelines, and implement preventive measures to eradicate the virus and improve outcomes for children with asthma.

CLINICS CARE POINTS

- The COVID-19 pandemic has caused catastrophic impact on health and well-being of humans globally.
- Unlike children, adults with chronic illnesses and other health risk factors had poorer outcomes.
- Current evidence suggests most children with chronic asthma were able to maintain asthma control during the pandemic.
- It is important to adhere to recommendations of international and national asthma guidelines for treatment of both acute exacerbation and chronic asthma.
- A multipronged measure including stepped pharmacotherapy based on asthma severity is necessary to maintain asthma control in children during the pandemic.
- Current evidence suggests favorable outcomes with inhaled corticosteroids and biologics used in treatment of asthma.
- It is important to implement CDC guidelines on SARS-CoV-2 infection control and vaccinations when available.

DISCLOSURE

The authors have nothing to disclose.

REFERENCES

1. Kahn JS, Mcintosh K. History and recent advances in coronavirus discovery. Pediatr Infect Dis J 2005;24(Suppl):S223–6.
2. Platto S, Xue T, Carafoli E. COVID-19: an announced pandemic. Cell Death Dis 2020;11:799–812.
3. COVID-19 Stats. COVID-19 Incidence, by Age Group -United States, March 1–November 14, 2020. MMWR Morb Mortal Wkly Rep 2021;69:1664.
4. Centers for Disease Control and Prevention. Coronavirus disease 2019 (COVID-19): people who are at high risk 2020. Available at: https://www.cdc.gov/coronavirus/2019-ncov/need-extra-precautions/asthma.html.
5. Novak N, Cabanillas B. Viruses and asthma: the role of common respiratory viruses in asthma and its potential meaning for SARS-CoV-2. Immunology 2020; 161(2):83–93.
6. Singh SP, Pritam M, Pandey B, et al. Microstructure, pathophysiology, and potential therapeutics of COVID-19: A comprehensive review. J Med Virol 2020.

7. Camiolo M, Gauthier M, Kaminski N, et al. Expression of SARS-CoV-2 receptor ACE2 and coincident host response signature varies by asthma inflammatory phenotype. J Allergy Clin Immunol 2020;146(2):315–24.e7.

8. Wakabayashi M, Pawankar R, Narazaki H, et al. Coronavirus disease 2019 and asthma, allergic rhinitis: molecular mechanisms and host-environmental interactions. Curr Opin Allergy Clin Immunol 2021;21(1):1–7.

9. Jackson DJ, Busse WW, Bacharier LB, et al. Association of respiratory allergy, asthma, and expression of the SARS-CoV-2 receptor ACE2. J Allergy Clin Immunol 2020;146(1):203–6.e3.

10. Bunyavanich S, Do A, Vicencio A. Nasal gene expression of angiotensin-converting enzyme 2 in children and adults. JAMA 2020;323(23):2427–9.

11. Yamaya M, Nishimura H, Deng X, et al. Inhibitory effects of glycopyrronium, formoterol, and budesonide on coronavirus HCoV-229E replication and cytokine production by primary cultures of human nasal and tracheal epithelial cells. Respir Investig 2020;58(3):155–68.

12. Peters MC, Sajuthi S, Deford P, et al. Covid-19-related genes in sputum cells in asthma. Relationship to demographic features and corticosteroids. Am J Respir Crit Care Med 2020;202(1):83–90.

13. Skevaki C, Karsonova A, Karaulov A, et al. Asthma-associated risk for COVID-19 development. J Allergy Clin Immunol 2020;146(6):1295–301.

14. Papadopoulus NG, Custovic A, Deschildre A, et al. Pediatric Asthma in Real Life collaborators. Impact of COVID-19 on pediatric burden of asthma: Practice adjustments and disease burden. J Allergy Clin Immunol Pract 2020;8:2594–9.

15. Green I, Merzon E, Vinker S, et al. Covid-19 susceptibility in bronchial asthma. J Allergy Clin Immunol Pract 2021;9(2):684–92.e1.

16. Abe K, Miyawaki A, Nakamura M, et al. Trends in hospitalizations for asthma during the COVID-19 outbreak in Japan. J Allergy Clin Immunol Pract 2021;9(1):494–6.e1.

17. Ruano FJ, Somoza Álvarez ML, Haroun-Díaz E, et al. Impact of the COVID-19 pandemic in children with allergic asthma. J Allergy Clin Immunol Pract 2020;8(9):3172–4.e1.

18. Robinson LB, Fu X, Bassett IV, et al. COVID-19 severity in hospitalized patients with asthma: A matched cohort study. J Allergy Clin Immunol Pract 2021;9(1):497–500.

19. Lieberman-Cribbin W, Rapp J, Alpert N, et al. The impact of asthma on mortality in patients with covid-19. Chest 2020;158(6):2290–1.

20. Zheng F, Liao C, Fan Q-H, et al. Clinical characteristics of children with coronavirus disease 2019 in hubei, china. Curr Med Sci 2020;40(2):275–80.

21. Sun D, Li H, Lu X-X, et al. Clinical features of severe pediatric patients with coronavirus disease 2019 in Wuhan: a single center's observational study. World J Pediatr 2020;16(3):251–9.

22. Castro-Rodriguez JA, Forno E. Asthma and COVID-19 in children: A systematic review and call for data. Pediatr Pulmonol 2020;55(9):2412–8.

23. Wisniewski JA, McLaughlin AP, Stenger PJ, et al. A comparison of seasonal trends in asthma exacerbations among children from geographic regions with different climates. Allergy Asthma Proc 2016;37(6):475–81.

24. Larsen K, Zhu J, Feldman LY, et al. The annual september peak in asthma exacerbation rates. Still a reality? Ann Am Thorac Soc 2016;13(2):231–9.

25. Castro CR, Tarabichi Y, Gunzler DD, et al. Seasonal trends in asthma exacerbations: Are they the same in asthma subgroups? Ann Allergy Asthma Immunol 2019;123(2):220–2.

26. Van Bever HP, Chng SY, Goh DY. Childhood severe acute respiratory syndrome, coronavirus infections and asthma. Pediatr Allergy Immunol 2004;15(3):206–9.
27. Kenyon CC, Hill DA, Henrickson SE, et al. Initial effects of the COVID-19 pandemic on pediatric asthma emergency department utilization. J Allergy Clin Immunol Pract 2020;8(8):2774–6.e1.
28. Taquechel K, Diwadkar AR, Sayed S, et al. Pediatric asthma health care utilization, viral testing, and air pollution changes during the covid-19 pandemic. J Allergy Clin Immunol Pract 2020;8(10):3378–87.e11.
29. Bandi S, Nevid MZ, Mahdavinia M. African American children are at higher risk of COVID-19 infection. Pediatr Allergy Immunol 2020;31(7):861–4.
30. Bailey LC, Razzaghi H, Burrows EK, et al. Assessment of 135 794 pediatric patients tested for severe acute respiratory syndrome coronavirus 2 across the united states. JAMA Pediatr 2021;175(2):176–84.
31. Secord E, Poowuttikul P, Pansare M, et al. Pediatric emergency visits for asthma drop significantly with covid 19 school closure. J Allergy Clin Immunol 2021; 147(2):AB150.
32. Leeb RT, Price S, Sliwa S, et al. Covid-19 trends among school-aged children - united states, march 1-september 19, 2020. MMWR Morb Mortal Wkly Rep 2020;69(39):1410–5.
33. American Telemedicine Association. ATA commends. Congress for giving HHS authority to waive restrictions on telehealth for Medicare beneficiaries in response to the COVID-19 outbreak. Arlington (VA): American Telemedicine Association; 2020. Available at: www.americantelemed.org/press-releases/ata-commends-congress-for-waiving-restrictionson-telehealth-for-medicare-beneficiaries-in-res ponse-to-the-covid-19-outbreak/. Accessed March 16, 2020.
34. Centers for Medicare & Medicaid Services. Coverage and payment related to COVID-19 Medicare. 2020. Available at: https://www.cms.gov/files/document/ 03052020-medicare-covid-19-fact-sheet.pdf. Accessed: March 15, 2020.
35. Hollander JE, Carr BG. Virtually perfect? Telemedicine for Covid-19. N Engl J Med 2020;382:1679–81.
36. Shaker MS, Oppenheimer J, Grayson M, et al. COVID-19: pandemic contingency planning for the allergy and immunology clinic. J Allergy Clin Immunol Pract 2020;8:1477–88.e5.
37. Cardinale F, Ciprandi G, Barberi S, et al. Consensus statement of the Italian society of pediatric allergy and immunology for the pragmatic management of children and adolescents with allergic or immunological diseases during the COVID19 pandemic. Ital J Pediatr 2020;46:84.
38. Kaye L, Theye BA, Smeenk I, et al. Changes in medication adherence among patients with asthma and COPD during the COVID-19 pandemic. J Allergy Clin Immunol Pract 2020;8:2384–5.
39. Oreskovic NM, Kinane TB, Aryee E, et al. The unexpected risks of covid-19 on asthma control in children. J Allergy Clin Immunol Pract 2020;8(8):2489–91.
40. Cazeiro C, Silva C, Mayer S, et al. Inhaled corticosteroids and respiratory infections in children with asthma: a meta-analysis. Pediatrics 2017;139(3).
41. Bradding P, Richardson M, Hinks TSC, et al. ACE2, TMPRSS2, and furin gene expression in the airways of people with asthma-implications for COVID-19. J Allergy Clin Immunol 2020;146(1):208–11.
42. GINA interim guidance on COVID-19 and asthma. Available at: https://ginasthma. org/wp-content/uploads/2020/12. Accessed: January12, 2020.
43. AAAAI. Asthma and COVID-19 2020. Available at: https://www.aaaai.org/ask-the-expert/covid. Accessed: December 20, 2020.

44. Morais-Almeida M, Aguiar R, Martin B, et al. COVID-19, asthma, and biological therapies: What we need to know. World Allergy Organ J 2020;13:100–26.
45. Cazzola M, Ora J, Bianco A, et al. Guidance on nebulization during the current COVID-19 pandemic. Respir Med 2020;176:106236.
46. Mei-Zahav M, Amirav I. Aerosol treatments for childhood asthma in the era of COVID-19. Pediatr Pulmonol 2020;55(8):1871–2.
47. Camargo CA Jr, Rachelefsky G, Schatz M. Managing asthma exacerbations in the emergency department: Summary of the National Asthma Education and Prevention Program Expert Panel Report 3 guidelines for the management of asthma exacerbations. J Allergy Clin Immunol 2009;124(2):S5–14.
48. Crimi C, Impellizzeri P, Campisi R, et al. Practical considerations for spirometry during the COVID-19 outbreak: Literature review and insights. Pulmonology 2020.

Clinical Patterns and Morphology of COVID-19 Dermatology

Ritesh Agnihothri, MD, Lindy P. Fox, MD*

KEYWORDS

• COVID-19 • SARS-CoV-2 • Dermatology • Morphology

KEY POINTS

- Numerous skin manifestations associated with COVID-19 have been reported. Dermatologists should be aware of these cutaneous manifestations, which may help with diagnosis, management, and prognosis.
- The most commonly reported cutaneous manifestations associated with COVID-19 infection include pernio (chilblain)-like acral lesions, morbilliform (exanthematous) rash, urticaria, vesicular (varicella-like) eruptions, and vaso-occlusive lesions (livedo racemosa, retiform purpura).
- It is important to consider COVID-19 on the differential diagnosis for these disease entities in the proper clinical context, as dermatologic findings of COVID-19 can be a presenting sign in an otherwise minimally or asymptomatic individual.

INTRODUCTION

In December 2019, unexplained pneumonia cases were reported in Wuhan, China. The new pathogen, named SARS-CoV-2 (severe acute respiratory syndrome coronavirus 2), was isolated from samples of the respiratory tract of infected patients, and the resulting disease was called COVID-19 (coronavirus disease 2019). The virus traveled rapidly throughout the globe and was characterized as a pandemic by the World Health Organization on March 11, 2020.

It was soon recognized that COVID-19 patients were experiencing myriad clinical manifestations involving multiple organ systems (including the central nervous, gastrointestinal, and cardiovascular systems), as well as viral illness-induced coagulopathy.[1–4] Initial case series rarely documented skin changes, possibly due to the lack of dermatologists caring for patients with COVID-19 infection as well as the inability to perform complete skin examinations in critically ill patients. Dermatologists also experienced significant challenges collecting samples and taking clinical images while maintaining strict infection prevention techniques, particularly with a widespread limited supply of personal protective equipment.[5] In an early cohort study of 1099

This article previously appeared in *Dermatologic Clinics*, Volume 39, Issue 4, October 2021.
Department of Dermatology, University of California San Francisco, 1701 Divisadero Street, 3rd Floor, San Francisco, CA 94115, USA
* Corresponding author.
E-mail address: lindy.fox@ucsf.edu

Clinics Collections 12 (2022) 263–284
https://doi.org/10.1016/j.ccol.2021.12.027
2352-7986/22/© 2021 Elsevier Inc. All rights reserved.

patients with laboratory-confirmed COVID-19, only 2 patients were noted to have "skin rash."[6]

Shortly thereafter, small cohorts of patients were being reported to have cutaneous findings possibly associated with COVID-19 infection.[7,8] The reported findings ranged from those more commonly seen in viral infections, such as morbilliform eruptions and urticaria, to more unique, such as pernio and varicelliform eruptions. A large case series describing patterns of skin manifestations among 375 patients highlighted 5 predominant morphologic patterns: maculopapular, urticarial, pernio-like, vesicular, and livedoid.[9] This series also provided for the first time, a temporal relationship between cutaneous lesions, systemic symptoms, as well as severity of disease. As COVID-19 testing was initially only available to those with severe disease, the true incidence of cutaneous manifestations with COVID-19 infection is not yet known. The pandemic has encouraged broad collaboration among physicians and scientists around the world,[10] facilitated by multiple registries, which are helping us increase our understanding of dermatologic manifestations in patients with COVID-19.[11,12]

Virology/Immunology

SARS-CoV-2 is a single-stranded RNA virus composed of 16 nonstructural proteins, each of which plays a specific role in replication.[13] SARS-CoV-2 binds to angiotensin-converting enzyme 2 (ACE2) receptors, which is known to be found in the lungs (surfactant producing alveolar type 2 cells) as well as the cardiovascular, gastrointestinal, pulmonary, and renal systems.[14] Expression of ACE2 in the skin is highest in keratinocytes, followed by sweat glands. The widespread expression of ACE2 in the skin is just one of the potential reasons for cutaneous manifestations seen with COVID-19 infection.[15,16]

Pernio (chilblain)-Like Acral Lesions

Since the outbreak of SARS-CoV-2, reports of pernio-like acral lesions have rapidly accumulated. Pernio (chilblains) is an idiopathic cold-sensitive inflammatory disorder that manifests as pink to violaceous macules, papules, plaques, or nodules at sites of cold exposure, commonly on the fingers or toes.[17] Chilblains may be idiopathic or may be associated with autoimmune conditions (ie, chilblains lupus), hematologic malignancies, genetic mutations, and less commonly infections, such as Epstein-Barr virus (EBV).[18] When EBV-associated, cold agglutinins are thought to play a role in pathogenesis.[18] Skin findings may be accompanied by pruritus, pain, burning, and sometimes blistering or ulceration. When making a diagnosis of chilblains, it is important to rule out Parvovirus B19 infection, which can present with acral purpuric lesions.

The first report of pernio-like lesions thought to be associated with COVID-19 was of an Italian adolescent (with family members suspected of having COVID-19 infection) who developed purpuric lesions on the feet before developing systemic symptoms such as fever and myalgias.[19] Reports of young adults with skin lesions on hands and feet identical to chilblains began appearing, seemingly later in the course of their infection.[9] Analysis of Google Trends data, which illustrates popularity of search trends over a period in a particular location, demonstrated that there were sharp increases in search terms including chilblains, fingers, and toes in early 2020.[20,21] As this phenomenon became better known and circulated on social media, it was colloquialized as "COVID-toes," although the precise relationship with SARS-CoV-2 continues to be elucidated. The association was first suspected for multiple reasons: there was a spike in cases during the pandemic, at an atypical time of year for symptoms to occur (spring), in temperate areas, and in patients typically at low risk (ie, no known comorbid conditions associated with chilblains such as autoimmunity,[22] connective tissue disease such as lupus erythematosus, Raynaud phenomenon/syndrome, or a history of chilblains).

Before the pandemic, pernio was uncommon; one case series reported an average of 9 to 10 diagnoses per year across an entire tertiary academic center.[18] Since the onset of the pandemic, studies from around the world have reported numerous individuals with pernio-like lesions thought to be associated with COVID-19 infection. In a French retrospective study on skin manifestations during the early COVID-19 outbreak, pernio-like lesions were noted in 38.3% (106 of 277) of dermatologic outpatients.[23] More recently, an international registry of COVID-19 dermatologic manifestations has recorded 619 cases of pernio in patients with suspected or confirmed COVID-19 infection.[24] Patients with pernio-like lesions are noted to present with pruritus and pain of their toes (less often fingers or heels), which progresses to pink-red papules or plaques and then to violaceous purpuric lesions.[25] Rarely, pernio-like lesions have been reported in other acral sites, such as on the ear.[26] In addition to pernio-like lesions, variations in morphologies have been reported, including erythema multiforme (EM)-like (round, maculopapular, or targetoid lesions), punctiform purpuric lesions, diffuse vascular erythema, and edema of the dorsum/sole of foot or palms.[27] Patients with COVID-19 who develop pernio have relatively mild courses; with 2% to 16% of patients with pernio-like lesions being hospitalized.[9,28–32] This can be compared to other dermatologic manifestations associated with more severe disease such as retiform purpura, where 100% of patients were hospitalized, with 82% of patients developing acute respiratory distress syndrome.[28] Pernio-like acral lesions should be recognized as distinct from acroischemic lesions. The two terms were initially used synonymously, but acroischemic lesions are now known to represent a separate manifestation seen among critically ill patients with hypercoagulopathy and/or disseminated intravascular coagulation.[8]

Histopathology of pernio-like lesions is similar to that of idiopathic or systemic disease-associated chilblains. Pathology frequently contains vascular changes, dermal edema, and a superficial and deep perivascular lymphocytic infiltrate. In select reports, immunohistochemistry has confirmed vasculitis of dermal vessels, deposition of immunoglobulins or complement on dermal vessels, and platelet aggregation.[22,31] When histologic findings of pernio-like lesions in multiple reports were reviewed, it appears that these lesions are primarily inflammatory, nonischemic, and not reflective of systemic coagulopathy, unlike retiform purpura or acral ischemia.[28] Furthermore, the microthrombi seen in a small subset of patients with chilblains are likely secondary to the inflammation and clinically correlate with a bullous or necrotic phenotype.[33]

In a study of dermoscopy features of COVID-19–related chilblains in children and adolescents, dermoscopic findings were found to correlate with clinical and histopathologic findings of COVID-19–related chilblains. For example, the background color noted on dermoscopy is an indicator of vascular macules, hemosiderin, and inflammatory cells in the dermis; gray areas may be indicative of an ischemic phenomenon, and globules likely representing damaged vessels with extravasated red cells. The specificity of these findings, however, is unclear as there is no dermoscopic study of primary chilblains or chilblains secondary to other causes.[34,35]

Overall, pernio-like lesions are typically seen in patients with relatively mild COVID-19 disease courses and resolve within 2 to 8 weeks (median 12 days in laboratory-confirmed cases).[32,36,37] However, persistent and recurrent lesions have been reported. Recent data illustrate a subset of patients with "long COVID" in the skin who had dermatologic signs of COVID-19 that persisted longer than 60 days, including 7 of 103 cases of pernio.[37] Recurrent pernio-like lesions in the absence of reinfection have also been noted, with patients who complained of pernio in the fall experiencing an absence of symptoms in the summer, despite surges of COVID-19 infections in the warmer months.[24] Of note, pernio lesions in type I interferonopathies are also known to flare with cold exposure.[38]

There are increasing number of reports suggesting a direct association between pernio-like lesions and SARS-CoV-2. Positive anti–SARS-CoV-2 immunostaining and viral spike protein have been demonstrated in lesional skin biopsy specimens (endothelial cells and eccrine glands) in adult and pediatric patients with pernio-like lesions.[39–41] However, owing to lack of specificity, some authors have suggested that these findings be interpreted with caution.[42–44]

The pathogenesis of pernio-like lesions is not well understood but is thought to be predominantly an inflammatory process similar to idiopathic and autoimmune-related chilblains. The striking similarity of pernio-like lesions to those observed in type 1 interferonopathies (ie, Aicardi-Goutieres syndrome and STING-associated vasculopathy) has raised the suspicion of the important role of interferon (IFN) despite the absence of other manifestations of interferonopathies in patients with COVID-19 infection.[45–47] One group demonstrated induction of the type I IFN pathway in lesional sections of COVID-19–associated chilblain-like lesions.[48] Type I interferon is known to have an important role in the pathogenesis of lupus erythematosus.[49,50] Furthermore, interferons are also thought to induce microangiopathic changes contributing to the development of chilblains lupus.[46,47]

As mounting evidence suggests a direct association with SARS-CoV-2, pernio-like lesions are currently believed to represent a postviral or late-onset finding after COVID-19 infection, especially in those who can mount a robust IFN response. In a report by Freeman and colleagues, 80 of 318 cases developed pernio-like lesions after the onset of other symptoms of COVID-19 infection; a similar finding has been noted in at least one other study.[9,32] Conversely, pernio-like lesions have also been reported to occur concurrently with RT-PCR test positivity.[32,51] Negative nasopharyngeal reverse-transcription polymerase chain reaction (RT-PCR) or anti–SARS-CoV-2 serologies in many patients[52–58] created uncertainty early in the pandemic regarding the precise relationship.[39,54,57–59] Indeed, some patients who were RT-PCR negative after developing pernio, were later found to have positive COVID-19 antibodies (immunoglobulin M, G, or A).[24,26,32,60,61]

What was initially surprising, however, was that serologic testing for IgM or IgG antibodies was often negative. There is increased understanding of this mechanism:

I. Early in the pandemic, interpretation of RT-PCR/antibody results in patients with skin rash and probable COVID-19 was difficult due to lack of understanding of timing and antibody kinetics. Much of the available antibody data were drawn from patients with more severe illness as widespread testing was not available. Many patients with pernio-like lesions were undergoing serologic evaluation for SARS-CoV-2 antibodies early in the disease course. In one study, patients had antibody testing between 3 and 30 days after pernio developed, with most evaluated less than 15 days after pernio onset.[57] It is now appreciated that delayed antibody development after infection with SARS-CoV-2 is common.[62] In one early report, positive antibodies were detected a median of 30 days from disease onset, beyond the typical 14- to 21-day testing window.[63]

II. Population level antibody testing from the past year has revealed that there is a relationship between disease severity and the level of SARS-CoV-2 antibodies. In one particular hospital, for both IgG and IgA isotypes, patients with moderate/severe infection had significantly higher antibody titers within the first 1.5 months after diagnosis compared to those with milder disease.[64] As previously discussed, it is now well-established that those with COVID-19 who develop chilblains have relatively mild clinical courses and may not mount a marked antibody response, similar to others with minimal symptoms of infection.[60] Despite a more muted antibody response, data suggest that patients with milder SARS-CoV-2 infection are able to elicit in vitro neutralizing antibodies (preventing the virus from entering epithelial cells).[65] Negative RT-PCR on nasopharyngeal swabs is supportive of the notion that pernio-like lesions are a late symptom of COVID-19.[28]

III. Most serologic testing for SARS-CoV-2 currently is against SARS-CoV-2 IgM and IgG. It is appreciated that the host immune response to SARS-CoV-2 infection includes synthesis of several types of virus-specific antibodies including IgM, IgG, and IgA.[66,67] There are also reports that some patients with pernio-like lesions have positive serology for anti–SARS-CoV-2 IgA.[55,60] The authors postulated that children with mild or asymptomatic infection may develop an IgA humoral response, rather than IgG. Secretory IgA plays a vital role in host protection of mucosal surfaces by preventing entry and subsequent infection by respiratory viruses including influenza; elevated levels are also associated with improved influenza vaccine efficacy.[68] With SARS-CoV-2, a pathogen that first interacts with the immune system at mucosal surfaces/lungs due to person-to-person respiratory transmission, a robust IgA response appears before IgG. IgA serum levels reach their peak earlier than IgG (10–14 days) suggesting that both IgA and IgG are part of the initial humoral immune response. Given that currently widely used commercial antibody tests do not look for IgA, a "negative antibody test" may not truly reflect the absence of prior infection and/or antibody production.

IV. The kinetics of early interferon production may determine overall COVID-19 disease severity and antibody production. Interferons are early antiviral response proteins that interfere with intracellular viral replication, recruit other cells for antiviral response, and cause "flu-like symptoms" such as fever and muscle pain. It is thought that robust production of interferon-I is associated with early viral control, suppressed antibody response, and mild COVID-19 infection. This may be an additional explanation for why some patients fail serologic detection.[69] Conversely, patients with severe COVID-19 have notably depressed/absent interferon responses or interferon deficiency that can lead to severe, life-threatening COVID-19 infection.[70–73] Several authors hypothesize that chilblains, specifically, could be the cutaneous expression of a strong type I interferon response.[74–77] This could therefore explain the absence of antibodies in patients with chilblains.

There is a correlation between the severity of COVID and the timing of appearance of COVID-antigen–specific CD4 T-cells in circulation. Patients with the early expansion of antigen-specific CD4 T-cells (2 days after symptom onset) seem to have mild COVID and those who have a late response (CD4 appearance >20 days after symptoms) have severe disease, suggesting that an early CD4 T-cell response is important in fighting SARS-CoV-2 infection.[78] Sekine and colleagues have demonstrated T-cell immunity to SARS-CoV-2 in those with mild COVID-19 infection who were also subsequently seronegative.[79]

Morbilliform Eruptions

Morbilliform (maculopapular) eruptions frequently arise as a result of viral infections or adverse drug reactions, and are the most commonly reported cutaneous manifestation of COVID-19 with a prevalence as high as 47%.[7,9,23,28,80] Predominantly involving the trunk, the rash has been noted either at disease onset, or more frequently, after hospital discharge, with a reported median duration of 7 days.[7,37,81] Morbilliform eruptions are associated with intermediate severity of disease.[82] It is difficult to definitively associate morbilliform eruptions with SARS-CoV-2 infection as many reported patients may have received concomitant drug therapy for their infection. Although medications given as a part of COVID-19 treatment (ie, ribavarin, IVIG, and antiretroviral drugs) may cause morbilliform eruptions, this manifestation has been noted in patients with no new medications.[83,84] Taking a detailed history is critical, and it is important to consider COVID-19 testing in patients when the eruption is not better explained by medications or other infections.

Urticarial Eruptions

Urticaria (hives) is a common feature among COVID-19 patients who experienced rashes. Acute urticaria, defined as a self-limited lesion lasting less than 6 weeks, has been reported as a presenting sign of COVID-19 infection, although it can also occur later in the disease course.[7,9,23,28,45] COVID-associated urticaria has also been reported to present with fever as an early prodromal sign in otherwise asymptomatic individuals.[85–87] Acute urticaria can be triggered by infections, medications, insect bites/stings, and type I immune reactions. It has been hypothesized that viral IgM/IgG can cross-react with mast cell IgE and cause mast cell degranulation, which could explain urticaria in the setting of COVID-19 infection.[88] It is important to note that urticaria is also a possible side-effect for numerous medications used to treat COVID-19.[84] COVID-19–associated urticarial eruptions are reported to last a median of 4 days with a maximum duration of 28 days.[37] Although the specificity of urticaria to COVID-19 infection is low, in patients with new onset urticaria developing during the pandemic, one should consider evaluation for COVID-19 infection with RT-PCR and serologic studies.

Vesicular Eruptions

Vesicles are fluid-filled collections in the epidermis less than ½ cm in diameter. Vesicles can be caused by a variety of viral infections including varicella-zoster, herpes simplex, echovirus, and coxsackievirus infections.[89] Most patients with COVID-19 presenting with varicella-like exanthem also have general respiratory and general symptoms of COVID-19 infection. One Italian study including 22 patients reported vesicular, varicelliform lesions, which developed on average 3 days after onset of COVID-19 symptoms.[90] Although more often being reported as developing early after onset of systemic signs of COVID-19 infection (up to 79.2%),[91] 15% of patients in one study developed this rash before other symptoms.[9] The papulovesicular exanthems noted in association with COVID-19 infection differ from true varicella infection with their truncal involvement, scattered distribution, and minimal pruritus.[90] Vesicular lesions are thought to be associated with moderate severity of COVID-19.[9,91] In the appropriate clinical context, COVID-19 testing (in addition to HSV/VZV PCR) should be performed in a patient presenting with varicelliform cutaneous eruption.

Two morphologies of COVID-associated vesicular eruption have been described: localized, monomorphic lesions typically involving the trunk or back, and a more diffuse polymorphic eruption notable for small papules, vesicles, and pustules of varying sizes.[91] The distribution of lesions involving the trunk and back mimics Grover disease (transient acantholytic dermatosis), a benign condition seen in older Caucasian men with crusted papules and papulovesicles on the trunk and back. COVID-19–associated varicella-like exanthem can share some histologic similarity to Grover disease. In one report of 3 cases, a prominent nonballooning acantholysis with intraepidermal vesicle and eosinophilic dyskeratosis without nuclear atypia was noted, leading to the suggestion that this entity would be better termed "COVID-19–associated acantholytic rash."[92] Conversely, in other histologic reports of COVID-19–associated vesicular eruptions, histology was consistent with viral infection, with vacuolar degeneration of the basal layer with multinucleate, hyperchromatic keratinocytes and dyskeratotic cells.[90,93]

Erythema Multiforme-like Lesions

EM is an acute, typically self-limited hypersensitivity reaction involving the skin and mucous membranes presenting with concentric three-ring targetoid plaques on acral surfaces. It is clinically characterized as presenting with acute onset of concentric (targetoid) plaques. In adults, more than 90% of EM is thought to be triggered by infection, particularly the herpes simplex virus. EM-like eruptions of targetoid lesions with either truncal or acral predominance have been observed in association with SARS-CoV-2 infection in adults and children.[9,94–97] Children with COVID-19 who develop EM generally have mild respiratory/gastrointestinal symptoms or are otherwise asymptomatic.[98] In one series, 2 of 4 children with suspected COVID-related EM underwent skin biopsies with positive immunohistochemistry staining of endothelium to SARS-CoV-2 spike protein.[99] Another study reported 4 hospitalized women with COVID-19 infection who developed pink truncal papules evolving to targetoid lesions, which resolved in all 4 patients within 2 to 3 weeks.[94] A 60-year-old woman with fixed urticarial eruption (nonevanescent) underwent skin biopsy, which was notable for slight vacuolar-type interface dermatitis with necrotic keratinocytes and no eosinophils, most consistent with an EM-like pattern, highlighting that not all EM-like lesions present as targets.[100]

Pityriasis Rosea-like Eruption

Pityriasis rosea (PR) is a common papulosquamous eruption presenting with ovoid patches and plaques with fine collarettes of scale. In classic cases, a solitary lesion (herald patch) precedes the development of a more diffuse eruption. Lesions are classically formed along skin fold lines on the trunk. PR-like eruptions have been noted to be occurring in greater frequency and in association with SARS-CoV-2 infection.[101–107] An atypical digitate papulosquamous variant in an elderly patient with COVID-19 infection has also been reported.[108] Although the exact cause of typical PR is unclear, viral etiologies, including human herpesvirus (HHV)-6 and 7 have been favored. Reactivation of HHV-6 and EBV has been demonstrated in one patient with COVID-19 infection and PR.[109] A recent report demonstrated 2 patients with PR-like rash and urticaria-like rash with COVID-19 infection with SARS-CoV-2 spike protein present in the endothelium of dermal blood vessels of affected skin.[110] It is unclear if the increased incidence of PR is due to direct viral infection of SARS-CoV-2, reactivation of HHV-6/7, or other factors. Testing for infection is recommended in a patient who presents with this characteristic eruption in the appropriate clinical context.

Pediatric COVID-19

Despite more than 3.85 million testing positive for COVID-19 since the onset of the pandemic, children have been relatively spared from severe COVID-19–related complications, with less frequent infection, less severe respiratory sequelae, and generally a milder course.[111,112] This milder course is attributed to children having fewer predisposing factors for severe disease (ie, cardiovascular disease, diabetes mellitus), healthy vascular endothelium, strong antiviral innate immunity, and fewer ACE receptors in nasal and lung epithelium, making viral entry and infection more difficult.[113]

In children, cutaneous signs of COVID-19 may be the predominant or only clue of infection and, in fact, are not uncommon. Cutaneous lesions of COVID-19 occur in more than 8% of hospitalized children[114] and are the 7th most common extrapulmonary manifestation.[115] There are several case reports and case series of various cutaneous eruptions in COVID-positive children. Children with COVID-19 and skin manifestations carry an overall better prognosis than those without.[116]

Multisystem Inflammatory Syndrome in Children (MIS-C)

Since April 2020, there have been multiple reports worldwide of severe pediatric disease several weeks (median 25 days) after SARS-CoV-2 infection with fevers, multiorgan involvement, and characteristics of Kawasaki disease (KD).[117–119] This syndrome has been called MIS-C and is thought to be a postviral consequence of COVID-19 infection. There is confirmed laboratory evidence of COVID-19 infection in 99% of cases, antibody testing is positive, and RT-PCR tends to be negative. The US Centers for Disease Control and Prevention (CDC) has developed a case definition of MIS-C (Table 1).[120]

MIS-S shares some features of KD and toxic shock syndrome, including fever and skin, mucous membrane, and distal extremity changes. However, it is considered a distinct disease. In contrast to KD, MIS-C is being seen in older children and adolescents (median age 9 years) and non-Hispanic black and Hispanic children, whereas KD more commonly affects children younger than 5 years who are of East Asian descent. In addition, children with MIS-C experience more gastrointestinal symptoms and less than 50% meet formal criteria for KD.[121,122]

The pathogenesis of MIS-C is thought to be multifactorial, including the robust immune system of children, immune complex activation, and the superantigen activity of SARS-CoV-2 spike protein all leading to cytokine storm and systemic inflammation.[123–125] MIS-C cases and deaths unfortunately continue to accumulate; although most children with this condition require intensive care, patients with MIS-C carry a good prognosis, with current mortality estimated at 2%.

Although many studies have described cutaneous involvement with MIS-C, the type of rash, distribution, and clinical course needs to be studied further. Greater than 50% of cases of MIS-C are reported to have mucocutaneous changes. Reported mucocutaneous findings include morbilliform, scarlatiniform, urticarial, and reticulated patterns, as well as periorbital edema, malar rash, and reticulated exanthems similar to erythema infectiosum.[126] In addition, distal extremity changes, oral mucous membrane changes, conjunctivitis, and purpura are reported.[127] The molecular mechanisms underlying the relationship between COVID-19 and MIS-C are poorly understood. There are increasing numbers of adults being reported to have COVID-19–associated MIS-C, characterized by multiorgan dysfunction (particularly cardiac) in the absence of severe respiratory illness.[128,129]

Vascular Lesions

Petechiae and purpura

Petechiae and purpura (visible hemorrhage into the skin or mucous membranes) are among the less commonly described cutaneous manifestations of COVID-19 infection. The first COVID-19–associated cutaneous manifestation with purpuric features was reported by Joob and colleagues, who described a petechial rash misdiagnosed as dengue in a COVID-19 patient.[132] Only 3% of patients in a French study of 277 patients had petechial skin lesions.[23] Petechial eruptions can have many etiologies including platelet deficiency or dysfunction, disorders of coagulation, and loss of vascular wall integrity. This morphology is associated with certain viral infections including enterovirus, parvovirus B19, and dengue virus.[133] COVID-19–associated petechial and purpuric lesions have been noted on acral surfaces, intertriginous regions, extremities, or diffusely.[9,23,134–136] When secondary to vasculitis, lesions can progress to form blisters.[137] Henoch-Schonlein Purpura and IgA vasculitis has been reported to be triggered by SARS-CoV-2 infection.[138–140]

Table 1
Case definition for Multisystem Inflammatory Syndrome in Children (MIS-C) associated with COVID-19 infection[120]

Criteria	Additional Information	
Age <21 y		
Fever	Fever ≥38.0°C for ≥24 h, or report of subjective fever lasting ≥24 h	
Laboratory evidence of inflammation	Including, but not limited to, one or more of the following: an elevated CRP, ESR, fibrinogen, procalcitonin, D-dimer, ferritin, LDH, or IL-6, elevated neutrophils, reduced lymphocytes, and low albumin	
Multisystem (≥2) organ involvement (cardiac, renal, respiratory, hematologic, gastrointestinal, dermatologic, or neurologic)	*Organ system*	*Examples of involvement*[130,131]
	Gastrointestinal	Abdominal pain, diarrhea, nausea, vomiting, abnormal hepatobiliary markers
	Hematologic	Fever, myalgias, lymphadenopathy, fatigue, abnormal blood counts
	Neurologic	Headache, irritability, altered mental status, dizziness
	Dermatologic	Cutaneous eruption, conjunctivitis, edema, mucositis
	Respiratory	Dyspnea, upper respiratory infection-like signs, cough, wheezing, respiratory failure, pulmonary infiltrates
	Cardiovascular	Shock, chest pain, myocarditis, coronary artery dilatation/aneurysm, elevated cardiac enzyme markers
	Renal	Acute kidney injury
No alternative plausible diagnoses; AND		
Positive for current or recent SARS-CoV-2 infection by RT-PCR, serology, or antigen test; or exposure to a suspected or confirmed COVID-19 case within the 4 wk before the onset of symptoms.		

Abbreviations: CRP, C-reactive protein; ESR, erythrocyte sedimentation rate; IL-6, interleukin 6; LDH, lactic acid dehydrogenase.

Livedo reticularis-like lesions

Livedo reticularis (LR) is a transient finding that classically presents with a blue-purple reticulated vascular pattern. LR results from alterations in vascular flow, which results in accumulation of deoxygenated blood in the cutaneous venous plexis. LR has been observed in association with COVID-19 infection.[141–143] Although cases of LR were grouped with more severe necrosis in a major early study,[9] more recent reports estimate that this manifestation was present in 3.5% of patients.[28]

Fixed livedo racemosa, retiform purpura, and necrotic vascular lesions

Vaso-occlusive lesions (livedo racemosa, thrombotic retiform purpura, and acral ischemia) have been noted in elderly, critically ill patients with severe COVID-19 infection.[9,28,144] These clinical entities exist at the opposite end of the disease severity spectrum compared to perniosis, which occurs in those with mild or asymptomatic disease. Patients with this clinical finding have been noted to have markedly elevated D-dimer levels and disseminated intravascular coagulation.[8,144] Skin biopsy of a COVID patient with retiform purpuric patches showed multiple occlusive thrombi in most small vessels of the superficial and mid-dermis.[145] Direct immunofluorescence in this patient was notable for IgM, C3 and C9 deposition within dermal vessel walls.[145] In a subsequent study of a series of COVID patients with retiform purpura, terminal complements C5b-9 and other complement components were found in the microvasculature. This may be suggestive of systemic complement activation and pathophysiology similar to atypical hemolytic uremic syndrome or other microthrombotic syndromes.[144] Pauci-inflammatory purpuric (most often on buttocks) pressure ulcers have also been noted in several critically ill COVID patients with limited mobility, incontinence, and malnutrition.[146] Histopathology of these purpuric pressure ulcers were consistent with pressure necrosis (epidermal necrosis, eccrine gland necrosis); SARS-CoV-2 RNA in-situ hybridization of all 4 skin biopsies was negative. The reported patients did not have any laboratory evidence of coagulopathy such as disseminated intravascular coagulation.[146] It is important to recognize that this clinical finding is distinct from the thrombotic vasculopathy noted by Magro and colleagues[144]

In a recent review of the literature, vaso-occlusive lesions were found to be the least commonly reported cutaneous manifestation with COVID-19 infection but may portend a worse prognosis with the highest mortality rate of all COVID-associated cutaneous manifestations (18.2%).[82,147]

OTHER REPORTED CUTANEOUS MANIFESTATIONS/ASSOCIATIONS

Cutaneous Manifestation	Subtype, if Applicable	Morphology	Additional Clinical Findings
Alopecia	Androgenetic alopecia	Hair loss from the anterior hairline moving posteriorly or thinning at the vertex scalp	Associated with worse clinical outcomes in some studies[148,149]
	Telogen effluvium	Diffuse hair shedding 2–3 mo after a stressor[150,151]	
Gianotti-Crosti-like rash		Pruritic erythematous papules and vesicles on elbows, anterior thighs, and bilateral popliteal fossa coalescing into plaques.[152]	Rash started 18 d after onset of symptoms, 13 d after +COVID test, and 3 d after resolution of all respiratory and systemic symptoms.
SDRIFE-like		Erythematous rash on bilateral axillae and antecubital fossae, which subsequently extended to trunk and inner thighs[153,154]	

(continued on next page)

(continued)			
Cutaneous Manifestation	**Subtype, if Applicable**	**Morphology**	**Additional Clinical Findings**
Grover-disease-like		Red papules and papulovesicles distributed on the trunk[155] Note: some evidence suggests clinical overlap with vesicular, or "varicella-like" eruptions	
Erythema elevatum diutinum-like		Firm symmetric smooth nodules on extensor surfaces, particularly joints[156]	
Reactive infectious mucocutaneous eruption (formerly known as *Mycoplasma*-induced rash and mucositis)		Shallow erosions of the vermilion lips, hard palate, periurethral glans penis.[157]	Reported patient with +COVID PCR 1 wk before rash onset, and again positive at rash onset. Mycoplasma PCR negative, IgM negative, IgG positive (consistent with past exposure).
Enanthems (eruptions of the mucous membranes)		83% (5 patients) with petechial enanthem ± macular enanthem[158]	Recorded from a group of 21 patients with COVID-19 and skin rash ranging from papulovesicular, purpuric periflexural, and erythema multiforme-like.
Oral lesions		Aphthous-like, ulcerations, and macules, tongue depapillation, angular cheilitis, ulcers, blisters, white plaques, dark pigmentations.[159]	Etiology postulated to be multifactorial. Hypotheses include direct action of SARS-CoV-2 on oral mucosal cells, coinfection, immunity impairment, or adverse drug reactions[160]
Acute genital ulcers (Lipschütz ulcers)		Necrotic ulcers with raised, sharply demarcated borders of the labia minora with no evidence of "kissing lesions."[161]	Single oral aphtha was also observed, with no cutaneous involvement
Transient rash in newborns		Transient "rash" (morphology not described) in babies born to mothers with COVID-19.[162] Mottling noted in a neonate with sepsis and +COVID-19.[163]	

Abbreviation: SDRIFE, symmetric drug-related intertriginous and flexural exanthema.

DISCUSSION

As the novel SARS-CoV-2 virus rapidly spread throughout the world, the scientific and medical community has worked with remarkable pace to understand its full clinical effects. Early in the pandemic, scarcity of diagnostic assays limited our ability to confirm infection in patients presenting with an array of cutaneous manifestations. Most young patients presenting with pernio-like lesions had mild clinical courses, which precluded them from having access to COVID-19 testing early in the pandemic when diagnostic resources were limited.

Viral infections are known to produce a variety of clinical findings due not only to their direct action on human cells but also to the host immune response and resulting inflammatory cascade. Further complicating the clinical picture, patients with COVID-19 infections were often treated with a multitude of medications, many of which can be associated with the reported cutaneous manifestations. Now with relative widespread availability of RT-PCR assays and serologic testing, we are beginning to understand the utility and limitations of testing (including timing in relation to a patient's infection course and imperfect sensitivities and specificities of available tests).[62,164] It is now understood that a negative swab or antibody test at one point in time does not necessarily rule out SARS-CoV-2 as a causative agent.[164] Data derived from a UK COVID Symptoms Study app suggest that those with cutaneous rash are more likely to test positive for SARS-CoV-2 (odds ratio 1.67).[165] Although less prevalent than fever, the authors also found rash to be more specific for COVID-19 infection, which lends support to the diagnostic value of cutaneous manifestations of SARS-CoV-2 infection.[165]

The most commonly reported cutaneous manifestations associated with COVID-19 infection include pernio-like, urticarial, morbilliform, and retiform purpura. As previously discussed, identifying cutaneous eruptions and their possible association with SARS-CoV-2 infection can allow for early identification of infection, sometimes even before onset of more classic symptoms such as respiratory distress.[82] As seen in **Fig. 1**, Jamshidi and colleagues in their systematic review found that vesicular and urticarial eruptions are seen early relative to other COVID-19 symptoms. Maculopapular, papulosquamous, vascular lesions tend to occur around the time that a patient is symptomatic. Pernio-like lesions occur later in the disease course.[82] Certain cutaneous morphologies are noted to correlate to severity of illness and overall prognosis. According to a study by Galvan and colleagues, pernio-like, vesicular, urticarial, maculopapular, and livedoid/necrotic lesions were associated with progressively increasing disease severity.[9] This has been corroborated by another study by Freeman and colleagues, which demonstrated cutaneous manifestations associated with a spectrum of severity, with pernio-like lesions noted in mild disease, vesicular/urticarial/macular erythema/morbilliform eruption in intermediate severity, and retiform purpura in critically ill patients.[28] Similarly, pernio-like lesions and morbilliform eruptions are associated with the highest survival rates (98.7% and 98.2%, respectively), whereas vaso-occlusive lesions are associated with the lowest survival rate of 78.9%.[147] It is important to consider SARS-CoV-2 infection in the differential diagnosis of a patient presenting with these lesions (ie, new onset pernio-like lesions, vesicular or morbilliform eruption) in the appropriate clinical context, as cutaneous manifestations may be present in otherwise asymptomatic individuals, or present before developing other symptoms of infection.

The coronavirus pandemic has been found to disproportionally affect people of color in both the United States and the United Kingdom, yet registry data on cutaneous manifestations in this population is lacking.[28] A systematic review of literature describing cases of cutaneous manifestations associated with COVID-19 found a

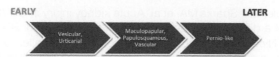

Fig. 1. Timing of skin lesions relative to other COVID-19 symptoms.[82]

significant paucity of reports and photographs of manifestations in skin of color, and no published photos of cutaneous manifestations in Fitzpatrick type V or VI skin.[166] A recent study suggests there are geographic differences in the morphology and prevalence of COVID-19–associated skin manifestations.[147] More work must be done to better understand the true prevalence of skin findings in COVID-19 across all populations and ethnicities.

SUMMARY

The clinical phenotype of COVID-19 includes a broad spectrum of cutaneous manifestations of varying degrees of severity and specificity. Although initially thought to be an infection with primarily internal/systemic manifestations, COVID-19 has taught us that dermatologists play an important role in the treatment of COVID-19 patients, as well as in the broad scientific collaboration to learn more about the pathophysiology of infection. Widespread availability of COVID-19 tests, as well as improved diagnostic assays, will further assist our understanding of how skin manifestations are related to this viral infection, and parse out potential confounding factors such as concurrent pharmacotherapy or lifestyle changes.

CLINICS CARE POINTS

- Cutaneous manifestations of COVID-19 are generally benign and self-limited. These manifestations have prognostic significance depending on type of skin lesion. Pernio (chilblain)-like acral lesions are generally associated with mild disease; retiform purpura is typically seen in patients on the severe end of the disease severity spectrum.

- Cutaneous manifestations may be present in otherwise asymptomatic individuals, or present before developing other symptoms of infection.

- With increased access to diagnostic testing, we are beginning to understand the utility and limitations of currently available assays.

DISCLOSURE

The authors have nothing to disclose.

REFERENCES

1. Hajifathalian K, Mahadev S, Schwartz RE, et al. SARS-COV-2 infection (coronavirus disease 2019) for the gastrointestinal consultant. World J Gastroenterol 2020;26(14):1546–53.
2. Helms J, Kremer S, Merdji H, et al. Neurologic Features in Severe SARS-CoV-2 Infection. N Engl J Med 2020;382(23):2268–70.
3. Bikdeli B, Madhavan MV, Jimenez D, et al. COVID-19 and Thrombotic or Thromboembolic Disease: Implications for Prevention, Antithrombotic Therapy, and Follow-Up: JACC State-of-the-Art Review. J Am Coll Cardiol 2020;75(23): 2950–73.

4. Batlle D, Soler MJ, Sparks MA, et al. Acute kidney injury in COVID-19: Emerging evidence of a distinct pathophysiology. J Am Soc Nephrol 2020;31(7):1380–3.
5. Fernandez-Nieto D, Ortega-Quijano D, Segurado-Miravalles G, et al. Comment on: Cutaneous manifestations in COVID-19: a first perspective. Safety concerns of clinical images and skin biopsies. J Eur Acad Dermatol Venereol 2020;34(6): e252–4.
6. Guan W, Ni Z, Hu Y, et al. Clinical Characteristics of Coronavirus Disease 2019 in China. N Engl J Med 2020;382(18):1708–20.
7. Recalcati S. Cutaneous manifestations in COVID-19: a first perspective. J Eur Acad Dermatol Venereol 2020;34(5):e212–3.
8. Zhang Y, Cao W, Xiao M, et al. Clinical and coagulation characteristics in 7 patients with critical COVID-2019 pneumonia and acro-ischemia. Zhonghua Xue Ye Xue Za Zhi 2020;41(4):302–7.
9. Galván Casas C, Català A, Carretero Hernández G, et al. Classification of the cutaneous manifestations of COVID-19: a rapid prospective nationwide consensus study in Spain with 375 cases. Br J Dermatol 2020;183(1):71–7.
10. Robinson PC, Yazdany J. The COVID-19 Global Rheumatology Alliance: collecting data in a pandemic. Nat Rev Rheumatol 2020;16(6):293–4.
11. Freeman EE, McMahon DE, Fitzgerald ME, et al. The American Academy of Dermatology COVID-19 registry: Crowdsourcing dermatology in the age of COVID-19. J Am Acad Dermatol 2020;83(2):509–10.
12. Freeman EE, McMahon DE, Hruza GJ, et al. International collaboration and rapid harmonization across dermatologic COVID-19 registries. J Am Acad Dermatol 2020;83(3):e261–6.
13. Chen Y, Liu Q, Guo D. Emerging coronaviruses: Genome structure, replication, and pathogenesis. J Med Virol 2020;92(4):418–23.
14. Prompetchara E, Ketloy C, Palaga T. Immune responses in COVID-19 and potential vaccines: Lessons learned from SARS and MERS epidemic. Asian Pac J Allergy Immunol 2020;38(1):1–9.
15. Li MY, Li L, Zhang Y, et al. Expression of the SARS-CoV-2 cell receptor gene ACE2 in a wide variety of human tissues. Infect Dis Poverty 2020;9(1). https://doi.org/10.1186/s40249-020-00662-x.
16. Xue X, Mi Z, Wang Z, et al. High Expression of ACE2 on Keratinocytes Reveals Skin as a Potential Target for SARS-CoV-2. J Invest Dermatol 2021;141(1): 206–9.e1.
17. Hedrich CM, Fiebig B, Hauck FH, et al. Chilblain lupus erythematosus - A review of literature. Clin Rheumatol 2008;27(8):949–54.
18. Cappel JA, Wetter DA. Clinical characteristics, etiologic associations, laboratory findings, treatment, and proposal of diagnostic criteria of pernio (chilblains) in a series of 104 patients at Mayo Clinic, 2000 to 2011. Mayo Clin Proc 2014;89(2): 207–15.
19. Mazzotta F, Troccoli T. Acute Acro-ischemia in the Child at the time of COVID-19, vol. 30, 2020. https://doi.org/10.26326/2281-9649.30.2.2102.
20. Kluger N, Scrivener JN. The use of Google Trends for acral symptoms during COVID-19 outbreak in France. J Eur Acad Dermatol Venereol 2020;34(8): e358–60.
21. Hughes M, Rogers S, Lepri G, et al. Further evidence that chilblains are a cutaneous manifestation of COVID-19 infection. Br J Dermatol 2020;183(3):596–8.
22. Kanitakis J, Lesort C, Danset M, et al. Chilblain-like acral lesions during the COVID-19 pandemic ("COVID toes"): Histologic, immunofluorescence, and

immunohistochemical study of 17 cases. J Am Acad Dermatol 2020;83(3): 870–5.

23. de Masson A, Bouaziz JD, Sulimovic L, et al. Chilblains is a common cutaneous finding during the COVID-19 pandemic: A retrospective nationwide study from France. J Am Acad Dermatol 2020;83(2):667–70.

24. Freeman EE, McMahon DE, Lipoff JB, et al. Cold and COVID: recurrent pernio during the COVID-19 pandemic. Br J Dermatol 2021. https://doi.org/10.1111/bjd.19894.

25. Hubiche T, Cardot-Leccia N, Le Duff F, et al. Clinical, Laboratory, and Interferon-Alpha Response Characteristics of Patients with Chilblain-like Lesions during the COVID-19 Pandemic. JAMA Dermatol 2020. https://doi.org/10.1001/jamadermatol.2020.4324.

26. Proietti I, Tolino E, Bernardini N, et al. Auricle perniosis as a manifestation of Covid-19 infection. Dermatol Ther 2020;33(6). https://doi.org/10.1111/dth.14089.

27. Le Cleach L, Dousset L, Assier H, et al. Most chilblains observed during the COVID-19 outbreak occur in patients who are negative for COVID-19 on PCR and serology testing. Br J Dermatol 2020. https://doi.org/10.1111/bjd.19377.

28. Freeman EE, McMahon DE, Lipoff JB, et al. The spectrum of COVID-19–associated dermatologic manifestations: An international registry of 716 patients from 31 countries. J Am Acad Dermatol 2020;83(4):1118–29.

29. Fernandez-Nieto D, Jimenez-Cauhe J, Suarez-Valle A, et al. Characterization of acute acral skin lesions in nonhospitalized patients: A case series of 132 patients during the COVID-19 outbreak. J Am Acad Dermatol 2020;83(1):e61–3.

30. Andina D, Noguera-Morel L, Bascuas-Arribas M, et al. Chilblains in children in the setting of COVID-19 pandemic. Pediatr Dermatol 2020;37(3):406–11.

31. Kolivras A, Dehavay F, Delplace D, et al. Coronavirus (COVID-19) infection–induced chilblains: A case report with histopathologic findings. JAAD Case Rep 2020;6(6):489–92.

32. Freeman EE, McMahon DE, Lipoff JB, et al. Pernio-like skin lesions associated with COVID-19: A case series of 318 patients from 8 countries. J Am Acad Dermatol 2020;83(2):486–92.

33. Baeck M, Herman A, Peeters C, et al. Are chilblains a skin expression of COVID-19 microangiopathy? J Thromb Haemost 2020;18(9):2414–5.

34. Navarro L, Andina D, Noguera-Morel L, et al. Dermoscopy features of COVID-19-related chilblains in children and adolescents. J Eur Acad Dermatol Venereol 2020;34(12):e762–4.

35. Piccolo V, Bassi A, Argenziano G, et al. Dermoscopy of chilblain-like lesions during the COVID-19 outbreak: A multicenter study on 10 patients. J Am Acad Dermatol 2020;83(6):1749–51.

36. Marzano AV, Genovese G, Moltrasio C, et al. The clinical spectrum of COVID-19-associated cutaneous manifestations: an Italian multicentre study of 200 adult patients. J Am Acad Dermatol 2021. https://doi.org/10.1016/j.jaad.2021.01.023.

37. McMahon DE, Gallman AE, Hruza GJ, et al. Long COVID in the skin: a registry analysis of COVID-19 dermatological duration. Lancet Infect Dis 2021. https://doi.org/10.1016/s1473-3099(20)30986-5.

38. Orcesi S, La Piana R, Fazzi E. Aicardi-Goutires syndrome. Br Med Bull 2009; 89(1):183–201.

39. Colmenero I, Santonja C, Alonso-Riaño M, et al. SARS-CoV-2 endothelial infection causes COVID-19 chilblains: histopathological, immunohistochemical and

ultrastructural study of seven paediatric cases. Br J Dermatol 2020;183(4): 729–37.

40. Santonja C, Heras F, Núñez L, et al. COVID-19 chilblain-like lesion: immunohistochemical demonstration of SARS-CoV-2 spike protein in blood vessel endothelium and sweat gland epithelium in a polymerase chain reaction-negative patient. Br J Dermatol 2020;183(4):778–80.

41. Gambichler T, Reuther J, Stücker M, et al. SARS-CoV-2 spike protein is present in both endothelial and eccrine cells of a chilblain-like skin lesion. J Eur Acad Dermatol Venereol 2021;35(3):e187–9.

42. Ko CJ, Harigopal M, Damsky W, et al. Perniosis during the COVID-19 pandemic: Negative anti-SARS-CoV-2 immunohistochemistry in six patients and comparison to perniosis before the emergence of SARS-CoV-2. J Cutan Pathol 2020; 47(11):997–1002.

43. Baeck M, Hoton D, Marot L, et al. Chilblains and COVID-19: why SARS-CoV-2 endothelial infection is questioned. Br J Dermatol 2020;183(6):1152–3.

44. Brealey JK, Miller SE. SARS-CoV-2 has not been detected directly by electron microscopy in the endothelium of chilblain lesions. Br J Dermatol 2021; 184(1):186.

45. Bouaziz JD, Duong TA, Jachiet M, et al. Vascular skin symptoms in COVID-19: a French observational study. J Eur Acad Dermatol Venereol 2020;34(9):e451–2.

46. Rodero MP, Crow YJ. Type I interferon–mediated monogenic autoinflammation: The type i interferonopathies, a conceptual overview. J Exp Med 2016;213(12): 2527–38.

47. Papa R, Volpi S, Gattorno M. Monogenetic causes of chilblains, panniculitis and vasculopathy: The Type I interferonopathies. G Ital di Dermatologia e Venereol 2020;155(5):590–8.

48. Aschoff R, Zimmermann N, Beissert S, et al. Type I Interferon Signature in Chilblain-Like Lesions Associated with the COVID-19 Pandemic. Dermatopathology 2020;7(3):57–63.

49. Saeed M. Lupus pathobiology based on genomics. Immunogenetics 2017; 69(1):1–12.

50. Ivashkiv LB, Donlin LT. Regulation of type i interferon responses. Nat Rev Immunol 2014;14(1):36–49.

51. Guarneri C, Venanzi Rullo E, Gallizzi R, et al. Diversity of clinical appearance of cutaneous manifestations in the course of COVID-19. J Eur Acad Dermatol Venereol 2020;34(9):e449–50.

52. Baeck M, Peeters C, Herman A. Chilblains and COVID-19: further evidence against a causal association. J Eur Acad Dermatol Venereol 2021;35(1):e2–3.

53. Colonna C, Genovese G, Monzani NA, et al. Outbreak of chilblain-like acral lesions in children in the metropolitan area of Milan, Italy, during the COVID-19 pandemic. J Am Acad Dermatol 2020;83(3):965–9.

54. Denina M, Pellegrino F, Morotti F, et al. All that glisters is not COVID: Low prevalence of seroconversion against SARS-CoV-2 in a pediatric cohort of patients with chilblain-like lesions. J Am Acad Dermatol 2020;83(6):1751–3.

55. El Hachem M, Diociaiuti A, Concato C, et al. A clinical, histopathological and laboratory study of 19 consecutive Italian paediatric patients with chilblain-like lesions: lights and shadows on the relationship with COVID-19 infection. J Eur Acad Dermatol Venereol 2020;34(11). https://doi.org/10.1111/jdv.16682.

56. Garcia-Lara G, Linares-González L, Ródenas-Herranz T, et al. Chilblain-like lesions in pediatrics dermatological outpatients during the COVID-19 outbreak. Dermatol Ther 2020;33(5). https://doi.org/10.1111/dth.13516.

57. Herman A, Peeters C, Verroken A, et al. Evaluation of Chilblains as a Manifestation of the COVID-19 Pandemic. JAMA Dermatol 2020;156(9):998–1003.

58. Stavert R, Meydani-Korb A, de Leon D, et al. Evaluation of SARS-CoV-2 antibodies in 24 patients presenting with chilblains-like lesions during the COVID-19 pandemic. J Am Acad Dermatol 2020;83(6):1753–5.

59. Roca-Ginés J, Torres-Navarro I, Sánchez-Arráez J, et al. Assessment of Acute Acral Lesions in a Case Series of Children and Adolescents during the COVID-19 Pandemic. JAMA Dermatol 2020;156(9):992–7.

60. Hubiche T, Le Duff F, Chiaverini C, et al. Negative SARS-CoV-2 PCR in patients with chilblain-like lesions. Lancet Infect Dis 2020. https://doi.org/10.1016/s1473-3099(20)30518-1.

61. Papa A, Salzano AM, Di Dato MT, et al. Images in Practice: Painful Cutaneous Vasculitis in a SARS-Cov-2 IgG-Positive Child. Pain Ther 2020;9(2):805–7.

62. Sethuraman N, Jeremiah SS, Ryo A. Interpreting Diagnostic Tests for SARS-CoV-2. JAMA - J Am Med Assoc 2020;323(22):2249–51.

63. Freeman EE, McMahon DE, Hruza GJ, et al. Timing of PCR and antibody testing in patients with COVID-19–associated dermatologic manifestations. J Am Acad Dermatol 2021;84(2):505–7.

64. Ma H, Zeng W, He H, et al. Serum IgA, IgM, and IgG responses in COVID-19. Cell Mol Immunol 2020;17(7):773–5.

65. Robbiani DF, Gaebler C, Muecksch F, et al. Convergent antibody responses to SARS-CoV-2 in convalescent individuals. Nature 2020;584(7821):437–42.

66. Long QX, Liu BZ, Deng HJ, et al. Antibody responses to SARS-CoV-2 in patients with COVID-19. Nat Med 2020;26(6):845–8.

67. Sterlin D, Mathian A, Miyara M, et al. IgA dominates the early neutralizing antibody response to SARS-CoV-2. Sci Transl Med 2021;(577):13.

68. Abreu RB, Clutter EF, Attari S, et al. IgA Responses Following Recurrent Influenza Virus Vaccination. Front Immunol 2020;11:902.

69. Baeck M, Herman A. COVID toes: Where do we stand with the current evidence? Int J Infect Dis 2021;102:53–5.

70. Hadjadj J, Yatim N, Barnabei L, et al. Impaired type I interferon activity and inflammatory responses in severe COVID-19 patients. Science 2020;369(6504):718–24.

71. Meffre E, Iwasaki A. Interferon deficiency can lead to severe COVID. Nature 2020;587(7834):374–6.

72. Magro CM, Mulvey JJ, Laurence J, et al. The differing pathophysiologies that underlie COVID-19-associated perniosis and thrombotic retiform purpura: a case series. Br J Dermatol 2021;184(1):141–50.

73. Park A, Iwasaki A. Type I and Type III Interferons – Induction, Signaling, Evasion, and Application to Combat COVID-19. Cell Host Microbe 2020;27(6):870–8.

74. Lipsker D. A chilblain epidemic during the COVID-19 pandemic. A sign of natural resistance to SARS-CoV-2? Med Hypotheses 2020;144:109959.

75. Battesti G, El Khalifa J, Abdelhedi N, et al. New insights in COVID-19–associated chilblains: A comparative study with chilblain lupus erythematosus. J Am Acad Dermatol 2020;83(4):1219–22.

76. Damsky W, Peterson D, King B. When interferon tiptoes through COVID-19: Pernio-like lesions and their prognostic implications during SARS-CoV-2 infection. J Am Acad Dermatol 2020;83(3):e269–70.

77. Rodríguez-Villa Lario A, Vega-Díez D, González-Cañete M, et al. Histological findings in chilblain lupus-like COVID lesions: in search of an answer to understand their aetiology. J Eur Acad Dermatol Venereol 2020;34(10):e572–4.

78. Sette A, Crotty S. Adaptive immunity to SARS-CoV-2 and COVID-19. Cell 2021; 184(4):861–80.

79. Sekine T, Perez-Potti A, Rivera-Ballesteros O, et al. Robust T Cell Immunity in Convalescent Individuals with Asymptomatic or Mild COVID-19. Cell 2020; 183(1):158–68.e14.

80. Najarian DJ. Morbilliform exanthem associated with COVID-19. JAAD Case Rep 2020;6(6):493–4.

81. Rubio-Muniz CA, Puerta-Peña M, Falkenhain-López D, et al. The broad spectrum of dermatological manifestations in COVID-19: clinical and histopathological features learned from a series of 34 cases. J Eur Acad Dermatol Venereol 2020;34(10):e574–6.

82. Jamshidi P, Hajikhani B, Mirsaeidi M, et al. Skin Manifestations in COVID-19 Patients: Are They Indicators for Disease Severity? A Systematic Review. Front Med 2021;8:634208.

83. Reymundo A, Fernáldez-Bernáldez A, Reolid A, et al. Clinical and histological characterization of late appearance maculopapular eruptions in association with the coronavirus disease 2019. A case series of seven patients. J Eur Acad Dermatol Venereol 2020;34(12):e755–7.

84. Türsen Ü, Türsen B, Lotti T. Cutaneous side-effects of the potential COVID-19 drugs. Dermatol Ther 2020;33(4). https://doi.org/10.1111/dth.13476.

85. Hassan K. Urticaria and angioedema as a prodromal cutaneous manifestation of SARS-CoV-2 (COVID-19) infection. BMJ Case Rep 2020;13(7). https://doi.org/10.1136/bcr-2020-236981.

86. van Damme C, Berlingin E, Saussez S, et al. Acute urticaria with pyrexia as the first manifestations of a COVID-19 infection. J Eur Acad Dermatol Venereol 2020;34(7):e300–1.

87. Quintana-Castanedo L, Feito-Rodríguez M, Valero-López I, et al. Urticarial exanthem as early diagnostic clue for COVID-19 infection. JAAD Case Rep 2020; 6(6):498–9.

88. Imbalzano E, Casciaro M, Quartuccio S, et al. Association between urticaria and virus infections: A systematic review. Allergy Asthma Proc 2016;37(1):18–22.

89. Drago F, Ciccarese G, Gasparini G, et al. Contemporary infectious exanthems: An update. Future Microbiol 2017;12(2):171–93.

90. Marzano AV, Genovese G, Fabbrocini G, et al. Varicella-like exanthem as a specific COVID-19–associated skin manifestation: Multicenter case series of 22 patients. J Am Acad Dermatol 2020;83(1):280–5.

91. Fernandez-Nieto D, Ortega-Quijano D, Jimenez-Cauhe J, et al. Clinical and histological characterization of vesicular COVID-19 rashes: a prospective study in a tertiary care hospital. Clin Exp Dermatol 2020;45(7):872–5.

92. Mahé A, Birckel E, Merklen C, et al. Histology of skin lesions establishes that the vesicular rash associated with COVID-19 is not 'varicella-like. J Eur Acad Dermatol Venereol 2020;34(10):e559–61.

93. Trellu LT, Kaya G, Alberto C, et al. Clinicopathologic Aspects of a Papulovesicular Eruption in a Patient with COVID-19. JAMA Dermatol 2020;156(8):922–4.

94. Jimenez-Cauhe J, Ortega-Quijano D, Carretero-Barrio I, et al. Erythema multiforme-like eruption in patients with COVID-19 infection: clinical and histological findings. Clin Exp Dermatol 2020;45(7):892–5.

95. Gargiulo L, Pavia G, Facheris P, et al. A fatal case of COVID-19 infection presenting with an erythema multiforme-like eruption and fever. Dermatol Ther 2020;33(4). https://doi.org/10.1111/dth.13779.

96. Bapst T, Romano F, Romano F, et al. Special dermatological presentation of pae-diatric multisystem inflammatory syndrome related to COVID-19: Erythema mul-tiforme. BMJ Case Rep 2020;13(6):e236986.

97. Janah H, Zinebi A, Elbenaye J. Atypical erythema multiforme palmar plaques lesions due to Sars-Cov-2. J Eur Acad Dermatol Venereol 2020;34(8):e373–5.

98. De Giorgi V, Recalcati S, Jia Z, et al. Cutaneous manifestations related to coro-navirus disease 2019 (COVID-19): A prospective study from China and Italy. J Am Acad Dermatol 2020;83(2):674–5.

99. Torrelo A, Andina D, Santonja C, et al. Erythema multiforme-like lesions in chil-dren and COVID-19. Pediatr Dermatol 2020;37(3):442–6.

100. Rodríguez-Jiménez P, Chicharro P, De Argila D, et al. Urticaria-like lesions in COVID-19 patients are not really urticaria – a case with clinicopathological cor-relation. J Eur Acad Dermatol Venereol 2020;34(9):e459–60.

101. Kutlu Ö, Metin A. Relative changes in the pattern of diseases presenting in dermatology outpatient clinic in the era of the COVID-19 pandemic. Dermatol Ther 2020;33(6). https://doi.org/10.1111/dth.14096.

102. Merhy R, Sarkis A, Stephan F. Pityriasis rosea as a leading manifestation of COVID-19 infection. J Eur Acad Dermatol Venereol 2020. https://doi.org/10.1111/jdv.17052.

103. Ehsani AH, Nasimi M, Bigdelo Z. Pityriasis rosea as a cutaneous manifestation of COVID-19 infection. J Eur Acad Dermatol Venereol 2020;34(9):e436–7.

104. Dursun R, Temiz SA. The clinics of HHV-6 infection in COVID-19 pandemic: Pity-riasis rosea and Kawasaki disease. Dermatol Ther 2020;33(4). https://doi.org/10.1111/dth.13730.

105. Veraldi S, Spigariolo CB. Pityriasis rosea and COVID-19. J Med Virol 2020. https://doi.org/10.1002/jmv.26679.

106. Veraldi S, Romagnuolo M, Benzecry V. Pityriasis rosea-like eruption revealing COVID-19. Australas J Dermatol 2020. https://doi.org/10.1111/ajd.13504.

107. Martín Enguix D, Salazar Nievas M del C, Martín Romero DT. Pityriasis rosea Gi-bert type rash in an asymptomatic patient that tested positive for COVID-19. Med Clínica (English Ed 2020;155(6):273.

108. Sanchez A, Sohier P, Benghanem S, et al. Digitate Papulosquamous Eruption Associated with Severe Acute Respiratory Syndrome Coronavirus 2 Infection. JAMA Dermatol 2020;156(7):819–20.

109. Drago F, Ciccarese G, Rebora A, et al. Human herpesvirus-6, -7, and Epstein-Barr virus reactivation in pityriasis rosea during COVID-19. J Med Virol 2020. https://doi.org/10.1002/jmv.26549.

110. Welsh E, Cardenas-de la Garza JA, Cuellar-Barboza A, et al. SARS-CoV-2 Spike Protein Positivity in Pityriasis Rosea-like and Urticaria-like Rashes of COVID-19. Br J Dermatol 2021. https://doi.org/10.1111/bjd.19833.

111. Children and COVID-19: State-Level Data Report. Available at: https://services.aap.org/en/pages/2019-novel-coronavirus-covid-19-infections/children-and-covid-19-state-level-data-report/. Accessed May 13, 2021.

112. Assaker R, Colas AE, Julien-Marsollier F, et al. Presenting symptoms of COVID-19 in children: a meta-analysis of published studies. Br J Anaesth 2020;125(3):e330–2.

113. Zimmermann P, Curtis N. Why is COVID-19 less severe in children? A review of the proposed mechanisms underlying the age-related difference in severity of SARS-CoV-2 infections. Arch Dis Child 2020. https://doi.org/10.1136/archdischild-2020-320338.

114. Kilani MM, Odeh MM, Shalabi M, et al. Clinical and laboratory characteristics of SARS-CoV2-infected paediatric patients in Jordan: serial RT-PCR testing until discharge. Paediatr Int Child Health 2021;41(1):83–92.

115. Pousa PA, Mendonça TSC, Oliveira EA, et al. Extrapulmonary manifestations of COVID-19 in children: a comprehensive review and pathophysiological considerations. J Pediatr (Rio J 2021;97(2):116–39.

116. Rekhtman S, Tannenbaum R, Strunk A, et al. Mucocutaneous disease and related clinical characteristics in hospitalized children and adolescents with COVID-19 and multisystem inflammatory syndrome in children. J Am Acad Dermatol 2021;84(2):408–14.

117. Galeotti C, Bayry J. Autoimmune and inflammatory diseases following COVID-19. Nat Rev Rheumatol 2020;16(8):413–4.

118. Verdoni L, Mazza A, Gervasoni A, et al. An outbreak of severe Kawasaki-like disease at the Italian epicentre of the SARS-CoV-2 epidemic: an observational cohort study. Lancet 2020;395:1771–8.

119. Feldstein LR, Tenforde MW, Friedman KG, et al. Characteristics and Outcomes of US Children and Adolescents with Multisystem Inflammatory Syndrome in Children (MIS-C) Compared with Severe Acute COVID-19. JAMA - J Am Med Assoc 2021;325(11):1074–87.

120. Information for Healthcare Providers about Multisystem Inflammatory Syndrome in Children (MIS-C) | CDC. Available at: https://www.cdc.gov/mis-c/hcp/. Accessed May 13, 2021.

121. Multisystem Inflammatory Syndrome in Children (MIS-C) | CDC. Available at: https://www.cdc.gov/mis-c/. Accessed May 13, 2021.

122. Yasuhara J, Watanabe K, Takagi H, et al. COVID-19 and multisystem inflammatory syndrome in children: A systematic review and meta-analysis. Pediatr Pulmonol 2021;56(5):837–48.

123. Yonker LM, Neilan AM, Bartsch Y, et al. Pediatric Severe Acute Respiratory Syndrome Coronavirus 2 (SARS-CoV-2): Clinical Presentation, Infectivity, and Immune Responses. J Pediatr 2020;227:45–52.e5.

124. Roe K. A viral infection explanation for Kawasaki disease in general and for COVID-19 virus-related Kawasaki disease symptoms. Inflammopharmacology 2020;28(5):1219–22.

125. Multisystem Inflammatory Syndrome in Children in the United States. N Engl J Med 2020;383(18):1793–6.

126. Young TK, Shaw KS, Shah JK, et al. Mucocutaneous Manifestations of Multisystem Inflammatory Syndrome in Children during the COVID-19 Pandemic. JAMA Dermatol 2020. https://doi.org/10.1001/jamadermatol.2020.4779.

127. Whittaker E, Bamford A, Kenny J, et al. Clinical Characteristics of 58 Children with a Pediatric Inflammatory Multisystem Syndrome Temporally Associated with SARS-CoV-2. J Am Med Assoc 2020;324(3):259–69.

128. Shaigany S, Gnirke M, Guttmann A, et al. An adult with Kawasaki-like multisystem inflammatory syndrome associated with COVID-19. Lancet 2020; 396(10246):e8–10.

129. Morris SB, Schwartz NG, Patel P, et al. Morbidity and Mortality Weekly Report Case Series of Multisystem Inflammatory Syndrome in Adults Associated with SARS-CoV-2 Infection-United Kingdom and United States. 2020. Available at: https://www.cdc.gov/mis-c/pdfs/hcp/mis-c-form-fillable.pdf. Accessed May 13, 2021.

130. Feldstein LR, Rose EB, Horwitz SM, et al. Multisystem Inflammatory Syndrome in U.S. Children and Adolescents. N Engl J Med 2020;383(4):334–46.

131. Ahmed M, Advani S, Moreira A, et al. Multisystem inflammatory syndrome in children: A systematic review. EClinicalMedicine 2020;26. https://doi.org/10.1016/j.eclinm.2020.100527.
132. Joob B, Wiwanitkit V. COVID-19 can present with a rash and be mistaken for dengue. J Am Acad Dermatol 2020;82(5):e177.
133. McGrath A, Barrett MJ. Petechiae 2020.
134. Askin O, Altunkalem RN, Altinisik DD, et al. Cutaneous manifestations in hospitalized patients diagnosed as COVID-19. Dermatol Ther 2020;33(6). https://doi.org/10.1111/dth.13896.
135. Karaca Z, Yayli S, Çalışkan O. A unilateral purpuric rash in a patient with COVID-19 infection. Dermatol Ther 2020;33(4). https://doi.org/10.1111/dth.13798.
136. Silva DHM, Oppenheimer AR, Cunha T do AC. Purpuric rash on the legs of a patient with coronavirus disease. Rev Soc Bras Med Trop 2020;53:e20200464.
137. Negrini S, Guadagno A, Greco M, et al. An unusual case of bullous haemorrhagic vasculitis in a COVID-19 patient. J Eur Acad Dermatol Venereol 2020;34(11):e675–6.
138. Suso AS, Mon C, Oñate Alonso I, et al. IgA Vasculitis With Nephritis (Henoch—Schönlein Purpura) in a COVID-19 Patient. Kidney Int Rep 2020;5(11):2074–8.
139. AlGhoozi DA, AlKhayyat HM. A child with Henoch-Schonlein purpura secondary to a COVID-19 infection. BMJ Case Rep 2021;14(1). https://doi.org/10.1136/bcr-2020-239910.
140. Jacobi M, Lancrei HM, Brosh-Nissimov T, et al. Purpurona: A Novel Report of COVID-19-Related Henoch-Schonlein Purpura in a Child. Pediatr Infect Dis J 2021;40(2):e93–4.
141. García-Gil MF, Monte Serrano J, Lapeña-Casado A, et al. Livedo reticularis and acrocyanosis as late manifestations of COVID-19 in two cases with familial aggregation. Potential pathogenic role of complement (C4c). Int J Dermatol 2020;59(12):1549–51.
142. Khalil S, Hinds BR, Manalo IF, et al. Livedo reticularis as a presenting sign of severe acute respiratory syndrome coronavirus 2 infection. JAAD Case Rep 2020;6(9):871–4.
143. Manalo IF, Smith MK, Cheeley J, et al. A dermatologic manifestation of COVID-19: Transient livedo reticularis. J Am Acad Dermatol 2020;83(2):700.
144. Magro C, Mulvey JJ, Berlin D, et al. Complement associated microvascular injury and thrombosis in the pathogenesis of severe COVID-19 infection: A report of five cases. Transl Res 2020;220:1–13.
145. Bosch-Amate X, Giavedoni P, Podlipnik S, et al. Retiform purpura as a dermatological sign of coronavirus disease 2019 (COVID-19) coagulopathy. J Eur Acad Dermatol Venereol 2020;34(10):e548–9.
146. Chand S, Rrapi R, Lo JA, et al. Purpuric ulcers associated with COVID-19: A case series. JAAD Case Rep 2021;11:13–9.
147. Tan SW, Tam YC, Oh CC. Skin manifestations of COVID-19: A worldwide review. JAAD Int 2021;2:119–33.
148. Wambier CG, Vaño-Galván S, McCoy J, et al. Androgenetic alopecia in COVID-19: Compared to age-matched epidemiologic studies and hospital outcomes with or without the Gabrin sign. J Am Acad Dermatol 2020;83(6):e453–4.
149. Wambier CG, McCoy J, Goren A. Male balding as a major risk factor for severe COVID-19: A possible role for targeting androgens and transmembrane protease serine 2 to protect vulnerable individuals. J Am Acad Dermatol 2020;83(6):e401–2.
150. Olds H, Liu J, Luk K, et al. Telogen effluvium associated with <scp>COVID</scp>-19 infection. Dermatol Ther 2021;e14761. https://doi.org/10.1111/dth.14761.

151. Domínguez-Santás M, Haya-Martínez L, Fernández-Nieto D, et al. Acute telogen effluvium associated with SARS-CoV-2 infection. Aust J Gen Pract 2020;49. https://doi.org/10.31128/ajgp-covid-32.
152. Brin C, Sohier P, L'honneur AS, et al. An isolated peculiar gianotti-crosti rash in the course of a covid-19 episode. Acta Derm Venereol 2020;100(16):1–2.
153. Chicharro P, Rodríguez-Jiménez P, Muñoz-Aceituno E, et al. SDRIFE-like rash associated with COVID-19, clinicopathological correlation. Australas J Dermatol 2020. https://doi.org/10.1111/ajd.13444.
154. Mahé A, Birckel E, Krieger S, et al. A distinctive skin rash associated with coronavirus disease 2019? J Eur Acad Dermatol Venereol 2020;34(6):e246–7.
155. Boix-Vilanova J, Gracia-Darder I, Saus C, et al. Grover-like skin eruption: another cutaneous manifestation in a COVID-19 patient. Int J Dermatol 2020; 59(10):1290–2.
156. Català A, Galván-Casas C, Carretero-Hernández G, et al. Maculopapular eruptions associated to COVID-19: A subanalysis of the COVID-Piel study. Dermatol Ther 2020;33(6). https://doi.org/10.1111/dth.14170.
157. Holcomb ZE, Hussain S, Huang JT, et al. Reactive Infectious Mucocutaneous Eruption Associated With SARS-CoV-2 Infection. JAMA Dermatol 2021;157(5). https://doi.org/10.1001/jamadermatol.2021.0385.
158. Jimenez-Cauhe J, Ortega-Quijano D, De Perosanz-Lobo D, et al. Enanthem in Patients with COVID-19 and Skin Rash. JAMA Dermatol 2020;156(10):1134–6.
159. Brandini DA, Takamiya AS, Thakkar P, et al. Covid-19 and oral diseases: Crosstalk, synergy or association? Rev Med Virol Published Online 2021. https://doi.org/10.1002/rmv.2226.
160. La Rosa GRM, Libra M, De Pasquale R, et al. Association of Viral Infections With Oral Cavity Lesions: Role of SARS-CoV-2 Infection. Front Med 2021;7. https://doi.org/10.3389/fmed.2020.571214.
161. Falkenhain-López D, Agud-Dios M, Ortiz-Romero PL, et al. COVID-19-related acute genital ulcers. J Eur Acad Dermatol Venereol 2020;34(11):e655–6.
162. Zimmermann P, Curtis N. COVID-19 in Children, Pregnancy and Neonates: A Review of Epidemiologic and Clinical Features. Pediatr Infect Dis J 2020;39(6):469–77.
163. Kamali Aghdam M, Jafari N, Eftekhari K. Novel coronavirus in a 15-day-old neonate with clinical signs of sepsis, a case report. Infect Dis (Auckl) 2020;52(6):427–9.
164. Freeman EE, McMahon DE, Fox LP. Emerging Evidence of the Direct Association Between COVID-19 and Chilblains. JAMA Dermatol 2020. https://doi.org/10.1001/jamadermatol.2020.4937.
165. Visconti A, Bataille V, Rossi N, et al. Diagnostic value of cutaneous manifestation of SARS-CoV-2 infection. Br J Dermatol 2021;(5):184. https://doi.org/10.1111/bjd.19807.
166. Lester JC, Jia JL, Zhang L, et al. Absence of images of skin of colour in publications of COVID-19 skin manifestations. Br J Dermatol 2020;183(3):593–5.

Postscript
Women's Health and the Era After COVID-19

Denisse S. Holcomb, MD[a],*, William F. Rayburn, MD, MBA[b]

KEYWORDS

- COVID-19 • Future • Medical education • Obstetrics & gynecology
- Practice change • Safety • Telehealth • Vaccinations

KEY POINTS

- Disruptive changes from the COVID-19 pandemic has led to a heightened focus on safety in the office, on labor and delivery, and in the operating room.
- Greater utilization of telehealth has gained more acceptance in all aspects of women's health care.
- The lack of pregnant and lactating women enrolled in COVID-19 clinical trials has raised public concerns.
- Virtual meetings are common and have led to significant changes in patient care and education delivery.
- More attention toward marginalized communities and needs of the diverse women's health care workforce will create opportunities for improvement.

You can't solve a problem in the same level that it was created. You have to rise above it to the next level.

—Albert Einstein

INTRODUCTION

This issue of the *Obstetrics and Gynecology Clinics of North America* was planned in 2019 before the emergence of the coronavirus disease 2019 (COVID-19) in December 2019 in the Hubei Province, China.[1] As COVID-19 was declared a pandemic by the World Health Organization on March 11, 2020, health care systems were required to rapidly adapt given safety concerns for both patients and health care personnel. In the field of obstetrics and gynecology, these concerns led to the postponement of well-women visits, adjustments of the prenatal and postpartum visit schedule, implementation of telehealth visits, cancellation of elective gynecologic surgeries, patient symptom prescreening before visits, and other adaptations.[2–4]

This article previously appeared in *Obstetrics and Gynecology Clinics*, Volume 48, Issue 4, December 2021.

[a] Department of Obstetrics and Gynecology, University of Texas Southwestern Center, Dallas, TX, USA; [b] Department of Obstetrics and Gynecology, University of New Mexico School of Medicine, Albuquerque, NM, USA

* Corresponding author. 5939 Harry Hines Boulevard, Dallas, TX 75390.

E-mail address: denisse.holcomb@utsouthwestern.edu

Clinics Collections 12 (2022) 285–293
https://doi.org/10.1016/j.ccol.2021.12.020
2352-7986/22/© 2021 Elsevier Inc. All rights reserved.

In response to changes resulting from the pandemic, the authors elected to end this issue with a commentary on lessons learned that may impact the future of our specialty. We do not claim to be experts, but we did endure this experience while providing patient care. Preparing this postscript created an opportunity to reflect, add perspective, and begin to navigate several directions from this experience that would affect the future of our practices.

CHANGES IN OUTPATIENT SETTINGS
Abbreviating the Prenatal Schedule

Precautions about minimizing direct exposure to potentially infected patients prompted a reevaluation of the conventional prenatal visit schedule comprised of 12 to 14 visits.[3,5,6] Throughout the country, obstetricians have adopted either abbreviated or hybrid schedules, comprised of both in-person and telehealth visits. This pandemic-shifted paradigm from the traditional prenatal schedule has been endorsed by American College of Obstetricians and Gynecologists (ACOG). Although a revision of this standard prenatal schedule has long been overdue and supported by numerous studies, it took a worldwide pandemic to prompt change.[7–9] Since implementation, many groups have documented patient support of these changes. As society continues to conform to decreased in-person visits, it is difficult to imagine a world where this is reverted following the COVID-19 pandemic. The authors anticipate that this rightsizing of maternity care will continue in the postpartum period that may extend to a 12-month period.

Telehealth

In response to COVID-19, obstetrician and gynecologist (ob-gyn) practices rapidly adapted by quickly implementing telehealth visits. Publication of the *Obstetrics and Gynecology Clinics of North America* issue pertaining to telehealth in obstetrics and gynecology (Telemedicine and Connected Health in Obstetrics and Gynecology, *Obstet Gynecol Clin*, volume 42.2, June 2020) was well timed. Interim measures by the Centers for Medicare and Medicaid Services (CMS) and the Department of Health and Human Services helped decrease barriers to the speedy adoption of telehealth services.[10,11] Physicians suddenly found themselves able to see new patients via telehealth, provide audio-only visits when most convenient to patients, get reimbursed for these visits at the same rates as in-person visits, and see patients across state lines without barriers.[11,12] Longer-term policies adopted by CMS and across all payors will be essential to allow this improved access to care and thus help reduce travel, especially from rural locations.

Outpatient Gynecology

As the pandemic commenced in the United States, attention focused on limiting outpatient clinic visits. Gynecologists quickly had to consider how to prevent barriers to contraception in this new paradigm. ACOG quickly provided guidance on the use of telehealth visits for contraceptive counseling and prescribing; they also recommended filling contraceptives for a full year and to consider proactively prescribing emergency contraception to those patients that desired it.[4] ACOG also recommended that long acting reversible contraception (LARC) methods continue to be offered. It remains to be seen what the long-term effects of such strategies are.

Mental Health

The COVID-19 pandemic has had a great impact on patients in myriad ways. Social isolation, economic hardship, limited resources, uncertainty of the future, and illness or even death of close family members are all factors that have contributed to the nearly 3-fold higher prevalence of depression symptoms noted in the United States as compared with the pre-COVID era.[13] As we continue to move past this pandemic, we must remember to address both the physical and the emotional needs of our patients to improve recognition of potential mental illness. Health care systems and professional organizations will need to come up with innovative ways to increase access to mental health resources for all patients in order to meet the increasing demand.

CHANGES IN HOSPITAL SETTINGS
Labor and Delivery

The labor and delivery (L&D) unit is the most frequent site for direct hospitalization in obstetrics. As L&Ds throughout the country struggled to keep up with steady obstetric volumes despite quarantine efforts and social distancing mandates, attention was directed at maintaining a safe environment for both patients and hospital personnel. From employee and patient screening efforts, use of personal protection equipment (PPE) for hospital personnel, universal mask mandates for patients and visitors, and universal COVID-19 testing for patients in labor, we have learned a great deal about infectious disease transmission best practices.[14,15] Those practices developed during the past 2 years will continue in some ways. Visitors will likely continue to be limited, and some form of universal infection screening will persist despite many persons being asymptomatic. Vigilant use of PPE, performance of frequent handwashing, and universal precautions will likely continue more than before the pandemic.

Gynecology

The COVID-19 pandemic led to recommendations that nonemergent elective medical and surgical services be canceled or delayed, to reduce exposures and allow for preservation of PPE for emergency procedures.[16,17] National guidance prompted hospitals to adopt universal preoperative COVID-19 testing to allow for extra protective measures used during aerosolizing procedures in the event of COVID-19 exposure. As the number of cases slowly declined and PPE manufacturing continued to improve, resumption of elective surgical procedures commenced. We expect an uptick of gynecologic cases as patients return to their gynecologists. As we move forward past this pandemic, we suspect that presurgical screening for infectious disease will remain.

MEDICAL EDUCATION

The COVID-19 pandemic has dramatically impacted the educational experience for trainees at all levels. For medical students, opportunities for direct patient care were placed at a standstill to preserve precious PPE.[18] Didactic sessions became virtual (live or recorded), and small group teaching was limited because of the absence of patient assignments. An assessment from this lack of direct patient contact will be necessary to determine whether a student's knowledge base was undermined as a result. The interview process for students applying for obstetrics and gynecology residencies was converted to virtual experiences to reduce exposure to potentially infected individuals. As the COVID-19 pandemic recedes, we should consider whether residency interviews should remain virtual, given its advantages, such as reduced cost and decreased time away from elective courses.

The importance of resident and fellow safety, supervision, and work hour requirements will continue to be closely scrutinized.[19] Lessons were learned from the COVID-19 experience about team building and interprofessional education. Any impact on suspending normal block rotations and deploying residents and fellows to cover obstetric services and urgent gynecologic cases will warrant examination. Close attention will need to be paid to the impact of suspending elective surgical procedures on resident surgical experience and education. As graduating residents join practices, postgraduate training workshops and seminars in addition to targeted mentorship programs may help provide support for this cohort of obstetrician/gynecologists as they enter the workforce.

Virtual conferences, rather than onsite regional or national meetings, are likely to remain as a popular option. Some hybrids of virtual learning (synchronous and asynchronous) with in-person teaching will be necessary, bringing both benefits and challenges. The mode of delivery will depend on the educational activity to address the practical needs of learners to better close their knowledge gap and improve their performance. Furthermore, special attention should be paid to provide training in telemedicine for trainees of all levels, as this is most likely to remain substantial means of health care delivery.[20]

Although unclear at this time, it will be interesting to discover how the American Board of Obstetrics and Gynecology will alter its approach to certification and recertification of graduating ob-gyn residents and those in practice. Whether the COVID-19 pandemic will affect the timing and administration of written and oral examinations and collection of cases remains to be seen. The requirement of answering questions pertaining to select medical journal articles will probably remain a popular means of focused learning at the home or office for continuing education credit.

RESEARCH
Research in Women's Health

Viral infection outbreaks from the HIV, Zika, and COVID-19 prompted needs for immediate and long-term research that impacted women's health. More unique to the coronavirus pandemic was social distancing, with many research activities being suspended early.[21] Reduced productivity was seen. Research meetings became mostly virtual, and many national scientific organizations either canceled their in-person meetings or replaced them with virtual meetings. As we move past this pandemic, it is likely that virtual meetings as a mode for data exchange will persist. Furthermore, lessons were learned during COVID-19 about the need for research practices to be prompter and more nationwide.

Coronavirus 2019 Vaccination Trials

The COVID-19 pandemic shed light on the everyday exclusion of pregnant and lactating women in clinical trials of therapeutics and vaccines, prompting uncertainty in counseling patients.[22] At the time of publication, Whitehead and Walker[22] reported nearly universal exclusion of pregnant women from more than 300 trials for COVID-19 treatments. Even before this pandemic, infectious diseases like Zika and HIV virus have placed the practice of excluding pregnant women into question.[23] In 2016, the Task Force on Research Specific to Pregnant Women and Lactating Women provided a proactive protocol to allow for the safe inclusion of pregnant and breastfeeding women in clinical trials.[24] Several years later, this pandemic has provided us with yet another example of the consequences of such exclusions.

As numerous pharmaceutical companies early in the pandemic joined the race for COVID-19 vaccination Food and Drug Administration (FDA) authorization, it became clear that pregnant and lactating women were being excluded. Despite the paucity of data on the current FDA-authorized vaccines available, ACOG, the Society for Maternal Fetal Medicine, and the Centers for Disease Control and Prevention (CDC) recommended that the COVID-19 vaccines not be withheld from pregnant or lactating women who meet criteria for vaccination based on the Advisory Council for Immunization Practices recommendations.[25,26] Minimal data from animal studies on messenger RNA vaccines and inadvertently vaccinated pregnant people have demonstrated no harmful effects.[27,28] Since the FDA began to issue emergency use authorizations to pharmaceutical companies for COVID-19 vaccines,[28,29] we have had to counsel our patients through a process of shared decision making, citing the limited data available as well as the science basis for vaccine efficacy and potential harms of being infected during pregnancy. As the Pfizer COVID-19 vaccine undertakes a global clinical trial on pregnant women in the upcoming year, perhaps other drug companies will follow suit.[30]

SERVICE TO AT-RISK AND MARGINALIZED COMMUNITIES

Responses during the COVID-19 crisis affected all communities, particularly those already experiencing structural, societal, economic, and health inequities. From the onset of the pandemic, health disparities were noted for those locations that reported data on race and ethnicity, with African Americans and Latinos carrying a disproportionate burden of adverse outcomes.[31] Reasons for these inequalities are likely multifaceted, including social determinants of health, racism, discrimination, economic disadvantages, health care access, and preexisting comorbidities.[32]

Interest in diversity, equity, and inclusiveness has accelerated a culture of belongingness and inclusiveness over the past 2 years. The pandemic should encourage the development of government-sponsored registries in the collection, evaluation, and reporting of COVID-19–specific data, including race and ethnicity. These data would aid in understanding of whether infection-induced morbidity and mortality relate to economic or racial inequities in maternal health access, preventive services including contraception, and health outcomes. Planning and prioritization of resources can thus result from evaluating crisis responses on marginalized communities. Innovative solutions to promote the health of incarcerated, emotionally challenged, or homeless people and to avoid suspension of medically inappropriate restrictions may arise from the COVID-19 experience.

INVESTING IN THE WOMEN'S HEALTH WORKFORCE

Like all physicians, particularly those who were procedure based, ob-gyns had reductions in revenue production as elective surgeries, office visits, and staff availability declined early during the pandemic.[33] New and existing financial relief programs are important and require periodic examination.[34] Medicaid physicians need support through appropriate reimbursement, including maternity care and participation by all willing and qualified providers. Equitable reimbursement and coverage are necessary to scale-up ob-gyn's telehealth use for essential health services, such as prenatal and postpartum physical and mental health services.

Expansion of physician license portability and multistate licensure privileges would be appropriate to consider more seriously. Liability of health care professionals needed to be protected in providing services within the scope of authority under COVID-19 emergency. This could expand to other conditions and circumstances associated with the public health emergencies.[35] As safer working conditions continue, protection from retaliation for reporting unsafe practices are necessary to support health care professionals.

The pandemic has weighed emotionally on most health care workers throughout the country. Long work hours, PPE shortages, increased patient deaths in hospitals, fear of infecting loved ones, and decisions on reallocation of health resources have contributed to psychological stressors that all physicians have faced.[36] As we move past this pandemic, we must remember to address what our workforce has endured to allow for rebuilding and healing. Education on psychosocial issues during COVID-19 should be provided to not only patients but also health care workers by professional organizations and health systems alike.

Obstetrics and gynecology has the highest proportion of female physicians. The COVID-19 pandemic has further impacted the balance of household duties and childcare that disproportionately fall on female health care professionals compared with their male colleagues. This was particularly pronounced when the country's K-12 education was largely accessible only through virtual learning at home.[37] The stress of advancing professionally and practicing, while attempting to meet the emotional and educational needs of their children, created significant professional and personal conflicts and impacted further on any burnout. For ob-gyn faculty, an understanding and the support from their department chairs and division directors are necessary in making accommodations to ensure an appropriate work-life balance that does not significantly derail academic career development.[38,39] An opportunity exists for academic and community departments of obstetrics and gynecology to take a lead in developing innovative strategies and serve as role models to handle these fundamental changes now and in the future.

ETHICAL CONSIDERATIONS

As the COVID-19 pandemic evolved, ob-gyns faced numerous ethical questions related to how they would practice within the social and political confines of our country. Early on, patients often received conflicting information about the coronavirus and would turn to their physicians for further guidance. Physicians, in turn, had to quickly modify their existing patient care infrastructures to meet the demands of a newly evolving pandemic. Even when expert opinion and guidance were provided from the CDC, there still existed a lack of information on how to optimize patient care in the context of COVID-19.

Box 1
Ethical questions affecting obstetricians and gynecologists during the COVID-19 pandemic

How can ob-gyns navigate the competing interests of providing the best care for individual patients with the responsibility of safeguarding public health?

What principles can help health care systems allocate limited health care resources?

What are the ethical considerations and implications of postponing nonurgent surgical procedures and clinic visits?

What are the ethical considerations associated with caring for patients without adequate PPE available?

How can ob-gyns maintain rapport with patients through telehealth?

What are ethical considerations regarding enrolling pregnant patients in vaccinations trials for COVID-19?

What are ethical considerations in caring for patients who refuse preprocedure COVID-19 testing?

Data from American College of Obstetricians and Gynecologists. COVID-19 FAQs for obstetricians-gynecologists, ethics. Washington, DC: ACOG; 2020.

This rapidly evolving situation led to the development of protocols that attempted to meet the health care needs of patients. Frequently ethical dilemmas were also encountered. Examples of frequently asked questions to ACOG, as shown in **Box 1**, required frequent updated responses.[40] As we move past the COVID-19 pandemic, ob-gyns will have gained knowledge on how to balance patient care and public safety simultaneously. We will also feel better prepared to respond to such ethical dilemmas that may be encountered in future public health emergencies.

SUMMARY

Despite the challenges faced by women's health care communities during the COVID-19 pandemic, we will continue to meet the needs of our patients and families. Every health care organization faces crises at one time or another, but the ones who weather them best have a clear sense of mission, have strong leadership in place, and communicate regularly with staff, patients, and the community throughout the pandemic. As a second year of transition draws to a close, we encourage you and your health care team to take the opportunity to pause, reflect, and appreciate the important contributions you have made. A commitment to change during and after this shift to a "new normal" will require outcome measures. Lessons learned from this pandemic in patient care, medical education, technology and clinical research, marginalized communities, and our workforce will serve us in accelerating efforts to provide high-quality care to our patients and fulfillment to our profession.

DISCLOSURE

The authors have no financial disclosures or conflicts of interest to report.

REFERENCES

1. World Health Organization. Timeline: WHO's COVID-19 response. Available at: https://www.who.int/emergencies/diseases/novel-coronavirus-2019/interactive-timeline/#!. Accessed February 28, 2021.
2. American College of Obstetricians and Gynecologists. Novel coronavirus 2019 (COVID-19) practice advisory. Available at: https://www.acog.org/clinical/clinical-guidance/practice-advisory/articles/2020/03/novel-coronavirus-2019. Accessed February 28, 2021.
3. American College of Obstetricians and Gynecologists. COVID-19 FAQs for obstetrician-gynecologists, obstetrics. Available at: https://www.acog.org/clinical-information/physician-faqs/covid-19-faqs-for-ob-gyns-obstetrics. Accessed February 24, 2021.
4. American College of Obstetricians and Gynecologists. COVID-19 FAQs for obstetrician-gynecologists, gynecology. Available at: https://www.acog.org/clinical-information/physician-faqs/covid19-faqs-for-ob-gyns-gynecology. Accessed February 24, 2021.
5. Peahl AF, Smith RD, Moniz MH. Prenatal care redesign: creating flexible maternity care models through virtual care. Am J Obstet Gynecol 2020;223(3):389.e1–10.
6. Duzyj CM, Thornburg LL, Han CS. Practice modification for pandemics. Obstet Gynecol 2020;136(2):237–51.
7. Peahl AF, Heisler M, Essenmacher LK, et al. A comparison of international prenatal care guidelines for low-risk women to inform high-value care. Am J Obstet Gynecol 2020;222:505–7.

8. Dowswell T, Carroli G, Duley L, et al. Alternative versus standard packages of antenatal care for low-risk pregnancy. Cochrane Database Syst Rev 2015; 2015:CD000934.

9. Butler Tobah YS, LeBlanc A, Branda ME, et al. Randomized comparison of a reduced-visit prenatal care model enhanced with remote monitoring. Am J Obstet Gynecol 2019;221:638. e1-8.

10. Centers for Medicare & Medicaid Services. Medicare telemedicine health care provider fact sheet. Available at: https://www.cms.gov/newsroom/fact-sheets/medicare-telemedicine-health-care-provider-fact-sheet. Accessed February 23, 2021.

11. U.S. Department of Health and Human Services Office for Civil Rights (OCR). Notification of enforcement discretion for telehealth remote communications during the COVID-19 nationwide public health emergency. Available at: https://www.hhs.gov/hipaa/for-professionals/special-topics/emergency-preparedness/notification-enforcement-discretion-telehealth/index.html. Accessed February 23, 2021.

12. Wosik J, Fudim M, Cameron B, et al. Telehealth transformation: COVID-19 and the rise of virtual care. J Am Med Inform Assoc 2020;27(6):957–62.

13. Ettman CK, Abdalla SM, Cohen GH, et al. Prevalence of depression symptoms in US adults before and during the COVID-19 pandemic. JAMA Netw Open 2020; 3(9):e2019686.

14. Sutton D, Fuchs K, D'Alton M, et al. Universal screening for SARS-CoV-2 in women admitted for delivery. N Engl J Med 2020;382:2163–4.

15. Jamieson DJ, Steinberg JP, Martinello RA, et al. Obstetricians on the coronavirus disease 2019 (COVID-19) front lines and the confusing world of personal protective equipment. Obstet Gynecol 2020;135:1257–63.

16. CMS. Non-emergent, elective medical services, and treatment recommendations. Available at: https://www.cms.gov/files/document/cms-non-emergent-elective-medical-recommendations.pdf. Accessed February 25, 2021.

17. American College of Surgeons Joint statement: road map for resuming elective surgery after COVID-19 pandemic. Available at: https://www.facs.org/covid-19/clinical-guidance/roadmap-elective-surgery. Accessed February 25, 2021.

18. Rose S. Medical student education in the time of COVID-19. JAMA 2020;323(21): 2131–2.

19. Accreditation Council for Graduate Medical Education. ACGME resident/fellow education and training considerations related to coronavirus (COVID-19). Available at: https://www.acgme.org/Newsroom/Newsroom-Details/ArticleID/10085/ACGME-Resident-Fellow-Education-and-Training-Considerations-related-to-Coronavirus-COVID-19. Accessed February 28, 2021.

20. Edirippulige S, Armfield NR. Education and training to support the use of clinical telehealth: a review of the literature. J Telemed Telecare 2017;23(2):273–82.

21. Alvarez RD, Goff BA, Chelmow D, et al. Reengineering academic departments of obstetrics and gynecology to operate in a pandemic world and beyond: a joint American Gynecological and Obstetrical Society and Council of University Chairs of Obstetrics and Gynecology statement. Am J Obstet Gynecol 2020;223:383–8.

22. Whitehead CL, Walker SP. Consider pregnancy in COVID-19 therapeutic drug and vaccine trials. Lancet 2020;395(10237):e92.

23. Cohen J. Zika rewrites maternal immunization ethics. Science 2017; 357(6348):241.

24. Eunice Kennedy Shriver National Institute of Child Health and Human Development. Task force on research specific to pregnant women and lactating women

(PRGLAC). December 29. 2020. Available at: https://www.nichd.nih.gov/about/advisory/PRGLAC. Accessed February 24, 2021.

25. Centers for Disease Control and Prevention. Vaccination considerations for people who are pregnant or breastfeeding. Available at: https://www-cdc-gov.libproxy.unm.edu/coronavirus/2019-ncov/vaccines/recommendations/pregnancy.html. Accessed February 20, 2021.

26. American College of Obstetricians and Gynecologists. Practice advisory. Vaccinating pregnant and lactating patients against COVID-19. Available at: https://www.acog.org/clinical/clinical-guidance/practice-advisory/articles/2020/12/vaccinating-pregnant-and-lactating-patients-against-covid-19. Accessed February 27, 2021.

27. Dashraath P, Nielsen-Saines K, Madhi SA, et al. COVID-19 vaccines and neglected pregnancy. Lancet 2020;396(10252):e22.

28. FDA. Emergency use authorization (EUA). Pfizer-BioNTech COVID-19 vaccine/BNT162b2. Available at: https://www-fda-gov.libproxy.unm.edu/emergency-preparedness-and-response/coronavirus-disease-2019-covid-19/pfizer-biontech-covid-19-vaccine. Accessed February 25, 2021.

29. Emergency Use Authorization (EUA). Moderna COVID-19 vaccine/mRNA-1273. Available at: https://www-fda-gov.libproxy.unm.edu/emergency-preparedness-and-response/coronavirus-disease-2019-covid-19/moderna-covid-19-vaccine. Accessed February 25, 2021.

30. Pfizer. Pfizer and Biontech commence global clinical trial to evaluate COVID-19 vaccine in pregnant women. Available at: https://www.pfizer.com/news/press-release/press-release-detail/pfizer-and-biontech-commence-global-clinical-trial-evaluate. Accessed February 28, 2021.

31. Webb Hooper M, Nápoles AM, Pérez-Stable EJ. COVID-19 and racial/ethnic disparities. JAMA 2020 23;323(24):2466–7.

32. Yancy CW. COVID-19 and African Americans. JAMA 2020;323(19):1891–2.

33. Rubin R. COVID-19's crushing effects on medical practices, some of which might not survive. JAMA 2020;324(4):321–3.

34. American College of Obstetricians and Gynecologists. Financial support for physicians and practices during the COVID-19 pandemic. Available at: https://www.acog.org/practice-management/payment-resources/resources/financial-support-for-physicians-and-practices-during-the-covid-19-pandemic. Accessed February 28, 2021.

35. CMS. COVID-19 emergency declaration blanket waivers for health care providers. Available at: https://www.cms.gov/files/document/summary-covid-19-emergency-declaration-waivers.pdf. Accessed February 28, 2021.

36. Pfefferbaum B, North CS. Mental health and the Covid-19 pandemic. N Engl J Med 2020;383(6):510–2.

37. Black E, Ferdig R, Thompson LA. K-12 virtual schooling, COVID-19, and student success. JAMA Pediatr 2021;175(2):119–20.

38. Gabster BP, van Daalen K, Khatt R, et al. Challenges for the female academic during the COVID-19 pandemic. Lancet 2020;395:1968–70.

39. Brubaker L. Women physicians and the COVID-19 pandemic. JAMA 2020;324:835–6.

40. American College of Obstetricians and Gynecologists. COVID-19 FAQs for obstetricians-gynecologists, ethics. Washington, DC: ACOG; 2020. Available at: https://www.acog.org/clinical-information/physician-faqs/covid-19-faqs-for-ob-gyns-ethics. Accessed February 24, 2021.

The Impact of the COVID-19 Pandemic on Breast Imaging

Phoebe E. Freer, MD, FSBI

KEYWORDS

- COVID-19 • Pandemic • Breast cancer • Breast imaging • Delayed care
- Radiology finances

KEY POINTS

- The COVID-19 pandemic starting in the United States in 2020 has had practice-changing effects on cancer care, clinical workflow, education, research, and radiology finances.
- Significant volume reductions and delays occurred to breast imaging, with screening mammography being the hardest hit.
- Long-term outcomes from changes in breast cancer management algorithm during the pandemic are yet to be determined.
- Increased telehealth and telecommuting will likely continue after the pandemic is over in some fashion.
- Radiology practices and hospitals sustained large financial ramifications from the effects of the pandemic.

INITIAL RESPONSE: ROUTINE HEALTH CARE DEFERRED

The approach to the handling of COVID-19 has been fluid, as understanding of the pathophysiology, clinical spectrum and severity of illness, and possible preventions and treatment of the virus have evolved.[1,2]

Early Response: Concerns for Mammography in COVID-19

Shortly after the first outbreaks in the United States on the Diamond Princess Cruise Ship, in Seattle and New York, on the heels of large outbreaks in China and Italy, the main prevention strategy of "social distancing" was adopted by the World Health Organization.[3] By April 2020, 33 states had state mandated "stay-at-home-orders." The Centers for Disease control (CDC) issued recommendations to reschedule nonurgent patient care and delay screenings in an effort to minimize risks to patients and health care workers (HCWs).[4] Although social distancing measures varied regionally,

This article previously appeared in *Radiologic Clinics*, Volume 59, Issue 1, January 2021..
Breast Imaging, Department of Radiology and Imaging Sciences, University of Utah Health / Huntsman Cancer Institute, 30 North 1900 East #1A071, Salt Lake City, UT 84132, USA
E-mail address: Phoebe.Freer@hsc.utah.edu

most of the school systems, churches, and businesses were closed in March or April 2020, often moving to virtual encounters. Leaders in breast imaging and radiology departments discussed the best ways to protect patients, protect HCWs, and conserve personal protective equipment (PPE) and ventilators to be used for patients with COVID-19.[5] Many sites began rescheduling screening mammography patients, some diagnostic or biopsy cases, or even delaying breast surgeries in an ad hoc fashion. Varied interpretations of the CDC, WHO, and the varied state policies led to nonuniform disruptions in patient care, in some cases varying within the same large cities.[6]

On March 24th, news reports of potential danger to mammography technologists from work exposures were released, with a death of a mammography technologist in Georgia from COVID-19, a possible work exposure.[7] HCWs were confirmed to be high risk for COVID-19 infections (up to 10%) from initial data in early outbreaks in China, Italy, and Spain.[8] The *National Comprehensive Cancer Network* (NCCN) issued guidelines for health care worker safety early in the pandemic, based on WHO recommendations.[9] In a study rating different professions' risk of contracting COVID-19 from work, radiology technologists were one of the highest (a score or 84 out of 100), and then sonographers (80 out of 100).[10] Mammography technologists likely have an even higher risk, as they are unable to maintain social distancing (2 m or 6 feet) during positioning.

Quickly, breast radiologists and technologists had palpable concerns regarding the need to protect HCWs and patients during screening, and firm statements were released by national organizations with the American Society of Breast Surgeons (ASBrS) and American College of Radiology (ACR) Joint Statement on Breast Screening Exams During the COVID-19 Pandemic and the Society of Breast Imaging Statement on Breast Imaging during the COVID-19 Pandemic, all released later in March, 2020, and recommending to "postpone all breast screening exams (to include screening mammography, ultrasound, and MRI) effective immediately" as well as to discontinue routine and nonurgent breast health appointments.[11,12]

Moreover, shortages of PPE existed, and so technologist and radiologists could not uniformly be masked, with only 35.3% (60 of 170) of radiology practices stating they had an adequate supply and 29.4% reporting that PPE supplies were low and needed to rationed.[13]

A More Standardized Approach to Deferred Care

By March, the Canadian Society of Breast Imaging and Canadian Association of Radiologists Joint Position Statement on COVID-19 recommended that all screening mammography and MR imaging be deferred for at least 6 to 8 weeks and suggested triaging the diagnostic cases, deferring ones that were not highly suspicious for cancer.[14] The Society of Breast Imaging followed suit with a statement that was broader and less prescriptive but also recommended delaying screening by "several weeks or a few months."[15] Other international societies published similar statements.[16,17]

Multidisciplinary care algorithms changed the management of breast cancer during the pandemic in response to need to balance the urgency of care against the risks to patients and HCWs secondary to potential COVID-19 exposures. Surgeries were postponed both to limit COVID-19 transmission as well as to preserve resources such as ventilators, PPE, and hospital beds. The American College of Surgeons (ACS) and the Society of Surgical Oncology released triage guidelines recommending an interim cancellation of most routine surgeries, while still performing breast surgeries for those in more urgent cases.[18,19] Some centers, such as Magee-Breast Cancer Program and Johns Hopkins published multidisciplinary algorithms of how best to triage patients with breast cancer, broken down by subtypes program.[20,21] Other published tools suggested risk-stratifying patients for breast surgery with the purpose of causing few deleterious effects in patients recommended for postponement.[22]

In early April, a multidisciplinary group of breast cancer experts in the United States formed the COVID-19 Pandemic Breast Cancer Consortium and released its recommendations for prioritization, treatment, and triage of patients with breast cancer during the COVID-19 pandemic. The panel represents a joint collaboration from the ASBrS, the National Accreditation Program for Breast Centers (NAPBC), the NCCN, the Commission on Cancer, and ACR.[23] The main goals of the Consortium recommendations were to "preserve hospital resources for virus-inflicted patients by deferring BC treatments without significantly compromising long-term outcomes for individual BC patients". Patients were placed into categories based on severity of symptoms or illnesses with algorithms for chemotherapy and surgery outlined based on disease process.

REOPENING OF ROUTINE CARE

By July 2020, as the pandemic proved lasting and PPE supplies improved nationwide, consensus guidelines shifted to avoid delays in care and focused instead on how to better protect patients and workers.[24] Leaders in breast cancer made evidence-based pleas to cease labeling patients with cancer as a high-risk population in order to avoid delays in their diagnosis and treatment.[25] Numerous consensus statements and guidelines regarding how to best balance the risks of COVID-19 transmission to patients and HCWs against the risks of delaying care have been published.[26] The European Society for Medical Oncology Guidelines include increasing telehealth appointments (noting in person visits are needed for new patients with cancer or urgent infections/postoperative complications) and specific guidance for management and advised that the risk/benefit balance for most patients favored continued administration of systemic therapies and chemotherapies, with additional precautions when possible (eg, choosing less immunosuppressive therapies, regimens requiring fewer appointments).[25] Numerous other guidance documents have emerged fluidly including from American Society of Clinical Oncology (ASCO) and an online resource from ASCO, and others globally.[17,27–32]

Although the recommendations for the management of breast cancer change the order and timing of breast cancer treatments, the goals have remained to change these algorithms in ways that do not affect long-term outcomes or changes for a cure. For example, surgery should remain the primary option for small triple-negative breast cancers that did not require chemotherapy based on pre-COVID-19 algorithms.[33] In addition, patients with progressive disease on medical therapy should have surgery. Further patients who are competing their neoadjuvant regimens or patients who did not respond to neoadjuvant therapy should receive surgery.[33]

Prophylactic measures were implemented with guidance from the CDC, for protecting patients and HCWs, including social distancing where possible, masking both patients and HCWs, decreasing the number of scheduled patients, increasing space in waiting areas, and implementing disinfection protocols. Nearly all imaging centers implemented preappointment screening for symptoms of COVID-19, most requiring temperature screening at some point during the pandemic and a few even required COVID-19 negative testing before a breast interventional procedure (although many centers required COVID-19 negative testing before breast surgeries).[34]

CHANGES IN FOOD AND DRUG ADMINISTRATION INSPECTIONS DURING COVID-19

Initially, the FDA halted inspections of mammography facilities required by the Mammographic Quality Standards Act in mid-March, 2020. In addition, the ACR granted automatic extensions and halted in-person inspections for sites where accreditation was expiring.[35] As the reopening phase began, the FDA announced that it would restart inspections at facilities in locations that were not as affected by the pandemic on July 20th, although it did not actually start them then. It recommended that state inspections could start based on individual state guidance at the end of June 2020, guided by an advisory system to take into account the extent of the outbreak in that location combined with how critical the inspection would be.[36]

BREAST CANCER AS A COMORBIDITY FOR COVID-19 SEVERE OUTCOMES/ FATALITIES

Initially, concern existed that patients with breast cancer, especially advanced or metastatic breast cancer, may be more susceptible to severe outcomes with COVID-19. Many of the most common chemotherapy regimens used to treat breast cancer are known to cause immunosuppression. Further, patients undergoing cancer care have more visits and therefore more exposures to HCWs and patients, potentially making them more at risk of being infected with COVID-19.[37,38] Initial studies from Wuhan, China showed worse outcomes from COVID-19 in patients with cancer and suggested caution with cancer care during the pandemic.[38–40] In one study of 1524 patients from the Wuhan outbreak, patients with cancer had more than double the risk of contracting COVID-19 than patients without (odds ratio [OR], 2.31; 95% confidence interval [CI], 1.89 to 3.02).[37] In another early study from the Wuhan experience, the relative risk of dying or being admitted to the intensive care unit with COVID-19 in patients with cancer was 5.4 (95% CI 1.8–16.2).[38] Moreover, patients with cancer had a higher relative risk of requiring intubation, across all age ranges.[38] The mortality rate of COVID-19 in patients with cancer has ranged from 11% to 28% in reported studies,[41–43] compared with the 1.4% mortality rate reported in the general population from the initial Wuhan studies.[44] However, not all patients with cancer have the same risks, as a patient with an early stage breast cancer may not have the COVID-19 risks as a patient with end-of-life stage IV breast cancer. This was confirmed by one study of 900 patients with cancer and COVID-19 that found that having active cancer that was progressing (as opposed to remission) and having a worse performance status were associated with increased risk of mortality.[43]

As the pandemic has unfolded, registries for patients with cancer and COVID-19 have been developed in an attempt to better understand the risk to patients with cancer, as initial reports on outcomes were limited to single institutional or smaller studies. An international database was established to study the risks of COVID-19 on patients with cancer from the United States, Canada, and Spain with underlying cancer (the COVID-19 and Cancer Consortium Database or CCC19).[43] And ASCO developed its own registry to be able to share data rapidly and contribute to evidence-based decision-making for patients with cancer during the pandemic.[45]

Initial reports from mid-March through mid-April of the CCC19, including more than 900 patients with cancer (21% breast cancer) and COVID-19 found that although the 30-day all-cause mortality for the entire population with cancer and COVID-19 was high, associated with both general and cancer-specific risk factors, the actual risk in patients with solid tumors (ie, breast cancer) was not significantly higher.[45] This study also confirmed recent cancer surgery did not affect the mortality rate from concurrent infections with COVID-19.[45] A large cohort study of 800 patients with cancer with COVID-19 in the United Kingdom (UK Coronavirus Cancer Monitoring Project), at a similar time frame of the pandemic, found that although the mortality rate was

28%, when adjusted for age and other comorbidities, the presence of cancer alone did not increase the mortality from COVID-19.[46] Importantly, the use of chemotherapy before COVID-19 infection did not affect mortality, neither did the use of hormonal, targeted, and, immune therapies, or radiation.[46]

Thus, although it may be possible that some patients with cancer have a propensity toward worse outcomes with COVID-19, it does not seem likely that cancer treatments such as chemotherapy, hormonal therapy, radiation, and surgery predispose patients to more serious outcomes from COVID-19. If care is taken for protective measures for the patients and HCWs as outlined in different care algorithms, breast cancer treatment should continue during the pandemic, especially in light of the unknown timeframe of the crisis.

EFFECTS OF DELAYING CARE ON PATIENTS WITH BREAST CANCER

Not only did multidisciplinary care algorithms force patients into delaying care during the pandemic but patients also self-selected to delay care. Nearly 4 out of 10 patients said the economic changes from the pandemic affected their ability to pay for medical care.[47] A survey by ACEP demonstrated almost one-third of patients (29%) delayed or avoided going to the emergency room in March/April 2020 in order to avoid COVID-19 exposures.[48] Four out of five patients were fearful of contracting the virus from a patient or HCW if they did go.[48] Greater than 81% of survey participants acknowledged practicing social distancing.[48] In an Italian study, during the height of the outbreak, there was a significant increase in patients refusing to undergo diagnostic appointments and breast biopsies at a major cancer center.[49]

In another 600 breast care patients surveyed, almost 80% stated they had routine and follow-up appointments delayed, two-thirds had reconstruction surgery delayed, and 60% had delayed diagnostic imaging.[50] Therapies that required in-person visits to the hospital (radiation, chemotherapy infusion, and surgical lumpectomies) were more likely to be delayed than those that could be obtained through telehealth appointments or a prescription pick-up.[50] Medicare and Medicaid Services and private insurers expanded telehealth benefits to patients covering increased virtual visits.[51] On average, about 30% of patients experienced delays in the mainstays of breast cancer treatment including lumpectomies, radiation therapy, and chemotherapy.[50] Breast cancer surgeries declined significantly during the early parts of the global pandemic.[52] In data from 55 breast centers in 27 states, it was noted that the average decline in breast surgery clinic appointments over the first few weeks was 21% with a nadir of 40% from baseline and a near 20% decline in new breast cancer surgery consultations in the surgery clinics.[52] Similarly, breast cancer genetics appointments declined, ranging between 25% and 30%.[52] In one study from Wuhan, China, more than half of the patients receiving radiation therapy were unable to complete their regimens during the lockdowns.[53] The pandemic increased the use of neoadjuvant and hormonal therapies before surgery, as well as increased genotypic profiling, secondary to deferrals of surgeries.[21] In another study from the Netherlands one-third of patients noted that the pandemic affected their cancer care, with most of these noting a shift to telehealth consultations.[54] Chemotherapy was also affected in about one-third of these patients.[54]

The long-term physical and psychosocial ramifications of these delays remain to be determined. One study demonstrated that more than half of the patients with cancer were concerned the delays or discontinuation of care during the pandemic affected their outcomes.[54] Oncologic patients noted anxieties regarding whether they were at increased risk of worse outcomes with COVID-19, as well as anger and worry from delays or interruptions in their care during COVID-19. Some patients even stated that the changes in their care encountered sounded "like a death sentence" or made them "feel like my care and health aren't important to you".[55] These patient perceptions, whether accurate or not, will need to be addressed as the pandemic unfolds.[55,56]

The mental health effects of limiting care during this pandemic, and potentially in future crises, on both cancer specialists and patients, who are used to unlimited resources for health care, may be far reaching. Having consensus guidelines to guide fair decision-making and developing empathic communication with regard to these issues is important.[57] Education and shifts in mindsets to prioritize the maximum health benefit for the community over the individual may be necessary in a country used to unlimited resources. Guidelines have been developed for low resource communities that may prove useful.[58,59]

It is unclear what effects these COVID-19 provoked changes in cancer screening and management will have on long-term cancer outcomes. In the United States, an estimated additional 87,001 deaths occurred in March and most of April 2020 compared with the last 6 years, of which 35% (30,755) were not directly attributable to COVID-19 (and in 14 states, >50% of excess deaths frame were not attributable).[60] Almost half (48%) of US people surveyed had a family member who had delayed medical care during the pandemic, with 10% stating that that member's medical condition worsened during the delay.[61] One modeling study of 6281 new stage 1 to 3 cancer cases in the United Kingdom who were delayed multidisciplinary workup during the pandemic suggested that an additional 181 lives and 3316 life years would be lost with a conservative estimate of only 25% of cases backlogged for 2 months.[62]

During the early phases of the pandemic, the number of new cancers diagnosed decreased.[63,64] This drop was likely secondary to patients not presenting for care and not a true drop in incidence. Thus, these cancers will come to the radar eventually at a greater size or stage than they would have with earlier detection, which may affect prognosis. A model that assumed only a 6-month disruption of care during the pandemic estimated the potential excess deaths from breast and colorectal cancer secondary to the pandemic disruptions in care demonstrates an excess of more than 10,000 deaths in the next decade, peaking in the first few years.[65] This model does not account for the increased morbidity, with possible more extensive surgeries including more mastectomies or more need for chemotherapy secondary to later presentations of disease.

Previous studies have demonstrated worsened outcomes during economic downturns, and in times of stress, and so it is likely the effects on breast cancer detection and management combined with the economic and societal effects of the pandemic will lead to effects on long-term outcomes.[66] It is also plausible that if there are not measurable deleterious effects from these delays, then reimbursements for care may be renegotiated or guidelines may shift to reduce care.

EFFECTS ON HOSPITALS AND RADIOLOGISTS OF CHANGES IN CARE

The COVID-19 pandemic has had marked economic effects on the health care system, academic radiology departments, and radiology practices. A survey conducted by ACR and the Radiology Business Management Association reported that 97.4% of 228 radiology practices (urban, academic, and rural) experienced declines in imaging volume in March/April 2020, with a drop of greater than 90% of elective procedures and 60% of urgent procedures.[13] One-third of academic radiology chairs reported a near two-thirds decrease in volume with some reporting an 80% drop in hard hit areas.[34] Greater than 82% of chairs had at least a 50% decrease in total radiology volume at the nadir.[34]

Breast imaging was disproportionately affected by postponed cases. The largest health care system in New York reported a drop of 88% affecting all modality types, with mammography use plummeting by 94%, MR imaging 74%, and ultrasound 64%.[67] In another study of 6 academic medical centers across the United States, 3 centers in regions with lower rates of COVID-19, radiology volumes declined steeply from calendar week 11 to 16 with a range of 40% to 70% total volume drop at the lowest drop.[68] Of those drops, screening mammography was among the most significant drop, as well as slowest in recovering. The reduction in screening mammography went as far as 99% in weeks 15 and 16. Diagnostic mammography volumes did not drop as dramatically, however still hit a low of 85% volume decrease at the nadir in week 16.[68]

On gradual reopenings of care (in May–July in most centers), a significant backlog of past studies had built. In addition, significant changes in scheduling with increased evening or weekend hours, changes in protocols for shorter MR imaging scan times,[68] and off-loading studies from hospitals and cancer centers to protect higher risk patients were required to allow for more spacing. Changes to patient registration and check-in, prescreening for symptoms, PPE requirements, and disinfection protocols were instituted briskly. One hundred percent of academic radiology departments reported reorganizing the waiting rooms and dressing areas to comply with social distancing mandates.[34]

Radiology practices restructured reading rooms and implemented home PACS. Some practices shifted rapidly to home PACS, moving from100% of radiologists onsite to 80% reading from home within a few weeks.[69] However, for breast imaging, this process is more complicated and expensive due to quality compliance requirements, the need for high-resolution monitors, and the need to be on site for diagnostic and interventions and happened at much lower levels. Telehealth increased in general, for patient surgery, oncology, and genetics appointments, as well as for virtual multidisciplinary tumor boards, leading to fewer in person multidisciplinary consults. Educational conferences and lectures moved to virtual platforms such as Webex, Microsoft Teams, and Zoom.[13,70] The effect of increased telecommuting and telehealth remain unclear. Telecommuting may increase radiologist morale, flexibility, and even potentially productivity, or alternatively it may decrease collaborations, interfacing with multidisciplinary colleagues, educational value, or productivity.[71] About half of the radiologists surveyed nationwide believed that teleradiology would continue and lead to increased efficiency.[13]

The marked reductions in volume have devastating financial implications to practices. Half of the health care practices in California furloughed or laid off employees and almost two-thirds reduced staff hours.[61,72] In academic practices, a quarter had furloughed or laid off staff.[34] Significant reductions in radiologist and staff incomes (in about 50% of practices in one survey), personal and academic protected time, research endeavors, workload, hours, professional funds, bonuses and financial incentives, and retirement allocations occurred amid hiring freezes and workspaces changes.[13] In a survey of 228 practices from across the country, there were mean reductions in both receipts and gross charges on average about 50%,[13] and greater than 70% of respondents reported applying for some sort of governmental financial relief. Although emergency governmental funds for financial relief were dispensed to hospitals and health care organizations through The Coronavirus Aid, Relief, and Economic Security Act and the Paycheck Protection Program and Health Care Enhancement Act (on the order of nearly $200 billion dollars), these funds are likely not enough to prevent lasting financial implications from the significant disruptions in volume and care.[73,74] Although practices are recovering, some near fully, as of September 2020, the anticipated time to full recovery remains unknown.

Effects on radiologist's mental health through this crisis have been significant. More than 60% of 600 radiologists in 44 states rated their anxiety as a 7 out of 10 during the pandemic.[75] In addition to having work and economic worries, some radiologists and staff were redeployed in the early days in hotspots to better serve COVID-19 patient care. In addition, many radiologists have had increased burdens at home with unexpected need to provide childcare and teaching duties for virtual schooling amid school and childcare care closures.[76] In addition, more than one-third of radiologists thought that they did not have adequate teleradiology capabilities during the pandemic, and about half said they did not have adequate PPE for themselves or their patients.[75] Mental stress regarding personal and family health, disruptions to travel and schedule, and family members with lost jobs or decreased income also affects the potential for long-term burnout in radiologists to increase, and mitigation strategies for burnout should be used.[77]

DELAYS IN CLINICAL RESEARCH EDUCATION AND ACADEMIC MEETINGS

Radiology education has also been significantly disrupted during the COVID-19 pandemic, including the need for redeployment, changes to reading rooms and social distancing, and cessation of in person conferences and didactic learning.[78] Some radiologists, especially residents early in training, were redeployed to other areas, particularly hard-hit urban environments such as New York and Boston, with some medical students even graduating early to join the front lines in caring for COVID-19–infected patients. Approximately 40% of radiologists in one survey thought that the shift to socially distant interpretations and conferences had a deleterious effect on resident and fellow education.[13]

Hundreds of scientific and medical conferences including dozens of radiology conferences were canceled or moved to virtual formats.[79] Significant impacts on networking, collaboration, committee work, vendor marketing, scientific presentations, and sharing of research are likely that may affect scientific progress as well as career choices.[80] Many radiologists were placed on institutional or state travel bans. Virtual grand rounds and virtual interviews both for education and for hiring were implemented during the pandemic. The cost and time savings of such virtual practices may prove to be practice changing after the pandemic is over.

Initially, most academic centers and universities suspended research, especially all trials involving patients or in-person interactions.[81] Guidance on how best to preserve clinical trials, and maintain integrity for those interrupted, was offered by the senior editorial staff at JAMA.[82] The FDA offered direction for those trials that may be disrupted.[83] Additional suggestions on how to avoid overestimation of disease-free survival if patients skip assessments and to report results from data during the pandemic separately from date before the pandemic continue to be offered.[82,83] In contrast, the National Cancer Institute intentionally kept functioning at 100% and stressed the importance of maintaining research to allow patients to have access to clinical trials and to maintain scientific progress, as well as to study the effects of COVID-19 in patients with cancer.[84] The National Cancer Institute (NCI) showed increased flexibility for prior minor infractions (such tests as a missed blood draw), recognizing that they may be necessary during COVID-19 to help maintain social distancing best practices for the patient. Some of the flexibility extended to clinical trials during the pandemic such as virtual, instead of in-person, visits for enrollment or assessments, the ability to receive tests and laboratory draws at sites closer to the patient that are not part of the trial sites, and decreases in the administrative tasks required prepandemic may carry over to the postpandemic world, perhaps making clinical trials more accessible to the general population.[85]

Of note, the pandemic led to the creation of unique opportunities for the creation of collaborative, crowdsourced research endeavors and databases, including the COVID-19 and Cancer Consortium, among others, collecting real-time data for observational trials.[86]

LONG-TERM RAMIFICATIONS AND REBUILDING

The final economic costs of the pandemic on the health care industry will likely be colossal. One study proposes the direct medical costs will approach $165 billion dollars if only 20% of the population is infected (53.8 million symptomatic cases) and would continue to cost up to a total of almost $215 billion in indirect costs in the year after discharge.[87] This figure will increase if the percent infected increased greater than that. Nationally, there has been significant deleterious effects on the economy including almost 17 million Americans filing for unemployment in a 3-week period over March/April alone, although with claims decreasing continually since that peak.[88,89] Whether or not COVID-19 will continue to circulate in the population with annual or seasonal outbreaks or whether this will be an outbreak that has mostly cycled through the population with a return to closer to normal by 2022 or so remains unclear and debated yet at the time of this writing.

What is clear is that without a vaccine and other treatments, social distancing and PPE with masks and other protections for HCWs are likely to remain the primary weapons against the virus and will likely continue to play a part in daily life and in radiology practices and patient care in breast imaging centers for a while yet to come. What the future looks like on the other side of the pandemic remains unclear but will involve significant effects on both COVID-19– and non-COVID-19–related health outcomes, mental health outcomes, the national and global economy, radiology practices and breast centers, and on cancer outcomes, screening rates, and cancer management and treatment protocols.

REFERENCES

1. Holshue ML, DeBolt C, Lindquist S, et al. First Case of 2019 Novel Coronavirus in the United States. N Engl J Med 2020;382:929–36.
2. Coronavirus Resource Center. Johns Hopkins University School of Medicine. Available at: https://coronavirus.jhu.edu. Accessed September 10, 2020.
3. World Health Organization. Responding to community spread of COVID-19: interim guidance, 7 March 2020. World Health Organization. Available at: https://apps.who.int/iris/handle/10665/331421. Accessed September 10, 2020.
4. Framework for Healthcare Systems Providing Non-COVID-19 Clinical Care During the COVID-19 Pandemic. Available at: https://www.cdc.gov/coronavirus/2019-ncov/hcp/framework-non-COVID-care.html. Updated June 30th. Accessed September 10, 2020.
5. Moy L, Toth HK, Newell MS, et al. Response to COVID-19 in Breast Imaging. J Breast Imaging 2020;2(3):180–5.
6. Sharpe RE Jr, Kuszyk BS, Mossa-Basha M, For the RSNA COVID-19 Task Force. Special Report of the RSNA COVID-19 Task Force: The Short- and Long-Term

Financial Impact of the COVID-19 Pandemic on Private Radiology Practices. Radiology 2020. https://doi.org/10.1148/radiol.2020202517.

7. The coronavirus claims two Georgia health care workers. 2020. Available at: https://www.ajc.com/news/virus-claims-two-georgia-healthcare-workers/XTijtgzE6z2gcoZ7QLvPZN/. Accessed September 8, 2020.

8. Nguyen LH, Drew DA, Graham MS, et al. Risk of COVID-19 among front-line health-care workers and the general community: a prospective cohort study. Lancet Public Health 2020;5:e475–83.

9. Cinar P, Kubal T, Freifeld A, et al. Safety at the Time of the COVID-19 Pandemic: How to Keep our Oncology Patients and Healthcare Workers Safe. J Natl Compr Canc Netw 2020;1–6. https://doi.org/10.6004/jnccn.2020.7572.

10. Lu M. The front line: visualizing the occupations with the highest COVID-19 risk. 2020. Available at: https://www.visualcapitalist.com/the-front-line-visualizing-the-occupations-with-the-highest-COVID-19-risk/. Accessed September 9, 2020.

11. ASBrS and ACR Joint Statement on Breast Screening Exams During the COVID-19 Pandemic. 2020. Available at: https://www.sbi-online.org/Portals/0/Position%20Statements/2020/society-of-breast-imaging-statement-on-breast-imaging-during-COVID19-pandemic.pdf. Accessed September 9, 2020.

12. Society of Breast Imaging Statement on Breast Imaging during the COVID-19 Pandemic. 2020. Available at: https://www.sbi-online.org/Portals/0/Position%20Statements/2020/society-of-breast-imaging-statement-on-breast-imaging-during-COVID19-pandemic.pdf. Accessed September 9, 2020.

13. Malhotra A, Wu X, Fleishon HB, et al. Initial Impact of Coronavirus Disease 2019 (COVID-19) on Radiology Practices: An ACR/RBMA Survey [published online ahead of print, 2020 Aug 4]. J Am Coll Radiol 2020. https://doi.org/10.1016/j.jacr.2020.07.028.

14. Canadian Society of Breast Imaging and Canadian Association of Radiologists Joint Position Statement on COVID-19. 2020. Available at: https://csbi.ca/wp-content/uploads/2020/03/Covid-19-statement-CSBI_CAR-1.pdf. Accessed. September 14, 2020.

15. Society of Breast Imaging Statement on Screening in a Time of Social Distancing. 2020. Available at: https://www.sbi-online.org/Portals/0/Position%20Statements/2020/SBI-statement-on-screening-in-a-time-of-social-distancing_March-17-2020.pdf. Accessed September 10, 2020.

16. Pediconi F, Mann RM, Gilbert FJ, et al. on behalf of the EUSOBI Executive Board. EUSOBI recommendations for breast imaging and cancer diagnosis during and after the COVID-19 pandemic. 2020. Available at: https://www.eusobi.org/content-eusobi/uploads/EUSOBI-Recommendations_Breast-Imaging-during-COVID.pdf. Accessed September 9, 2020.

17. Pediconi F, Galati F, Bernardi D, et al. Breast imaging and cancer diagnosis during the COVID-19 pandemic: recommendations from the Italian College of Breast Radiologists by SIRM. Radiol Med 2020;125(10):926–30.

18. American College of Surgeons. COVID-19: Guidance for Triage of Non-Emergent Surgical Procedures. 2020. Available at: https://www.facs.org/covid-19/clinical-guidance/triage. Accessed September 10, 2020.

19. Bartlett DL, Howe JR, Chang G, et al. Management of Cancer Surgery Cases During the COVID-19 Pandemic: Considerations. Ann Surg Oncol 2020;27:1717–20.

20. Soran A, Brufsky A, Gimbel M, et al. Breast Cancer Diagnosis, Treatment and Follow-Up During COVID-19 Pandemic. Eur J Breast Health 2020;16(2):86–8.

21. Sheng JY, Santa-Maria CA, Mangini N, et al. Management of Breast Cancer During the COVID-19 Pandemic: A Stage- and Subtype-Specific Approach

[published online ahead of print, 2020 Jun 30]. JCO Oncol Pract 2020. https://doi.org/10.1200/OP.20.00364.

22. Smith BL, Nguyen A, Korotkin JE, et al. A system for risk stratification and prioritization of breast cancer surgeries delayed by the COVID-19 pandemic: preparing for re-entry. Breast Cancer Res Treat 2020. https://doi.org/10.1007/s10549-020-05792-2.

23. Dietz JR, Moran MS, Isakoff SJ, et al. Recommendations for prioritization, treatment, and triage of breast cancer patients during the COVID-19 pandemic the COVID-19 pandemic breast cancer consortium. Breast Cancer Res Treat 2020. https://doi.org/10.1007/s10549-020-05644-z.

24. American College of Surgeons, American Society of Anesthesiologists. Association of periOperative Registered Nurses, American Hospital Association. Joint Statement: Roadmap for Resuming Elective Surgery after COVID-19 Pandemic. 2020. Available at: https://www.facs.org/covid-19/clinical-guidance/roadmap-elective-surgery. Accessed September 9, 2020.

25. Curigliano G, Banerjee S, Cervantes A, et al. Managing cancer patients during the COVID-19 pandemic: an ESMO multidisciplinary expert consensus [published online ahead of print, 2020 Jul 31]. Ann Oncol 2020. https://doi.org/10.1016/j.annonc.2020.07.010.

26. Hanna TP, Evans GA, Booth CM. Cancer, COVID-19 and the precautionary principle: prioritizing treatment during a global pandemic. Nat Rev Clin Oncol 2020; 17:268–70.

27. Chan JJ, Sim Y, Ow SGW, et al. The impact of COVID-19 on and recommendations for breast cancer care: the Singapore experience. Endocr Relat Cancer 2020;27(9):R307–27.

28. Curigliano G, Cardoso MJ, Poortmans P, et al. Recommendations for triage, prioritization and treatment of breast cancer patients during the COVID-19 pandemic. Breast 2020;52:8–16.

29. de Azambuja E, Trapani D, Loibl S, et al. ESMO Management and treatment adapted recommendations in the COVID-19 era: Breast Cancer. ESMO Open 2020;5(Suppl 3):e000793.

30. ESMO. The ESMO-MCBS Score Card esmo.org. 2020. Available at: https://www.esmo.org/guidelines/esmo-mcbs/esmo-magnitude-of-clinical-benefit-scale. Accessed September 9, 2020.

31. ASCO Special Report: A Guide to Cancer Care Delivery During the COVID-19 Pandemic. 2020. Available at: https://www.asco.org/sites/new-www.asco.org/files/content-files/2020-ASCO-Guide-Cancer-COVID19.pdf. Accessed September 9, 2020.

32. ASCO Coronavirus Resources. Available at: https://www.asco.org/asco-coronavirus-information. Accessed September 10, 2020.

33. Spring LM, Specht MC, Jimenez RB, et al. Case 22-2020: A 62-Year-Old Woman with Early Breast Cancer during the Covid-19 Pandemic. N Engl J Med 2020; 383(3):262–72.

34. Siegal DS, Wessman B, Zadorozny J, et al. Operational Radiology Recovery in Academic Radiology Departments After the COVID-19 Pandemic: Moving Toward Normalcy. J Am Coll Radiol 2020;17(9):1101–7.

35. ACR Response to COVID-19. 2020. Available at: https://accreditationsupport.acr.org/support/solutions/articles/11000084016-acr-response-to-covid-19-created-03-20-2020-?_ga=2.106697866.821974201.1585157241-178615201.1580929929. Accessed September 10, 2020.

36. Coronavirus (COVID-19) Update: FDA prepares for resumption of domestic inspections with new risk assessment system. 2020. Available at: https://www.fda.gov/news-events/press-announcements/coronavirus-covid-19-update-fda-prepares-resumption-domestic-inspections-new-risk-assessment-system. Accessed September 8, 2020.

37. Yu J, Ouyang W, Chua MLK, et al. SARS-CoV-2 Transmission in patients with cancer at a tertiary care hospital in Wuhan, China [published online March 25]. JAMA Oncol 2020. https://doi.org/10.1001/jamaoncol.2020.0980.

38. Liang W, Guan W, Chen R, et al. Cancer patients in SARS-CoV-2 infection: a nationwide analysis in China. Lancet Oncol 2020;21(3):335–7.

39. Zhang L, Zhu F, Xie L, et al. Clinical characteristics of COVID-19-infected cancer patients: a retrospective case study in three hospitals within Wuhan, China. Ann Oncol 2020;31(7):894–901.

40. Wu Z, McGoogan JM. Characteristics of and important lessons from the coronavirus disease 2019 (COVID-19) outbreak in China: Summary of a report of 72314 cases from the Chinese Center for Disease Control and Prevention. JAMA 2020; 323(13):1239–42.

41. Mehta V, Goel S, Kabarriti R, et al. Case fatality rate of cancer patients with COVID-19 in a New York hospital system. Cancer Discov 2020. https://doi.org/10.1158/2159-8290.CD-20-0516.

42. Miyashita H, Mikami T, Chopra N, et al. Do patients with cancer have a poorer prognosis of COVID-19? An experience in New York City. Ann Oncol 2020. https://doi.org/10.1016/j.annonc.2020.04.006.

43. Kuderer NM, Choueiri TK, Shah DP, et al. Clinical impact of COVID-19 on patients with cancer (CCC19): a cohort study [published correction appears in Lancet. 2020;396(10253):758]. Lancet 2020;395(10241):1907–18.

44. Guan WJ, Ni ZY, Hu Y, et al. Clinical characteristics of coronavirus disease 2019 in China. N Engl J Med 2020;382:1708–20.

45. American Society of Clinical Oncology. ASCO Survey on COVID-19 in Oncology (ASCO) Registry. Available at: https://www.asco.org/asco-coronavirus-information/coronavirus-registry. Accessed September 10, 2020.

46. Lee LY, Cazier JB, Angelis V, et al. COVID-19 mortality in patients with cancer on chemotherapy or other anticancer treatments: a prospective cohort study [published correction appears in Lancet. 2020;396(10250):534]. Lancet 2020; 395(10241):1919–26.

47. Printz C. When a global pandemic complicates cancer care: Although oncologists and their patients are accustomed to fighting tough battles against a lethal disease, Coronavirus Disease 2019 (COVID-19) has posed an unprecedented challenge. Cancer 2020;126(14):3171–3.

48. American College of Emergency Physicianns COVID-19. 2020. Available at: https://www.emergencyphysicians.org/globalassets/emphysicians/all-pdfs/acep-mc-COVID19-april-poll-analysis.pdf. Accessed September 8, 2020.

49. Vanni G, Materazzo M, Pellicciaro M, et al. Breast Cancer and COVID-19: The Effect of Fear on Patients' Decision-making Process. In Vivo 2020;34(3 Suppl): 1651–9.

50. Papautsky EL, Hamlish T. Patient-reported treatment delays in breast cancer care during the COVID-19 pandemic. Breast Cancer Res Treat 2020. https://doi.org/10.1007/s10549-020-05828-7.

51. Medicare telemedicine health care provider fact sheet. 2020. Available at: https://www.cms.gov/newsroom/fact-sheets/medicare-telemedicine-health-care-provider-fact-sheet. Accessed September 8, 2020.

52. Yin K, Singh P, Drohan B, et al. Breast imaging, breast surgery, and cancer genetics in the age of COVID-19 [published online ahead of print, 2020 Aug 4]. Cancer 2020. https://doi.org/10.1002/cncr.33113.

53. Xie C, Wang X, Liu H, et al. Outcomes in Radiotherapy-Treated Patients With Cancer During the COVID-19 Outbreak in Wuhan, China [published online ahead of print, 2020 Jul 30]. JAMA Oncol 2020;e202783. https://doi.org/10.1001/jamaoncol.2020.2783.

54. de Joode K, Dumoulin DW, Engelen V, et al. Impact of the coronavirus disease 2019 pandemic on cancer treatment: the patients' perspective. Eur J Cancer 2020;136:132–9.

55. Gharzai LA, Resnicow K, An LC, et al. Perspectives on Oncology-Specific Language During the Coronavirus Disease 2019 Pandemic: A Qualitative Study [published online ahead of print, 2020 Aug 6]. JAMA Oncol 2020;e202980. https://doi.org/10.1001/jamaoncol.2020.2980.

56. Oncology Language for the COVID-19 Pandemic. 2020. Available at: https://www.nccn.org/covid-19/pdf/Oncology%20Langauge-Communicating%20Changes%20in%20Delivery%20of%20Care.pdf. Accessed September 8, 2020.

57. Emanuel EJ, Persad G, Upshur R, et al. Fair Allocation of Scarce Medical Resources in the Time of Covid-19. N Engl J Med 2020;382(21):2049–55.

58. DeBoer RJ, Fadelu TA, Shulman LN, et al. Applying Lessons Learned From Low-Resource Settings to Prioritize Cancer Care in a Pandemic. JAMA Oncol 2020; 6(9):1429–33.

59. Yip CH, Anderson BO. The Breast Health Global Initiative: clinical practice guidelines for management of breast cancer in low- and middle-income countries. Expert Rev Anticancer Ther 2007;7(8):1095–104.

60. Woolf SH, Chapman DA, Sabo RT, et al. Excess Deaths From COVID-19 and Other Causes, March-April 2020. JAMA 2020;324(5):510–3.

61. Hamel L, Kearney A, Kirsinger A, et al. KFF Health Tracking Poll. 2020. Available at: https://www.kff.org/report-section/kff-health-tracking-poll-late-april-2020-economic-and-mental-health-impacts-of-coronavirus/. Accessed September 10, 2020.

62. Sud A, Torr B, Jones ME, et al. Effect of delays in the 2-week-wait cancer referral pathway during the COVID-19 pandemic on cancer survival in the UK: a modelling study. Lancet Oncol 2020. https://doi.org/10.1016/s1470-2045(20)30392-2.

63. IJzerman M, Emery J. Is a delayed cancer diagnosis a consequence of COVID-19?. 2020. Available at: https://pursuit.unimelb.edu.au/articles/is-a-delayed-cancer-diagnosis-a-consequence-of-covid-19. Accessed September 9, 2020.

64. Kaufman HW, Chen Z, Niles J, et al. Changes in the Number of US Patients With Newly Identified Cancer Before and During the Coronavirus Disease 2019 (COVID-19) Pandemic. JAMA Netw Open 2020;3(8):e2017267.

65. Sharpless NE. COVID-19 and cancer. Science 2020;368(6497):1290.

66. Maruthappu M, Watkins J, Noor AM, et al. Economic downturns, universal health coverage, and cancer mortality in high-income and middle-income countries, 1990-2010: a longitudinal analysis. Lancet 2016;388(10045):684–95.

67. Naidich JJ, Boltyenkov A, Wang JJ, et al. Impact of the Coronavirus Disease 2019 (COVID-19) Pandemic on Imaging Case Volumes. J Am Coll Radiol 2020;17(7): 865–72.

68. Norbash AM, Moore AV Jr, Recht MP, et al. Early-Stage Radiology Volume Effects and Considerations with the Coronavirus Disease 2019 (COVID-19) Pandemic: Adaptations, Risks, and Lessons Learned. J Am Coll Radiol 2020;17(9):1086–95.

69. Sammer MBK, Sher AC, Huisman TAGM, et al. Response to the COVID-19 Pandemic: Practical Guide to Rapidly Deploying Home Workstations to

Guarantee Radiology Services During Quarantine, Social Distancing, and Stay Home Orders [published online ahead of print, 2020 Jun 30]. AJR Am J Roentgenol 2020;1–4. https://doi.org/10.2214/AJR.20.23297.

70. Madox W. Coronavirus has sparked a teleradiology revolution. Available at: https://www.dmagazine.com/healthcare-business/2020/2004/coronavirus-has-sparked-a-teleradiology-revolution/. Accessed September 10, 2020.

71. Simons J. IBM, a pioneer of remote work, calls workers back to the office: Big Blue says move will improve collaboration and accelerate the pace of work. Wall St J 2017. Available at: https://www.wsj.com/articles/ibm-a-pioneer-of-remote-work-calls-workers-back-to-the-office-14 95108802. Accessed September 9, 2020.

72. Thousands of healthcare workers are laid off or furloughed as coronavirus spreads. Los Angeles Times 2020;. https://www.latimes.com/california/story/2020-05-02/coronavirus-california-healthcare-workers-layoffs-furloughs. Accessed September 8, 2020.

73. Coronavirus Aid, Relief, and Economic Security (CARES) Act. Pub L No 116-136 (2020).

74. Paycheck Protection Program and Health Care Enhancement Act. Pub L No 116-139 (2020).

75. Demirjian NL, Fields BKK, Song C, et al. Impacts of the Coronavirus Disease 2019 (COVID-19) pandemic on healthcare workers: A nationwide survey of United States radiologists. Clin Imaging 2020;68:218–25.

76. Shanafelt T, Ripp J, Trockel M. Understanding and Addressing Sources of Anxiety Among Health Care Professionals During the COVID-19 Pandemic. JAMA 2020;323(21):2133–4.

77. Restauri N, Sheridan AD. Burnout and Posttraumatic Stress Disorder in the Coronavirus Disease 2019 (COVID-19) Pandemic: Intersection, Impact, and Interventions. J Am Coll Radiol 2020;17(7):921–6.

78. Alvin MD, George E, Deng F, et al. The Impact of COVID-19 on Radiology Trainees. Radiology 2020;296(2):246–8.

79. Kalia V, Srinivasan A, Wilkins L, et al. Adapting Scientific Conferences to the Realities Imposed by COVID-19. Radiol Imaging Cancer 2020;2(4):e204020.

80. Evens R. The impact of a pandemic on professional meetings. Radiol Imaging Cancer 2020;2(3).

81. Vagal A, Reeder SB, Sodickson DK, et al. The Impact of the COVID-19 Pandemic on the Radiology Research Enterprise: Radiology Scientific Expert Panel. Radiology 2020;296(3):E134–40.

82. McDermott MM, Newman AB. Preserving clinical trial integrity during the coronavirus pandemic. JAMA 2020. https://doi.org/10.1001/jama.2020.4689.

83. FDA guidance on conduct of clinical trials of medical products during COVID-19 pandemic: guidance for industry, investigators, and institutional review boards. US Food and Drug Administration. 2020. Available at: https://www.fda.gov/media/136238/download. Accessed September 11, 2020.

84. Eary J, Shankar L. COVID-19 Update from the NCI Cancer Imaging Program. Radiol Imaging Cancer 2020;2(3):e204017.

85. Nabhan C, Choueiri TK, Mato AR. Rethinking Clinical Trials Reform During the COVID-19 Pandemic. JAMA Oncol 2020;6(9):1327–9.

86. COVID-19 and Cancer Consortium Registry (CCC19). ClinicalTrials.gov identifier: NCT04354701. 2020. Available at: https://www.clinicaltrials.gov/ct2/show/NCT04354701?term=NCT04354701&draw=2&rank=1. Accessed September 11, 2020.

87. Bartsch SM, Ferguson MC, McKinnell JA, et al. The Potential Health Care Costs And Resource Use Associated With COVID-19 In The United States. Health Aff (Millwood) 2020;39(6):927–35.
88. Department of Labor. 2020. Available at: https://www.dol.gov/ui/data.pdf. Accessed September 10, 2020.
89. Cavallo JJ, Forman HP. The Economic Impact of the COVID-19 Pandemic on Radiology Practices. Radiology 2020;296(3):E141–4.

The Future of Endoscopic Operations After the Coronavirus Pandemic

Klaus Mergener, MD, PhD, MBA

KEYWORDS

- Coronavirus • COVID-19 pandemic • Gastroenterology • GI endoscopy
- Practice management

KEY POINTS

- Modern GI practices have a high overhead structure and are thus vulnerable to sudden interruptions in cash flow.
- Professional management and constant vigilance are necessary to respond quickly to new developments and adapt expense and revenue structures as needed.
- Procedure backlogs from COVID shutdowns have resulted in delayed GI care that needs to be addressed in a structured fashion, with higher-risk patients prioritized for examinations.
- The pandemic accelerated the implementation of telemedicine programs, and these services will continue to be used in the postpandemic era.
- A crisis presents challenges but also opportunities, and the sense of accomplishment from having navigated this crisis will result in a strong culture of teamwork.

INTRODUCTION

The coronavirus disease 2019 (COVID-19) pandemic represents an unprecedented global health crisis that has challenged GI practices and endoscopy operations in major and unforeseen ways. As of March 1, 2021, there were 115 million confirmed cases of COVID-19 and more than 2.5 million deaths globally, with almost 30 million cases and more than 527,000 deaths in the United States alone.[1]

Rapidly implemented global shutdowns of everyday life and business, including medical operations, resulted in sudden delays in our ability to diagnose and treat GI illnesses and perform cancer screening. As the country is moving toward a full reopening supported by rapidly evolving vaccination programs and scientific discoveries related to the prevention and management of COVID-19, medical practices are

This article previously appeared in *Gastrointestinal Endoscopy Clinics*, Volume 31, Issue 4, October 2021.

Division of Gastroenterology, University of Washington, 1917 Warren Avenue North, Seattle, WA 98109, USA

E-mail address: klausmergener@aol.com

Twitter: @kmergener (K.M.)

Clinics Collections 12 (2022) 311–323

https://doi.org/10.1016/j.ccol.2021.12.022

2352-7986/22/© 2021 Elsevier Inc. All rights reserved.

wrestling with the challenge of a complete retooling of their operations with the goal of quickly returning to providing high-quality care to large numbers of patients safely and effectively.

At the same time, assessment has begun of the long-term impact that the current pandemic may have on future practice operations: What will postpandemic GI care look like, and how soon will we get there? Will we return to prepandemic operations in all aspects of our work, or will some elements of GI practice be changed forever? If so, what are those elements, and what are the implications for GI leaders as they look to position their groups for continued success? This chapter provides an overview of the impact of the pandemic on US-based GI practices and discusses some key "lessons learned" that may affect future operations.

THE PREPANDEMIC STATE OF GI PRACTICE

Before discussing the ongoing impact of COVID-19 on GI groups and endoscopy operations, it is useful to briefly take stock of the recent history and challenges encountered by GI practices prior to 2020.

Gastroenterologists have enjoyed great success due to the large burden of GI disease and thus high demand for GI services. In our health care system, with its predominantly fee-for-service reimbursement, procedural specialties have fared well economically. Still, there have been considerable and mounting challenges to the current GI practice model[2]: Reimbursement for endoscopic procedures has declined significantly in recent years while practice costs have continued to skyrocket. Many primary care providers have become employed by payers or large health systems, thereby affecting patient referral patterns for specialty services. Hospital and payer consolidation has resulted in a rapidly changing landscape where small practices often lose leverage in contract negotiations. Disruptive technologies such as nonendoscopic tests for cancer screening and advances in radiology have the potential to further challenge a specialty that is now heavily reliant on revenue from endoscopic procedures.

At the same time, gastroenterologists have been resilient in meeting current challenges. Moving many endoscopic services from the hospital to physician-owned ambulatory endoscopy centers has allowed physicians to increase efficiencies and capture income from facility fees. Adding ancillary revenue streams such as pathology, anesthesia services, infusion, and imaging centers has allowed some groups to compensate for the continued decline in professional fees.[2]

As a result, the prepandemic GI practice had evolved from a low-overhead hospital-based operation to a high-overhead business with high capital investments and thus a significant dependence on efficient, high-throughput endoscopy services to generate constant cash flow in support of its cost structure. While this potential vulnerability was not lost on astute practice managers, there was no reason to believe that smoothly running endoscopy services would experience a sudden interruption and downturn in procedure volumes.

THE COVID-19 PANDEMIC

Such was the situation in late December 2019 when the first report arrived at the World Health Organization (WHO) from Wuhan, China, about a new type of pneumonia of unknown cause.[3] The ensuing weeks and months brought the most rapid progress of science ever accomplished in the history of infectious diseases: The responsible agent for COVID-19 was identified as a novel beta-coronavirus, now termed severe acute respiratory syndrome coronavirus 2 (SARS-CoV-2).[4] The virus was isolated on January 7, the full genome sequence was published on January 10, and the first fully validated polymerase chain reaction (PCR) testing protocol was shared with the WHO on January 13, 2020. Since then, the molecular structure of this virus has been determined, PCR, antigen, and antibody tests have been developed, and numerous studies have been performed to elucidate the mechanism of viral transmission, the immunologic response of the host, disease characteristics, treatment options, and vaccine development. Several key findings from this research provide important insights into the anticipated impact of COVID-19 on GI practices and endoscopic operations going forward.[4,5]

Virus Structure and Transmission

The genetic sequence and structure of SARS-Co-V-2 are similar to those of other human coronaviruses. A lipid bilayer envelope makes the virus particle susceptible to regular detergents, thereby facilitating virus deactivation with standard cleaning procedures such as those used during regular endoscope reprocessing. The spike glycoprotein (S-protein) is embedded in the viral envelope and mediates host cell binding and entry. S-protein has been identified as the main target in current vaccine development efforts,[6] and monoclonal anti-S antibodies have been produced as one of the first therapeutic agents to combat COVID-19 illness.[7] The 30 kb single-strand RNA genome of SARS-CoV-2 encodes several other structural and nonstructural proteins, including a replication proofreading apparatus. While this might be expected to reduce the rate of virus mutations compared with other RNA viruses, there have been numerous reports in recent months of emerging virus variants that appear to confer higher transmissibility.[8] The full impact of these mutations on the epidemiology of COVID-19 and the effectiveness of vaccination programs remains incompletely understood, but this will be a major determinant of what GI practice operations will look like in the near to medium term.

SARS-CoV-2 infects epithelial cells in the respiratory and GI tracts and possibly other target cells. The incubation period ranges from 2 to 14 days, and symptomatic individuals are most contagious immediately before and within the first 5 days of symptom onset with a rapid decline of viral load thereafter.[9] A key determinant of the high transmissibility is that an estimated 40% to 50% of all COVID-19 infections are transmitted by individuals who are either presymptomatic or remain entirely asymptomatic during the course of their own infection.[10,11] This has important implications for the implementation of safety measures in the endoscopy unit because simple screening for COVID-19 symptoms will miss a large percentage of SARS-CoV-2 carriers. Virus transmission occurs at close range (within 2 m) via respiratory droplets expelled during coughing or sneezing but also via aerosol transmission, that is, microdroplets small enough to remain suspended in the air for 30 minutes or longer and expose individuals at distances beyond 2 m, often in poorly ventilated indoor settings without sufficient air exchange.[12] Infection via contaminated surfaces appears to play only a minor role, and the relative contributions of these different modalities are not fully known at present.[13] The role of fecal–oral transmission received considerable attention during the early stages of the pandemic but appears to be minimal if it occurs at all.[14,15] Although SARS-CoV-2 infects GI epithelial cells, and viral RNA can be identified in stool specimens via PCR testing, studies using viral culture have not consistently identified infectious particles in stool, and no credible reports exist in the English literature of clinically relevant fecal–oral transmission.

Propagation of the Pandemic and Initial Impact on Endoscopy Centers

Since its initial appearance in late 2019, COVID-19 has spread around the globe at an alarming pace. The first US case was reported in a Washington state resident who returned from Wuhan, China, on January 15, 2020. On January 31, 2020, WHO issued a global health emergency, and on March 11, WHO declared COVID-19 a pandemic. With cases rising rapidly, travel restrictions, business shutdowns, and stay-at-home orders followed within a few days. By the end of March 2020, endoscopy volumes for elective procedures had fallen to less than 10% of baseline volumes.[16-18]

At that point, endoscopy unit managers were confronted with a sudden and profound decrease in cash flow for these very cash-dependent operations. Strategies had to be developed quickly to (1) reduce expenses and (2) repair revenues. For the rapid reduction of expenses, the main cost drivers had to be identified and addressed: (1) staff costs needed to be reduced via layoffs and furloughs; (2) accounts payable such as rent and other contracts needed to be renegotiated as much as feasible; and (3) efforts to reduce operational costs/waste needed to be intensified. Revenue repair focused on the following items: (1) rapid implementation of telehealth capabilities, including training of patients and staff on IT platforms; (2) procurement of sufficient personal protective equipment (PPE) and retooling of workflows in the endoscopy center to allow at least partial resumption of elective operations as soon as state regulations allowed; (3) development of communication tools to (a) inform patients of the steps taken to maintain a safe environment in GI practice and endoscopy unit and (b) to keep staff up to date on the rapid implementation of these changes.

Since April 2020, the pandemic has progressed in a typical manner through phases of deceleration and acceleration. On April 7, daily case numbers reached the first peak of 35,000 before decreasing and then rising again to well over 80,000 cases per day in late July.[1] Another decrease was followed by an even larger third wave that peaked at more than 250,000 daily cases in early January 2021. At the time of this writing in March 2021, daily case numbers have again decreased and leveled off at a still concerningly high trough level of 45,000 to 50,000/d, with the direction of the next trend yet to be determined. Significant variability of this dynamic from state to state and the lack of a standardized federal approach to reopening and shutdown orders have resulted in a varied approach to and timing of reopening of endoscopy centers depending on their geographic location and local circumstances. At the 1-year mark of the COVID-19 pandemic on March 10, 2021, there is hope that the end of the pandemic can be reached by the end of summer 2021, mainly thanks to the rollout of a comprehensive vaccination program that has now begun.[19]

The Promise of COVID Vaccines

Initial COVID containment efforts focused on nonpharmacologic interventions to include social distancing, contact tracing, and isolation, the use of personal protective equipment (PPE) to include face masks, and handwashing and environmental cleaning. These efforts have now been significantly augmented by the development, approval, and rollout of COVID-19 vaccinations. Vaccines typically require years of research and testing before reaching clinical practice, but in early 2020, almost immediately after the identification of the molecular virology of SARS-CoV-2, scientists embarked on a race to produce safe and effective coronavirus vaccines in record time. By fall 2020, more than 150 vaccine candidates were in various stages of development.[6,20]

In the United States, 3 vaccines have now received emergency use authorization from the Food and Drug Administration.[21] While storage requirements and the number of necessary inoculations vary between products, all 3 vaccines result in a humoral and T-cell-mediated immune response against epitopes of the viral S-protein. Clinical trials to date have shown surprisingly high efficacy rates upwards of 85% to 94% for all 3 products,[22] with "efficacy" defined as a reduction in the rate of acquiring severe

COVID-19 disease. Importantly, and relevant to the risk of vaccinated individuals to still carry and transmit SARS-CoV-2 virus in endoscopy units, there is now emerging evidence that vaccinations also result in a marked decrease in viral load of up to 20-fold and therefore a projected lower risk of infection transmission.[23,24] While many details remain to be worked out, including the duration of protective immunity after vaccination and thus the need for and timing of possible future booster immunizations, the more immediate hope relates to continuing with rapid vaccine administration, currently occurring at a rate of 2 million individuals per day in the United States,[25] in order to reach "herd immunity." This term refers to the percentage of a population that must acquire immunity to an infectious agent in order for the transmission of the agent to slow and eventually seize. In the case of SARS-CoV-2, many experts predict that "herd immunity" requires that at least 70% of the population has become immune to COVID-19 through either vaccination or natural infection.[26] It is important to note that the "end of the COVID-19 pandemic" should not be envisioned as flipping a switch but rather as a stepwise process whereby, after reaching herd immunity, non-pharmacologic interventions to prevent COVID-19 transmission may be gradually lifted but could remain in effect in some areas or be implemented again at a later time depending on local disease prevalence. In addition, because not all individuals will have received or agreed to receive COVID vaccination, endoscopy units may still have to consider testing protocols or contact safety measures in nonvaccinated individuals in the event of persistently high case numbers in some geographic areas.

INITIAL REOPENING STRATEGIES AND SHORT-TERM IMPACT ON ENDOSCOPY OPERATIONS

The rapid spread of the COVID-19 pandemic in spring 2020 forced GI practice leaders to quickly develop contingency plans for their operations in order to provide uninterrupted GI care wherever feasible, maintain the solvency of the practice, and plan for a return to prepandemic patient volumes as soon as possible.[17,27] Many of these strategies have a budgetary impact, as they either require a financial investment or result in lower endoscopy unit throughput. Planning for the gradual resumption of services began during the first pandemic wave and was periodically updated as states proceeded through reopening and repeated shutdown mandates over the course of the pandemic. The American Society for Gastrointestinal Endoscopy (ASGE)[28] and several other professional organizations have produced guidance documents to provide gastroenterologists with recommendations to employ to mitigate infection risk and optimize endoscopy operations under these unique circumstances.[29–31]

Changes in Workflow

Creating a safe environment in the endoscopy unit for patients, staff, and providers should always remain the top priority for GI leaders. Preprocedure screening now includes a COVID symptom questionnaire, which should be mandatory for patients before any endoscopy and for staff at the beginning of each workday.[28] Symptom screening will miss asymptomatic and presymptomatic carriers, but positive responses in these questionnaires should prompt removal of the individual from care areas and self-quarantine or hospital referral as needed. Many practices have now included similar COVID-related questions in the postprocedure questionnaires typically used to assess patient satisfaction. Such questionnaires can be distributed and returned before and after endoscopy appointments, avoiding delays in workflows on the day of the procedure. Lobby, admittance area, and recovery bay capacities, as well as foot traffic, in the endoscopy center have been altered to accommodate the need for physical distancing, including fewer chairs in waiting areas, physical barriers (eg, plexiglass partitions) where physical distancing cannot be accomplished, and the implementation of unidirectional flow through the endoscopy unit wherever possible. Wearing a face mask that covers both mouth and nose has become mandatory for all patients, providers, and staff at all times, as it has been clearly shown to reduce the risk of COVID transmission.[32] A significant investment of both time and money is required for training patients and staff on the unit's COVID-19 protocols including new workflows, proper hand hygiene and disinfection procedures, timing of patient arrivals, discharge procedures, pickup by family members, etc.[28] Preprocedure office visits, generally poorly compensated but sometimes necessary in higher-risk patients referred for open-access procedures, are now commonly conducted via telemedicine.

Changes in the Endoscopy Room

Significant changes have been implemented in the endoscopy room as well in an attempt to minimize the risk of infection transmission.[33] All members of the endoscopy team need to wear a full set of PPE (gown, gloves, hair cover, eye protection), and the appropriate donning and doffing of PPE requires diligent training and frequent reinforcement.[28] Although the evidence supporting the use of a face mask to reduce the risk of infection is irrefutable, the decision regarding the choice of mask for endoscopy team members—specifically, whether to use N95 respirators versus regular surgical masks in the procedure room—is complex and not well supported by high-quality evidence. Some studies have shown surgical masks to be noninferior to N95 respirators in the prevention of viral infections like influenza,[34] but a recent systematic review and meta-analysis showed a benefit in using N95 respirators over standard masks in protecting health care workers from SARS-CoV-1.[35] While these devices are more costly than regular surgical masks, they should therefore be strongly considered (assuming no supply shortage) for team members in the endoscopy room, given that upper endoscopies are known to generate aerosols. While the advantage of N95 masks over surgical masks will diminish with decreasing prevalence of SARS-CoV-2, endoscopy units are well advised to err on the side of safety until vaccination efforts and testing can provide assurance of negligible COVID risk.

Some authors have suggested additional time for room aeration between individual endoscopic procedures even in ambulatory endoscopy settings, a recommendation that remains a topic of intense debate and has not been widely adopted. The rationale for increasing the number of air exchanges between cases rests on the notion of SARS-CoV-2 being transmitted via aerosols and thus remaining airborne for prolonged periods in indoor settings with poor ventilation. ASGE guidance notes that "rooms lacking negative pressure benefit from additional aeration time for adequate clearance of droplets/aerosols,"[28] and some authors have suggested that this extra time between procedures should be as long as 30 to 60 minutes per case, an approach that is economically prohibitive for busy endoscopy units. In the absence of definitive scientific evidence specific to the endoscopy unit, different centers have taken very different approaches, and more studies are required to inform these decisions. Because of the high susceptibility of coronaviruses to standard disinfectant solutions, no changes are recommended to established reprocessing procedures for endoscopes and accessories.[26] While infection transmission via contaminated surfaces may play a comparatively minor role in the spread of SARS-CoV-2, professional organizations recommend deep cleaning of high-touch surfaces in procedure rooms after each case.[28,29] No changes are recommended to "terminal cleaning" procedures for cleaning and disinfecting the endoscopy unit at the end of the day.[36]

Testing Strategies

Because asymptomatic SARS-CoV-2 infections are a frequent source for transmission, a preprocedure symptom-screen of all individuals presenting for endoscopy is insufficient to eliminate the risk of infection transmission in the endoscopy suite. Ideally, efforts to mitigate this risk require all patients (and staff) to demonstrate either the presence of convalescent antibodies to SARS-CoV-2 or a negative molecular test within 48 hours of a scheduled procedure (or in the case of staff, with some regularity—eg, weekly). Many endoscopy units have implemented a universal testing strategy for patients, especially because the cost of testing is currently borne by government agencies in most states. Performing such a test close to the date of a procedure is important to avoid a negative test result during the early incubation period with subsequent high viral loads at the time of the procedure. While a well-timed universal testing strategy may be desirable, several obstacles have made widespread implementation of such an approach difficult. First, sufficient test capacities were not available during the early stages of the pandemic, and reports persist of periodic test shortages in some geographic areas. Second, test results need to be available at the time of the procedure, as cancellations will result in a significant number of unused endoscopy slots and thus considerable inefficiencies. In addition, test accuracies are not perfect. The Infectious Diseases Society of America suggests against universal testing when PPE is readily available, noting significant rates of false-negative tests and thus lower negative predictive value in areas of high disease prevalence.[37] Testing is favored if PPE is limited. The American Gastroenterological Association has published a detailed decision-making guide related to preprocedure testing, taking into account the test used, prevalence of the disease, and several other factors.[38] While this guide provides a detailed framework for decision-making, its algorithm is complex, and its application in everyday GI practice is therefore somewhat limited. With the increasing availability of point-of-care (POC) antigen tests and the development of new rapid turnaround molecular tests, and with the pandemic beginning to recede, the approach to preprocedure testing can be expected to undergo further changes. It appears likely that testing will eventually be employed in a more focused and targeted manner—for example, POC testing for individuals who are unable to produce proof of up-to-date vaccination or immunity to SARS-CoV-2.[39]

LONG-TERM IMPACT OF COVID-19 ON ENDOSCOPY OPERATIONS
Macroeconomic Considerations

The COVID-19 pandemic has led to record job losses. In April and May 2020 alone, more than 36 million Americans filed for unemployment benefits, levels not seen since the Great Depression.[40] While some unemployed individuals will have switched to an employed spouse's coverage, gotten on a parent's plan, or stayed covered by their previous employer through a COBRA package, many likely turned to coverage through health insurance exchanges, got on a Medicaid plan, or became uninsured. The end result of these shifts in the insurance market is projected to be an overall increase in the percentage of individuals who lose coverage or have to switch to insurance products that reimburse providers at lower rates for some services. What's more, financial hardships encountered during the pandemic may motivate people to postpone elective medical services such as screening exams or forgo them altogether, resulting in decreased practice revenues.

The federal government has enacted several pieces of legislation to provide relief to individuals and corporations affected by the COVID-19 pandemic. These provisions have been largely financed through borrowing, thereby increasing the US national debt. While these interventions were thought to be necessary to stimulate the economy and avoid a depression, the resulting increase in the national debt will put additional pressure on future annual budgets, including allocations for Medicare, Medicaid, and other health insurance programs. The prepandemic changes related to decreasing reimbursements for physician and facility services can therefore be expected to accelerate further. At the same time, costs will continue to increase. While innovations in care delivery or new endoscopic techniques or technologies may result in as yet unpredictable paradigm shifts and open new opportunities for GI endoscopists, the more immediate change will relate to the need to manage ever-decreasing profit margins. Hospitals and health systems have some ability to navigate this situation by shifting costs among their diversified services or pursuing further consolidation to gain negotiating clout and demand higher pricing. On the other hand, single-specialty GI groups have only limited ways to respond. They will need to intensify prepandemic efforts to contain costs, reduce waste and optimize efficiencies.[2] Paradoxically, practices that entered the pandemic year with suboptimal management and a low efficiency/high-cost structure may be expected to have the most room for improvement, provided that they recognize the need to quickly adopt professional management. One approach to cost containment relates to sharing resources across a larger organization, that is, merging with other GI practices. This trend had already begun prior to the pandemic and was partially fueled by private equity-funded practice roll-up models. It is anticipated that these mergers into ever larger, often multistate practices will continue and that other partners, such as payers and/or health systems, will also demonstrate an increasing interest in practice partnerships or opportunities to acquire GI practices outright. As was the case before COVID-19, there will not be a "one-size-fits-all" solution, and the best way forward for an individual practice will vary by region and market.[2]

Minimizing the Impact of Delayed GI Care

One critically important issue with long-term impact relates to the procedure backlog that has accumulated as a result of endoscopy center shutdowns. Colonoscopy is the most commonly performed GI endoscopy procedure, and its widespread use has been a major factor in the decline of colorectal cancer (CRC) in this country.[41] It is well documented that the risk of being diagnosed with CRC in general, and with advanced-stage CRC in particular, increases significantly if screening is delayed or is not completed in a timely manner after an initial positive stool test.[42–44] For example, Corley and colleagues[45] reported a 3.2-fold increase in CRC detected in fecal immunochemistry test (FIT)-positive patients when colonoscopy was delayed for more than 12 months. Modeling studies to estimate the potential impact of COVID-19-related disruptions to screening on CRC incidence and mortality have found that this disruption will have a marked and prolonged impact on CRC incidence and deaths between 2020 and 2050 attributable to missed screening.[46] Early reports of "real-world data" match the near-term predictions from these modeling studies. Using data sets from the National Health Service in England, Morris and colleagues[47] calculated a relative reduction of 22% in the number of CRC cases detected and referred for treatment in that country for the April to October 2020 time frame compared with the prior year.

With endoscopy units shut down for several weeks in 2020, some practices have accumulated procedure backlogs of several thousand procedures. It is crucial for these practices to explore ways to increase procedure capacities, for example, by extending work hours or offering weekend endoscopy times. Higher-risk patients, such as those with symptoms or a positive FIT test should be prioritized to minimize the risk of delayed cancer diagnoses. Efforts need to be increased to minimize vacant procedure slots due to last-minute cancellations or poor colon preparation and to avoid nonindicated procedures in order to preserve valuable procedure time for examinations on individuals with a higher risk of harboring GI pathology. Importantly, because patients may still be reluctant to return to medical facilities because they may perceive a continued high risk of contracting COVID-19, enhanced communication efforts are necessary to inform patients and referring providers of the safety of GI endoscopic services and the benefits of undergoing potentially life-saving procedures. Ongoing monitoring of screening participation rates will demonstrate the effects of changing patient behaviors and will identify needs for further patient education. Previous studies have shown that mass media campaigns can improve screening participation, have positive effects on long-term health impacts, and are highly cost-effective.[48]

The Role of Telemedicine

The pandemic accelerated the implementation of telemedicine programs by many years.[49] Before COVID-19, most practices had barely begun experimenting with virtual visits, and most payers provided very low reimbursement rates for these services, if they paid at all. When telehealth in a typical practice suddenly grew from a few visits to many thousand visits per month, physicians, patients, and payers became increasingly aware of its significant benefits. Patients appreciate the option of a virtual visit, especially those individuals who live far away or have mobility issues. Physicians can more easily conduct interactions with patients who do not always require physical examinations—for example, follow-up discussions after procedures or certain preprocedure screening assessments.[50] Additional services such as professional translators can be provided with greater ease in the virtual world. Provided that reimbursement for such virtual visits will remain adequate, it can be anticipated that a significant percentage of physician–patient visits will continue to be conducted via telemedicine. Practices are therefore well advised to continue to invest in their IT infrastructures. The leap to telemedicine in spring 2020 was fast-tracked and could not always include the level of "at-the-elbow" support that is typically employed for this level of change. Practices will need to continue to optimize workflows and staff and provider training to provide patients with the best possible experience in these virtual encounters.

Pandemic Disruption as an Opportunity

Winston Churchill is credited with the quote "Never let a good crisis go to waste."[51] For GI groups, the COVID-19 pandemic of 2020–2021 was an unprecedented crisis that challenged all aspects of practice operations in unforeseen ways and brought some practices to the brink of insolvency. At the same time, after an initial phase of stress and struggle, the majority of GI practices have been able to pivot and adjust to the new realities, often with a massive team effort. Going forward, this should create a sense of shared mission and be reflected on by the entire team as a proud accomplishment. The most successful groups will have used this crisis to question restrictive routines and identify opportunities for creative change and innovation, an effort that may well leave them better positioned for the challenges of the future.

There are valuable lessons to be drawn from the pandemic: First, despite being well-positioned and in demand, our specialty is not immune to sudden and unexpected calamities. While COVID-19 represents the first global pandemic of our professional careers, it may not be the last. As noted in a recent review by Morens and Fauci,[52] our modern way of life, with increased global travel, crowded cities, and a changing environment, promotes the emergence of new infectious diseases and lays the foundation for rapid global spread. Practices should continue to expect the unexpected, remain on alert, and invest in professional management and an infrastructure that allows them to respond rapidly to new developments. Second, the basic tenets of practice management hold as true in calm as they do in crisis. Groups that enter a difficult period with a solid organizational infrastructure and sound financial health are likely to fare better than those who fail to continuously improve and optimize their operations. A solid foundation is most useful in times of earthquake. Third, and most importantly, although GI represents a specialty with a strong procedural focus, and the modern endoscopy unit is geared toward throughput and efficiency, the pandemic has provided a powerful reminder that at its core, GI endoscopy, and the entire practice of gastroenterology, is a team sport. GI leaders are well advised to invest in their staff at all levels of the organization, creating a sense of coherence and shared mission and a culture of teamwork. The most successful GI practices are taking great care of people, and they do so in large part by taking care of the people who take care of people! With these learnings incorporated into the postpandemic GI practice, the future of our specialty continues to be bright!

CLINICS CARE POINTS

- Continue to monitor and follow GI society guidelines for changes in practice workflows and endoscopic operations during the COVID pandemic to keep patients and staff safe.

- Prioritize higher-risk patients and develop additional procedure capacities to quickly reduce procedure backlogs and avoid long waiting times for patients with potential significant GI diseases.

- Invest in IT and telemedicine capabilities and continue to offer this service to patients postpandemic to support timely medical care.

DISCLOSURE

The author has nothing to disclose.

REFERENCES

1. Worldometer COVID-19 tracker. Available at: https://www.worldometers.info/. Accessed March 1, 2021.
2. Mergener K. Impact of health care reform on the independent GI practice. Gastrointest Endosc Clin N Am 2012;22(1):15–27.
3. Zhu N, Zhang D, Wang W, et al. A novel coronavirus from patients with pneumonia in China, 2019. N Engl J Med 2020;382:727–33.
4. Cevik M, Kuppalli K, Kindrachuk J, et al. Virology, transmission, and pathogenesis of SARS-CoV-2. BMJ 2020;371:m3862.
5. Hu B, Guo H, Zhou P, et al. Characteristics of SARS-CoV-2 and COVID-19. Nat Rev Microbiol 2021;19:141–54.
6. Krammer F. SARS-CoV-2 vaccines in development. Nature 2020;586:516–27.
7. Cohen MS. Monoclonal antibodies to disrupt progression of early COVID-19 infection. N Engl J Med 2021;384:289–91.
8. Baric RS. Emergence of a highly fit SARS-CoV-2 variant. N Engl J Med 2020;383: 2684–6.
9. Meyerowitz EA, Richterman A, Gandhi RT, et al. Transmission of SARS-CoV-2: a review of viral, host and environmental factors. Ann Intern Med 2021;174:69–79.

10. Buitrago-Garcia D, Egli-Gany D, Counotte MJ, et al. Occurrence and transmission potential of asymptomatic and presymptomatic SARS-CoV-2 infections: a living systematic review and meta-analysis. PLoS Med 2020;17(9):e1003346.
11. Meyerowitz EA, Richterman A, Bogoch II, et al. Towards an accurate and systematic characterisation of persistently asymptomatic infection with SARS-CoV-2. Lancet Infect Dis 2020;21(6):e163–9.
12. Leung NHL, Chu DKW, Shiu EYC, et al. Respiratory virus shedding in exhaled breath and efficacy of face masks. Nat Med 2020;26(5):676–80.
13. Kissler SM, Tedijanto C, Goldstein E, et al. Projecting the transmission dynamics of SARS-CoV-2 through the postpandemic period. Science 2020;368:860–8.
14. Gu J, Han B, Wang J. COVID-19: gastrointestinal manifestations and potential fecal-oral transmission. Gastroenterology 2020;158:1518–9.
15. Repici A, Aragona G, Cengia G, et al. Low risk of COVID-19 transmission in GI endoscopy. Gut 2020;69:1925–7.
16. Parasa S, Reddy N, Faigel DO, et al. Global impact of the COVID-19 pandemic on endoscopy: an international survey of 252 centers from 55 countries. Gastroenterology 2020;159:1579–81.
17. Forbes N, Smith ZL, Spitzer RL, et al. Changes in gastroenterology and endoscopy practices in response to the COVID-19 pandemic: results from a North American survey. Gastroenterology 2020;159:772–4.e13.
18. Repici A, Pace F, Gabbiadini R, et al. Endoscopy units and the coronavirus disease 2019 outbreak: a multicenter experience from Italy. Gastroenterology 2020; 159:363–6.
19. Available at: https://news.harvard.edu/gazette/story/2020/12/anthony-fauci-offers-a-timeline-for-ending-covid-19-pandemic/. Accessed March 7, 2021.
20. Krammer F. Pandemic vaccines: how are we going to be better prepared next time? Med 2020;1:28–32.
21. Available at: https://www.fda.gov/emergency-preparedness-and-response/coronavirus-disease-2019-covid-19/covid-19-vaccines. Accessed March 4, 2021.
22. Forni G, Mantovani A. COVID-19 vaccines: where we stand and challenges ahead. Cell Death Differ 2021;28:626–39.
23. Levine-Tiefenbrun M, Yelin I, Katz R, et al. Decreased SARS-CoV-2 viral load following vaccination. MedRxiv 2021. https://doi.org/10.1101/2021.02.06.21251283.
24. Petter E, Mor O, Zuckerman N, et al. Initial real-world evidence for lower viral load of individuals who have been vaccinated by BNT162b2. MedRxiv 2021. https://doi.org/10.1101/2021.02.08.21251329.
25. Available at: https://www.nytimes.com/interactive/2020/us/covid-19-vaccine-doses.html. Accessed March 8, 2021.
26. Omer SB, Yildirim I, Forman HP. Herd immunity and implications for SARS-CoV-2 control. JAMA 2020;324:2095–6.
27. Repici A, Maselli R, Colombo M, et al. Coronavirus (COVID-19) outbreak: what the department of endoscopy should know. Gastrointest Endosc 2020;92:192–7.
28. American Society for Gastrointestinal Endoscopy. Guidance for resuming GI endoscopy and practice operations after the COVID-19 pandemic. Gastrointest Endosc 2020;92:743–7.
29. British Society of Gastroenterology. Endoscopy activity and COVID-19: British Society of Gastroenterology and Joint Advisory Group Guidance 2020. Available at: https://www.bsg.org.uk/covid-19-advice/endoscopy-activity-and-covid-19-bsg-and-jag-guidance/. Accessed March 7, 2021.

30. Gralnek IM, Hassan C, Beilenhoff U, et al. ESGE and ESGENA position statement on gastrointestinal endoscopy and the COVID-19 pandemic. Endoscopy 2020; 52:483–90.

31. American Society for Gastrointestinal Endoscopy. Gastroenterology professional society guidance on endoscopic procedures during the COVID-19 pandemic 2020. Available at: https://www.asge.org/home/resources/key-resources/covid-19-asge-updates-for-members/gastroenterology-professional-society-guidance-on-endoscopic-procedures-during-the-covid-19-pandemic. Accessed March 7, 2021.

32. Chu DK, Akl EA, Duda S, et al. Physical distancing, face masks, and eye protection to prevent person-to-person transmission of SARS-CoV-2 and prevent COVID-19: a systematic review and meta-analysis. Lancet 2020;395:1973–87.

33. Cennamo V, Bassi M, Landi S, et al. Redesign of a GI endoscopy unit during the COVID-19 emergency: a practical model. Dig Liver Dis 2020;52:1178–87.

34. Long Y, Hu T, Liu L, et al. Effectiveness of N95 respirators versus surgical masks against influenza: a systematic review and meta-analysis. J Evid Based Med 2020;13:93–101.

35. Offeddu V, Yung CF, Low MSF, et al. Effectiveness of masks and respirators against respiratory infections in healthcare workers: a systematic review and meta-analysis. Clin Infect Dis 2017;65:1934–42.

36. Petersen BT, Cohen J, Hambrick RD, et al. Multisociety guideline on reprocessing flexible GI endoscopes: 2016 update. Gastrointest Endosc 2017;8:282–94.

37. IDSA guidelines on the diagnosis of COVID-19: molecular diagnostic testing. Available at: https://www.idsociety.org/COVID19guidelines/dx. Accessed March 1, 2021.

38. Sultan S, Siddique SM, Altayar O, et al. AGA Institute rapid review and recommendations on the role of pre-procedure SARS-CoV-2 testing and endoscopy. Gastroenterol 2020;159:1935–48.

39. Brown RCH, Kelly D, Wilkinson D, et al. The scientific and ethical feasibility of immunity passports. Lancet Infect Dis 2020;21(3):e58–63.

40. US Department of Labor. Unemployment insurance weekly claims. 2020. Available at: https://www.dol.gov/sites/dolgov/files/OPA/newsreleases/ui-claims/20201122.pdf. Accessed March 6, 2021.

41. Nishihara R, Wu K, Lochhead P, et al. Long-term colorectal-cancer incidence and mortality after lower endoscopy. N Engl J Med 2013;369:1095–105.

42. Lee YC, Fann JC-Y, Chiang T-H, et al. Time to colonoscopy and risk of colorectal cancer in patients with positive results from fecal immunochemical tests. Clin Gastroenterol Hepatol 2019;17:1332–40.

43. Rutter CM, Kim JJ, Meester RGS, et al. Effect of time to diagnostic testing for breast, cervical, and colorectal cancer screening abnormalities on screening efficacy: a modeling study. Cancer Epidemiol Biomarkers Prev 2018;27:158–64.

44. Meester RG, Zauber AG, Doubeni CA, et al. Consequences of increasing time to colonoscopy examination after positive result from fecal colorectal cancer screening test. Clin Gastroenterol Hepatol 2016;14:1445–51.

45. Corley DA, Jensen CD, Quinn VP, et al. Association between time to colonoscopy after a positive fecal test result and risk of colorectal cancer and cancer stage at diagnosis. JAMA 2017;317:1631–41.

46. De Jonge L, Worthington J, Van Wifferen F, et al. Impact of the COVID-19 pandemic on faecal immunochemical test-based colorectal cancer screening programmes in Australia, Canada and the Netherlands: a comparative modelling study. Lancet Gastroenterol Hepatol 2021;6:304–14.

47. Morris EJA, Goldacre R, Spata E, et al. Impact of the COVID-19 pandemic on the detection and management of colorectal cancer in England: a population-based study. Lancet Gastroenterol Hepatol 2021;6(3):199–208.
48. Worthington J, Lew J-B, Feletto E, et al. Improving Australian National Bowel Cancer Screening Program outcomes through increased participation and cost-effective investment. PLoS One 2020;15:e0227899.
49. Keihanian T, Sharma P, Goyal J, et al. Telehealth utilization in gastroenterology clinics amid the COVID-19 pandemic: impact on clinical practice and gastroenterology training. Gastroenterology 2020;159:1598–601.
50. Dobrusin A, Hawa F, Gladshteyn M, et al. Gastroenterologists and patients report high satisfaction rates with telehealth services during the novel coronavirus 2019 pandemic. Clin Gastroenterol Hepatol 2020;18:2393–7.
51. Available at: https://realbusiness.co.uk/as-said-by-winston-churchill-never-waste-a-good-crisis/. Accessed March 7, 2021.
52. Morens DM, Fauci AS. Emerging pandemic diseases: how we got to COVID-19. Cell 2020;182:1077–92.

The Epidemiology of Acute Respiratory Distress Syndrome Before and After Coronavirus Disease 2019

Kathryn W. Hendrickson, MD[a,b], Ithan D. Peltan, MD, MSc[a,c], Samuel M. Brown, MD, MS[a,b],*

KEYWORDS

- ARDS • Epidemiology • Incidence • Subtypes • Mortality • COVID-19

KEY POINTS

- Acute respiratory distress syndrome (ARDS) is heterogeneous.
- ARDS has high incidence among intensive care unit patients.
- ARDS has high morbidity and mortality.
- Improved supportive care has decreased ARDS incidence and mortality.
- Coronavirus Disease 2019–associated ARDS is a syndrome within the known ARDS spectrum.

INTRODUCTION

Acute respiratory distress syndrome (ARDS) occurs when a diverse array of triggers cause acute, bilateral pulmonary inflammation and increased pulmonary capillary permeability leading to acute hypoxemic respiratory failure. Pulmonary biopsy (or autopsy) classically demonstrates diffuse alveolar damage (DAD).[1] Recognizing that ARDS is a syndrome and that research and benchmarking require reproducible definitions, a 2011 consensus conference in Berlin proposed a practical, updated definition (the "Berlin Definition"),[2] In summary, this requires,

This article previously appeared in *Critical Care Clinics*, Volume 37, Issue 4, October 2021.
[a] Division of Pulmonary and Critical Care Medicine, Department of Medicine, University of Utah School of Medicine, 26 North 1900 East, Salt Lake City, UT 84112, USA; [b] Division of Pulmonary and Critical Care Medicine, Department of Medicine, Intermountain Medical Center; [c] Pulmonary Division, Department of Medicine, Intermountain Medical Center, 5121 South Cottonwood Street, Murray, UT 84107, USA
* Corresponding author. Pulmonary Division, Department of Medicine, Intermountain Medical Center, 5121 South Cottonwood Street, Murray, UT 84107.
E-mail address: Samuel.Brown@imail.org

Clinics Collections 12 (2022) 325–338
https://doi.org/10.1016/j.ccol.2021.12.023
2352-7986/22/© 2021 Elsevier Inc. All rights reserved.

1. An acute process developing within 1 week of a known clinical insult or new or worsening respiratory symptoms;
2. Radiographic images showing bilateral opacities not fully explained by effusions, lobar or lung collapse, or nodules; and
3. Impairment in oxygenation as measured by a $Pao_2/Fio_2 \leq 300$ mm Hg in the presence of a positive end-expiratory pressure (PEEP) of at least 5 cm H2O.

Despite many advances in the understanding of ARDS, morbidity and mortality remain high with few targeted therapies. In this epidemiologic review, we consider the etiology, subtypes and phenotypes, incidence, mortality, long-term outcomes, and the relationship(s) between Coronavirus Disease 2019 (COVID-19) and prepandemic ARDS.

ETIOLOGY

Admitting that patients would not have survived long enough to be diagnosed with ARDS before the widespread use of intensive care unit (ICU) ventilators for hypoxemic respiratory failure, Ashbaugh and colleagues first reported on ARDS as a distinct syndrome in a 1967 series of 12 patients.[3] Despite suffering from heterogeneous primary insults, the patients all developed similar patterns of acute-onset respiratory failure with bilateral infiltrates and decreased pulmonary compliance accompanied by autopsy findings of acute inflammation and hyaline membranes.[3]

This initial report captured the heterogeneity of ARDS that continues to present challenges in diagnosis and treatment. Pneumonia is the most common trigger for ARDS, although nonpulmonary sepsis, aspiration pneumonitis, and trauma are also common. An assortment of less common triggers have been identified including pancreatitis and blood transfusion. Clinical syndromes compatible with ARDS but with no identifiable trigger are referred to as acute interstitial pneumonia (AIP) or sometimes Hamman-Rich syndrome rather than ARDS and may represent a response to an array of sometimes overlapping pulmonary insults.[1,4-15] In both ARDS and, presumptively, AIP, an insult elicits an inflammatory response which leads to increased-permeability pulmonary edema creating the hypoxemia and bilateral opacities on imaging required for diagnosis.[16,17] In its most severe forms, DAD results pathologically.

ARDS resulting from direct pulmonary insult such as pneumonia manifests pathologically as alveolar collapse, fibrinous exudate, and edema of the alveolar walls to a greater degree than ARDS resulting from nonpulmonary causes such as pancreatitis.[18] This may represent a spectrum of severity or alternative pathophysiological processes. What is less clear is why some patients with inciting conditions develop ARDS while others do not, and whether differences in genotype, phenotype, or therapeutic context play a role remains unclear.

Chronic conditions including obesity and diabetes have been associated with a decreased incidence of ARDS. In diabetes, some hypothesize that this observed association reflects a decreased inflammatory response among diabetics.[19,20] A potential association with obesity is less clear.[21-23] Importantly, collider bias may in fact account for the observed associations.[24]

On the contrary, chronic alcohol use has been associated with higher risk of ARDS. Kaphalia and Calhoun[25] found that chronic alcohol use leads to pulmonary immune dysfunction, epithelial dysfunction, and the inability to handle reactive oxygen species leading to the high permeability pulmonary edema and hyaline membrane formation seen in ARDS. Smoking is also associated with higher risks of ARDS. Not only are patients who smoke more likely to get pneumonia they also have higher rates of ARDS triggered by nonpulmonary causes.[26,27] Cigarette smoking may thus increase the risk of the inflammatory cascade that results in ARDS. Interestingly, ozone exposure (but no other known pollutants) is also associated with increased risk of ARDS.[28] Consistently, older age,[8] non-white race (likely a surrogate for "social determinants of disease"),[29] and some genetic variants[30] have been described as host factors associated with risk of developing ARDS.

Although age is a risk factor for developing ARDS, it has not consistently been found to be associated with increased mortality. The multinational LUNG-SAFE (The Large Observational Study to Understand the Global Impact of Severe Acute Respiratory Failure) study showed older age to be a risk factor for mortality[31]; however, when controlling for risk, severity, and comorbidity, the independent relationship between age and mortality in ARDS is not consistent.[8] The association of race and ethnicity with ARDS mortality was studied in a retrospective cohort study in 2009 using patient data from three ARDS network randomized control trials. Black race and Hispanic ethnicity were found to have not only higher rates of ARDS than white individuals but higher mortality as well. The causes of race- and ethnicity-related differences are not well understood and likely vary between groups but, in all cases, likely derive substantially from "social determinants of disease" rather than genetic factors. For instance, the fact that higher mortality in Black patients resolves with adjustment for illness severity suggests barriers that hinder Black individuals from seeking early care, physician delay in diagnosis, and other factors worsen the severity mix in these groups.[29]

SUBTYPES

A defining characteristic of ARDS is its heterogeneity, from Ashbaugh's initial publication to the present day.[32,33] Traditional categorizations (as, eg, in the Berlin definition) are based on severity of hypoxemia, which correlates with mortality and the extent of DAD on pathologic examination.[34,35] The effects of some potential ARDS therapies may also vary with hypoxemia severity. For example, in 2018, Guo and colleagues[36] published a systemic review and meta-analysis showing a likely trend toward improved outcomes in patients receiving a high-PEEP protocol. For patients with a Pao_2/Fio_2 (P/F) ratio ≤ 200, there was a slightly lower risk of death; however, in patients with a P/F ratio 201 to 300, there was a possible higher risk of death. Of note this mortality benefit has not been seen in any individual randomized control trials[37–39] and remains a controversial topic. Another example is the 2019 study of therapeutic neuromuscular blockade to improve outcomes in ARDS. Although a previous trial hinted at decreased mortality in patients with P/F ratio less than 130,[40] this larger trial concluded no mortality benefit.[41]

ARDS can also be subdivided based on the initial insult, whether pulmonary (pneumonia, pulmonary contusion, and aspiration) or extrapulmonary (nonthoracic trauma, nonpulmonary sepsis, and transfusion).[7,42,43] Several pathologic, biologic, and physiologic differences have been identified on this basis.[18,44–47] However, in practice, it is difficult to differentiate between the two groups based on substantial overlap.[13] These pathologic, biologic, and physiologic differences are heavily influenced by underlying lung function and architecture, smoking status, chronic diseases, and other conditions, which inflate the heterogeneity of ARDS. No mortality difference has been found between the two groups, likely related to the complexities of the overlap between the two groups.[48]

More recently, "machine learning"-style techniques have been used to identify distinct subtypes. Post-hoc analysis (using latent class analysis) of the ARMA (ARDSnet: Ventilation with Lower Tidal Volumes as Compared with Traditional Tidal Volumes for Acute Lung Injury and the Acute Respiratory Distress Syndrome) and ALVEOLI (Assessment of Low Tidal Volume and Elevated End-Expiratory Pressure to Obviate Lung Injury) trials revealed two phenotypes of ARDS.[37,49] Relative to phenotype 1, phenotype 2 was hyperinflammatory, with higher plasma levels of inflammatory biomarkers, a higher prevalence of vasopressor use, lower serum bicarbonate, and a higher prevalence of sepsis found in phenotype 2 than in phenotype 1.[50] Critically, in terms of its clinical utility, this hyperinflammatory phenotype was also associated with higher mortality. Phenotype may also predict response to therapies: A post-hoc analysis of a randomized controlled trial of statin therapy for ARDS suggested benefit for hyperinflammatory patients.[51] It will be important with the expanding use of novel statistical techniques for subtyping to ground them in reality and validate them in both prospective cohorts and within prespecified subgroups in prospective trials.

INCIDENCE

The incidence of ARDS varies globally by over 400%.[52] It is important to acknowledge in this context that ARDS as a syndrome reflects both patient physiology and clinical context. For example, where patients with hypoxemic respiratory failure are not routinely intubated (as may occur in certain institutional settings in USA/Europe or in low- and middle-income country settings with limited supplies of ventilators and/or resources and personnel for ICU-level care), ARDS incidence may appear lower than it actually is. Similarly, routine use of high-tidal-volume ventilation among patients at risk may increase the incidence of ARDS in a given setting. With those caveats in mind, incidence ranges from 10.1/100,000/y in Brazil in 2014 to 82/100,000/y in the United States in 2005 (**Table 1**).[5,7,8,10] Between-study differences in case ascertainment and local context may drive these observed differences.[53,54] Some studies, for instance, relied on clinician diagnosis while others used billing codes, both of which may be inaccurate. Both methods are likely to undercount ARDS cases, as only 60% of ARDS cases were appropriately identified by clinicians in one large study.[1] Differences in the prevalence of ARDS risk factors may account for some of the variation as well.

Likely the highest quality evidence on ARDS incidence and management patterns originates from LUNG-SAFE, a prevalence study conducted during a 4-week period in 459 ICUs in 50 countries. Overall, 10% of all ICU patients and 23% of mechanically ventilated patients met ARDS criteria, yielding an ICU incidence of 5.5 cases per ICU bed per year.

In 2011, the Prevention and Early Treatment of Acute Lung Injury (PETAL) Network developed the Lung Injury Prediction Score (LIPS) to help identify patients in the emergency department with high risk of developing ARDS. ARDS predictors included in the final score both triggers (ie, shock, aspiration, lung contusion) and risk modifiers (ie, smoking, diabetes mellitus, acidosis). This tool also works in hospitalized patients as a quick and effective way of identifying high-risk patients.[55–57] Hopes that this score would help enrich enrollment in trials of therapeutics to decrease incidence and death from ARDS, however, have so far not borne fruit. For instance, the LIPS-A trial, in which aspirin was tested as a possible intervention in this subgroup of patients, showed no difference in rates of ARDS and rates of death after receiving aspirin versus placebo.[58]

Between 2001 and 2008, rates of ARDS fell by half in two ICUs in Rochester, Minnesota, in a population-based, retrospective cohort study of the epidemiology of ARDS patients admitted during that time period. Severity of acute illness, greater number of comorbidities, and major predisposing conditions in patients with ARDS increased while mortality stayed the same during this time. Interestingly, the reduction in incidence occurred exclusively in patients with hospital-acquired ARDS. As noted by the authors, during this time, a separate hospital-wide program to limit risk factors for ARDS was undertaken which can explain this reduction in hospital-acquired ARDS. This indicates that ARDS may, in part, be a preventable hospital-acquired

Table 1
Main epidemiologic studies on ARDS incidence after AECC definition

Authors, Year of Publication [Reference]	Study Period	Country or Countries	Incidence of All ARDS Categories (per 100,000 Person-Years-Population-Based Studies) or Percentage (%, Hospitalization-Based Studies)	Incidence of Moderate and Severe ARDS Categories (per 100,000 Person-Years-Population-Based Studies) or Percentage (%, Hospitalization-Based Studies)
Sigurdsson et al,[15] 2013	1988–2010	Iceland		3.65–9.63
Nolan et al,[4] 1997	1990–1994	Australia		7.3–9.3
Luhr et al,[5] 1999	1997	Scandinavia (Sweden, Denmark, Iceland, Norway)	17.9	13.5
Bersten et al,[6] 2002	1999	Australia (South, Western, and Tasmania)	34	28
Brun-Buisson et al,[13] 2004	1999	Europe	7.1% (of all ICU admissions)	6.1% (of all ICU admissions)
Rubenfeld et al,[7] 2005	1999–2000	King County, WA, USA	78.9	58.7
Manzano et al,[8] 2005	2001	Granada, Spain	25.5	23
Sakr et al,[92] 2005	2002	Europe	12.5% (of all ICU admissions), 19.1% (of all mechanically ventilated patients)	10.6% (of all ICU admissions), 16.5% (of all mechanically ventilated patients)
Li et al,[9] 2011	2001–2008	Olmsted County, MN		81 (in 2001), 38.3 (in 2008)
The Irish Critical Care Trials Group,[14] 2008	2006	Ireland	19%	
Caser et al,[10] 2014	2006–2007	Vitoria Region, Brazil	10.1	6.3
Linko et al,[11] 2009	2007	Finland	10.6	5
Villar et al,[12] 2011	2008–2009	Spain		7.2
Bellani et al,[1] 2016	2014	50 Countries	10.4% of all ICU admissions, 5.5 cases per ICU bed per year	

ARDS was defined using the Berlin definition nomenclature: All ARDS categories include mild, moderate, and severe ARDS.

complication.[9] Multiple additional studies have shown that using LTVV in all visitors to the hospital and ICU have decreased incidence of ARDS arguing for the use of LTVV in all patients and not only on those with respiratory failure.[59,60]

ACUTE RESPIRATORY DISTRESS SYNDROME-ASSOCIATED MORTALITY

Despite improved mortality rates, ARDS continues to be a syndrome of high mortality. As noted previously, P/F ratio correlates with ARDS outcome, prompting the authors of the Berlin Criteria to maintain the traditional severity categories in their updated consensus definition. Mortality in cohorts analyzed by the Berlin Criteria authors was 34.9% (95% confidence interval [CI]: 24%-30%) in mild ARDS, 40.3% (95% CI: 29%-34%) in moderate ARDS, and 46.1% (95% CI: 29%-34%) in severe ARDS, as defined by P/F thresholds of 300, 200, and 100.[2] The LUNG-SAFE study reported similar findings, with 28-day mortality of 29.6% (95% CI: 26.2%-33.0%) in mild ARDS, 35.2% (95% CI: 32.4%-38.1%) in moderate ARDS, and 40.9% (95% CI: 36.8%-45.1%) in severe ARDS using the same P/F thresholds used in the Berlin definition.[1]

Reported ARDS mortality has decreased over recent decades. Compared to the late 1990s, when independent studies reported ARDS mortality of 58% to 59%,[4,13] mortality in contemporary studies is much lower (**Figs. 1** and **2**). ARDS mortality in 2014 in LUNG-SAFE was 10.4%,[1] and 28% in the LOTUS-FRUIT U.S. multicenter study conducted by the PETAL Network in 2019.[61] While imperfect,[62] death certificate data also suggest decreasing risk of death for ARDS patients, with annual attributable mortality in one U.S. death certificate analysis decreasing from 5.01 per 100,000 people in 1999 to 2.82 per 100,000 population in 2013.[63] While changes in ascertainment (diagnosing more patients with less-severe ARDS) and decreasing use of mechanical ventilation for patients near the end of life may contribute to this trend, it appears likely that increasing the use of LTVV since the publication of the seminal ARMA trial in 2000 is a key factor driving improved outcomes in ARDS.[49] In fact, among patients who do

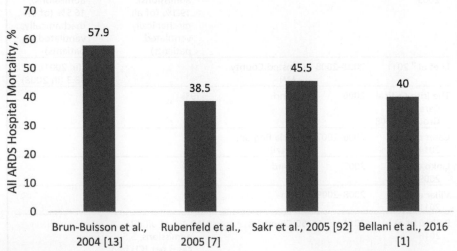

Fig. 1. Estimated overall hospital mortality rates for patients with ARDS of any severity. Hospital mortality reported in the main epidemiologic studies in all ARDS categories (mild, moderate, and severe). On the X-axis, the studies are chronologically ordered based on the study period.

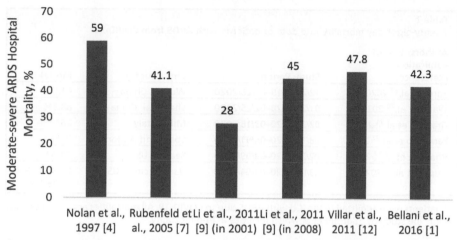

Fig. 2. Estimated mortality rates for patients with moderate-severe ARDS. Hospital mortality reported in the subgroups of moderate-severe ARDS. Moderate-severe ARDS hospital mortality in the study by Li *and colleagues* [2011] is reported in two different years of study, 2001 and 2008. On the X-axis, the studies are chronologically ordered based on the study period.

receive low tidal volume ventilation, there has been no change in mortality.[64] It is also important to note that, in some settings, apparent stability of crude ARDS mortality may mask changes in case mix (increasing illness severity and comorbidities) and therefore improving risk-adjusted mortality.[9]

LONG-TERM OUTCOMES

Despite the significant lung injury experienced during the course of a patient's illness with ARDS, postillness pulmonary function tests showed normalization at 5 years after ICU.[65] Despite this normalization in lung function, reported quality-of-life scores and exercise tolerance, measured by 6-minute walk test, remain lower than average at 5 years. Multiple factors likely contribute to this including persistent weakness and neuropsychologic impairments. These neuropsychologic issues are heterogeneous and affect both the patient and their caregivers.[65] These patients also accrue larger health care costs after hospitalization because of increased utilization of the health care system. ARDS is one of the most common reasons for admission to a long-term ventilator rehabilitation unit.[66]

COVID-19

The severe acute respiratory distress syndrome-associated coronavirus-2 was first identified in December 2019 in Wuhan, Hubei, China, as the agent causing what is now called COVID-19.[67] COVID-19 was officially declared a pandemic by the World Health Organization on March 11, 2020. As of November 21, 2020, 57,274,018 confirmed cases have been reported with 1,368,000 deaths worldwide.[68] While it is increasingly clear that COVID-19 is a multisystem disease, the primary manifestation is a viral pneumonia that, in some patients, progresses to ARDS, often complicated by protracted illness or death.

Mortality estimates for COVID-19-associated ARDS vary widely, ranging from 3.4% to 88.3% (**Table 2**).[69–74] These estimates are affected by the studied population,

Table 2
Twenty-eight-day mortality rate data of patients with ARDS from COVID-19

Authors, Year of Publication [Reference]	Study Period	City, Country	Mortality
Yang et al,[69] 2020	12/24/2019–01/26/2020	Wuhan, China	61.5%
Wang et al,[70] 2020	01/25/2020–02/25/2020	Shanghai, China	88.3%
Grasselli et al,[71] 2020	02/20/2020–03/18/2020	Milan, Italy	26%
Ferrando et al,[72] 2020	03/12/2020–06/01/2020	Spain and Andora	36%
Bhatraju et al,[74] 2020	02/24/2020–03/09/2020	Seattle, USA	50%*
Gupta et al,[73] 2020	03/04/2020–04/04/2020	Various cities, USA	6.6%-80.8% (35.4%)

All patients were admitted to the ICU with ARDS due to COVID-19. All mortalities are 28-d mortality except the study by *Batraju et al which includes a 14-d mortality.

health system factors (thresholds for hospitalization varied across cohorts substantially), therapeutic context (Early in the pandemic, large numbers of potentially toxic therapies were administered in cocktails.), institutional context (the degree to which the studied health care systems were strained by the pandemic surge), and patient-level risk factors (some sites predominantly cared for patients in nursing homes). For example, patients admitted to hospitals with fewer ICU beds had higher risk of death likely because of less training and comfort of caregivers in treating ARDS as well as limited resources in these settings, particularly in the pandemic context. Critically, some early mortality studies had insufficient follow-up to provide accurate estimates of morality, excluding patients without a final outcome (discharge or death) and thereby inflating mortality estimates by excluding patients alive and still in the hospital.

The question of whether and how COVID-19-associated ARDS differs from prior forms of ARDS has been surprisingly contentious.[75] Early anxiety about abrupt decompensation specific to this condition, the risk of aerosolization and consequent transmission to caregivers with high-flow nasal cannula oxygen, and lack of effective therapeutics all played a role, as did clinician perceptions that some patients with COVID-19 exhibit "happy hypoxemia" and/or higher-than-expected lung compliance for their degree of hypoxemia.[76] The opinion that ARDS resulting from COVID-19 might be exceptional and clinicians' frustration over the lack of proven treatments were sometimes associated with calls for application of therapies previously shown ineffective in general ARDS and even for the use of high-tidal-volume ventilation. Spring and summer 2020 witnessed a vigorous debate on the issues, with some thought leaders arguing for novel supportive care, and others arguing that standard supportive care for ARDS represented the best approach.[77,78]

While some prognostic factors differ and time from COVID-19 symptom onset to full ARDS is sometimes slightly longer than with some classic ARDS etiologies,[79] most evidence to date suggests that ARDS in COVID-19 lacks important differences from the syndrome generally. Contradicting the postulated "L-type" (high compliance) and "H-type" (low compliance) dichotomy advanced by some as unique to COVID-19 ARDS,[76,80] the spectrum of lung compliance in COVID-19 ARDS appears similar to that observed in prior studies of general ARDS.[81] Pathologic analysis also shows findings similar to ARDS generally, demonstrating hyaline membrane formation, edema, and DAD.[82] We therefore manage COVID-19 ARDS with the package of evidence-based care that we apply to ARDS generally, including strict adherence to low-tidal-volume ventilation,[49] consideration of prone positioning,[83] and high PEEP for more severe ARDS,[36] conservative fluid management,[84] protocolized spontaneous breathing and awakening trial,[85] and early mobilization.[86] It is nevertheless plausible that, given its homogeneous trigger and potentially more homogeneous inflammatory phenotype, ARDS resulting from COVID-19 could respond to therapies that failed trials enrolling patients with a heterogeneous array of triggers and endotypes. The apparent efficacy of steroid therapy in several (imperfect) trials,[87,88] a treatment for which trials in general ARDS population had repeatedly yielded conflicting evidence,[89–91] may be one early example of this phenomenon.

SUMMARY

ARDS remains a common, deadly problem among critically ill patients around the world. It is a syndrome of significant heterogeneity, with sub-phenotypes requiring further characterization and tools for prompt clinical identification. COVID-19 has brought new challenges including a large, and relatively homogeneous, population of ARDS patients but does not seem to cause a truly unique respiratory failure syndrome distinct from ARDS generally nor even engender a truly homogenous subtype of ARDS. Further advances in ARDS care will likely require improved understanding of the epidemiology of this syndrome and its subtypes as well as innovative trials of focused therapeutics. Given the high mortality of the syndrome and its long-term morbidity, ongoing study into treatment and care of patients with ARDS is paramount.

CLINICS CARE POINTS

- Although acute respiratory distress syndrome (ARDS) has a high incidence among intensive care unit patients, with high morbidity and mortality, it remains underdiagnosed.
- The Berlin criteria were created to help clearly identify patients with ARDS.
- Supportive measures with low-tidal-volume ventilation, prone positioning, conservative fluid management strategies, high PEEP for severe disease, protocolized spontaneous breathing and awakening trials, and early mobilization have lowered the morbidity and mortality of ARDS and are the cornerstone of therapy.
- COVID-19-associated ARDS is a syndrome on the ARDS spectrum and should therefore be treated with the same strategies as classic ARDS while we await results of ongoing trials.

DISCLOSURE

K.W. Hendrickson declares no disclosures. I.D. Peltan reports receiving research support from the National Institutes of Health, Centers for Disease Control, Janssen Pharmaceuticals, and Immunexpress, Inc. and support to institution from Regeneron and Asahi Kasei Pharma. S.M. Brown-please see pdf in Other Content tab.

REFERENCES

1. Bellani G, et al. Epidemiology, patterns of care, and mortality for patients with acute respiratory distress syndrome in intensive care units in 50 countries. JAMA 2016;315(8):788–800.
2. Force ADT, et al. Acute respiratory distress syndrome: the Berlin definition. JAMA 2012;307(23):2526–33.
3. Ashbaugh DG, et al. Acute respiratory distress in adults. Lancet 1967;2(7511):319–23.

4. Nolan S, et al. Acute respiratory distress syndrome in a community hospital ICU. Intensive Care Med 1997;23(5):530–8.
5. Luhr OR, et al. Incidence and mortality after acute respiratory failure and acute respiratory distress syndrome in Sweden, Denmark, and Iceland. The ARF Study Group. Am J Respir Crit Care Med 1999;159(6):1849–61.
6. Bersten AD, et al. Incidence and mortality of acute lung injury and the acute respiratory distress syndrome in three Australian States. Am J Respir Crit Care Med 2002;165(4):443–8.
7. Rubenfeld GD, et al. Incidence and outcomes of acute lung injury. N Engl J Med 2005;353(16):1685–93.
8. Manzano F, et al. Incidence of acute respiratory distress syndrome and its relation to age. J Crit Care 2005;20(3):274–80.
9. Li G, et al. Eight-year trend of acute respiratory distress syndrome: a population-based study in Olmsted County, Minnesota. Am J Respir Crit Care Med 2011; 183(1):59–66.
10. Caser EB, et al. Impact of distinct definitions of acute lung injury on its incidence and outcomes in Brazilian ICUs: prospective evaluation of 7,133 patients*. Crit Care Med 2014;42(3):574–82.
11. Linko R, et al. Acute respiratory failure in intensive care units. FINNALI: a prospective cohort study. Intensive Care Med 2009;35(8):1352–61.
12. Villar J, et al. The ALIEN study: incidence and outcome of acute respiratory distress syndrome in the era of lung protective ventilation. Intensive Care Med 2011;37(12):1932–41.
13. Brun-Buisson C, et al. Epidemiology and outcome of acute lung injury in European intensive care units. Results from the ALIVE study. Intensive Care Med 2004;30(1):51–61.
14. Irish Critical Care Trials, G. Acute lung injury and the acute respiratory distress syndrome in Ireland: a prospective audit of epidemiology and management. Crit Care 2008;12(1):R30.
15. Sigurdsson MI, et al. Acute respiratory distress syndrome: nationwide changes in incidence, treatment and mortality over 23 years. Acta Anaesthesiol Scand 2013; 57(1):37–45.
16. Bachofen M, Weibel ER. Structural alterations of lung parenchyma in the adult respiratory distress syndrome. Clin Chest Med 1982;3(1):35–56.
17. Tomashefski JF Jr. Pulmonary pathology of the adult respiratory distress syndrome. Clin Chest Med 1990;11(4):593–619.
18. Hoelz C, et al. Morphometric differences in pulmonary lesions in primary and secondary ARDS. A preliminary study in autopsies. Pathol Res Pract 2001;197(8): 521–30.
19. Moss M, et al. Diabetic patients have a decreased incidence of acute respiratory distress syndrome. Crit Care Med 2000;28(7):2187–92.
20. Rubenfeld GD, Herridge MS. Epidemiology and outcomes of acute lung injury. Chest 2007;131(2):554–62.
21. Ni YN, et al. Can body mass index predict clinical outcomes for patients with acute lung injury/acute respiratory distress syndrome? A meta-analysis. Crit Care 2017;21(1):36.
22. Zhi G, et al. Obesity paradox" in acute respiratory distress syndrome: a systematic review and meta-analysis. PLoS One 2016;11(9):e0163677.
23. McCallister JW, Adkins EJ, O'Brien JM Jr. Obesity and acute lung injury. Clin Chest Med 2009;30(3):495–508, viii.

24. Stensrud MJ, Valberg M, Aalen OO. Can collider bias explain paradoxical associations? Epidemiology 2017;28(4):e39–40.

25. Kaphalia L, Calhoun WJ. Alcoholic lung injury: metabolic, biochemical and immunological aspects. Toxicol Lett 2013;222(2):171–9.

26. Calfee CS, et al. Cigarette smoke exposure and the acute respiratory distress syndrome. Crit Care Med 2015;43(9):1790–7.

27. Hsieh SJ, et al. Prevalence and impact of active and passive cigarette smoking in acute respiratory distress syndrome. Crit Care Med 2014;42(9):2058–68.

28. Ware LB, et al. Long-term ozone exposure increases the risk of developing the acute respiratory distress syndrome. Am J Respir Crit Care Med 2016;193(10): 1143–50.

29. Erickson SE, et al. Racial and ethnic disparities in mortality from acute lung injury. Crit Care Med 2009;37(1):1–6.

30. Meyer NJ, Christie JD. Genetic heterogeneity and risk of acute respiratory distress syndrome. Semin Respir Crit Care Med 2013;34(4):459–74.

31. Laffey JG, et al. Potentially modifiable factors contributing to outcome from acute respiratory distress syndrome: the LUNG SAFE study. Intensive Care Med 2016; 42(12):1865–76.

32. Calfee CS, et al. Trauma-associated lung injury differs clinically and biologically from acute lung injury due to other clinical disorders. Crit Care Med 2007; 35(10):2243–50.

33. Tejera P, et al. Distinct and replicable genetic risk factors for acute respiratory distress syndrome of pulmonary or extrapulmonary origin. J Med Genet 2012; 49(11):671–80.

34. Villar J, et al. A universal definition of ARDS: the PaO2/FiO2 ratio under a standard ventilatory setting–a prospective, multicenter validation study. Intensive Care Med 2013;39(4):583–92.

35. Thille AW, et al. Comparison of the Berlin definition for acute respiratory distress syndrome with autopsy. Am J Respir Crit Care Med 2013;187(7):761–7.

36. Guo L, et al. Higher PEEP improves outcomes in ARDS patients with clinically objective positive oxygenation response to PEEP: a systematic review and meta-analysis. BMC Anesthesiol 2018;18(1):172.

37. Brower RG, et al. Higher versus lower positive end-expiratory pressures in patients with the acute respiratory distress syndrome. N Engl J Med 2004;351(4): 327–36.

38. Meade MO, et al. Ventilation strategy using low tidal volumes, recruitment maneuvers, and high positive end-expiratory pressure for acute lung injury and acute respiratory distress syndrome: a randomized controlled trial. JAMA 2008; 299(6):637–45.

39. Mercat A, et al. Positive end-expiratory pressure setting in adults with acute lung injury and acute respiratory distress syndrome: a randomized controlled trial. JAMA 2008;299(6):646–55.

40. Papazian L, et al. Neuromuscular blockers in early acute respiratory distress syndrome. N Engl J Med 2010;363(12):1107–16.

41. National Heart L, et al. Early neuromuscular blockade in the acute respiratory distress syndrome. N Engl J Med 2019;380(21):1997–2008.

42. Shaver CM, Bastarache JA. Clinical and biological heterogeneity in acute respiratory distress syndrome: direct versus indirect lung injury. Clin Chest Med 2014; 35(4):639–53.

43. Bernard GR, et al. The American-European Consensus Conference on ARDS. Definitions, mechanisms, relevant outcomes, and clinical trial coordination. Am J Respir Crit Care Med 1994;149(3 Pt 1):818–24.
44. Pelosi P, et al. Pulmonary and extrapulmonary acute respiratory distress syndrome are different. Eur Respir J Suppl 2003;42:48s–56s.
45. Gattinoni L, et al. Acute respiratory distress syndrome caused by pulmonary and extrapulmonary disease. Different syndromes? Am J Respir Crit Care Med 1998; 158(1):3–11.
46. Albaiceta GM, et al. Differences in the deflation limb of the pressure-volume curves in acute respiratory distress syndrome from pulmonary and extrapulmonary origin. Intensive Care Med 2003;29(11):1943–9.
47. Calfee CS, et al. Distinct molecular phenotypes of direct vs indirect ARDS in single-center and multicenter studies. Chest 2015;147(6):1539–48.
48. Agarwal R, et al. Is the mortality higher in the pulmonary vs the extrapulmonary ARDS? A meta analysis. Chest 2008;133(6):1463–73.
49. Acute Respiratory Distress Syndrome, N, et al. Ventilation with lower tidal volumes as compared with traditional tidal volumes for acute lung injury and the acute respiratory distress syndrome. N Engl J Med 2000;342(18):1301–8.
50. Calfee CS, et al. Subphenotypes in acute respiratory distress syndrome: latent class analysis of data from two randomised controlled trials. Lancet Respir Med 2014;2(8):611–20.
51. Calfee CS, et al. Acute respiratory distress syndrome subphenotypes and differential response to simvastatin: secondary analysis of a randomised controlled trial. Lancet Respir Med 2018;6(9):691–8.
52. Pham T, Rubenfeld GD. Fifty years of research in ARDS. The epidemiology of acute respiratory distress syndrome. A 50th birthday review. Am J Respir Crit Care Med 2017;195(7):860–70.
53. Ferguson ND, et al. Acute respiratory distress syndrome: underrecognition by clinicians and diagnostic accuracy of three clinical definitions. Crit Care Med 2005; 33(10):2228–34.
54. Frohlich S, et al. Acute respiratory distress syndrome: underrecognition by clinicians. J Crit Care 2013;28(5):663–8.
55. Gajic O, et al. Early identification of patients at risk of acute lung injury: evaluation of lung injury prediction score in a multicenter cohort study. Am J Respir Crit Care Med 2011;183(4):462–70.
56. Trillo-Alvarez C, et al. Acute lung injury prediction score: derivation and validation in a population-based sample. Eur Respir J 2011;37(3):604–9.
57. Soto GJ, et al. Lung injury prediction score in hospitalized patients at risk of acute respiratory distress syndrome. Crit Care Med 2016;44(12):2182–91.
58. Kor DJ, et al. Effect of aspirin on development of ARDS in at-risk patients presenting to the emergency department: the LIPS-A randomized clinical trial. JAMA 2016;315(22):2406–14.
59. Serpa Neto A, et al. Association between use of lung-protective ventilation with lower tidal volumes and clinical outcomes among patients without acute respiratory distress syndrome: a meta-analysis. JAMA 2012;308(16):1651–9.
60. Writing Group for the, P.I, et al. Effect of a low vs intermediate tidal volume strategy on ventilator-free days in intensive care unit patients without ARDS: a randomized clinical trial. JAMA 2018;320(18):1872–80.
61. Lanspa MJ, et al. Prospective assessment of the feasibility of a trial of low-tidal volume ventilation for patients with acute respiratory failure. Ann Am Thorac Soc 2019;16(3):356–62.

62. Falci L, et al. Examination of cause-of-death data quality among New York city deaths due to cancer, pneumonia, or diabetes from 2010 to 2014. Am J Epidemiol 2018;187(1):144–52.
63. Cochi SE, et al. Mortality trends of acute respiratory distress syndrome in the United States from 1999 to 2013. Ann Am Thorac Soc 2016;13(10):1742–51.
64. Walkey AJ, et al. Acute respiratory distress syndrome: epidemiology and management approaches. Clin Epidemiol 2012;4:159–69.
65. Herridge MS, et al. Functional disability 5 years after acute respiratory distress syndrome. N Engl J Med 2011;364(14):1293–304.
66. Mamary AJ, et al. Survival in patients receiving prolonged ventilation: factors that influence outcome. Clin Med Insights Circ Respir Pulm Med 2011;5:17–26.
67. Zhu N, et al. A novel coronavirus from patients with pneumonia in China, 2019. N Engl J Med 2020;382(8):727–33.
68. Available at: https://www.who.int/emergencies/diseases/novel-coronavirus-2019? gclid=EAIaIQobChMIoNWJg6m86wIVjcDACh2RZAFnEAAYASAAEgI7APD_BwE. Accessed August 27, 2020.
69. Yang X, et al. Clinical course and outcomes of critically ill patients with SARS-CoV-2 pneumonia in Wuhan, China: a single-centered, retrospective, observational study. Lancet Respir Med 2020;8(5):475–81.
70. Wang Y, et al. Clinical course and outcomes of 344 intensive care patients with COVID-19. Am J Respir Crit Care Med 2020;201(11):1430–4.
71. Grasselli G, et al. Baseline characteristics and outcomes of 1591 patients infected with SARS-CoV-2 admitted to ICUs of the Lombardy region, Italy. JAMA 2020;323(16):1574–81.
72. Ferrando C, et al. Clinical features, ventilatory management, and outcome of ARDS caused by COVID-19 are similar to other causes of ARDS. Intensive Care Med 2020;46(12):2200–11.
73. Gupta S, et al. Factors associated with death in critically ill patients with coronavirus disease 2019 in the US. JAMA Intern Med 2020;180(11):1436–47.
74. Bhatraju PK, et al. Covid-19 in critically ill patients in the seattle region - case series. N Engl J Med 2020;382(21):2012–22.
75. Barbeta E, et al. SARS-CoV-2-induced acute respiratory distress syndrome: pulmonary mechanics and gas-exchange abnormalities. Ann Am Thorac Soc 2020; 17(9):1164–8.
76. Marini JJ, Gattinoni L. Management of COVID-19 respiratory distress. JAMA 2020;323(22):2329–30.
77. Matthay MA, Aldrich JM, Gotts JE. Treatment for severe acute respiratory distress syndrome from COVID-19. Lancet Respir Med 2020;8(5):433–4.
78. Wiersinga WJ, et al. Pathophysiology, transmission, diagnosis, and treatment of coronavirus disease 2019 (COVID-19): a review. JAMA 2020;324(8):782–93.
79. Li X, Ma X. Acute respiratory failure in COVID-19: is it "typical" ARDS? Crit Care 2020;24(1):198.
80. Gattinoni L, et al. COVID-19 pneumonia: different respiratory treatments for different phenotypes? Intensive Care Med 2020;46(6):1099–102.
81. Panwar R, et al. Compliance phenotypes in early acute respiratory distress syndrome before the COVID-19 pandemic. Am J Respir Crit Care Med 2020;202(9): 1244–52.
82. Calabrese F, et al. Pulmonary pathology and COVID-19: lessons from autopsy. The experience of European Pulmonary Pathologists. Virchows Arch 2020; 477(3):359–72.

83. Guerin C, Reignier J, Richard JC. Prone positioning in the acute respiratory distress syndrome. N Engl J Med 2013;369(10):980–1.
84. National Heart L, et al. Comparison of two fluid-management strategies in acute lung injury. N Engl J Med 2006;354(24):2564–75.
85. Girard TD, et al. Efficacy and safety of a paired sedation and ventilator weaning protocol for mechanically ventilated patients in intensive care (Awakening and Breathing Controlled trial): a randomised controlled trial. Lancet 2008; 371(9607):126–34.
86. Taito S, et al. Early mobilization of mechanically ventilated patients in the intensive care unit. J Intensive Care 2016;4:50.
87. RECOVERY Collaborative Group, Horby P, Lim WS, et al. Dexamethasone in hospitalized patients with Covid-19. N Engl J Med 2021;384(8):693–704. https://doi.org/10.1056/NEJMoa2021436.
88. Prescott HC, Rice TW. Corticosteroids in COVID-19 ARDS: evidence and Hope during the pandemic. JAMA 2020;324(13):1292–5.
89. Schein RM, et al. Complement activation and corticosteroid therapy in the development of the adult respiratory distress syndrome. Chest 1987;91(6):850–4.
90. Peter JV, et al. Corticosteroids in the prevention and treatment of acute respiratory distress syndrome (ARDS) in adults: meta-analysis. BMJ 2008;336(7651): 1006–9.
91. Villar J, et al. Dexamethasone treatment for the acute respiratory distress syndrome: a multicentre, randomised controlled trial. Lancet Respir Med 2020; 8(3):267–76.
92. Sakr Y, et al. High tidal volume and positive fluid balance are associated with worse outcome in acute lung injury. Chest 2005;128(5):3098–108.

The COVID-19 Patient in the Surgical Intensive Care Unit

Ian Monroe, MD, Matthew Dale, MD, PhD, Michael Schwabe, MD, Rachel Schenkel, MD, Paul J. Schenarts, MD*

KEYWORDS

- COVID-19 • SARS-CoV-2 • Critical care management
- Multiple organ system failure • Respiratory failure • ARDS

KEY POINTS

- The COVID-19 pandemic continues to surge around the globe. Nonintensive care–trained surgeons may be called on to deploy into the critical care unit to care for these complex patients.
- Acute respiratory failure is the most common manifestation of severe COVID-19 infection.
- COVID 19 may be considered an endothelial disease, causing pathologic changes in the brain, heart, lungs, gastrointestinal tract, and kidneys.
- Our understanding of the pathophysiology and treatment of COVID-19 in the critical care setting continues to evolve at a rapid pace.

Coronaviruses, a name derived from their crownlike morphology observed on electron microscope, have been described in literature for over 70 years.[1] They are enveloped, positive single-stranded RNA viruses. These viruses are known to bind to host cells' membrane via a spike protein that facilitates fusion between the virus and host cell. On entry into the cell, their genome is replicated and packaged for delivery to other cells.[1,2]

Coronaviruses are known to cause a variety of symptoms. Many are nonspecific, including fever, cough, and generalized fatigue. They are often responsible for upper and lower respiratory tract infections that can vary from mild to severe, with acute hypoxic respiratory failure and acute respiratory distress syndrome (ARDS) being known sequalae of these respiratory infections.[1,3,4] Enteric, central nervous system (CNS), renal, cardiac, and hematologic diseases can also develop as a result of coronaviruses.[5]

This article previously appeared in *Surgical Clinics*, Volume 102, Issue 1, February 2022.
Department of Surgery, Creighton University, School of Medicine, Medical Education Building, Suite 501, 7710 Mercy Road, Omaha, NE 68124-2368, USA
* Corresponding author.
E-mail address: pjschenartsmd@gmail.com

Clinics Collections 12 (2022) 339–359
https://doi.org/10.1016/j.ccol.2021.12.024
2352-7986/22/© 2021 Elsevier Inc. All rights reserved.

Within the last 2 decades, multiple variants have been responsible for widespread outbreaks of primarily respiratory infections, including SARS-CoV and MERS-CoV in 2003 and 2012, respectively.[2,3]

In 2019, reports of a new variant called SARS-CoV-2 began circulating, and its resulting disease was named COVID-19.[6] By March 2020, the World Health Organization declared this infection a global pandemic.[7] At the time of this submission, COVID-19 infected more than 230 million people, of which approximately 4.7 million have died.[8] Despite other counties having larger populations, the United States accounts for the greatest number of deaths (more than 43 million).[8]

Because the number of patients with COVID-19 has surged, noncritical care–trained and even junior physicians have been redeployed from their normal area of practice into the intensive care unit (ICU) to mange patients with this complex disease.[9–11] Organizations such as the Society for Critical Care Medicine,[12] The American Thoracic Society,[13] and universities[14] have rushed to fill this educational and experience gap with "just-in-time" training.

There is a high likelihood that surgical intensivists and noncritical care–trained surgeons may be called up to provide critical care for patients who would typically be cared for in a medical ICU. The purpose of this article, therefore, is to provide an overview of the pathophysiology, disease manifestations, and treatment options for patients with COVID-19 admitted to a surgical ICU. To accomplish this, an organ-based, systematic approach will be used. Despite the importance of long-term complications of this infection,[15] the primary focus of this article is critical care.

It is important for the reader to understand that the concepts and strategies presented here are based on the best available current information. Given the rapid evolution of our understanding of this complex disease, updated recommendations may occur between manuscript submission and publication.

THE NEUROLOGIC SYSTEM

During the COVID-19 epidemic, one of the first known neurologic changes was anosmia, leading to a worry in otherwise asymptomatic individuals of an upcoming worse symptomatic infection. With ongoing publications, additional neurologic manifestations have been identified and are still being reported. Anosmia, encephalopathy, and stroke were the most common neurologic syndromes associated with SARS-CoV-2 infection.[16] Dizziness, fatigue, headache, nausea, and confusion have also been reported. Postinfectious complications of acute demyelinating encephalomyelitis, generalized myoclonus, acute transverse myelitis, Guillain–Barré syndromes, and variants have been reported.[17] With the vast array of symptoms reported in lethal and nonlethal COVID-19 infections, an infection with the SARS-CoV-2 virus must be included in the differential diagnosis. Imaging studies of patients with anosmia and COVID-19 revealed hyperintensity and swelling of the olfactory bulb, consistent with inflammation.[18] Biopsy samples of anosmic patients showed SARS-CoV-2 infection in the olfactory epithelium with associated local inflammation.[18]

Theories behind the mechanism of SARS-CoV-2 to cause neurologic changes are ongoing. Entry into the CNS may be due to a "trojan horse" theory, where the SARS-CoV-2 virus directly attaches to inflammatory cells such as lymphocytes, granulocytes, and monocytes, which all express angiotensin-converting enzyme 2 (ACE2). The virus is then picked up by the lungs and transported throughout the body.[19] The virus is then either deposited into the CNS or targets vascular endothelial cells in the CNS causing coagulopathy and vascular endothelial cell dysfunction, with resulting small vessel occlusions and microhemorrhages contributing to subtle neurologic and neuropsychiatric changes.[20] Postmortem studies on cerebral pathology show that the virus can directly cross the blood-brain barrier, directly infiltrating astrocytes and microglia.[21] With the ACE2 receptor widely expressed in brain microvascular and endothelial cells, the SARS-CoV-2 spike protein can directly bind to the receptor and either damage the blood brain barrier or induce a cytokine storm causing inflammation and neuronal damage.[22,23] The subsequent neurologic changes may also be secondary due to direct retrograde travel of the SARS-CoV-2 virus up the axons to reach the CNS.[24]

The long-term sequalae of COVID-19 infections are needing continued evaluation. With the exaggerated response of the CNS to infection leading to meningitis, encephalitis, and meningoencephalitis, continued neurologic manifestations are likely to be associated with a COVID-19 infection if otherwise unexplained.[25] A high proportion of patients with COVID-19 in the ICU develop delirium, suggesting microvascular and inflammatory pathologies to cause neurologic changes.[26] The long recovery of anosmic patients points toward long-term neurologic changes. The more severely affected patients with strokes, microvascular changes, and brain damage may have ongoing chronic issues, and further studies will elucidate associations with the COVID-19 pandemic.

THE CARDIAC SYSTEM

There is an emerging body of evidence to show that cardiac involvement is not uncommon among patients with COVID-19.[27–29] The range of cardiac manifestations of the COVID-19 disease is quite broad and requires a high degree of suspicion in order to diagnose and adequately treat the cardiac manifestations of COVID-19. Here, the authors briefly summarize the proposed pathophysiology of COVID-19 cardiac involvement, discuss the range of cardiac manifestations of the SARS-CoV-2 virus, and briefly discuss potential treatment options relevant to the surgeon caring for patients with COVID-19.

Cardiac Pathophysiology

As described in the pulmonary section of this publication, the SARS-CoV-2 virus binds to ACE2 receptors in type 1 and type 2 pneumocytes as well as other ACE2-expressing cell types, then subsequently enter those ACE2-expressing cells.[30] The ACE2 receptor is found in high amounts in pericytes within adult human hearts, indicating that the heart itself is susceptible to infection by the SARS-CoV-2 virus.[31,32] Indeed, there is evidence to suggest that COVID-19 causes viral myocarditis via direct myocardial cell injury.[33] Compared with patients who have no underlying comorbidities, patients with cardiovascular disease, diabetes, chronic obstructive pulmonary disease, hypertension, and cancer have been shown to have a higher incidence of severe/fatal COVID-19 disease. It has been shown that patients with conditions that result in high levels of activation of the renin-angiotensin system, such as heart failure, hypertension, and atherosclerosis, have higher expression of ACE2 receptors on their cardiac pericytes, possibly predisposing them to more severe manifestations of cardiac disease.[31,32]

In addition to direct infection, COVID-19 is known to cause a systemic inflammatory response in severe disease states, which results in high levels of circulating cytokines that cause injury to a host of tissues, including the reticuloendothelial system as well as cardiomyocytes.[27–30] Endothelial dysfunction is a well-established mechanism of myocardial ischemia and dysfunction, and damage to the endothelial system caused by this cytokine storm may result in increased metabolic demand and decreased cellular perfusion to the stressed myocardium, depressing cardiac systolic function and inducing myocardial ischemia. The systemic inflammation/endothelial dysregulation seen in COVID-19 has also been linked to plaque rupture and acute coronary syndromes in patients with underlying coronary artery disease.[28,34]

Patients with COVID-19 are also at risk of secondary cardiac complications. Medications used to treat COVID, such as steroids, antivirals, and other immunologic drugs, can have cardiotoxic effects. All patients with severe illness, including patients with COVID-19, are at risk for electrolyte disturbances that may trigger arrythmias. Given the interaction of the SARS-CoV-2 virus with the renin-angiotensin-aldosterone *system* system, hypokalemia is of particular concern and is well known to increase susceptibility to a variety of arrythmias.[28,35]

Cardiac Manifestations and Treatments

Acute coronary syndrome

There have been some studies that have shown an association between COVID-19 and acute coronary syndrome (ACS).[36,37] In some case series, patients presented with classic ST-segment elevation myocardial infarction (STEMI) symptoms without prior COVID-19 symptoms, suggesting that their ACS was not caused by severe systemic inflammation.[38] The pathophysiology of how COVID-19 may lead to ACS is still uncertain; however, it seems to involve endothelial damage with resultant subendocardial microthrombi (in the case of nonepicardial obstruction) or systemic inflammation leading to plaque rupture or coronary spasm (in the case of epicardial coronary vessel obstruction).[39]

The treatment of ACS in the setting of COVID-19 illness is similar to the algorithm for ACS from any other cause. In the case of STEMI presentation, early cardiac catheter laboratory activation and coronary angiography is essential. A thorough workup including electrocardiogram, cardiac biomarkers, coagulation studies, and possibly echocardiography all may be indicated. In patients with demand-induced cardiac ischemia (type II NSTEMI), treatment should focus on optimizing myocardial oxygen delivery and reducing myocardial oxygen demand by treating the underlying disease process. Referral to centers capable of angiography/percutaneous coronary intervention is essential for patients with any history of coronary artery disease who have severe COVID-19 features.

Heart failure

Multiple studies that have emerged over the last 18 months have described a link between COVID-19 and new-onset heart failure. Studies have shown that among patients with severe COVID-19, 23% to 33% of patients developed new-onset cardiomyopathy, depressed ejection fraction, or cardiogenic shock.[40–42]

In some of the early studies out of Wuhan, China, nearly 50% of the patients who died of COVID-19 developed heart failure.[42] COVID-19 is well known to cause hypoxia and acute lung injury, resulting in significant pulmonary hypertension, and this can lead to development of right heart failure, and the clinician caring for COVID-19 patient must maintain a high degree of suspicion for developing right ventricular failure.

Workup for potential COVID-19–induced heart failure consists of obtaining a congestive heart failure peptide, troponin biomarkers, transthoracic or transesophageal echocardiography, and in some cases cardiac MRI. For patients with suspected right ventricular failure, hemodynamic monitoring via a pulmonary arterial catheter may be indicated.

Treatment of COVID-19–induced heart failure is similar to that of other types of acute heart failure. Limiting preload as well as reducing afterload, particularly in patients with right heart failure, is essential. Inotropic agents such as epinephrine or dobutamine can be used to increase the contractile function of the myocardium. In patients with right ventricular failure, particularly due to pulmonary hypertension, milrinone seems to be an effective medication at reducing the pulmonary vasoconstriction while significantly increasing the contractile force of the right ventricle. Inhaled vasodilators such as epoprostenol may also be used to reduce the afterload experienced by the right heart. In severe cases, venoarterial extracorporeal membranous oxygenation (ECMO) may be used to provide both hemodynamic and ventilatory support; however, the indications for initiation of VA-ECMO in patients with COVID-19 are highly individualized and beyond the scope of this publication.

Arrythmia/sudden cardiac death

As described earlier, COVID-19 can cause injury to the heart via several mechanisms, including hypoxia, exacerbation of underlying coronary artery disease, direct cellular damage, and systemic inflammation.[36] All types of cardiac injury can induce an arrythmia within the cardiac conduction system. Patients with COVID-19 are particularly prone to deviations in serum potassium levels due to the interaction of the SARS-CoV-2 virus with the renin-angiotensin-aldosterone pathway.[36]

Various types of arrhythmias have been seen in patients with COVID-19, including high-grade atrioventricular blocks, supraventricular tachyarrythmias, and ventricular tachyarrhythmias.[43] It is imperative that clinicians be mindful of the proclivity for patients with COVID-19 to develop arrythmias, particularly in light of the various QT-prolonging medications that may be given to these patients. Cardiac monitoring with telemetry is essential, and regular assessment of the QTc is imperative.

Treatment of these cardiac arrythmias is no different than if they were to arise in a non–COVID-19 patient. Correction of underlying electrolyte derangements, hemodynamic stabilization, and possibly correction of the arrythmia are all warranted.

Thromboembolism/hypercoagulability

Studies have shown that COVID-19 tends to cause a hypercoagulable state in affected patients.[44] The hypercoagulability is likely caused by a combination of severe systemic inflammation, extensive cytokine release, and endothelial damage, all of which produce additive effects in patients with baseline hypercoagulable comorbidities.[45,46] This hypercoagulable state can lead to multiple pulmonary emboli and subsequent right heart failure and can even lead to microthrombi within the myocardium itself, presenting as an acute STEMI.[44]

There is some early evidence to suggest that early anticoagulation is of benefit in patients with COVID-19.[47] Retrospective studies have suggested that use of enoxaparin or other low-molecular-weight heparins was associated with increased survival in patients with clinical coagulopathy or elevated D-dimer.[48] Recent studies are still mixed with regard to the optimal anticoagulation strategy. One recent study showed no benefit to intermediate-dose enoxaparin (1 mg/kg daily) compared with standard prophylactic dosing (40 mg daily),[49] whereas other observational studies have suggested a mortality benefit to treatment-dose anticoagulation, particularly in patients with more severe disease.[47] The European Heart Journal has proposed an algorithmic approach to the level of anticoagulation based on severity of disease, serum biomarkers, level of care, and presence of thromboembolism on point-of-care ultrasound.[50] In general, more severe cases of COVID-19 seem to necessitate higher levels of anticoagulation; however, the optimal strategy is still yet to be determined.[51,52]

THE PULMONARY SYSTEM
Pathophysiology of COVID-19–Induced Lung Injury

The role of angiotensin-converting enzyme 2 in the lung

ACE2 has been repeatedly demonstrated to be the host receptor of SARS-CoV-2. ACE2 is an essential component of the renin-angiotensin system (RAS). ACE is the enzyme responsible for catalyzing the conversion of angiotensin I to angiotensin II, which promotes the synthesis of aldosterone, vasoconstriction, and increased sodium reabsorption in the kidney's nephrons.[2,53] Meanwhile, ACE2 inactivates angiotensin II and cleaves it into angiotensin I. Therefore, ACE2 provides a counterbalance to ACE, thus regulating the effect of the RAS system on the body. ACE/ACE2 also play a role in the inflammation process, and a careful balance between proinflammatory and antiinflammatory pathways is maintained in healthy patients.[53] In contrast to its proinflammatory counterpart, the antiinflammatory responsibility of ACE2 provides necessary protection to the lung against injury.

In the lungs, ACE2 is expressed in the alveolar epithelial cells. It has mainly been detected in type II alveolar cells. The role of these cells includes surfactant production, movement of water across the epithelium, and restoration and regeneration of damaged lung alveolar epithelium.[54] The lung's substantial surface area and large concentration of ACE2 contribute to the lung's significant vulnerability to COVID-19 in comparison to other organs.

Sars-CoV-2 and receptor binding

The interaction between ACE2 and SARS-CoV-2 has been thoroughly investigated. Research into its binding kinetics show a 10 to 20x higher receptor preference for SARS-CoV-2 in comparison to SARS-CoV-1, which may provide insight into why the virus is so easily transmissible.[53] Similar to how other coronaviruses bind to host cells, it is thought the spike protein of SARS-CoV-2 interacts with ACE2, which initiates the release of viral RNA into the epithelial cells.[55]

Hyperinflammation, the cytokine storm, and fibrosis

Once SARS-CoV-2 binds to ACE2, the virus is replicated and cell apoptosis occurs. Consequently, proinflammatory cytokines are released, which upregulate the inflammatory reaction.[55,56] ACE2 is also downregulated, reducing its antiinflammatory capabilities in the lung. This local emission of cytokines, including tumor necrosis factor alpha, interleukin-1 (IL-1), IL-6, IL-8, and *monocyte chemoattractant protein 1*, is then released into systemic circulation. Homeostasis is progressively lost between proinflammatory and antiinflammatory pathways, which leads to widespread release of cytokines and damage to tissues, including the lung.[55,56] In addition, this cytokine storm also produces a collapse of T cells, and cellular-mediated adaptive immune response fails to produce meaningful protection for patients with COVID-19.[55] In the lung, ARDS is a common sequela after this widespread cytokine storm. Downregulation of ACE2 also leads to an increase in angiotensin II. Angiotensin II is proinflammatory and profibrotic, thus contributing to the development of pulmonary fibrosis.

Pathophysiologic Modulators of COVID-19 Severity in the Lungs

Age

Age is the strongest predictor of severity of COVID-19 disease in patients.[53] One study found that patients with COVID-19 younger than 60 years had a 1.38% mortality rate compared with 6.4% for those aged 60 years and older[57]; this may occur for a few reasons. First, ACE2 expression may increase with age, thus creating a greater susceptibility to COVID-19 in the elderly population.[58] Moreover, it is widely acknowledged that innate and adaptive immune responses weaken with aging, predisposing older populations to a more severe COVID-19 infection.

OBESITY

Evidence supports an association between obesity and higher mortality from COVID-19, with obese patients having 3.4-fold greater odds of developing severe COVID-19.[59] ACE2 is widely expressed in adipocytes. As a result, when SARS-CoV-2 binds to ACE2, the adipocytes release proinflammatory mediators that are then released systemically andaffect other organs, including the lungs. Furthermore, it is thought that ACE2 also downregulates pulmonary fibrosis, thus pulmonary fibrosis tends to develop more often in obese patients.[59,60]

Diabetes Mellitus

Diabetic patients have a 2.95x higher risk of mortality from COVID-19 in comparison with patients without diabetes, and they are more likely to develop a severe COVID-19 infection, with an odds ratio of 2.58 compared with nondiabetic patients.[61] Diabetes mellitus is known to involve a constant low-grade proinflammatory state that consequently compounds inflammatory damage on the lungs. Furthermore, hyperglycemia associated with diabetes mellitus promotes dysregulation of innate and adaptive immune responses. Studies have demonstrated a higher prevalence of ARDS in patients with hyperglycemia.[62]

Immunosuppression

Intuitively immunosuppression would be predicted to increase the risk of developing COVID-19. A recent metanalysis did not show any significant increased risk of COVID-19 infection for chronically immunosuppressed patients.[63] The pathophysiology of COVID-19 involves upregulation of proinflammatory pathways. However, with immunosuppressed patients, immunosuppressants modulate the proinflammatory pathways, which then limits the damage that COVID-19 can have on the lungs and the rest of the body. Although, the investigators did admit that their study may have been susceptible to selection bias, as immunosuppressed patients are more likely to adhere to precautions to limit transmission of SARS-CoV-2.[63]

MANAGEMENT OF COVID-19–INDUCED RESPIRATORY FAILURE

Management of acute respiratory failure due to COVID-19 may be thought of as a therapeutic pyramid,[64] staring with conventional oxygen therapy, progressing to high-flow nasal canula, noninvasive mechanical ventilation, intubation, conventional and if needed advanced mechanical ventilation, and ultimately extracorporeal membrane oxygenation.

High-Flow Nasal Cannula and Noninvasive Mechanical Ventilation

High-flow nasal cannula has emerged as treatment of hypoxic respiratory failure due to COVID-19. Although data continue to evolve, this technique seems to be an effective alternative to noninvasive mechanical ventilation, delay or reduce the need for intubation, and reduce mortality.[65,66]

Noninvasive ventilation, including continuous positive airway pressure and bilevel positive airway pressure, has been successfully and safely used to treat moderate-to-severe acute hypoxemic respiratory failure and ARDS.[67,68] Preventing the need for invasive ventilation and its potential complications, including ventilator associated pneumonia and lung injury, is undoubtedly beneficial. In patients with acute hypoxemic respiratory failure treated with noninvasive ventilation, only 28% of patients required eventual endotracheal intubation.[67] Meanwhile, noninvasive ventilation was successful in 48.1% of patients with ARDS secondary to COVID-19.[68]

Invasive Mechanical Ventilation

The next step up in the management of respiratory failure in patients with COVID-19 is intubation and conventional mechanical ventilation. Similar to other types of patients with ARDS, it is recommended that patients with CVOID-19 undergo traditional lung protective ventilation, as outlined in the ARDS net study published in 2000.[69] This type of ventilation is characterized by low tidal volume (4–8 mL/kg), high and individualized positive end-expiratoty pressure, and plateau pressures less than 30 cm H_2O.[69–71] It should be noted that although this approach is commonly used, some data suggest that it may also have detrimental effects.[72]

Extracorporeal Membrane Oxygenation

Should invasive mechanical ventilation failure occur, ECMO may be an option. However, evidence on the utilization of ECMO to treat the pulmonary complications of COVID-19 is inconclusive. A recent meta-analysis of 25 peer-reviewed journal articles on the subject showed that further research needs to be performed to determine the effectiveness of ECMO on COVID-19 pulmonary complications because a most of the available research are case reports or case series.[73]

Venovenous (VV) ECMO is the most common form of ECMO used in reported studies. Indications that were used to initiate VV-ECMO included refractory hypoxia and hypercapnia or single organ failure. Meanwhile, venoarterial ECMO was very rarely used in reported studies. Indications that were used included cardiogenic shock due to cardiac injury.[73] Because of the limited amount of data available, the investigators of the meta-analysis recommended caution with using ECMO in the setting of COVID-19 until studies with larger sample sizes are performed to investigate its efficacy.

FLUID MANAGEMENT IN PATIENTS WITH COVID-19 ACUTE RESPIRATORY DISTRESS SYNDROME

In ARDS, regardless of cause, fluid overload can detrimentally affect patients' outcomes, and, consequently, conscientious fluid management is essential. Positive pressure ventilation is known to contribute to pulmonary vasoconstriction, which produces fluid retention and interstitial edema.[70,71] As a result, restrictive fluid management is recommended, as it is associated with greater ventilator-free days.[74] Unfortunately, fluid management in patients with ARDS secondary to COVID-19 has not been thoroughly investigated.

PRONE POSITIONING

Prone positioning has long been used for ARDS and acute hypoxic respiratory failure.[75,76] Over the years, when and how to use this strategy has been refined.[77] Prone positioning has now been implemented as a treatment of COVID-19 respiratory sequelae.

Prone positioning is thought to improve oxygenation through several means. First, lung recruitment and perfusion are optimized. Second, the functional lung size is greatly improved. Third, evidenced on echocardiography, right heart strain is significantly reduced by decreasing overall pulmonary resistance.[70]

For awake, nonintubated patients, it has been demonstrated that simply giving these patients supplemental oxygen in the emergency department and placing them in prone position increases oxygen saturation from a median of 80% to 94%.[78] However, studies have shown that on resupination the increased oxygenation continues in only approximately one-half of patients.[79] Even more, studies have not demonstrated a significant difference in rates of intubation when comparing prone awake patients with supine awake patients, although a delay to intubation has been noted.[80,81] Also, significant changes in 28-day mortality were not evidenced when comparing proned versus supine patients.[81]

Prone positioning has also been used for intubated patients with COVID-19.[82] In ventilated patients, timing of initiating prone positioning is essential. If patients are placed into prone position early in the disease course, then they are less likely to experience in-hospital mortality.[83] Use of early use of the prone position seems to lead to better oxygenation and an earlier pulmonary recovery.

THE ENTERIC SYSTEM
The Gastrointestinal System and Nutrition

Although known primarily as a respiratory ailment, COVID-19 infection has been implicated in the dysfunction of every major organ system, and the gastrointestinal (GI) organs are no exception. An estimated 4% of patients with COVID infection present solely with GI complaints,[84] including diarrhea, abdominal pain, nausea and vomiting, and loss of appetite. Large meta-analyses with thousands of subjects have shown that prevalence of gastrointestinal symptoms among patients with COVID-19 ranged from 10% to 17.6%,[85] and one study found that patients who did present with GI symptoms (nausea, vomiting, or diarrhea) had significantly more severe symptoms of fever, fatigue, and shortness of breath[86] as well as delayed presentation.[87] These gastrointestinal symptoms begin to make sense when examining the pathophysiology of infection; ACE2 is a known cellular attachment receptor for the COVID-19 virion, and transmembrane protease serine 2 (TMPRSS2) has been shown to cleave the spike protein of COVID-19, together facilitating entry into the cell.[88,89] These effects are marked in the lung tissue, whose high expressions of ACE-2 and TMPRSS2 are likely responsible for the characteristic pulmonary symptoms of the disease. High expressions of ACE-2 and TMPRSS2 are also found throughout the gastrointestinal tract, especially in the small intestine and colon,[89] and may be the culprit behind the GI effects of COVID-19.

COVID-19 virions are known to be shed in stool, creating a potential reservoir of infectious virus particle.[90] Seventy percent of those with fecal RNA shedding testing fecal positive after their respiratory specimens cleared the virus,[88] leading to concerns that patients who test negative on a nasopharyngeal swab could still expose others to active disease through fecal-oral transmission. The Centers for Disease Control and Prevention recommends using separate bathrooms for COVID-19–positive patients.[91] COVID has been shown to replicate virus in enterocytes,[85] adding to the concern that endoscopies could be high-risk aerosolizing procedures. All major GI societies have recommended to delay any nonurgent endoscopies during the height of the pandemic.[92] Internationally, upper endoscopy and colonoscopy rates decreased by 85%,[84] concerning for delayed diagnoses or progression of cancer. It has been suggested that alternatives to endoscopy, such as FIT testing for colorectal cancer screening or calprotectin for inflammatory bowel disease (IBD) diagnosis, be used to reduce risk during the pandemic while minimizing harm from delaying endoscopic procedures. Modeling has found that widespread FIT testing would prevent 90% of life years lost due to cancer diagnosis delay.[84] Coronaviruses are known to be transmittable through a fecal-oral routes; one study in mice found exaggerated symptoms and pathology in infected mice that had been treated with a proton pump inhibitors. This group of mice demonstrated increased pulmonary inflammation histologically,[93] raising questions about proton pump inhibitor usage and infectivity in humans but further research is needed. ACE2 and TMPRSS2 both are key receptors involved in cellular entry of COVID-19 virions; ACE2 is overexpressed in states of bowel inflammation,[94] and TMPRSS2 is overexpressed in the ileal inflammation,[84] possibly increasing the likelihood of cellular entry and infection. Direct absorptive enterocyte injury due to COVID-related inflammation can lead to malnutrition and secretory diarrhea.[87] Malnutrition, whether from enterocyte injury or from poor oral intake during acute illness, can lead to atrophied lymphoid tissue and increased bacterial translocation.[95] Loss of appetite is noted to be common ($\sim 26\%$)[94] during COVID infections with a high prevalence of gustatory dysfunction, which may contribute to this[90]; early enteral nutrition is recommended in patients with COVID by the American and European Societies for Parental and Enteral Nutrition, even in proned patients.[95] There are multiple cytokines released in the course of infection that are known to alter gut microbiota[94]; some patients demonstrate decreased intestinal probiotics[92] and increased opportunistic gut bacteria that have been known to cause bacteremia, changes that were shown to persist even after clearance of COVID-19.[85]

GI bleeding does not seem to be increased among patients with COVID but a study among New York patients with GI bleeds found that they tended to have significantly poorer outcomes during the pandemic, possibly related to patient's reluctance to present to hospital during an outbreak along with an increased threshold to perform endoscopy in the setting of widespread COVID-19.[84]

A special population to consider in the COVID era is patients with IBD. ACE2 expression has been shown to be elevated during active IBD.[94] An analysis of patients on the SECURE-IBD registry found that in patients with IBD, steroid and mesalamine use has been shown to be associated with higher rates of mortality from COVID-19, with almost 20% of patients with COVID who require steroid use for their IBD experiencing ICU admission, mechanical ventilation, or death as part of their clinical course of COVID-19.[84] In contrast, only 2% to 3% of patients on biological monotherapy for their IBD experienced these adverse events.

The Liver

In the setting of patients without preexisting liver disease, COVID-19–associated liver injury tends to be mild in most cases. Elevated aspartate transaminase/alanine aminotransferase has been found to be the most common hepatic manifestation of the disease at an estimated rate of 20% to 30%.[92]. However, Hajifathalian and colleagues[96] reported that an association between risk of ICU admission/mortality and the presence of acute liver injury on admission. Potential mechanisms to explain this process include drug-induced liver injury, direct COVID-induced hepatitis/myositis, and ACE2-mediated binding and damage. ACE2 receptors were found to be high in cholangiocytes,[97] and although normally were low in hepatocytes their expression has been shown to be inducible by hypoxia and inflammation or preexisting liver disease,[98] hypoxic injury, indirect injury due to systemic inflammation and cytokines, ventilator-associated hepatic congestion, and aggravation of preexisting viral hepatitis.[99] Remdesivir has been found in a large trial (n = 1073) to increase liver enzymes[88] with 2.5% and 3.6% of patients in the 5- and 10-day courses, respectively, discontinuing treatment due to these elevated liver enzymes.[100]

Other drugs commonly used in the off-label treatment of COVID-19 such as hydroxychloroquine, corticosteroids, and acetaminophen also have known hepatotoxic potential.[98] Systemic inflammatory response syndrome–induced markers of cholestasis, such as bile duct proliferation, bile plugs, and inflammatory infiltrates, have been found in autopsy studies of patients with COVID.[98] Beyond the frequently encountered mild acute liver injury, COVID-19 can have severe implications for patients with preexisting liver problems. Chronic liver disease was associated with a 60% increased risk of mortality from COVID-19, and frequent hepatic decompensation has been reported among this population during acute infection.[84]

Chronic liver disease can also affect COVID treatment options for patients; for example, patients with decompensated cirrhosis are recommended to not receive remdesivir, one of the only antivirals approved to treat COVID-19.[84]

The pandemic has also affected liver transplant programs around the globe; for prospective transplant candidates, it is recommended that transplant be limited to high MELD score patients or those with high risk of decompensation/hepatocellular carcinoma progression, especially given the decreased number of organs procured during the pandemic.[101] It is also unanimously recommended to continue immunosuppressive therapy in postliver transplant patients throughout the COVID pandemic, given the increased risk for rejection.[101]

The Pancreas

Pancreatic acinar cells do express ACE2 receptors, and it was theorized that this could lead to direct viral-mediated pancreatic damage, but despite several early reports of COVID-associated acute pancreatitis, acute pancreatitis seems to be a rare finding in people infected with COVID. One retrospective study of 63,000 patients with COVID in Spain found an incidence of only 0.07% of acute pancreatitis among these patients.[102] However, patients with COVID were much more likely to be diagnosed with idiopathic pancreatitis versus gallstone or alcoholic pancreatitis (69% compared with 21%), although this was thought to be related to pancreatitis due to widespread multiorgan failure. Many early studies did not use uniform definitions of pancreatitis but instead used elevated serum amylase as an indicator even in the absence of abdominal symptoms.[103] Amylase was found to be elevated in 17.9% of severe COVID cases versus only 1.9% of nonsevere COVID-19 cases, although most of these had no other signs of pancreatitis[104]; elevated amylase is not specific for pancreatitis and could be elevated due to cytokine storm or multiorgan failure that can be seen in severe COVID infection. Lung injury and increased intestinal permeability seen in the setting of COVID infection both could also cause increased serum amylase levels. Pancreatic cancer has been associated with increased ACE2 expression, possibly raising the baseline risk for infection among patients with pancreatic adenocarcinoma.[104] Similar to other cancers, the immunosuppressive effects of chemotherapy can worsen the effects of COVID; one study found a 40% rate of severe adverse events, including death, associated with pancreatic cancer among patients with COVID-19 as opposed to just 8% among those without cancer.[105]

THE RENAL SYSTEM

Acute kidney injury in the setting of COVID-19 may be the result of direct viral injury to the kidney[106] and/or dysfunctions in other organ systems that secondarily affect the kidney.[107] Although exact pathophysiologic mechanisms remain controversial,[108] the development of acute kidney injury or worsening of chronic kidney disease is associated with a worse prognosis.[109] Treatment approaches used for acute kidney injury in patients with COVID-19 are similar to those used in non–COVID-19 patients.[110]

THE VASCULAR AND HEMATOLOGICAL SYSTEMS

During normal times of health, the vascular endothelium has many roles: immune competence, inflammatory equilibrium, maintaining tight junctional barriers, and aiding in hemodynamic stability. It is well known that the vascular endothelium also plays a significant role in the thrombotic and fibrinolytic pathways. During the COVID-19 epidemic, studies have been able to elucidate many vascular complications associated with infection with this novel virus apart from the known respiratory problems. Thromboembolic complications have been reported affecting not just the vasculature of the lungs[111] but also the brain,[112] heart,[113] and extremities.[114] The incidence of thrombotic complications in the ICU ranges from 16% to 69%.[114] Current clinical data indicate both deep vein thrombosis and pulmonary embolisms are the most frequent thrombotic events.[115,116] The mechanisms by which this occurs is related to the damage caused by virus on endothelial cells and subsequent inflammatory reaction and activation of the coagulation cascade. The vascular endothelial cells have vast expression of ACE2, including alveolar cells of the lung.[117] Entry of the SARS-CoV-2 virus into the endothelial cell occurs by binding of the spike (S) protein to the ACE2 receptors, where the SARS-CoV-2 virus has a nearly 10-fold greater affinity for ACE2 versus its SARS-CoV-1, also known as severe acute respiratory syndrome.[118] This entry into the endothelial cell then triggers activation of the immune system followed by cytokine release and subsequent activation of macrophages. This hyperinflammatory state leads to expression of IL-1, IL-6, damage-associated molecular patterns, and recruitment of macrophages to the infected cells leading to endothelial injury. Damaged endothelial cells increase vascular permeability and activate the coagulation cascade.[119] In patients with COVID-19, this heightened innate immune system creates a prothrombotic state and endothelial cell injury. Injury then leads to plasminogen activator inhibitor-1 upregulation, which inhibits fibrinolysis. Tissue factor is increased, leading to procoagulation, as well as release of von Willebrand factor creating intraluminal thrombus. Studies have demonstrated an increase in fibrinogen levels as well.[120,121] D-dimer levels have been elevated, as well as fibrin degradation products increased.[122,123]

Autopsy reports in patients with COVID-19 revealed increased pulmonary endothelial inclusions and increased capillary microthrombi.[124,125] Questions on how to best treat this hypercoagulative state remain active. An observational study found a lower mortality and risk of intubation in patients with COVID-19 with either therapeutic or prophylactic anticoagulation compared with no anticoagulation.[126] No benefit was seen comparing prophylactic with therapeutic anticoagulation. A recent recommendation for patients with COVID-19 recommends prophylactic low-molecular-weight heparin given for all patients with COVID-19 in the absence of active bleeding, low platelet counts less than 25,000, and fibrinogen levels less than 0.5 g/L.[127]

Other hematologic issues may also occur in patients with COVID-19. Lymphopenia does develop in more than 50% of patients with COVID-19 infection.[128] The O and Rh blood groups may be associated with a slightly lower risk for SARS-CoV-2 infection and severe COVID-19 illness. However, the reasons why and the significance of this association have yet to be determined.[129]

PHARMACOLOGIC TREATMENTS AND CONVALESCENT PLASMA
Lopinavir-Ritonavir

Lopinavir-ritonavir is a protease inhibitor and nucleoside analogue combination medication primarily used to treat human immunodeficiency virus. It was theorized that its dual antiviral nature would be effective in treating COVID-19. However, a systematic risk-benefit analysis of 7 peer reviewed journal articles did not demonstrate a clear benefit to using this medication for severe COVID-19 infection. Dangerous side effects include prolonged QT interval and inhibitor of cytochrome P450.[130]

Chloroquine and Hydroxychloroquine

Chloroquine and hydroxychloroquine are medications that have multiple antiviral mechanisms, including inhibition of viral entry and release of virus into the cell, along with immunomodularity activities.[130] Despite its increase in popularity in 2020 as a treatment of COVID-19, data are inconclusive in terms of its potential benefit. Dangerous side effects include prolonged QT interval and hypoglycemia.[130–132]

Dexamethasone

Dexamethasone is a corticosteroid that has been used to treat COVID-19. A 10-day course has been demonstrated by multiple studies and trials, including the RECOVERY and CoDEX trials, to have a significant decrease in 28-day mortality, number of ventilator-free days, and incidence of hypoxia.[133,134] As a result, dexamethasone has become standard of care in the treatment of COVID-19.[135] Despite its benefit in the treatment of COVID-19, dexamethasone is also associated with several complications including glaucoma, hyperglycemia, and hypertension.[136]

Remdesivir

Remdesivir is an antiviral nucleoside analogue known to inhibit RNA polymerase that has also been used to treat COVID-19. It has been shown to significantly reduce recovery time and has been associated with higher odds of clinical improvement.[137–140] Side effects are generally mild, but more severe ones include hypotension and cardiac arrythmias.

CONVALESCENT PLASMA

Convalescent plasma treatment of infectious diseases is characterized by immediate immunity through the administration of passive antibodies.[141] A systematic report of 5 studies on convalescent plasma and COVID-19 demonstrated there may be clinical benefit, and it seems to be safe. Almost all patients who were administered convalescent plasma had symptomatic improvement, and zero mortality was reported.[142] However, a recommendation was made for a large multicenter clinical trial to provide stronger evidence. Recommendations for ideal plasma donors include donors who donate 28 days after the onset of symptoms and had fevers for more than 3 days.[143]

SUMMARY

COVID-19 continues to ebb and flow, as waves, across the globe. During times of surge, nonintensive care–trained surgeons may be deployed into a critical care setting, to care for patients who would normally be treated in a medical ICU. Although primarily a pulmonary disease, COVID-19 has many extrapulmonary manifestations. The interaction between different organ systems and COVID-19's effect on each create difficulty in managing these patients. This difficulty is further exacerbated by our incomplete understanding and constantly evolving guidelines. The authors wish health for our patients and safety for those who provide care at this historically challenging time.

CONFLICT OF INTEREST

None of the authors have any conflicts of interest related to this article.

REFERENCES

1. Weiss SR, Navas-Martin S. Coronavirus pathogenesis and the emerging pathogen severe acute respiratory syndrome coronavirus. Microbiol Mol Biol Rev 2005;69(4):635–64.
2. Rezaei M, Ziai SA, Fakhri S, et al. ACE2: Its potential role and regulation in severe acute respiratory syndrome and COVID-19. J Cell Physiol 2021;236(4): 2430–42.
3. Meyerholz DK, Perlman S. Does common cold coronavirus infection protect against severe SARS-CoV-2 disease? J Clin Invest 2021;131(1):e144807.
4. Gengler I, Wang JC, Speth MM, et al. Sinonasal pathophysiology of SARS-CoV-2 and COVID-19: A systematic review of the current evidence. Laryngoscope Investig Otolaryngol 2020;5(3):354–9.
5. Paules CI, Marston HD, Fauci AS. Coronavirus Infections-More Than Just the Common Cold. JAMA 2020;323(8):707–8.
6. Coronavirus disease (COVID-19) outbreak. World Health Organization. Available at: http://www.euro.who.int/en/health-topics/health-emergencies/coronavirus-COVID -19/novel-coronavirus-2019-ncov. Accessed on 15 Sept 2021.
7. 2019-nCoV outbreak is an emergency of international concern. World Health Organization. Available at: http://www.euro.who.int/en/health-topics/health-emergencies/international-health-regulations/news/news/2020/2/2019-ncov-outbreak-is-an-emergency-of-international-concern. Accessed on 17 Sept 2021.
8. COVID-19 live update. Available at: https://www.worldometers.info/coronavirus. Accessed on 21 Sept 2021.
9. Engberg M, Bonde J, Sigurdsson ST, et al. Training non-intensivist doctors to work with COVID-19 patients in intensive care units. Acta Anaesthesiol Scand 2021;65(5):664–73.
10. Dhar SI. An Otolaryngologist Redeployed to a COVID-19 Intensive Care Unit: Lessons Learned. Otolaryngol Head Neck Surg 2020;163(3):471–2.
11. Coughlan C, Nafde C, Khodatars S, et al. COVID-19: lessons for junior doctors redeployed to critical care. Postgrad Med J 2021;97(1145):188–91.
12. Critical Care for the Non-ICU Clinician. Available at: https://www.covid19.sccm.org/nonicu/. Accessed on 21 Sept 2021.
13. An international Virtual COVID-19 critical care training Forum for Healthcare Workers. Available at. https://www.atsjournals.org/doi/full/10.34197/ats-scholar.2020-0154IN. Accessed on 21 Sept 2021.
14. Critical Care Primer: Educational Resources for Non-ICU Clinicians. Available at: https://guides.himmelfarb.gwu.edu/criticalcareprimer. Accessed on 21 Sept 2021.
15. Higgins V, Sohaei D, Diamandis EP, et al. COVID-19: from an acute to chronic disease? Potential long-term health consequences. Crit Rev Clin Lab Sci 2021;58(5):297–310.

16.. Ellul MA, Benjamin L, Singh B, et al. Neurological associations of COVID-19. Lancet Neurol 2020;19(9):767–83.
17. Maury A, Lyoubi A, Peiffer-Smadja N, et al. Neurological manifestations associated with SARS-CoV-2 and other coronaviruses: A narrative review for clinicians. Rev Neurol (Paris) 2021;177(1–2):51–64.
18. Solomon T. Neurological Infection with SARS-CoV-2 - the Story so Far. Nat Rev Neurol 2021;17(2):65–6.
19. Wang F, Kream RM, Stefano GB. Long-Term Respiratory and Neurological Sequelae of COVID-19. Med Sci Monit 2020;26:e928996.
20. Beyrouti R, Adams ME, Benjamin L, et al. Characteristics of ischaemic stroke associated with COVID-19. J Neurol Neurosurg Psychiatr 2020;91(8):889–91.
21. Matschke J, Lütgehetmann M, Hagel C, et al. Neuropathology of patients with COVID-19 in Germany: a post-mortem case series. Lancet Neurol 2020; 19(11):919–29.
22. Pezzini A, Padovani A. Lifting the mask on neurological manifestations of COVID-19. Nat Rev Neurol 2020;16(11):636–44.
23. Tsai LK, Hsieh ST, Chang YC. Neurological manifestations in severe acute respiratory syndrome. Acta Neurol Taiwan 2005;14(3):113–9.
24. Li YC, Bai WZ, Hashikawa T. The neuroinvasive potential of SARS-CoV2 may play a role in the respiratory failure of COVID-19 patients. J Med Virol 2020; 92(6):552–5.
25. Yachou Y, El Idrissi A, Belapasov V, et al. Neuroinvasion, neurotropic, and neuro-inflammatory events of SARS-CoV-2: understanding the neurological manifestations in COVID-19 patients. Neurol Sci 2020;41(10):2657–69.
26. Helms J, Kremer S, Merdji H, et al. Delirium and encephalopathy in severe COVID-19: a cohort analysis of ICU patients. Crit Care 2020;24(1):491.
27. Zheng YY, Ma YT, Zhang JY, et al. COVID-19 and the cardiovascular system. Nat Rev Cardiol 2020;17(5):259–60.
28. Xiong TY, Redwood S, Prendergast B, et al. Coronaviruses and the cardiovascular system: acute and long-term implications. Eur Heart J 2020;41(19): 1798–800.
29. Clerkin KJ, Fried JA, Raikhelkar J, et al. COVID-19 and Cardiovascular Disease. Circulation 2020;141(20):1648–55.
30. Xu Z, Shi L, Wang Y, et al. Pathological findings of COVID-19 associated with acute respiratory distress syndrome. Lancet Respir Med 2020;8(4):420–2.
31. Chen L, Li X, Chen M, et al. The ACE2 expression in human heart indicates new potential mechanism of heart injury among patients infected with SARS-CoV-2. Cardiovasc Res 2020;116(6):1097–100.
32. Tikellis C, Thomas MC. Angiotensin-Converting Enzyme 2 (ACE2) Is a Key Modulator of the Renin Angiotensin System in Health and Disease. Int J Pept 2012;2012:256294.
33. Halushka MK, Vander Heide RS. Myocarditis is rare in COVID-19 autopsies: cardiovascular findings across 277 postmortem examinations. Cardiovasc Pathol 2021;50:107300.
34. Schoenhagen P, Tuzcu EM, Ellis SG. Plaque vulnerability, plaque rupture, and acute coronary syndromes: (multi)-focal manifestation of a systemic disease process. Circulation 2002;106(7):760–2.
35. Bansal M. Cardiovascular disease and COVID-19. Diabetes Metab Syndr 2020; 14(3):247–50.
36. Basu-Ray I, Almaddah Nk, Adeboye A, et al. Cardiac manifestations of Coronavirus (COVID-19) [Updated 2021 May 19]. In: StatPearls [Internet]. Treasure

Island (FL): StatPearls Publishing; 2021. Available at: https://www.ncbi.nlm.nih.gov/books/NBK556152/. Accessed on 21 Sept 2021.

37. Bangalore S, Sharma A, Slotwiner A, et al. ST-Segment Elevation in Patients with Covid-19 - A Case Series. N Engl J Med 2020;382(25):2478–80.

38. Stefanini GG, Montorfano M, Trabattoni D, et al. ST-Elevation Myocardial Infarction in Patients With COVID-19: Clinical and Angiographic Outcomes. Circulation 2020;141(25):2113–6.

39. Mahmud E, Dauerman HL, FGP Welt, et al. Management of acute myocardial infarction during the COVID-19 pandemic: A Consensus Statement from the Society for Cardiovascular Angiography and Interventions (SCAI), the American College of Cardiology (ACC), and the American College of Emergency Physicians (ACEP). Catheter Cardiovasc Interv 2020;96(2):336–45.

40. Zhou F, Yu T, Du R, et al. Clinical course and risk factors for mortality of adult inpatients with COVID-19 in Wuhan, China: a retrospective cohort study. Lancet 2020;395:1054–62.

41. Arentz M, Yim E, Klaff L, et al. Characteristics and Outcomes of 21 Critically Ill Patients With COVID-19 in Washington State. JAMA 2020;323(16):1612–4.

42. Chen T, Wu D, Chen H, et al. Clinical characteristics of 113 deceased patients with coronavirus disease 2019: retrospective study. BMJ 2020;368:m1091.

43. Kochav SM, Coromilas E, Nalbandian A, et al. Cardiac Arrhythmias in COVID-19 Infection. Circ Arrhythm Electrophysiol 2020;13(6):e008719.

44. Pellegrini D, Kawakami R, Guagliumi G, et al. Microthrombi as a Major Cause of Cardiac Injury in COVID-19: A Pathologic Study. Circulation 2021;143(10):1031–42.

45. Panigada M, Bottino N, Tagliabue P, et al. Hypercoagulability of COVID-19 patients in intensive care unit: A report of thromboelastography findings and other parameters of hemostasis. J Thromb Haemost 2020;18(7):1738–42.

46. Tang N, Li D, Wang X, et al. Abnormal coagulation parameters are associated with poor prognosis in patients with novel coronavirus pneumonia. J Thromb Haemost 2020;18(4):844–7.

47. Paranjpe I, Fuster V, Lala A, et al. Association of Treatment Dose Anticoagulation With In-Hospital Survival Among Hospitalized Patients With COVID-19. J Am Coll Cardiol 2020;76(1):122–4.

48. Tang N, Bai H, Chen X, et al. Anticoagulant treatment is associated with decreased mortality in severe coronavirus disease 2019 patients with coagulopathy. J Thromb Haemost 2020;18(5):1094–9.

49. INSPIRATION Investigators, Sadeghipour P, Talasaz AH, et al. Effect of Intermediate-Dose vs Standard-Dose Prophylactic Anticoagulation on Thrombotic Events, Extracorporeal Membrane Oxygenation Treatment, or Mortality Among Patients With COVID-19 Admitted to the Intensive Care Unit: The INSPIRATION Randomized Clinical Trial. JAMA 2021;325(16):1620–30.

50. Atallah B, Mallah SI, AlMahmeed W. Anticoagulation in COVID-19. Eur Heart J Cardiovasc Pharmacother 2020;6(4):260–1.

51. Hadid T, Kafri Z, Al-Katib A. Coagulation and anticoagulation in COVID-19. Blood Rev 2021;47:100761.

52. The Lancet Haematology. COVID-19 coagulopathy: an evolving story. Lancet Haematol 2020;7(6):e425.

53. Bourgonje AR, Abdulle AE, Timens W, et al. Angiotensin-converting enzyme 2 (ACE2), SARS-CoV-2 and the pathophysiology of coronavirus disease 2019 (COVID-19). J Pathol 2020;251(3):228–48.

54. Castranova V, Rabovsky J, Tucker JH, et al. The alveolar type II epithelial cell: a multifunctional pneumocyte. Toxicol Appl Pharmacol 1988;93(3):472–83.
55. Singh SP, Pritam M, Pandey B, et al. Microstructure, pathophysiology, and potential therapeutics of COVID-19: A comprehensive review. J Med Virol 2021; 93(1):275–99.
56. Ryabkova VA, Churilov LP, Shoenfeld Y. Influenza infection, SARS, MERS and COVID-19: Cytokine storm - The common denominator and the lessons to be learned. Clin Immunol 2021;223:108652.
57. Verity R, Okell LC, Dorigatti I, et al. Estimates of the severity of coronavirus disease 2019: a model-based analysis. Lancet Infect Dis 2020;20(6):669–77.
58. Chen Y, Li L. SARS-CoV-2: virus dynamics and host response. Lancet Infect Dis 2020;20(5):515–6.
59. Wang J, Sato T, Sakuraba A. Coronavirus Disease 2019 (COVID-19) Meets Obesity: Strong Association between the Global Overweight Population and COVID-19 Mortality. J Nutr 2021;151(1):9–10.
60. Kruglikov IL, Scherer PE. The Role of Adipocytes and Adipocyte-Like Cells in the Severity of COVID-19 Infections. Obesity (Silver Spring) 2020;28(7): 1187–90.
61. Wu J, Zhang J, Sun X, et al. Influence of diabetes mellitus on the severity and fatality of SARS-CoV-2 (COVID-19) infection. Diabetes Obes Metab 2020; 22(10):1907–14.
62. Fleming N, Sacks LJ, Pham CT, et al. An overview of COVID-19 in people with diabetes: Pathophysiology and considerations in the inpatient setting. Diabet Med 2021;38(3):e14509.
63. Tassone D, Thompson A, Connell W, et al. Immunosuppression as a risk factor for COVID-19: a meta-analysis. Intern Med J 2021;51(2):199–205.
64. Cinesi Gómez C, Peñuelas Rodríguez Ó, Luján Torné M, et al. Clinical consensus recommendations regarding non-invasive respiratory support in the adult patient with acute respiratory failure secondary to SARS-CoV-2 infection. Arch Bronconeumol 2020;56:11–8.
65. Matthay MA, Aldrich JM, Gotts JE. Treatment for severe acute respiratory distress syndrome from COVID-19. Lancet Respir Med 2020;8:433–4.
66. Chavarria AP, Lezama ES, Navarro MG, et al. High-flow nasal cannula therapy for hypoxemic respiratory failure in patients with COVID-19. Ther Adv Infect Dis 2021;8. 20499361211042959.
67. Franco C, Facciolongo N, Tonelli R, et al. Feasibility and clinical impact of out-of-ICU noninvasive respiratory support in patients with COVID-19-related pneumonia. Eur Respir J 2020;56(5):2002130.
68. Menzella F, Barbieri C, Fontana M, et al. Effectiveness of noninvasive ventilation in COVID-19 related-acute respiratory distress syndrome. Clin Respir J 2021; 00:1–9.
69. The Acute Respiratory Distress Syndrome Network: Ventilation with lower tidal volumes as compared with traditional tidal volumes for acute lung injury and the acute respiratory distress syndrome. N Engl J Med 2000;342:1301–8.
70. Welker C, Huang J, Gil IJN, et al. 2021 Acute Respiratory Distress Syndrome Update, With Coronavirus Disease 2019 Focus. J Cardiothorac Vasc Anesth 2021;(21):00188–9. S1053-S0770.
71. Griffiths MJD, McAuley DF, Perkins GD, et al. Guidelines on the management of acute respiratory distress syndrome. BMJ Open Respir Res 2019;6(1):e000420.
72. Tsolaki V, Zakynthinos GE, Makris D. The ARDSnet protocol may be detrimental in COVID-19. Crit Care 2020;24(1):351.

73. Haiduc AA, Alom S, Melamed N, et al. Role of extracorporeal membrane oxygenation in COVID-19: A systematic review. J Cardiovasc Surg 2020; 35(10):2679–87.

74. Vignon P, Evrard B, Asfar P, et al. Fluid administration and monitoring in ARDS: which management? Intensive Care Med 2020;46(12):2252–64.

75. Guérin C, Reignier J, Richard JC, et al, PROSEVA Study Group. Prone positioning in severe acute respiratory distress syndrome. N Engl J Med 2013; 368(23):2159–68.

76. Scholten EL, Beitler JR, Prisk GK, et al. Treatment of ARDS With Prone Positioning. Chest 2017;151(1):215–24.

77. Guérin C, Albert RK, Beitler J, et al. Prone position in ARDS patients: why, when, how and for whom. Intensive Care Med 2020;46(12):2385–96.

78. Caputo ND, Strayer RJ, Levitan R. Early Self-Proning in Awake, Non-intubated Patients in the Emergency Department: A Single ED's Experience During the COVID-19 Pandemic. Acad Emerg Med 2020;27(5):375–8.

79. Coppo A, Bellani G, Winterton D, et al. Feasibility and physiological effects of prone positioning in non-intubated patients with acute respiratory failure due to COVID-19 (PRON-COVID): a prospective cohort study. Lancet Respir Med 2020;8(8):765–74.

80. Padrão EMH, Valente FS, Besen BAMP, et al. Awake Prone Positioning in COVID-19 Hypoxemic Respiratory Failure: Exploratory Findings in a Single-center Retrospective Cohort Study. Acad Emerg Med 2020;27(12):1249–59.

81. Ferrando C, Mellado-Artigas R, Gea A, et al, COVID-19 Spanish ICU Network. Awake prone positioning does not reduce the risk of intubation in COVID-19 treated with high-flow nasal oxygen therapy: a multicenter, adjusted cohort study. Crit Care 2020;24(1):597.

82. Elharrar X, Trigui Y, Dols AM, et al. Use of Prone Positioning in Nonintubated Patients With COVID-19 and Hypoxemic Acute Respiratory Failure. JAMA 2020; 323(22):2336–8.

83. Mathews KS, Soh H, Shaefi S, et al. Prone Positioning and Survival in Mechanically Ventilated Patients With Coronavirus Disease 2019-Related Respiratory Failure. Crit Care Med 2021;49(7):1026–37.

84. Hunt RH, East JE, Lanas A, et al. COVID-19 and Gastrointestinal Disease: Implications for the Gastroenterologist. Dig Dis 2021;39(2):119–39.

85. Trottein F, Sokol H. Potential Causes and Consequences of Gastrointestinal Disorders during a SARS-CoV-2 Infection. Cell Rep 2020;32(3):107915.

86. Jin X, Lian JS, Hu JH, et al. Epidemiological, clinical and virological characteristics of 74 cases of coronavirus-infected disease 2019 (COVID-19) with gastrointestinal symptoms. Gut 2020;69(6):1002–9.

87. Patel KP, Patel PA, Vunnam RR, et al. Gastrointestinal, hepatobiliary, and pancreatic manifestations of COVID-19. J Clin Virol 2020;128:104386.

88. Thuluvath PJ, Alukal JJ, Ravindran N, et al. What GI Physicians Need to Know During COVID-19 Pandemic. Dig Dis Sci 2020;1–11.

89. Dong M, Zhang J, Ma X, et al. ACE2, TMPRSS2 distribution and extrapulmonary organ injury in patients with COVID-19. Biomed Pharmacother 2020;131: 110678.

90. Su S, Shen J, Zhu L, et al. Involvement of digestive system in COVID-19: manifestations, pathology, management and challenges. Therap Adv Gastroenterol 2020;13. 1756284820934626.

91. Soetikno R, Teoh AYB, Kaltenbach T, et al. Considerations in performing endoscopy during the COVID-19 pandemic. Gastrointest Endosc 2020;92(1):176–83.

92. Kopel J, Perisetti A, Gajendran M, et al. Clinical Insights into the Gastrointestinal Manifestations of COVID-19. Dig Dis Sci 2020;65(7):1932–9.

93. Zhou J, Li C, Zhao G, et al. Human intestinal tract serves as an alternative infection route for Middle East respiratory syndrome coronavirus. Sci Adv 2017;3(11): eaao4966.

94. Perisetti A, Gajendran M, Mann R, et al. COVID-19 extrapulmonary illness - special gastrointestinal and hepatic considerations. Dis Mon 2020;66(9):101064.

95. Aguila EJT, Cua IHY, Fontanilla JAC, et al. Gastrointestinal Manifestations of COVID-19: Impact on Nutrition Practices. Nutr Clin Pract 2020;35(5):800–5.

96. Hajifathalian K, Krisko T, Mehta A, et al, WCM-GI research group*. Gastrointestinal and Hepatic Manifestations of 2019 Novel Coronavirus Disease in a Large Cohort of Infected Patients From New York: Clinical Implications. Gastroenterology 2020;159(3):1137–40.e2.

97. Galanopoulos M, Gkeros F, Doukatas A, et al. COVID-19 pandemic: Pathophysiology and manifestations from the gastrointestinal tract. World J Gastroenterol 2020;26(31):4579–88.

98. Nardo AD, Schneeweiss-Gleixner M, Bakail M, et al. Pathophysiological mechanisms of liver injury in COVID-19. Liver Int 2021;41(1):20–32.

99. Kunutsor SK, Laukkanen JA. Markers of liver injury and clinical outcomes in COVID-19 patients: A systematic review and meta-analysis. J Infect 2021; 82(1):159–98.

100. Goldman JD, Lye DCB, Hui DS, Marks KM, Bruno R, Montejano R, Spinner CD, Galli M, Ahn MY, Nahass RG, Chen YS, SenGupta D, Hyland RH, Osinusi AO, Cao H, Blair C, Wei X, Gaggar A, Brainard DM, Towner WJ, Muñoz J, Mullane KM, Marty FM, Tashima KT, Diaz G, Subramanian A; GS-US-540-5773.

101. Mohammed A, Paranji N, Chen PH, et al. COVID-19 in Chronic Liver Disease and Liver Transplantation: A Clinical Review. J Clin Gastroenterol 2021;55(3): 187–94.

102. de-Madaria E, Capurso G. COVID-19 and acute pancreatitis: examining the causality. Nat Rev Gastroenterol Hepatol 2021;18(1):3–4.

103. Jabłońska B, Olakowski M, Mrowiec S. Association between acute pancreatitis and COVID-19 infection: What do we know? World J Gastrointest Surg 2021; 13(6):548–62.

104. Samanta J, Gupta R, Singh MP, et al. Coronavirus disease 2019 and the pancreas. Pancreatology 2020;20(8):1567–75.

105. Patel R, Saif MW. Management of Pancreatic Cancer During COVID-19 Pandemic: To Treat or Not to Treat? JOP 2020;21(2):27–8.

106. Batlle D, Soler MJ, Sparks MA, et al. Acute kidney injury in COVID-19: emerging evidence of a distinct pathophysiology. J Am Soc Nephrol 2020;31(7): 1380-1383.

107. Ahmadian E, Hosseiniyan Khatibi SM, Razi Soofiyani S, et al. Covid-19 and kidney injury: Pathophysiology and molecular mechanisms. Rev Med Virol 2021; 31(3):e2176.

108. Lau WL, Zuckerman JE, Gupta A, et al. The COVID-Kidney Controversy: Can SARS-CoV-2 Cause Direct Renal Infection? Nephron 2021;145(3):275–9.

109. Titus T, Rahman A. SARS-CoV-2 and the kidney. Aust J Gen Pract 2021;50(7): 441–4.

110. Ronco C, Reis T, Husain-Syed F. Management of acute kidney injury in patients with COVID-19. Lancet Respir Med 2020;8(7):738–42.

111. Wichmann D, Sperhake JP, Lütgehetmann M, et al. Autopsy Findings and Venous Thromboembolism in Patients With COVID-19: A Prospective Cohort Study. Ann Intern Med 2020;173(4):268–77.
112. Oxley TJ, Mocco J, Majidi S, et al. Large-Vessel Stroke as a Presenting Feature of Covid-19 in the Young. N Engl J Med 2020;382(20):e60.
113. Juthani P, Bhojwani R, Gupta N. Coronavirus Disease 2019 (COVID-19) Manifestation as Acute Myocardial Infarction in a Young, Healthy Male. Case Rep Infect Dis 2020;2020:8864985.
114. Klok FA, Kruip MJHA, van der Meer NJM, et al. Confirmation of the high cumulative incidence of thrombotic complications in critically ill ICU patients with COVID-19: An updated analysis. Thromb Res 2020;191:148–50.
115. Gómez-Mesa JE, Galindo-Coral S, Montes MC, et al. Thrombosis and Coagulopathy in COVID-19. Curr Probl Cardiol 2021;46(3):100742.
116. Hanff TC, Mohareb AM, Giri J, et al. Thrombosis in COVID-19. Am J Hematol 2020;95(12):1578–89.
117. Letko M, Marzi A, Munster V. Functional assessment of cell entry and receptor usage for SARS-CoV-2 and other lineage B betacoronaviruses. Nat Microbiol 2020;5(4):562–9.
118. Wrapp D, Wang N, Corbett KS, et al. Cryo-EM structure of the 2019-nCoV spike in the prefusion conformation. Science 2020;367(6483):1260–3.
119. Siddiqi HK, Libby P, Ridker PM. COVID-19 - A vascular disease. Trends Cardiovasc Med 2021;31(1):1–5.
120. Han H, Yang L, Liu R, et al. Prominent changes in blood coagulation of patients with SARS-CoV-2 infection. Clin Chem Lab Med 2020;58(7):1116–20.
121. Goshua G, Pine AB, Meizlish ML, et al. Endotheliopathy in COVID-19-associated coagulopathy: evidence from a single-centre, cross-sectional study. Lancet Haematol 2020;7(8):e575–82.
122. Levi M, Thachil J, Iba T, et al. Coagulation abnormalities and thrombosis in patients with COVID-19. Lancet Haematol 2020;7(6):e438–40.
123. Helms J, Tacquard C, Severac F, et al. CRICS TRIGGERSEP Group (Clinical Research in Intensive Care and Sepsis Trial Group for Global Evaluation and Research in Sepsis). High risk of thrombosis in patients with severe SARS-CoV-2 infection: a multicenter prospective cohort study. Intensive Care Med 2020 Jun;46(6):1089–98.
124. Ackermann M, Verleden SE, Kuehnel M, et al. Pulmonary Vascular Endothelialitis, Thrombosis, and Angiogenesis in Covid-19. N Engl J Med 2020;383(2):120–8.
125. Varga Z, Flammer AJ, Steiger P, et al. Endothelial cell infection and endotheliitis in COVID-19. Lancet 2020;395(10234):1417–8.
126. Nadkarni GN, Lala A, Bagiella E, et al. Anticoagulation, Bleeding, Mortality, and Pathology in Hospitalized Patients With COVID-19. J Am Coll Cardiol 2020;76(16):1815–26.
127. Rosovsky RP, Sanfilippo KM, Wang TF, et al. Anticoagulation Practice Patterns in COVID-19: A Global Survey. Res Pract Thromb Haemost 2020;4(6):969–78.
128. Carpenter CR, Mudd PA, West CP, et al. Diagnosing COVID-19 in the Emergency Department: A Scoping Review of Clinical Examinations, Laboratory Tests, Imaging Accuracy, and Biases. Acad Emerg Med 2020;27(8):653–70.
129. Ray JG, Schull MJ, Vermeulen MJ, et al. Association Between ABO and Rh Blood Groups and SARS-CoV-2 Infection or Severe COVID-19 Illness : A Population-Based Cohort Study. Ann Intern Med 2021;174(3):308–15.

130. Osborne V, Davies M, Lane S, et al. Lopinavir-Ritonavir in the Treatment of COVID-19: A Dynamic Systematic Benefit-Risk Assessment. Drug Saf 2020; 43(8):809–21.
131. Meyerowitz EA, Vannier AGL, Friesen MGN, et al. Rethinking the role of hydroxychloroquine in the treatment of COVID-19. FASEB J 2020;34(5):6027–37.
132. Fteiha B, Karameh H, Kurd R, et al. QTc prolongation among hydroxychloroquine sulphate-treated COVID-19 patients: An observational study. Int J Clin Pract 2020;e13767.
133. Welker C, Huang J, Gil IJN, et al. 2021 Acute Respiratory Distress Syndrome Update, With Coronavirus Disease 2019 Focus. J Cardiothorac Vasc Anesth 2021;(21):00188. S1053-S0770.
134. Hosseinzadeh MH, Shamshirian A, Ebrahimzadeh MA. Dexamethasone vs COVID-19: An experimental study in line with the preliminary findings of a large trial. Int J Clin Pract 2020;e13943.
135. Tomazini BM, Maia IS, Cavalcanti AB, et al. COALITION COVID-19 Brazil III Investigators. Effect of Dexamethasone on Days Alive and Ventilator-Free in Patients With Moderate or Severe Acute Respiratory Distress Syndrome and COVID-19: The CoDEX Randomized Clinical Trial. JAMA 2020;324(13):1307–16.
136. Mattos-Silva P, Felix NS, Silva PL, et al. Pros and cons of corticosteroid therapy for COVID-19 patients. Respir Physiol Neurobiol 2020;280:103492.
137. Davies M, Osborne V, Lane S, et al. Remdesivir in Treatment of COVID-19: A Systematic Benefit-Risk Assessment. Drug Saf 2020;43(7):645–56.
138. Jiang Y, Chen D, Cai D, et al. Effectiveness of remdesivir for the treatment of hospitalized COVID-19 persons: A network meta-analysis. J Med Virol 2021; 93(2):1171–4.
139. Beigel JH, Tomashek KM, Dodd LE, et al. ACTT-1 Study Group Members. Remdesivir for the Treatment of Covid-19 - Final Report. N Engl J Med 2020; 383(19):1813–26.
140. Jorgensen SCJ, Kebriaei R, Dresser LD. Remdesivir: Review of Pharmacology, Pre-clinical Data, and Emerging Clinical Experience for COVID-19. Pharmacotherapy 2020;40(7):659–71.
141. Tiberghien P, de Lamballerie X, Morel P, et al. Collecting and evaluating convalescent plasma for COVID-19 treatment: why and how? Vox Sang 2020;115(6): 488–94.
142. Rajendran K, Krishnasamy N, Rangarajan J, et al. Convalescent plasma transfusion for the treatment of COVID-19: Systematic review. J Med Virol 2020;92(9): 1475–83.
143. Li L, Tong X, Chen H, et al. Characteristics and serological patterns of COVID-19 convalescent plasma donors: optimal donors and timing of donation. Transfusion 2020;60(8):1765–72.

Perspectives on the Impact of the COVID-19 Pandemic on the Sports Medicine Surgeon: Implications for Current and Future Care

Kyle N. Kunze, MD, Peter D. Fabricant, MD, MPH, Robert G. Marx, MD, MSc, Benedict U. Nwachukwu, MD, MBA*

KEYWORDS

- SARS-Cov-2 • COVID-19 • Sports medicine • Athletes • Orthopedics
- Practice management

KEY POINTS

- The COVID-19 (Coronavirus disease 2019) pandemic has presented considerable challenges for orthopedic sports medicine surgeons and their patients, requiring rapid adjustment.
- For sports medicine surgeons, major challenges have included navigating telemedicine, personal and institutional financial losses, and psychosocial impacts from providing care.
- For patients and athletes, major challenges have included delayed return to sport, incomplete or limited rehabilitation, and anxiety associated with traveling to health care settings.
- Clinicians must take the lessons learned thus far and continue to apply them now and for the future as a new normal evolves that consists of treating patients with injuries previously treated with traditionally normal methods.
- The authors speculate that practices will continue to adopt telemedicine as a standard of care, and distancing and transmission precautions will remain in place for the foreseeable future.

INTRODUCTION

The impact of the COVID-19 (Coronavirus disease 2019) pandemic has been immense and far reaching. At the time of this writing, almost 5 months after the effects of COVID-19 began to be recognized in the United States, the number of new cases remains uncontrolled in certain regions.[1] Coinciding with this pandemic have been numerous unforeseen effects, ranging from socioeconomic ramifications to significant changes in the ways in which clinicians routinely evaluate and treat patients.[2–4] At this

This article previously appeared in *Clinics in Sports Medicine*, Volume 40, Issue 1, January 2021.
Department of Orthopaedic Surgery, Hospital for Special Surgery, New York, NY, USA
* Corresponding author. Hospital for Special Surgery, 535 East 70th Street, New York, NY 10021.
E-mail address: nwachukwub@hss.edu

point, orthopedic surgeons, although returning to some degree of normalcy with regard to their practices, must be ready to permanently adapt the changes that this pandemic has imposed.

The subspecialty of sports medicine in particular has felt a significant impact. With essentially all sports, ranging from novice to professional levels, being canceled or postponed for the foreseeable future, it is difficult to conjecture what the future of sports participation will entail.[5] Patients with musculoskeletal injuries treated by sports medicine surgeons may have treatment delayed because of preventive measures introduced by health care institutions and prioritization of nonelective cases. From both patient and sports medicine surgeon perspectives, these barriers may also create significant financial crises. For example, restrictions on participation in sports and on performing elective surgeries may leave institutions with financial deficits or on the brink of bankruptcy.[4,6] Although many clinicians remain optimistic that these barriers will be gradually rescinded, it is only speculation as to whether and when health care practices will return to normal volumes and routines.

The COVID-19 pandemic has raised many questions that remain unanswered; however, the financial, psychosocial, and physical impacts are clear. This article highlights from both patient and physician perspectives the impact of the COVID-19 pandemic on sports medicine surgeons. These perspectives are reinforced using an evidence-based review of recent literature highlighting the various impacts of the pandemic. It is the primary aim of this article to enlighten both the academic community and general public as to how this pandemic has and continues to influence current sports medicine practice and thought, in addition to how it is poised to change future practice, perhaps permanently.

IMPACT ON SPORTS MEDICINE SURGEONS

The current health care landscape has transformed orthopedic sports medicine care. The global pandemic has required surgeons to cater to the musculoskeletal needs of their patients in a way that respects their overall health and mitigates the risk of COVID-19 transmission. Some of the ways that sports medicine surgeons and health care institutions have adapted to this landscape are highlighted here, along with a perspective on how this has affected care delivery.

Telemedicine: Treating Physical Problems Through Virtual Means

The use of telemedicine has been expanded to include a large portion of patient visits in order to respect the physical barriers instated by government and state officials such that the risk of COVID-19 transmission be minimized.[7,8] Specifically, the barriers associated with the provision of virtual musculoskeletal care have been removed in the wake of the COVID-19 global pandemic. Insurers now reimburse for telemedicine and legislature, which allows the provision of virtual care, even going as far as to allow the practice of telemedicine across state lines for some encounters in some jurisdictions. A health care industry analysis by Bestsenny and colleagues[9] suggested that in health care there had been a rapid adoption of telemedicine with high rates of both patient and provider satisfaction.

There are many benefits and challenges for sports medicine surgeons in engaging in virtual visits with patients. Major limitations to the use of telemedicine include technical difficulties resulting in lag or premature ending or disruption of a visit, concern for the quality of the encounter, and inability to perform a complete physical examination.[10] These limitations may negatively influence the diagnostic value of a new or return patient encounter. However, there are significant benefits to these visits, including decreased risk of COVID-19 transmission, saved travel time for patients, and potentially lower rates of no-shows.[11] A recent article by Tenforde and colleagues[12] sought to describe the results from a quality improvement initiative during a rapid adoptive phase of telemedicine for outpatient sports and musculoskeletal physicians where surveys were completed by 119 patients and 14 physiatrists. The investigators reported that telemedicine was primarily used for follow-up visits (70.6% of visits); patients rated their experience as excellent or very good between 91.6% and 95.0% of the time with regard to having concerns addressed, communication, treatment plan development, convenience, and satisfaction; the rate of no-show was only 2.7%; and the key barrier identified for the visits was technical issues.

Although telemedicine continues to expand and the efficiency and technical quality of visits will likely to continue to improve, the in-person physical examination is impossible to replicate, because this is a skill that is cultured and developed throughout training. Tanaka and colleagues[10] recently proposed a set of checklist items and systematic virtual examination techniques to help address these limitations. Their recommendations for a virtual checklist include (1) ensuring the camera is secured in a steady position; (2) numerous space and positioning guidelines for the knee, hip, shoulder, and elbow depending on the extremity that is the chief complaint; (3) lighting recommendations; (4) clothing recommendations depending on the extremity that is the chief complaint; and (5) ensuring that the location allows the patient to speak privately. For the systematic virtual examination, the investigators propose various maneuvers that patients can perform in conjunction with provider instruction in the comfort of their own homes, and provide approximate weights of household items that can be used during provocative strength tests. Because telemedicine is likely to remain common in the examination and evaluation of patients presenting for sports medicine evaluations, development of further examination maneuvers and new technology that will allow improved examinations will be imperative. Future directions may include standardized video instructions for patients, application of motion capture technology, and more reliance on diagnostic aids. Sports medicine surgeons will need to adapt their diagnostic algorithm in the virtual era in order to continue to provide the highest quality of care for their patients.

Financial Implications

High-volume orthopedic sports medicine centers have been forced to quickly absorb significant revenue losses that could not have been anticipated. Because these institutions were unprepared for such rapid financial losses, many are on the verge of bankruptcy and, for most, a large source of income (elective surgery) has been suddenly and dramatically curtailed.[4,13] As a result of financial pressures, many institutions have instituted pay decreases, furlough policies, and even orthopedic staff downsizing. In order to respond to these financial pressures and better align themselves with their institutional plight, hospital-employed surgeons may find themselves accepting pay decreases, and private-practice surgeons may seek out governmental loans to weather the financial storm. The elimination of elective surgery and by proxy income for sports medicine surgeons may have forced some to seek out alternative sources of income, including increased call and locum positions. As sports medicine surgeons return to a new normal, there is likely to be immense pressure to recoup the missed volume. However, the reality is that financial losses in the current fiscal year will have to be amortized in upcoming years and may have implications for surgeon decision making and workload.

The likely ripple effects of the current financial difficulties associated with COVID-19 are that financial disaster planning will become a part of institutional contingency planning. Specifically, institutions will pay increased attention to their cash flow, cash reserve, and maintaining a health account receivable. In addition, surgeons have become sensitized to the importance of having cash on hand to cover ongoing monthly expenditures in the absence of monthly income. Financial wisdom suggests 6 months of typical salary as appropriate liquidity.

Psychosocial Perspectives: Effects of Off-Service Deployment

With governmental and institutional focus on resuming patient care and returning to a new normal, the short-term and long-term effects of being immersed in a critical care environment may be overlooked. Many physicians were previously required to care for patients with COVID-19 or volunteered to do so, which has been shown to be a significant stressor and to impose a large psychological burden.[14,15] A recent worldwide study of the impact of COVID-19 on spine surgeons revealed that family health concerns and anxiety were common and significant stressors, and that loss of income, clinical practice, and extent of surgical management varied widely. It is plausible, and likely, that these trends exist for sports medicine surgeons as well. Because COVID-19 disproportionality affects individuals of an older age,[16–18] older sports medicine surgeons may be at risk of increased susceptibility and this too may have a psychological impact. Because sports medicine surgeons are required to be in hospital settings, this anxiety may be unavoidable and frequent. Such studies highlight the challenges experienced by orthopedic providers and the need for guidelines to be established for (1) psychosocial treatment of these providers, and (2) for anticipation of a second COVID-19 wave.

Research Productivity and Expectations

There has been a profound increase in research productivity during recent months, which coincides with diminishing clinical responsibilities. Furthermore, there is likely an academic "gold rush" to take advantage of the high rate of acceptance for articles pertaining to the COVID-19 pandemic. Gazendam and colleagues[19] recently described this phenomenon as the infodemic of journal publication. This group performed a systematic literature search and found that, over the 13-week period since the initial documentation of COVID-19, a total of 1741 articles pertaining to COVID-19 and severe acute respiratory syndrome–coronavirus-2 (SARS-CoV-2) were published in scientific journals, representing an exponential increase in academic productivity. This group also noted a short time from submission to publication, and a higher proportion of commentaries and opinion articles in journals with high impact factors.

Although a similar exploratory study has yet to be performed specifically for orthopedic research, similar trends are likely present. This trend would have benefits but also potentially negative consequences, if increased academic output is a function of sacrifices in quality. However, benefits of this trend include both personal and institutional gains in academic productivity and the potential to advance the field at a much more rapid pace. Institutions may seek to institute research infrastructures that give them the propensity to maintain the productivity observed during this era both now and in future years.

IMPACT ON PATIENTS AND ATHLETES

Although sports medicine surgeons have been greatly affected by the COVID-19 pandemic, challenges for their patients are also extensive and must be recognized.

Such challenges include enduring musculoskeletal pain and dysfunction in order to minimize travel and potential COVID-19 exposure, anxiety in association with traveling to and being in hospital settings, and return to sport. Some of these challenges, and the way in which sports medicine surgeons may contribute to addressing these challenges, are discussed here.

Anxiety, Pain, or Safety: Which Should Be Prioritized?

Patients have expressed significant concerns in coming into a hospital setting, whether this is for clinical evaluation or a surgical procedure. Although hospitals are prioritizing minimization of the risk of COVID-19 transmission, for patients not routinely part of hospital settings, this can be an overwhelming and anxiety-provoking experience.[20] In contrast, social isolation has been shown to be associated with increased anxiety and stress,[21] and the additional effects of musculoskeletal injuries in combination with this remains unknown. Because the balance of patient care, financial incentives, and COVID-19 risk is delicate, it will be imperative to appropriately counsel patients regarding this anxiety. The authors recommend taking advantage of clinical encounters in the telemedicine setting to prime patients to their experience in the hospital and to emphasize the precautions set in place to minimize the risk of COVID-19 transmission and the need to abide by these regulations. This approach may address anxiety through guiding expectations, addressing pain through conservative or surgical care in the inpatient setting, and ensuring the safety of all in these settings.

Returning to Sport, Eventually

Because amateur sporting events have been classified as low-priority events in the sequence of returning to a new normal, it is uncertain as to when, and the extent to which, sports will resume. Because athletes represent a large proportion of patients evaluated and treated by sports medicine surgeons, and because athletes remain sidelined, this has implications for both patients and providers.

There remain many questions for athletes. These questions include, (1) whether athletes who have contracted COVID-19 will experience long-term effects that influence their health and subsequently their game performance (and if so, what those long-term diseases and consequences are); (2) for those unaffected but that remain sidelined, how potential deconditioning or delayed treatment of a musculoskeletal injury will influence their propensity for return to sport and their performance; and (3) what the future of organized sports will look like. At the time of this writing, some professional sports, such as golf and mixed martial arts, have experienced some success in reinstating regular events because a surge of COVID-19 cases has not been observed (this may be a function of these sports being individual based). Hockey and basketball are sports with smaller teams, which may make this effort slightly less challenging than sports with large teams, especially because these sports were in the postseason. In order to facilitate a safe return to sport, some of these larger team sports organizations have explored the so-called bubble concept; however, professional baseball has experienced early setbacks, and other large spectator sports such as football may also if COVID-19 transmission cannot be adequately controlled. These complications indicate how difficult it will be for amateur sports, including high school and collegiate athletics, to resume regular schedules before the introduction of a widely available vaccine. It is hoped that future protocols can improve safety for these professional athletes and the staff that surround them.

It will be imperative for sports medicine surgeons to safely guide athletes to returning to sport, regardless of when that is or what it looks like. It will be essential for sports medicine surgeons and those involved in the care of athletes to counsel athletes to safely return to sport. In this way, clinicians may help their athletes to avoid injuries associated with returning to sport, such as ruptures of the Achilles tendon or anterior cruciate ligament. Close attention must be paid to fatigue and signs of imminent injury, such as pain with activity, and the athletes must be guided accordingly. Although clinicians are passionate about the return of sports and hope that athletes can soon return to doing what they love, their number 1 priority must be to facilitate a safe return.

The Impact of COVID-19 on Rehabilitation and Home Injury

Another unique cohort of patients being affected by the COVID-19 pandemic are those who underwent a surgical procedure in the period before the pandemic. These patients who required extensive rehabilitation and physical therapy were unable to receive it in most cases. Prohibiting this essential aspect of surgical recovery may predispose such patients to suboptimal outcomes compared with their counterparts who were able to successfully complete physical therapy and rehabilitation. It is also likely that such patients will endure a longer recovery than their counterparts accordingly. Sports medicine surgeons and physical therapists will need to be conscientious of this impact and help these patients experience the best clinical and functional outcomes possible.

As many individuals continue to seek ways of maintaining fitness and staying healthy during the pandemic, a trend in injuries related to home exercise programs may be observed. These patients may develop overuse tendinopathies of the biceps and rotator cuffs if they are not accustomed to performing these exercises regularly. As such, sports medicine surgeons are likely to continue to observe an increase in these types of injuries as long as gyms and fitness centers remain closed.

A TRANSIENT CHANGE OR NEW NORMAL?

There are many challenges that have been faced and new issues that will continue to be encountered as sports medicine surgeons care for patients and athletes in the midst of the evolving pandemic. Despite these challenges, they will endeavor to continue to provide the highest level of care to their patients and to get them back to what they love to do, whether that is walking along the river or hitting a buzzer beater. There will continue to be injuries regardless of the infectious burden imparted by COVID-19, and therefore clinicians have an obligation to their patients to find innovative and effective ways to treat them both mentally and physically. The rapidly evolving nature of the pandemic may make this process more challenging, because recommendations and epidemiologic data are dynamic; however, it is of the utmost importance to take the lessons learned thus far and continue to apply them now and for the future as a new normal evolves in the treatment of patients with injuries previously treated with traditionally normal methods. The changes that may be required cannot be predicted with any certainty, but the authors speculate that practices will continue to adopt telemedicine as a standard of care and that distancing and transmission precautions will remain in place for the foreseeable future.

DISCLOSURE

The authors have nothing to disclose.

REFERENCES

1. World Health Organization. Coronavirus disease 2019 (COVID-19). Situation Report April 29, 2020. Available at: https://nam03.safelinks.protection.outlook.

com/?url=https%3A%2F%2Fwww.who.int%2Fdocs%2Fdefault-source%
2Fcoronaviruse%2Fsituation-reports%2F20200429-sitrep-100-covid-19.pdf%
3Fsfvrsn%3Dbbfbf3d1_6&data=02%7C01%7Cr.mayakrishnan%40elsevier.com
%7C70ae398d1ef94726d77808d8566ccaac%
7C9274ee3f94254109a27f9fb15c10675d%7C0%7C0%
7C637354373097911192&sdata=baLhM3c%2FTL6Xpl4guVi5F3g%
2BLOp1JslnS3plsnpgRiw%3D&reserved=0. Accessed July 30, 2020.

2. Khalatbari-Soltani S, Cumming RC, Delpierre C, et al. Importance of collecting data on socioeconomic determinants from the early stage of the COVID-19 outbreak onwards. J Epidemiol Community Health 2020;74(8):620–3.

3. Nicola M, Alsafi Z, Sohrabi C, et al. The socio-economic implications of the coronavirus pandemic (COVID-19): A review. Int J Surg 2020;78:185–93.

4. Vaccaro AR, Getz CL, Cohen BE, et al. Practice management during the COVID-19 pandemic. J Am Acad Orthop Surg 2020;28(11):464–70.

5. Schellhorn P, Klingel K, Burgstahler C. Return to sports after COVID-19 infection. Eur Heart J 2020. https://doi.org/10.1093/eurheartj/ehaa448.

6. Khullar D, Bond AM, Schpero WL. COVID-19 and the financial health of US hospitals. JAMA 2020. https://doi.org/10.1001/jama.2020.6269.

7. Hollander JE, Carr BG. Virtually perfect? telemedicine for covid-19. N Engl J Med 2020;382(18):1679–81.

8. Loeb AE, Rao SS, Ficke JR, et al. Departmental experience and lessons learned with accelerated introduction of telemedicine during the COVID-19 crisis. J Am Acad Orthop Surg 2020;28(11):e469–76.

9. Bestsenny O, Gilbert G, Harris A, et al. Telehealth: a quarter-trillion-dollar post-COVID-19 reality? McKinsey & Company; 2020. Available at: https://nam03. safelinks.protection.outlook.com/?url=https:%2F%2Fwww.mckinsey.com%2F~% 2Fmedia%2FMcKinsey%2FIndustries%2FHealthcare%2520Systems%2520and% 2520Services%2FOur%2520Insights%2FTelehealth%2520A%2520quarter% 2520trillion%2520dollar%2520post%2520COVID%252019%2520reality% 2FTelehealth-A-quarter-trilliondollar-post-COVID-19-reality.pdf&data=02%7C01% 7Cr.mayakrishnan%40elsevier.com%7C70ae398d1ef94726d77808d8566ccaac% 7C9274ee3f94254109a27f9fb15c10675d%7C0%7C0% 7C637354373097911192&sdata=a4sen1492tt% 2B92rS2dcSwW8oup7ElenAd83LaoY9dqM%3D&reserved=0. Accessed July 30, 2020.

10. Tanaka MJ, Oh LS, Martin SD, et al. Telemedicine in the era of COVID-19: the virtual orthopaedic examination. J Bone Joint Surg Am 2020;102(12):e57.

11. Atanda A, Pelton M, Fabricant PD, et al. Telemedicine utilisation in a paediatric sports medicine practice: decreased cost and wait times with increased satisfaction. J ISAKOS 2018;3(2):94.

12. Tenforde AS, Iaccarino MA, Borgstrom H, et al. Telemedicine During COVID-19 for outpatient sports and musculoskeletal medicine physicians. PM R 2020. https://doi.org/10.1002/pmrj.12422.

13. Gilat R, Cole BJ. COVID-19, Medicine, and Sports. Arthrosc Sports Med Rehabil 2020;2(3):e175–6.

14. Elbay RY, Kurtulmus A, Arpacioglu S, et al. Depression, anxiety, stress levels of physicians and associated factors in Covid-19 pandemics. Psychiatry Res 2020;290:113130.

15. Lai J, Ma S, Wang Y, et al. Factors associated with mental health outcomes among health care workers exposed to coronavirus disease 2019. JAMA Netw Open 2020;3(3):e203976.

16. Imam Z, Odish F, Gill I, et al. Older age and comorbidity are independent mortality predictors in a large cohort of 1305 COVID-19 patients in Michigan, United States. J Intern Med 2020. https://doi.org/10.1111/joim.13119.
17. Lloyd-Sherlock PG, Kalache A, McKee M, et al. WHO must prioritise the needs of older people in its response to the covid-19 pandemic. BMJ 2020;368:m1164.
18. Mueller AL, McNamara MS, Sinclair DA. Why does COVID-19 disproportionately affect older people? Aging (Albany NY) 2020;12(10):9959–81.
19. Gazendam A, Ekhtiari S, Wong E, et al. The "infodemic" of journal publication associated with the novel coronavirus disease. J Bone Joint Surg Am 2020; 102(13):e64.
20. Vindegaard N, Benros ME. COVID-19 pandemic and mental health consequences: Systematic review of the current evidence. Brain Behav Immun 2020. https://doi.org/10.1016/j.bbi.2020.05.048.
21. Xiao H, Zhang Y, Kong D, et al. Social capital and sleep quality in individuals who self-isolated for 14 days during the coronavirus disease 2019 (COVID-19) Outbreak in January 2020 in China. Med Sci Monit 2020;26:e923921.

Virtual Care in the Veterans Affairs Spinal Cord Injuries and Disorders System of Care During the COVID-19 National Public Health Emergency

Daniel Barrows, LCSW, MHA[a],[1], Barry Goldstein, MD, PhD[a],[b],*

KEYWORDS

- Telehealth • Virtual health • Spinal cord injuries and disorders (SCI/D)
- Veterans Administration (VA) • Veterans Health Administration (VHA) • COVID-19

KEY POINTS

- Video-based telehealth and other forms of delivering care virtually are useful tools in the provision of care to individuals with spinal cord injuries and disorders (SCI/D).
- A wide range of services can be virtually delivered by SCI/D interdisciplinary team members, including education, counseling, reinforcement, monitoring, and information gathering.
- The Veterans Administration increased the use of virtual health during the COVID-19 National Health Emergency so that continuity of care could be maintained for Veterans with SCI/D.
- Telehealth supports care delivery to Veterans with SCI/D in a manner that is convenient and efficient.

INTRODUCTION

The Veterans Health Administration (VHA) is an international leader in the use of virtual health, including live video telehealth, asynchronous store-and-forward telehealth, remote patient monitoring, and mobile health. There are more than 9 million Veterans enrolled in the Department of Veterans Affairs (VA) health care system, and of those, approximately 6 million receive health care at VA medical centers and

This article previously appeared in *Physical Medicine and Rehabilitation Clinics*, Volume 32, Issue 2, May 2021.

[a] Spinal Cord Injuries and Disorders, National Program Office, Veterans Health Administration, 810 Vermont Avenue NW, Washington, DC 20571, USA; [b] Department of Rehabilitation Medicine, University of Washington, 325 9th Avenue, Box 359612, Seattle, WA 98104, USA
[1] Present address: 150 Muir Road (R-1, 117), Martinez, CA 94553.
* Corresponding author. 4820 Northeast 106th Street, Seattle, WA 98125.
E-mail address: barry.goldstein@va.gov

Clinics Collections 12 (2022) 369–383
https://doi.org/10.1016/j.ccol.2021.12.026
2352-7986/22/Published by Elsevier Inc.

community-based outpatient clinics throughout the United States each year.[1] Among these users of VA health care, 1.6 million Veterans (27.2%) received some type of virtual health care, and more than 4.8 million virtual visits were conducted between October 1, 2019 and September 30, 2020 (FY2020). Although this volume reflects higher use than in previous years, likely because of the COVID-19 pandemic, the VA has seen a steady and significant increase in the delivery of virtual care since 2009, when it aggressively implemented telehealth as part of the VA's Transformation 21 (T-21) Initiative, an effort aimed at modernizing VA care. The growth of virtual care services is illustrated in **Fig. 1**, which shows the percentage of VA's overall patient population served through virtual care modalities over the past 5 years.

Although the VA's T-21 Initiative ushered in the VA's modern age use of telehealth, the use of virtual care was not new to VA. As the nation's largest integrated health care system, the VA was an early adopter and innovator in implementing the use of telehealth technologies to expand access to health care services to Veterans across the country. For example, in collaboration with the University of Nebraska in 1968, neurologic and psychiatric services were provided by a 2-way closed-circuit television system to VA patients located at VA Medical Centers (VAMC) in Omaha, Lincoln, and Grand Island, Nebraska.[2] In 1970, a microwave bidirectional television system was set up between Massachusetts General Hospital and the Bedford VA Medical Center's psychiatric ward to deliver video-based care.[3] These early efforts were reflective of the VA's commitment to technological innovation in enhancing care to Veterans. The potential value of this increased access is important for many individuals and groups, including the most vulnerable Veterans. Virtual care can reduce disparities that result from physical disabilities, difficulties with transportation, geographic barriers, and scarce specialists. In using virtual care to address disparities and access barriers, a particularly important subgroup to consider is Veterans with spinal cord injuries and disorders (SCI/D) owing to the severity of disabilities associated with severe neurologic impairments, scarcity of knowledgeable SCI/D experts, and long distances to access care in VA SCI/D centers.

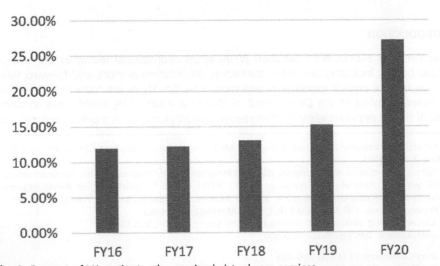

Fig. 1. Percent of VA patients who received virtual care services.

VETERANS ADMINISTRATION SPINAL CORD INJURIES AND DISORDERS SYSTEM OF CARE AND VIRTUAL CARE

VA has the largest integrated, comprehensive, single network of SCI/D care in the nation, providing a full range of primary and specialty care to Veterans with SCI/D. More than 25,000 (FY20: 25,187 in the SCI/D Registry) eligible Veterans receive health care and services within the VA SCI/D System of Care, which is designed to provide lifelong care for all eligible Veterans with SCI/D. This SCI/D System of Care is focused on the provision of care from initial spinal cord injury, or onset of spinal cord disease, throughout the entire lifespan and includes health care management, health promotion and disease prevention, sustaining care, management of new health problems, and long-term care. In addition, the VA's SCI/D System of Care is geographically dispersed throughout the nation, while maintaining integrated services and information systems. This dispersity allows continuity of care to be maintained even when Veterans move around the country, whether temporarily or permanently. At times, non-Veterans also receive care in the VA. For instance, rehabilitation is provided in the VA SCI/D System of Care to active-duty military service members with SCI/D, as established by a memorandum of agreement between the VA and Department of Defense.[4]

In the VA Spinal Cord Injury System of Care, the population served includes individuals with traumatic injuries and several nontraumatic spinal cord disorders, including multiple sclerosis, motor neuron disease, transverse myelitis, severe spondylotic cervical myelopathy, and spinal cord tumor. People with all levels of injury and severity are followed in the SCI/D System of Care, including individuals that are ventilator dependent and that need end-of-life care.[5]

The VA SCI/D System of Care is organizationally designed as a "hub-and-spokes" model in which 25 regional SCI/D centers (hubs), strategically located throughout the country, provide comprehensive primary and highly specialized care tailored to the needs of Veterans with SCI/D. Each of the regional SCI/D centers provides a full continuum of services, including acute rehabilitation, sustaining medical/surgical treatment, primary and preventive care, including annual evaluations, mental health services, provisions for prosthetics and durable medical equipment, and unique SCI/D care, such as ventilator management, respite care, and end-of-life care. Interconnected SCI/D programs and activities coordinate and extend care into the community, including SCI/D home care and other noninstitutional extended care programs. SCI/D centers are staffed by interdisciplinary teams (IDTs) of highly trained SCI/D health care clinicians, which include but are not limited to physicians; physician assistants; nurse practitioners; nurses; physical, occupational, recreation, and kinesiotherapists; psychologists; social workers; pharmacists; dietitians; and vocational counselors.

Each SCI/D center works with VAMC within a geographic catchment that does not have SCI/D centers, called VA SCI/D Spokes; smaller SCI/D teams in those VAMCs are called VA SCI/D Patient Aligned Care Teams. Approximately 110 spokes have dedicated SCI/D teams to deliver primary and basic SCI/D specialty care, and they work collaboratively with the respective SCI/D center to ensure that Veterans with SCI/D receive comprehensive care to address their diverse and complex needs. A spoke is often geographically closer and more accessible to a Veteran's place of residence.

Services in the VA SCI/D System of Care span clinical settings, including inpatient, outpatient, long-term, home, and telehealth care. There are also unique dedicated institutional SCI/D long-term care units at 6 of the VA SCI/D centers. An SCI/D National

Program Office provides operational, programmatic, administrative, management, and strategic oversight to the SCI/D System of Care and is organizationally aligned in VA Central Office.

In addition to the VA SCI/D System of Care infrastructure and services, there is an organized and accurate registry of Veterans with SCI/D. Standardized information about demographics, services and utilization, and outcomes is specified and collected for purposes of clinical care, operations, benchmarking, quality improvement, and research. The VA SCI/D registry is a standardized, automated database, which contains aggregated data created at the point of care. There are strict registry inclusion criteria, and the resultant data have been validated throughout the SCI/D System of Care. Using the registry, operational reports are created and made available through the VHA Support Service Center. A registry-based telehealth utilization report provides detailed reporting on telehealth usage among the VA's SCI/D patient population.

Although this comprehensive network of physical locations and infrastructure is in place to provide SCI/D care, health care delivery to this population is complicated by barriers related to underlying physical disabilities, complex comorbid conditions, sparse SCI/D specialty services in most communities, and the rural residence of many Veterans with SCI/D. The use of SCI/D virtual care allows for Veterans with SCI/D to have more frequent contact and communications with SCI/D specialists, especially when large geographic distances limit access to specialty care. Many benefits of virtual care extend to individuals with SCI/D, including improved access, better coordinated patient care, closer follow-up, improved access to specialists, and increased patient satisfaction with care, whereas other benefits, such as prevention of secondary conditions, reduction in emergency room utilization, and cost savings, are less certain.[6-10]

Health care access provided to Veterans in the VA SCI/D System of Care is significantly enhanced using a wide range of virtual care modalities. These modalities include synchronous modalities, such as live video telehealth, asynchronous activities, such as store-and-forward telehealth, interactive remote patient monitoring, secure messaging, and a variety of mobile applications designed to promote Veteran health through self-care coaching. Telehealth within the SCI/D System of Care is supported by the SCI/D National Program Office with a dedicated Telehealth Program Analyst responsible for oversight, program and policy development, training, and supporting field-based telehealth staff in the SCI/D System of Care.

Spinal Cord Injuries and Disorders Telehealth Coordinators

As part of the T-21 Initiative in 2009, VA telehealth was expanded to further develop people-centric, results-driven, and forward-looking systems. As part of this initiative, each of the VA's 25 SCI/D centers (hubs) was staffed with an SCI/D telehealth nurse coordinator, responsible for the implementation, oversight, expansion, and ongoing support of telehealth programs for the respective SCI/D center and its affiliated spokes. In most cases, the SCI/D Telehealth Coordinator is an experienced registered nurse, trained in the care of people with SCI/D as well as being technologically and telehealth proficient. These coordinators are responsible for establishing virtual care programs and ensuring that SCI/D virtual care modalities are effective and used efficiently by other members of the SCI/D IDT. Beyond the technical support and administrative oversight of telehealth operations, there are advantages in having a registered nurse function in this role. Because of their clinical expertise, the SCI/D telehealth coordinators are often involved in the direct provision of telehealth-based care to Veterans with SCI/D. For instance, some maintain a panel of Veterans with SCI/D that they regularly communicate with using video for follow-up care, education, and health maintenance. Other SCI/D telehealth coordinators monitor and coordinate care for patients who are participating in telehealth-based chronic disease management programs for conditions such as hypertension and diabetes. As members of the SCI/D clinical team, the telehealth coordinators participate in treatment planning and advance telehealth-based options to optimize patient care.

Utilization and Workload (Before and After the COVID National Public Health Emergency)

The implementation of telehealth use throughout the SCI/D System of Care has been an evolving process, particularly during the past 10 years. The use of telehealth and other virtual health modalities is not simply a case of what can or cannot be performed virtually. From the perspective of the health care clinician, initial adoption of telehealth was challenging, as it involved a cultural shift in the way care was delivered. Clinicians, especially those who work with complex patient populations, value in-person visits and sometimes question if high-quality care will be compromised without "hands-on" encounters with patients. Acute rehabilitation following the new onset of SCI/D remains an inpatient encounter rather than an attempt to do so virtually. There are many discrete clinical interactions with SCI/D patients that require an in-person, hands-on encounter, such as the detailed and standardized International Standards for Neurological Classification of Spinal Cord Injury. New onset of specific symptoms (eg, neurologic loss, fever, respiratory symptoms) continues to be evaluated in face-to-face visits rather than virtual visits.

Besides these specific examples, the use of telehealth is now used to supplement and support almost all aspects of delivering clinical care to Veterans with SCI/D. All SCI/D disciplines have used virtual care and telehealth to communicate with Veterans, particularly during the COVID pandemic. The virtual annual evaluation highlights evaluations by the SCI/D IDT. Because most SCI/D outpatient clinics closed during the early months of the pandemic, annual evaluations were often performed virtually. SCI/D providers, nurses, therapists, social workers, psychologists, dieticians, and pharmacists have conducted their portion of the annual evaluation using telehealth. More generally, virtual health has been effective in providing patient education, counseling, reinforcement, monitoring, straightforward observations, and information gathering.

During the COVID pandemic, there have been unique interactions that demonstrate the value of virtual health. A standardized, nationally approved SCI/D COVID-19 screen template was developed in the early months of the pandemic and has been used by SCI/D center and spokes teams to reach out to Veterans with SCI/D. Various SCI/D team members use telephone and telehealth to contact the Veteran and ask questions, including the primary qualifying SCI/D diagnosis, living setting, caregiver status, if the patient has new concerns, and if there are new or additional symptoms. Many sites proactively contacted all Veterans on their respective SCI/D registries.

SCI/D clinicians are using telehealth to problem solve and triage new problems. Evaluating new equipment problems, reviewing progress and/or new concerns with pressure injuries, and addressing medication issues are examples of the usefulness of telehealth in addressing new concerns. Telehealth has also been used for continuity, management of chronic problems, and/or continuing treatment, such as weight management, mental health counseling, diabetes follow-up, and a variety of educational programs.

The use of clinical video telehealth is especially useful to enhance encounters made by SCI/D home care nurses during their in-person visits with Veterans living in the community. During a home visit, the SCI/D nurse sometimes needs input from a provider; a simple video connection can bring in any type of specialist for consultation. In addition, store-and-forward telehealth is used during SCI/D home visits to transmit images of pressure injuries to consulting providers and ensure efficient care management. Often, this eliminates the need for travel, which is complicated if weight-bearing on the pressure injury is contraindicated. The VA has recently engaged in a pilot to enhance SCI/D home care using wearable technology that allows the transmission of vital signs, such as oxygen levels, heart rate, blood pressure, and temperature, allowing providers to virtually monitor a patient's condition and provide interventions when necessary.

An additional challenge to telehealth implementation is that Veterans with SCI/D often value the opportunity to come to the SCI/D center to see their providers and other Veterans in person. Many Veterans have been receiving care in the SCI/D System of Care for decades, and they develop trusting relationships with care providers. Veterans establish friendships and close relationships with peers. Although virtual care may offer convenience, improved access, lower costs and may be an appropriate modality for many SCI/D-related services, some Veterans still choose to have in-person visits for these other reasons.

The COVID-19 pandemic resulted in a monumental shift in both utilization and attitudes toward telehealth among providers and Veterans. Especially during the initial months of the pandemic, telehealth use became a fundamental tool in maintaining continuity of care for Veterans with SCI/D served by the VA. As illustrated in **Figs. 2–4**, there has been a remarkable increase in the number of Veterans with SCI/D who have participated in telehealth visits during FY2020. This increase is not surprising given that most routine outpatient in-person visits were canceled during the early months of the pandemic, and visits were shifted to virtual care. **Fig. 2** shows the percentage of Veterans listed on the SCI/D registry who have received telehealth services. The figure demonstrates the steady adoption of telehealth use within the SCI/D system of care in FY2016 to FY2019 and the dramatic increase experienced during the COVID-19 pandemic during FY20.

Fig. 3 shows the total number of telehealth visits provided to Veterans with SCI/D during the past 5 years, also illustrating the gradual increase in telehealth utilization in the previous 4 years, which greatly accelerated during FY20. In comparing FY2019 to FY20, there was more than a 400% increase in telehealth visits. This

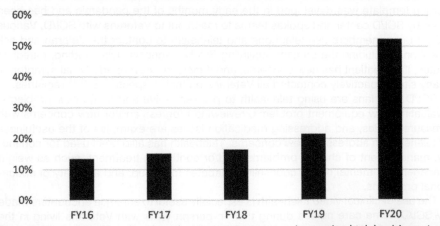

Fig. 2. Percent of Veterans listed on the VHA SCI/D registry who received telehealth services.

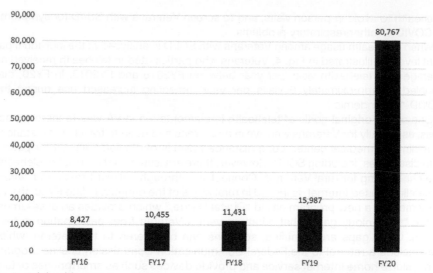

Fig. 3. Telehealth visits provided to Veterans listed on the VHA SCI/D registry.

increase in telehealth utilization during the COVID pandemic reflects the SCI/D System of Care effective response to the pandemic and new constraints on face-to-face visits because Veterans with SCI/D are at extremely high risk of complications following respiratory disease. People who live with SCI/D often develop respiratory complications and/or are at risk of complications, hospitalizations, or death from respiratory illnesses. Burns and colleagues[11] recently published research concerning a higher mortality for Veterans with SCI/D (19%) than the general Veteran population (7.7%) enrolled for VHA health care; both populations have a similar proportion of individuals aged 65 years or greater. The SCI/D Veteran case fatality rate with COVID-19 is 2.4 times the rate observed in the non-SCI/D Veteran population, with an absolute rate that is 11% greater (95% confidence interval: 5%–19%; Z score = 4.8; $P < .0002$). Because of the high risk for COVID-related complications, hospitalizations, and death, there were aggressive efforts to contact Veterans with SCI/D by clinicians using

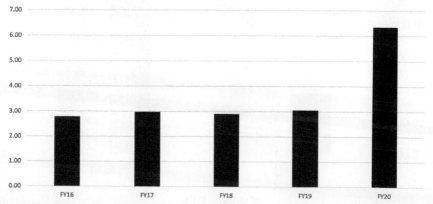

Fig. 4. Average number of telehealth visits per SCI/D patient listed on the VHA SCI/D registry who received telehealth.

telehealth to avoid in-person visits, and to screen Veterans with SCI/D for symptoms of COVID or other respiratory problems.

When telehealth usage among Veterans with SCI/D is analyzed at the individual patient level, as illustrated in **Fig. 4**, Veterans who participated in telehealth received an average of 3 telehealth visits per year between FY2016 and FY2019. In FY20, that doubled to approximately 6 visits per year, reflecting increased use during the COVID-19 pandemic.

One of the original goals of telehealth implementation in VA was to increase access, especially for Veterans who live in rural areas and need to travel long distances to a clinic or medical center. Long distance travel is particularly difficult for people with disabilities, including SCI/D. However, there are issues that can make telehealth use challenging for rural Veterans. Connectivity, through cellular broadband, wired, or satellite-based Internet, is limited in rural areas of the country. In late FY20, the VA implemented a new program called "Digital Divide," which provides an assessment of the "technology gaps" that might prevent a Veteran from participating in telehealth. Once gaps are identified, solutions can be offered to the Veteran, which may include a referral to the Federal Communication Commission Lifeline program to subsidize home Internet service and provide devices such as smartphones or tablets. In addition, the VA has a program to loan broadband-enabled iPads to Veterans who lack such devices. As technology advances and the availability of high-speed Internet options expands to more rural communities across the nation, it is expected that more Veterans will be able to take advantage of the improved access offered through virtual modalities.

Although one might expect that rural Veterans would be the primary users of VA telehealth services, urban Veterans also took advantage of virtual care services. In FY19, 21.98% of Veterans listed on the SCI/D registry and designated as "rural" took advantage of telehealth services, whereas 19.02% of those designated as "urban" did the same, reflecting a modest difference between the 2 groups. In FY20, as illustrated in **Fig. 5**, there was a small shift, likely because of the COVID-19 pandemic, with 46.1% of "rural" Veterans receiving telehealth services compared with 52.7% of their

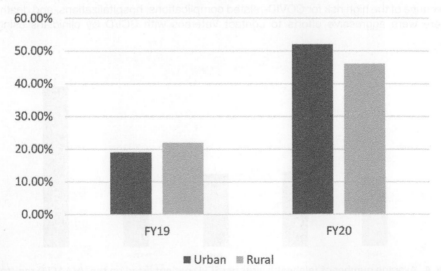

Fig. 5. Percent of SCI/D Veterans receiving telehealth services based on geography.

urban-residing counterparts. During the pandemic, other factors likely unrelated to geography prevented or discouraged Veterans with SCI/D from seeking in-person care, including closure of many SCI/D clinics, limiting admissions to inpatient SCI/D center beds, delaying elective procedures, and reluctance by Veterans with SCI/D to go in to clinics and medical centers.

In addition to the need to accurately identify the VA SCI/D population, which is provided by the SCI/D registry described earlier, tracking telehealth utilization is highly dependent on accurate and specific coding of SCI/D telehealth encounters. When telehealth was initially introduced throughout the SCI/D System of Care years ago, tracking implementation and utilization were complicated by the absence of a coding system to easily differentiate telehealth visits from in-person visits, and visits provided by SCI/D providers versus other VA providers. Differentiating between provider types was remedied with the development of an SCI/D-specific telehealth workload coding system, which now provides accurate tracking of workload, including the location and provider of care. The system requires providers to accurately code the encounter in the VA's electronic medical record system.

Although Veterans with SCI/D are often provided both SCI/D-specific primary and specialty care services by SCI/D-trained clinicians within the SCI/D System of Care, some Veterans with SCI/D receive care in non-SCI/D settings by non-SCI/D clinicians (eg, primary care, mental health services). **Fig. 6** illustrates that 57% of telehealth services provided to Veterans with SCI/D were SCI/D-specific, whereas the remaining 43% of the

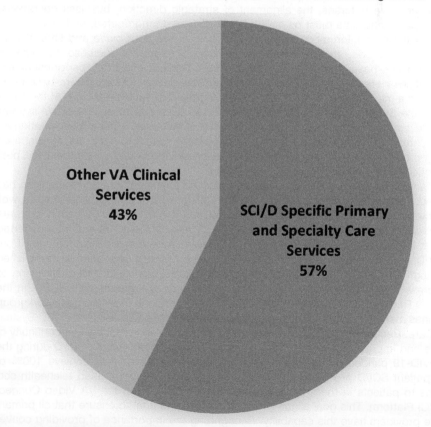

Fig. 6. VHA telehealth services delivered to Veterans with SCI/D in FY20.

services they received were provided in settings outside the SCI/D System of Care. In addition, Veterans with SCI/D may be enrolled and receive services from a VA facility's remote home monitoring program to manage chronic diseases, such as hypertension and diabetes, which is managed by nurses who may not be solely dedicated to SCI/D care.

The establishment of more effective workload tracking, combined with the ability to more accurately identify the VA's SCI/D patient population using the SCI/D registry, places the VA in a better position to use data more effectively to better understand the current state, establish improvement goals and performance benchmarks, and expand use of telehealth within the SCI/D Veteran population.

In summary, when comparing the VA's SCI/D cohort with the overall population of Veterans served by the VA, a greater percentage of Veterans with SCI/D (52.3%) took advantage of VA telehealth services compared with 27.9% of the overall VA patient population.

Performance Measurement

The VHA is the largest integrated health system in the United States. In 1995, under the leadership of the VHA Undersecretary for Health, Kenneth Kizer, MD, MPH, a major initiative was launched that included a focus on achievement of performance-based outcomes. This initiative has been evolving for years and has resulted in recognition of VA for leadership in clinical informatics and data-driven performance improvement. To best serve Veterans, the alignment of strategic direction, business operations, technology, and data must be methodically designed, aggregated, and managed to deliver the right information to the right people at the right place and time. During this same period, there have been significant efforts to increase the use of performance-based metrics for telehealth in VA. Beginning in FY11, performance expectations were set for all VHA facilities to achieve delivery of virtual care-based services to a minimum percentage of Veterans enrolled at each VA facility. At the same time, the SCI/D System of Care set performance targets to align with VA's goals and to increase telehealth utilization. As a result of these and other implementation efforts, steady growth in the use of telehealth has been seen over the years, as illustrated earlier in **Fig. 1**. Establishing standards and providing accurate data identified best practices and potential areas of improvement.

Maintaining relevant and achievable targets for telehealth use and expansion has faced challenges related to the competition for resources and provider time as well as the need to have adequate and cooperative buy-in from providers to incorporate telehealth use into their practice. The SCI/D System of Care has made a concerted effort to ensure that the establishment of performance metrics includes input from SCI/D subject matter experts in the field. Recently, this has been accomplished through the establishment of "think tanks" made up of field-based clinicians to address a wide variety of issues related to the care of Veterans with SCI/D. In the SCI/D Registry and Outcomes Think Tank, a performance measurement workgroup defines metrics to drive the enhancement and quality of services in the SCI/D System of Care. Recognizing the importance of virtual modalities in maintaining continuity of care and improving access to specialty services for Veterans with SCI/D during the COVID-19 pandemic, this group established an FY2021 goal to achieve 100% of outpatient SCI/D providers with capabilities to provide video-based telehealth services to patients in their home or other non-VA sites using the VA Video Connect (VVC) Platform. This goal aligns with a larger VA-wide goal to ensure that all primary care providers have this capability. Recognizing the importance of providing convenient access to specialty care for Veterans with SCI/D regardless of where they live and to address the varied needs that arise in this population, the goal in SCI/D goes a step further to ensure that *all* SCI/D clinicians have the capability to deliver virtual care, including physical and occupational therapists, pharmacists, social workers, mental health practitioners, and others who are delivering outpatient care to Veterans with SCI/D. The goal is to ensure that all SCI/D IDT clinicians are able to provide care, and Veterans with SCI/D have the choice to receive in-person or virtual care. In looking forward, the Think Tank workgroups are considering volume-based targets, which will aim to drive expanded use of telehealth to a larger percentage of Veterans with SCI/D and to ensure that facilities continue to offer telehealth-based services as a routine component of care for Veterans with SCI/D.

Technological Considerations

The initial implementation of telehealth within VA involved connecting 2 VA care sites by video. Within the SCI/D System of Care, this allowed Veterans with SCI/D to participate in visits, being present at the clinic or the SCI/D center. Telehealth visits between two VA care sites was particularly important for transitions of care. It also allowed Veterans to travel to a closer SCI/D spoke site location and still receive services from SCI/D specialists located at a distant SCI/D center in collaboration with the SCI/D spoke team. The technology and special telehealth equipment involved in these encounters are housed at VA clinics and SCI/D centers, operated by specially trained Telehealth Clinical Technicians and SCI/D Telehealth Coordinators. There are great coordinative advantages in these synchronous real-time video appointments between VA facilities and include activities such as discharge planning; specialty consultations, including pressure injury, neurogenic bladder, and pain management; preoperative planning; and wheelchair seating assessments. In general, Veterans and clinicians value these telehealth encounters, but coordination of the clinic-based telehealth visits is difficult, particularly when several clinicians participate. Challenges with clinic-to-clinic live video telehealth include coordination of appointments, equipment, space, and staff between 2 geographically separated teams.

Recognizing the potential to reach directly in to the Veterans' homes, VA has more recently released an application known as VVC, which allows Veterans to participate in virtual visits with a clinician using any video-enabled device, including a smartphone, tablet, or personal computer. VVC eliminates the need for the Veteran to travel and allows for direct conversation with the clinician. It also simplifies coordination for the visit in comparison with clinic-based telehealth. However, in implementing this program, challenges included a lack of technology, knowledge, and skills, especially for older Veterans, to participate in these types of visits. To solve this, the VA funded a program to loan Apple iPads, mentioned earlier, to Veterans who lacked their own devices. During the last quarter of calendar year 2020, the VA provided 57,000 of these devices to Veterans, and an additional 18,000 are on order. The program to provide tablets to Veterans solved many problems. However, Veterans with SCI/D may still have challenges or barriers in using iPads, particularly when hand function is impaired. A variety of strategies, tools, and modifications to use the devices have been used as needed by each individual Veteran with SCI/D. For instance, some Veterans require the activation of accessibility features built into the Apple iOS software to control the device with voice or a stylus. Simplification of multiple steps required to join an appointment has also been helpful for many Veterans with SCI/D. Devices can be set up in a mode known as "single use," which disables many of the features of an iPad in order to simplify its use for 1 application and minimizing multiple steps that normally would have to be taken to access the VVC application. In normal use, a Veteran receives an e-mail reminder about their upcoming video appointment, which contains a link to join the virtual meeting. However, some Veterans have been challenged with multiple steps required to join a VVC meeting, including use of a password to unlock the iPad, opening an e-mail application, finding the particular e-mail with their appointment, clicking the link to join the appointment, and then going through multiple steps to join the appointment. This challenge has been resolved with system modifications, which allow a provider to call the Veteran's specific device through the VVC application, only requiring a single click on the screen of the iPad by the Veteran.

The SCI/D Telehealth Coordinators and other SCI/D IDT members are invaluable in addressing barriers, training, education, positioning, adaptive equipment (eg, grips, stands, and styluses), and modifications of software settings to enable Veterans with SCI/D to more easily use VVC. Although the VA has set up a help desk hotline that operates on a 24-hour, 7-day-a-week schedule for Veterans who need assistance in setting up and using their VVC application, one of the limitations is that the technicians who staff the hotline are not trained to understand the unique physical limitations and challenges that are relevant to the use of technology by a person with SCI/D. Efforts are underway to address these limitations through increased training.

A more recent development, a mobile app called MyVA Images, is an example of the rapid advancement of virtual health apps that have tremendous potential for interactive asynchronous modalities. MyVA Images allows Veterans and/or their caregivers to securely submit still images or short video clips, in response to requests entered by providers to aid in evaluation and treatment. For example, a provider may request a photograph of an area of pressure injury for further evaluation and treatment. A gait video clip may be requested to further assess walking, mobility, and balance. Photographs of the environment may be requested to evaluate safety, accessibility, and barriers in the home. The MyVA Images App is in the pilot phase with expected wide rollout during 2021. Other mobile applications in use by VA provide self-management for pressure injuries, management of posttraumatic stress disorder, pain management, and coaching during quarantine and isolation during the COVID pandemic.

DISCUSSION

During the past several years, virtual health technologies have expanded rapidly, increasing access to health care in ways that were never before possible. For people with SCI/D and other severe disabilities, there is great potential in using telehealth to address needs and unique barriers to care. In addition, virtual health can be used during local, national, or international emergencies, when travel, access, systems, infrastructure, and in-person visits are affected.

The VA SCI/D System of Care has seen the unprecedented use of virtual health technologies during the COVID-19 health emergency. Because in-person visits were restricted, many disciplines from the SCI/D IDT used direct telehealth communication with Veterans with SCI/D to address a variety of needs and functions, including outreach to check on the status of each Veteran on the SCI/D Registry during the COVID pandemic; contact with Veterans with SCI/D to encourage flu vaccinations; follow-up of SCI/D complications (eg, pressure injuries, neurogenic bladder, and chronic pain); monitoring of chronic conditions, such as diabetes mellitus and hypertension; acute and subacute rehabilitation following onset of SCI/D by various members of the SCI/D IDT; medication reconciliation by SCI/D pharmacists; and annual evaluations.

Before and during the COVID-19 pandemic, many virtual health modalities have been used in the VA SCI/D System of Care. The greatest growth and use have been direct synchronous telehealth from clinicians to Veterans with SCI/D in their homes. Given the mobility challenges and vulnerability of Veterans with SCI/D to clinical complications, minimizing exposure during the COVID National Public Health Emergency to health threats experienced during in-person health care visits using telehealth in the home was and remains a top priority.

The advancement of technology during the past few years has also allowed expansion of virtual health to most Veterans with SCI/D, even in extremely rural environments, and expands the ability to provide what the Veteran needs at the right time while staying at home. During and following the pandemic, it is likely that continued rapid development and implementation of virtual health modalities and tools will occur.

There have been previous studies and articles about the use of telehealth in people with spinal cord injury.[7] Many of the studies were feasibility, observational, or pilot studies with small samples, primarily using telehealth communication directly to the consumer. Diverse questions were studied, and various outcome measures were used, most of which focused on the postrehabilitation period following an acute spinal cord injury. Other studies examined various modalities, often using asynchronous telehealth, including store-and-forward images of pressure injuries, Web-based treatments, and interactive home monitoring. In general, and anecdotally, there is wide acceptance of virtual health by many patients, consumers, caregivers, and clinicians. Nevertheless, there has been little systematic study of the use of virtual care modalities in the SCI/D population. Much work is needed to determine the relative benefits, effectiveness, costs, and obstacles to the wide use of virtual health as compared with face-to-face health care by the SCI/D community.

There is no doubt that virtual care will be part of the evolution of health care throughout the world for years to come. Many aspects of these technological advances have the potential to solve many access problems shared across disability groups. Changes have already begun. Data published by the Centers for Medicare and Medicaid Services demonstrated similar changes as evidenced in VA and in the SCI/D System of Care. Between 2014 and 2016, there was a 37.7% increase in the number of beneficiaries with disabilities using telehealth and a 53.7% increase in the total services used by these same beneficiaries.[12]

The COVID-19 pandemic has transformed health care as well as society and the economy. This current article focuses on the use of virtual health by Veterans with SCI/D during the COVID-19 National Public Health Emergency. A description of utilization and virtual modalities is provided comparing the current year with previous years of concerted efforts to provide virtual care to Veterans with SCI/D. This global health emergency has presented unprecedented challenges to in-person health care visits and catalyzed the rapid development of virtual care to meet and move beyond those challenges. During the COVID pandemic, VA telehealth and other virtual care modalities have been used to connect Veterans with SCI/D and IDT clinicians to maintain health, prevent complications, and address new issues because access to the VA SCI/D System of Care was significantly curtailed. In all likelihood, this situation will continue for several months or perhaps years. At the time of this writing, there is another surge that has resulted in record high numbers and rates for new daily cases, hospitalizations, and deaths. Reliance on virtual health modalities during the COVID pandemic will remain a priority in the VA SCI/D System of Care.

During the COVID-19 pandemic, there have been many advantages in the use of telehealth and other virtual modalities. Virtual care has provided a means of consistent communication, access, and continuity of care that overcome physical barriers during a time when in-person services were discontinued, "stay-at-home" orders were established, and physical distancing measures were used to reduce community and nosocomial spread. Secondary benefits included the conservation of personal protective equipment and decreased use of beds for other purposes to expand COVID units and to allow flexibility and adaptability to physical or geographic boundaries where there are surges.

Although the future utilization of VA SCI/D virtual care following the COVID-19 pandemic is unknown, telehealth use will probably be greater than prepandemic levels, now that a significant number of providers and Veterans have experienced its advantages. As with other technologic advancements, there is great potential for use of virtual health modalities by people with disabilities. Nevertheless, there remain broad questions about the development of virtual health and its application for people with disabilities. There is recent evidence that the digital divide remains large between Americans with and without a disability. The Pew Research Center recently found that disabled Americans are about 3 times as likely as those without a disability to say they never go online (23% vs 8%), One-in-four disabled adults say they have high-speed Internet at home, a smartphone, a desktop or laptop computer, *and* a tablet, compared with 42% of those who report not having a disability. Regardless of age, disabled Americans are adopting technology at lower rates, although the divide is even greater with older disabled Americans.[13] In the VA SCI/D System of Care, the average age of Veterans on the SCI/D Registry is 63 years of age, underscoring the complexities involved in a population of severely disabled that is in many cases older adults.

There are broad issues related to the development of virtual health for people with disabilities. There is a moral imperative to ensure that innovations in virtual care are available and accessible to people with disabilities. Although there is face validity to the potential benefits of virtual care for disabled Americans, advances in the field can paradoxically further heighten health and social disparities. Involving people with disabilities on the development, implementation, and study of virtual health is of the utmost importance.

There is much work left to do. There are still fundamental questions about effectiveness of virtual health, optimizing virtual care in the SCI/D community, addressing barriers, rigorously addressing satisfaction by Veterans and clinicians, and examining costs. Because Veterans with SCI/D is a well-defined population and there is a well-organized infrastructure for care, the VA SCI/D System of Care is an ideal setting to examine many of these questions.

CLINICS CARE POINTS

- Virtual health increases access and offers advantages for people with severe disabillties, such as spinal cord injuries and disorders.

- Virtual health increases access during periods of natural disasters and other public health emergencies, such as the COVID-19 pandemic.

- Telehealth offers advantages to prospectively contact people living in the community at high risk for complications, such as Veterans with spinal cord injuries and disorders during the COVID-19 pandemic.

- The Veterans Health Administration is an international leader in the use of virtual health and has greatly increased use of telehealth during the COVID National Public Health Emergency in the Spinal Cord Injuries and Disorders System of Care.

- There are some aspects of the spinal cord injuries and disorders examination that cannot be performed virtually, including the International Standards for Neurological Classification of Spinal Cord Injury.

- In the spinal cord injuries and disorders population, there are still fundamental questions about effectiveness of virtual health, how best to optimize care, limitations of telehealth, and how best to address barriers, rigorously addressing satisfaction by Veterans and clinicians and examining costs.

DISCLOSURE

The authors have nothing to disclose.

REFERENCES

1. How many Veterans receive healthcare at VA each year?. Available at: https://www.va.gov/health/aboutvha.asp#:~:text=The%20Veterans%20Health%20Administration%20(VHA,Veterans%20enrolled%20in%20the%20VA. Accessed December 15, 2020.
2. Wittson CL, Benschoter MS. Two-way television: helping the medical center reach out. Am J Psychiatry 1972;129(5):624–7.
3. Dwyer TF. Telepsychiatry: psychiatric consultation by interactive television. Am J Psychiatry 1973;130(8):865–9.
4. Memorandum of Agreement between Department of Veterans Affairs and Department of Defense for medical treatment provided to active duty service members with spinal cord injury, traumatic brain injury, blindness, or polytraumatic injuries (2009).
5. VHA Directive 1176(2): Spinal cord injuries and disorders system of care, September 30, 2019 (Revised February 7, 2020).
6. Careau E, Dussault J, Vincent C. Development of interprofessional care plans for spinal cord injury clients through videoconferencing. J Interprof Care 2010;24(1):115–8.
7. Irgens I, Rekand T, Arora M, et al. Telehealth for people with spinal cord injury: a narrative review. Spinal Cord 2018;56:643–55.
8. Woo C, Seton JM, Washington M, et al. Increasing specialty care access through use of an innovative home telehealth-based spinal cord injury disease management protocol (SCI DMP). J Spinal Cord Med 2016;39(1):3–12.
9. Coulter EH, McLean AN, Hasler JP, et al. The effectiveness and satisfaction of web-based physiotherapy in people with spinal cord injury: a pilot randomized controlled trial. Spinal Cord 2017;55:383–9.
10. Houlihan BV, Brody M, Everhart-Skeels S, et al. Randomized trial of a peer-led, telephone-based empowerment intervention for persons with chronic spinal cord injury improves health self-management. Arch Phys Med Rehabil 2017;98:1067–76.
11. Burns SP, Eberhart AC, Sippel JL, et al. Case-fatality with coronavirus disease 2019 (COVID-19) in United States Veterans with spinal cord injuries and disorders. Spinal Cord 2020;58(9):1040–1.
12. CMS. Information on Medicare telehealth report. Centers for Medicare & Medicaid Services. 2018. Available at: https://www.cms.gov/About-CMS/Agency-Information/OMH/Downloads/Information-on-Medicare-Telehealth-Report.pdf. Accessed December 15, 2020.
13. Pew Research Center. Disabled Americans are less likely to use technology. 2017. Available at: https://www.pewresearch.org/fact-tank/2017/04/07/disabled-americans-are-less-likely-to-use-technology/. Accessed December 15, 2020.